The Savvy Academic

The Savvy Academic

Publishing in the Social and Health Sciences

Seth J. Schwartz, PhD

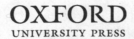

OXFORD

UNIVERSITY PRESS

OXFORD
UNIVERSITY PRESS

Oxford University Press is a department of the University of Oxford. It furthers
the University's objective of excellence in research, scholarship, and education
by publishing worldwide. Oxford is a registered trade mark of Oxford University
Press in the UK and certain other countries.

Published in the United States of America by Oxford University Press
198 Madison Avenue, New York, NY 10016, United States of America.

Library of Congress Cataloging-in-Publication Data
Names: Schwartz, Seth J., 1971– author.
Title: The savvy academic : publishing in the social and health sciences / Seth J. Schwartz.
Description: New York, NY : Oxford University Press, [2022] |
Includes bibliographical references and index.
Identifiers: LCCN 2021025243 (print) | LCCN 2021025244 (ebook) |
ISBN 9780190095918 (paperback) | ISBN 9780190095932 (epub) | ISBN 9780197612057
Subjects: LCSH: Social sciences—Research. | Social sciences—Authorship. |
Medical writing. | Medical sciences—Research. | Academic writing. | Scholarly publishing.
Classification: LCC H61.8 .S38 2021 (print) | LCC H61.8 (ebook) | DDC 808.06/661—dc23
LC record available at https://lccn.loc.gov/2021025243
LC ebook record available at https://lccn.loc.gov/2021025244

DOI: 10.1093/oso/9780190095918.001.0001

1 3 5 7 9 8 6 4 2

Printed by Marquis, Canada

This book is dedicated to all the people who taught me how to write. My mother, Eileen, used to sit with me for hours and help me choose the right words to convey the message I was trying to express. Mom always wanted to write children's stories, and although she never got to do that, she was the first person who gave me confidence in my writing skills. My father, Mort, read many of my graduate-school writings and gave me fantastic feedback. Dad is a deep thinker who always pushed me to see things in new ways. My undergraduate mentor, Dr. Richard (Dick) Dunham, wrote comments in red pen on the margins of the manuscript drafts I would give him. Many of Dick's ideas were so brilliant I wished I had thought of them—and we published some really amazing work together. My close colleague and friend Al Waterman and I would share drafts back and forth until we were both satisfied—and then we would submit for publication. Al was not a formal mentor of mine, but I learned so much about setting up a theoretical argument from writing with him. José Szapocznik, who hired me into my first faculty position, is probably the most critical and thorough editor with whom I have ever worked. I would send him a draft of a paper, and a few days later, I would find a printed copy in my mailbox, marked up in pencil with his edits and comments. I learned how to write for publication through José's careful (and sometimes overwhelming) editing. My wife, Lisa, spent a month of late nights reading one of my first publications and marking everything up with her red pen. When she returned the paper, there were more red markings than there were typed words on the page! But I cannot thank her enough for spending so much time and energy helping me improve my writing skills.

I also must acknowledge several colleagues who have helped me sharpen my writing skills. I met Byron Zamboanga at a conference in 2004, and he and I have published more than 80 articles together. His critical comments have always made me stop and think. Jennifer Unger was my co-principal investigator on my first large grant, and she has always made comments on my writing that forced me to be clearer and more complete in what I was saying. Marilyn Montgomery helped me publish one of my first major theoretical papers, and I really don't think I would have become the theorist I am today if not for her guidance. Koen Luyckx and Viv Vignoles were my co-editors on the first book I edited, and working with them really taught me how to see such a massive project through from start to finish. Jim Côté took the time to write with me even though he was a full professor and I was just getting started in my career. Jim showed me how to write between disciplines and how to engage readers from multiple fields. Veronica Benet-Martinez has given me amazingly challenging comments that have always improved the quality of our papers. There are so many other people I have forgotten to mention here, but who were just as important. I am in all of your debt.

Contents

Acknowledgments   ix
Note on Affiliations   xi
Prologue—Or How Did I Get Here?   xiii

Introduction: About Me, and About This Book   1

1. Getting Started and Selecting a Topic   20

2. Designing a Publishable Study   38

3. Key Principles in Ethical Data Analysis and Handling
   Conflicts of Interest   81

4. Developing an Outline   124

5. Getting Ready to Write   140

6. Principles of Good Writing   169

7. Plagiarism, Citations, and Paraphrasing   202

8. Writing a First Draft   226

9. Editing, Filling in Gaps, and Cutting   246

10. Selecting a Target Journal   281

11. Thinking Like a Reviewer   310

12. The Journal Review Process: Decision Letters,
    Reviewer Comments, and Author Responses   333

13. What to Do With Rejected Manuscripts   395

14. Working With Coauthors   417

15. Working With Public-Use and Proprietary Datasets   452

16. Publishing Non-Empirical Papers   470

17. Open-Access and Pay-to-Publish Journals   491

18. **Books and Book Chapters**   505

19. **Conclusion**   527

Index   529

Acknowledgments

I must thank several people for their contributions specifically to this book. Abby Gross and Nadina Persaud, my editors at Oxford University Press, are absolutely wonderful—and I am extremely blessed to have completed two books with them. Members of my research lab at the University of Miami read these chapters carefully and gave me critical feedback. These lab members include Tae Kyoung Lee, Melissa Castillo, Ivonne Calderón, Maria Duque, Mariya Petrova, Maria Fernanda Garcia, Carolina Scaramutti, Saskia Vos, and Sofia Puente-Duran. I also thank Ingrid Zeledon for her careful edits and comments.

I also would like to thank José Szapocznik, Al Waterman, Dick Dunham, Bill Kurtines, Marilyn Montgomery, and many other mentors for teaching me the skills and principles that I have included in this book. Jeff Arnett has served as a wonderful mentor for reviewing manuscripts and for serving as a journal editor. Much of the material I present in this book came from these amazing individuals.

Finally, I am deeply indebted to my wife, Lisa, and my daughters, Angelica and Alexia, for their support and patience throughout my career. These three strong, remarkable women inspire me and remind me about the most important things in life.

Note on Affiliations

I started this book in March 2019, while I was with the University of Miami. In January 2021, I moved to the University of Texas at Austin, where I completed the book. I believe that both universities should be acknowledged as supporting the completion of this project.

Prologue—Or How Did I Get Here?

"Why would you write a book telling people how to write?"

Those were the words of my 13-year-old daughter, Alexia, the day before I started writing this book. It's a good question, isn't it? Why would someone write a book to help others learn how to write? Doesn't everyone *already* know how to write? And the unspoken part of my daughter's question is this—what makes me think that I'm qualified to tell others how they should write their papers?

I started writing scholarly work long before I ever actually published my first journal article. I still remember it as though it were yesterday. It was September 1993, and I was only a few months removed from my college graduation. I wasn't accepted to any of the clinical psychology PhD programs I had applied to, so I had some time to figure out what I was going to do with the rest of my life.

My undergraduate mentor, Dr. Richard (Dick) Dunham, had invited me to come back to Florida State University, my alma mater, and work with him as a post-baccalaureate student. Dick was a deep thinker and a brilliant scholar. Seldom did I walk away from a meeting with him not feeling amazingly inspired. But Dick didn't like computers very much. He didn't even like typewriters. For most of his publications, he scribbled the text onto sheets of paper, and a student typed it up for him. Once word processors and personal computers started becoming common, Dick's publication rate slowed considerably. With one or two exceptions, the only papers he published during the last 10 years of his life were those that students initiated, where he could make edits and comments with his red pen.

Dick provided me with wonderful mentoring on thinking like a scholar, but I had to learn to write on my own. My PhD mentor, Dr. William (Bill) Kurtines, wasn't much different. Bill was a philosopher and theorist, but he didn't write all that much. It wasn't until I became an assistant professor that I really learned to write scholarly articles. But Dick really did help me to start thinking like a scholar.

Dick and I met regularly during the fall of 1993, and we decided that we were really interested in the concept of transcendence. Our definition of transcendence was this—how do people move to the next stage of their lives? How do children become adolescents, how do adolescents become young adults, and so on? Is there an "Ah, hah!" moment when the person knows that the transition has occurred, or is it something that one recognizes only retrospectively?

So, I started writing. The writing was not very good—certainly not by the standards of what is acceptable for publication in scholarly journals. But I was gaining experience writing scholarly papers. Dick and I eventually brought that paper to a point where we presented it at a conference and submitted it for publication. But the reviewers picked it apart, the editor rejected it, and despite our best intentions, that paper was never submitted for publication again. Looking back many years later, I believe the ideas were promising and maybe we should have pursued them further. I would go on to publish much more thoughtful and important papers, but none of them would have ever been written if not for that first paper I wrote with Dick Dunham between 1993 and 1995. It was my first attempt at scholarly writing—and gave me the *confidence* I needed to know that I could write scholarly articles.

When I started my first faculty position at the University of Miami in June 2001, I received a baptism by fire that transformed me from someone who hoped to publish into someone who knew he could publish. I had just completed a 1-year postdoctoral fellowship and began serving as a faculty-level assistant to Dr. José Szapocznik, who was the director of the university's Center for Family Studies. José was Principal Investigator (PI) on several federally funded grant projects—more than any one person could keep track of—and he needed help writing articles, reports, and other documents that he simply did not have time to write. Bill Kurtines, who had worked with José previously, gave me a glowing recommendation, and I became José's right-hand person.

I still remember the first article José asked me to work on. It was a family therapy outcome article that had been rejected by a top-tier journal and needed to be revised before it could be submitted elsewhere. Writing a paper about an intervention that had taken place before I started working at the Center was extremely challenging. I felt like a detective trying to solve a 30-year-old crime, piecing together information from several sources (including calling and meeting with people who no longer worked at the Center). There were several other authors on this article, and here I was—the new person who was just hired, writing an article about work that other people had done years earlier. The detective work I had to do before I was able to start writing emphasized to me that writing is often one of the *last* steps we take in the scientific research process. I stress this principle many times in this book.

When I finally sent José a draft of the article after another colleague and I had finished putting it together, he came back with a million comments. He picked apart my writing and questioned almost every word I had written. Initially, I was discouraged, but in the end, I learned to appreciate—and value—José's careful style of editing and commenting on drafts. There is an adage that we learn most efficiently by doing—and José's style was grounded in that line of thought. I was learning to write by working with a master who knew exactly what to say and how to say it. As I write this, nearly 20 years later, I am in José's debt for teaching me how to write like a scholar. And when I comment on other people's drafts, I channel my "inner José" and comment on as many issues as I can find. I learned from José that it is better to receive critical feedback from colleagues and mentors than from reviewers.

I learned many of the techniques I cover in this book from working closely with José for over 15 years. Some of them he taught me directly, some I came up with in the process of responding to his edits and comments, and some I learned from responding to reviewers who critiqued our papers. José was a heck of a mentor, and I thank him for everything he taught me. I would not be writing this book if not for him.

My goal in this book is to pass on the lessons I have learned during my writing career. I do so by providing straightforward advice, by recounting stories about my and my colleagues' successful and unsuccessful publishing experiences, and by providing words of caution about mistakes to avoid. I provide text from real papers and response letters that my colleagues and I have written. As many parents tell their children (and, indeed, as my wife and I tell our kids), there are important lessons to be learned from observing other people's experiences. We can choose to emulate others' behaviors and choices that yield results we would like to experience in our own lives—and to stay away from behaviors and choices that produce results we would rather avoid. In his social learning theory, Albert Bandura used the term *observational learning* to refer to the practice of copying behaviors that yield positive outcomes for others and avoiding behaviors that yield undesirable outcomes for others. Clearly, any book about writing adopts an observational learning approach. I share examples of what has worked (and what has not worked) in my career, and readers can benefit without having to make the same mistakes I made—while capitalizing on the strategies that have worked for me.

I invite you to learn from my publishing career. I use an easy-to-read, accessible, colloquial approach in writing the book—while at the same time presenting real scenarios that I have encountered. In many cases, my colleagues' identities are masked—and in some cases I refer to people using pseudonyms, such as "Dr. X" or "Dr. Y." Not all stories about publishing paint all the characters in a favorable light.

Although my writing style *in the book* is colloquial, the style that I am advising readers *to use in their own scholarly writing* is formal. To emphasize this point, I use a display format, italics, and underlining when I am suggesting specific writing tips or quoting excerpts from papers or response letters. I often italicize points that I consider to be especially important.

Most of all, I invite readers to try the strategies that I suggest here. What is essential in writing—or most anything else—is *confidence*. Albert Einstein once said, "Whether you think you can, or whether you think you cannot, you're right." Writing with confidence is not all that different from driving a car with confidence or hitting a baseball with confidence. If you believe you can do it, your chances of success are much higher than if you are doubting yourself. Confidence comes from success, such that the more I do something well, the more confident I am that I can *keep* doing it well. Once my first scholarly article was accepted for publication, I started publishing more and more—because I believed I could publish successfully.

A last note before I end this preface: no matter how good a writer you are, you will have papers rejected by journals. Many journals reject between 75% and 95% of manuscripts that are submitted for consideration. These rejection rates indicate that even papers that are quite good may not be accepted for publication in those journals. Writers need to develop a "thick skin" about getting rejected. Sometimes the editorial process is unfair (see Schwartz & Zamboanga, 2009)—but often there is not much that writers can do other than move on to the next journal. There are some cases where authors can challenge an editor's decision to reject their manuscript, but this strategy will fail more often than it succeeds. I write more about handling rejection in Chapters 11, 12, and 13, but for now what is most important is that rejection is a normal, and unavoidable, part of writing for publication.

With all these points made, let's proceed to the first chapter in the book!

Reference

Schwartz, S. J., & Zamboanga, B. L. (2009). The peer-review and editorial system: Ways to fix something that might be broken. *Perspectives on Psychological Science, 4*, 54–61.

Introduction

About Me, and About This Book

Before we get started, I should tell you a bit about myself. Why am I qualified to write a book about publishing? Why should you listen to me?

I could give you all of the typical, stock answers to these questions—and I will. But I will also tell you a number of stories about my writing career—stories that will help you understand how I acquired the skills and techniques I include in this book, and how I have used them successfully.

As of February 2021, I have published 312 journal articles, 31 book chapters, and two edited books (not including this one). Whereas the average faculty member produces five to six scholarly publications per year, between 2010 and 2020 I averaged 21 publications per year. I have published in some of the most prestigious journals in psychology and public health. According to Google Scholar, my h-index is 80, which means that 80 of my publications have been cited at least 80 times.

But none of that is why I think you should read this book.

I think you should read this book because of the *techniques* that yielded these publications—techniques that have as much to do with how to plan a study, conduct and interpret analyses, and collaborate with colleagues as they have to do with how to put together the written document.

If I didn't do that, and simply asked you to read my book because of how accomplished I am, then I would be wasting your time (not to mention my own). It would be like Tiger Woods writing a book about golf and not telling you about the skills he learned from constant practice, or like J. K. Rowling telling you all about Harry Potter, but not giving you a sense of how she put together the stories that have captivated millions of people around the world.

I'll give you an example that might help you understand my goals for this book. A couple of years ago, Howard Schultz, founder of Starbucks Coffee, published a book, *From the Ground Up*. In the book, Schultz spent a lot of time laying out key decisions he and his partners had to make while building Starbucks, and the "secret formula"—investing in their employees and remaining loyal to them—that propelled the company to such huge success.

The Savvy Academic. Seth J. Schwartz, Oxford University Press. © Oxford University Press 2022.
DOI: 10.1093/oso/9780190095918.003.0001

I read Schultz's book in 2019, and what kept me turning the pages was the inspiring and groundbreaking philosophy he developed and implemented. I am not interested in how much money Starbucks Coffee is worth or how famous Howard Schultz is. I'm interested in the skills and ideas he shared—skills and ideas that readers can apply to their own lives.

That is my point in writing this book. I share stories and anecdotes as well as provide direct examples of research principles and writing techniques. Readers who don't resonate with stories and anecdotes are certainly welcome to skip over this material—but I think that many readers will resonate with at least some of the stories and anecdotes I include.

How I Got Started in Academia

I utilize a fairly unusual tactic in this chapter. I tell my own academic story as a way of humanizing myself and illustrating my own journey toward becoming a well-published author. Many of my mentees and younger colleagues have told me that they don't think they could ever learn to write the way I write—and my response to them is that I wasn't always a skilled writer. In fact, I didn't always have the work ethic I have now. I have failed, been rejected, and fallen short of my goals many times in my career. By telling my academic story, I hope to convince you that you can reach—and surpass—where I am. As I like to tell people, if I can do it, then anyone can.

I was never a very good student in middle or high school. I generally didn't do my homework, goofed off in class, and was never my teachers' favorite student. Even throughout my first year and a half in college, I was skating by on my raw intelligence and my good memory. I am the first to admit that I was not putting forth my best effort.

Then along came Dick Dunham.

It was January 1991, the middle of my sophomore year at Florida State University in Tallahassee. I had just broken up with my girlfriend, and I was depressed. After spending the holidays with my family in South Florida, I returned to Tallahassee but very quickly became unsure whether I wanted to stay. I seriously considered dropping out of college—I even called my father and asked him whether there were any opportunities for me in the jewelry business that he and my grandfather were running. He urged me to stay in school. A couple of friends—one of whom I ended up dating briefly—convinced me to stick it out.

When I registered for classes, I strongly considered taking a course in the psychology of adolescence because I had always been fascinated by the teenage years—and I was still technically a teenager myself. But the class met at 8:00 a.m. three times per week, and I was not a morning person (I'm still not). My usual bedtime was between 3 and 5 a.m., and on many days I wouldn't wake up until 11 a.m. or noon. I wasn't sure whether to take the class because I didn't think I would be able to wake up early enough to make it.

But something told me to sign up for it.

On the first day of class, the instructor, Dr. Jeannie Kidwell, announced that she and her husband were holding a graduate seminar on Wednesday evenings. The seminar was on identity development—and I was immediately intrigued. Anyone who might be interested in attending the seminar was encouraged to speak to Dr. Kidwell after class.

I debated whether or not to approach her. Something told me I should, but a graduate seminar? I was only a 19-year-old college sophomore! And I wasn't exactly the most highly motivated student. But this nagging voice in my head kept telling me to talk to Dr. Kidwell.

Finally, during the second week of class, I mustered up the courage to speak with her after class. She was a pleasant, engaging woman, and she was also a licensed clinical psychologist—something I was pretty sure I wanted to be as well. So I told her I was interested in finding out more about the seminar. She beckoned me to follow her upstairs to her husband's office.

The office door opened, and there stood a broad-shouldered, imposing man. He was several inches taller than me, with white hair and a beard. He looked something like a cross between Moses and Santa Claus. He looked directly into my eyes with a stern face that reminded me of Poseidon, the Greek god of the sea. He introduced himself as Dr. Dunham. I was instantly intimidated. But there was something about him that drew me in.

I started attending the seminar that Drs. Kidwell and Dunham were offering—and I was the only person from Dr. Kidwell's class who had expressed interest. As an undergraduate, I was in over my head. But I was quickly bonding with Dr. Dunham. He had taken a liking to me despite my self-handicapping and my questionable work ethic. He clearly saw something in me that intrigued him—he saw potential in me that he wanted to bring out.

In the fall of 1991, Dick assigned me to work with another student who was an art therapist. This other student was in her late 40s and had returned to school after spending years in practice. Our goal was to integrate the identity work that the lab was doing with the other student's art therapy work. The project sounded interesting—but artists are not known for being overly structured, and I didn't yet have the leadership skills to pull off a project like that. We wound up going around in circles for most of a year and accomplished very little. Dick would later tell me that he knew the project would fail—but that he saw it as an important growth experience for me. Indeed it was.

In late 1991, Dick asked me to come to his office. He said he wanted to send me overseas to gain valuable research experience in a European lab. Psychology labs in many European countries—particularly Germany, the Netherlands, and the United Kingdom—were known for being especially rigorous. Dick networked through a colleague of his who had contacts in England and Wales, and he arranged for me to study at the University of Wales at Cardiff. I had never even heard of Cardiff, but apparently I was going to spend most of a year there. This was not a formal study-abroad arrangement between Florida State University and the University of Wales—Dick simply picked up the phone and called the head of the School of Psychology at Cardiff.

I lived in Cardiff between May and December 1992—and it was one of the most eye-opening experiences I have ever had. I worked in several research labs at the university, where I learned how to collect and analyze data and to program data-entry interfaces. This was long before the Internet was created, and long before data collection software like Qualtrics and RedCap were invented. I had to write the software myself—thank goodness I had minored in computer programming!

The Cardiff experience was my first foray into serious academic research. I also learned much about the world by living overseas for most of a year. Going to Tallahassee—8 hours' drive from home—had been difficult at first, but now being on the other side of the Atlantic really tested my ability to fend for myself. To my credit, I did very well there and learned a great deal. Many of the skills I learned there are still in my repertoire today.

But there was another major challenge coming. I was set to graduate from Florida State in May 1993, and if I wanted to pursue my dream of being an academic just like Dick, I had to get myself into graduate school. I had always wanted to be a clinical psychologist so that I could help people, so I decided to apply to some of the top clinical psychology PhD programs in the United States. However, as Dick had been warning me, I didn't have the résumé to be competitive for these programs. My grades were decent but not stellar. I had not published anything or presented research at conferences. My letters of recommendation, while solid, didn't jump off the page and scream "Admit this applicant now!" And perhaps most damning, many U.S. clinical psychology programs admit fewer than 5% of applicants. I had no shot at getting into any of the programs to which I had applied, but I put that out of my mind and refused to believe it. In short, I was being an ostrich—burying my head in the sand and hiding from reality.

One by one, the rejection letters started rolling in. Most of them were sent to my family's home. I received calls one after the other telling me that I had been rejected by Duke, North Carolina, Michigan, Southern California, Connecticut, Emory, and others. By the end of April, I had heard from all 13 schools I had applied to. I didn't get into any of them. I was shocked, disillusioned, and depressed. My dream of becoming a clinical psychologist was gone.

After spending the summer licking my wounds, I reluctantly returned to Tallahassee to work with Dick as a post-baccalaureate (non-degree-seeking) student. Following Dick's advice, I applied to—and was accepted into—a master's program in family and child sciences at Florida State. Drs. Ron and Ann Mullis would be my advisors. They were two of the kindest, most nurturing, and most amazing people with whom I had ever worked. They allowed me to continue working with Dick while I pursued my master's degree—and Ron, Dick, and I wound up publishing two articles together. I still keep in touch with Ron and Ann, who are now retired—and they have been nothing but wonderful and supportive.

I still remember Dick's words regarding the rejections I had received from the clinical psychology programs. "If you keep doing what you've been doing, the things that have been holding you back are going to keep holding you back." Those words have stuck with me ever since. I finally decided to wake up, get serious about my career, and stop blocking my own progress. The graduate school rejections turned out to be one of the best things that have ever happened to me. They forced me to pull my head out of the sand and start realizing my potential.

I also realized that clinical psychology was not as good a match for me as I thought it was. Dick was a practicing family therapist, and I helped him with one of his cases. I realized that I could never take on the kind of role that Dick was playing. It would leave me drained and despondent about the world. I loved science and loved numbers, and I loved trying to understand human behavior. I was born to be a social-science researcher. Paradoxically, by striking out in my efforts to get into clinical psychology, I wound up finding my true path—human development and developmental psychology. Sometimes failure can be a tremendous and enlightening gift.

Between 1993 and 1996, I went from being one of Dick's pet projects to being the assistant director of his lab. I collected three data sets during that time, and using the statistical knowledge I gained from my first formal statistics course, I analyzed the data myself and presented the results to Dick and to Ron. I presented some of this work at the inaugural conference of the Society for the Study of Identity Formation in February 1995, and it was there that I met Al Waterman, who would become a close friend and collaborator, and Bill Kurtines, who would wind up as my PhD advisor later on. I also met Jim Côté, with whom I have coauthored several articles and who has been an informal mentor to me. I was a major hit at my first academic conference, and I gained confidence in my ability to come up with research ideas, design research studies, collect and analyze data, and interpret and present results. I also presented the theoretical paper that Dick and I had been writing—the one I mention in the Prologue—and many years later, Al Waterman and Jim Côté would tell me that that rejected and unpublished paper is what impressed them most at that conference. It told them that I knew how to conceptualize and formulate ideas—a skill that has served me very well in my academic career.

In 1996, as I was preparing to finish my master's degree, I had a decision to make. Where would I pursue my doctoral degree? Gerald Adams, whom I met at the identity conference, invited me to apply to his developmental psychology PhD program at the University of Guelph in Ontario, Canada. I had also been in touch with Bill Kurtines, who was encouraging me to apply to his developmental psychology PhD program at Florida International University (FIU) in Miami. I applied to both, as well as to Ron and Ann's family and child sciences PhD program at Florida State and to the developmental psychology PhD program at the University of Miami. I wound up being accepted to all four of the PhD programs. I decided to enroll at FIU under Bill Kurtines' advisorship.

Relocating to Miami was a huge adjustment. Although I had lived in South Florida before, I had never lived in Miami—and Miami is culturally distinct from almost anywhere else in the United States. Three quarters of Miami residents are either immigrants or the children of immigrants, and as someone with no personal connection to immigration, I felt out of place. I had studied Spanish in college, but I didn't speak it fluently—so there were many parts of Miami where I could not communicate. I was definitely not used to this kind of environment.

As the years went by, however, I really fell in love with the culture of Miami—and this culture led to a major transformation in my scholarly writing and research interests. The stories that students told me about themselves and their parents braving life-threatening obstacles to reach the United States were awe-inspiring for me. One young man in one of my classes raised his hand and told the class that his parents had brought him to the United States from Cuba on a raft when he was a baby. A young woman told the class that her parents had fled drug-related violence in Colombia and had stowed away on a cargo flight to Miami—all while her mother was pregnant with her.

Another young lady told me that she and her family had ridden trains through Central America and swum the Rio Grande to get away from the Sandinista government in Nicaragua. I began to become interested in culture, in immigration, and in how people adjust to a new culture after they migrate.

A few years into my time in Miami, a colleague and I submitted a manuscript for publication attempting to replicate the factor structures of some personal identity measures using one of my Miami samples. An astute reviewer commented that, although the sample was 80% ethnic minorities, and although the majority of our sample was comprised of immigrants and children of immigrants, we didn't mention culture at all. At first, I bristled at this criticism of our work. Had the sample been 80% White, no one would have asked us to consider culture. But as I thought more about the reviewer's point, I realized that it was an opportunity to learn more about the lives of the immigrant students in my classes, the people I worked with in Bill Kurtines' lab, and the Miami community as a whole.

So I started reading up on the acculturation literature. It was fascinating! Studies on cultural adjustment supported what I was seeing in my own students. Many of them were completely bicultural—remaining faithful to their families' cultural heritage while also embracing the United States. I saw a huge amount of untapped potential in the acculturation literature— many of the studies were interesting but simplistic. For example, some of the work I was reading focused almost exclusively on language use—such as the "switch from Spanish to English" among Hispanic immigrants to the United States—but did not touch on people's values or sense of identity. Ethnic identity research—which examines how people define themselves as a member of their ethnic or racial group—generally was not touching on how people integrated their ethnic identity with their sense of attachment to the United States (or whichever other nation they resided in). After reading a few articles on acculturation and other forms of cultural adjustment, I was sold. I wanted to expand my work to include immigration, culture, and ethnicity as well as personal identity.

While I was pursuing my doctoral degree at FIU, I met an amazing and beautiful woman named Lisa Rodriguez. Lisa was a Miami native and was of Puerto Rican descent. The first time I saw her, I knew that she was my soulmate. We went on our first date on Valentine's Day 1998, and we were married in January 2000. Lisa was also strongly attached to the Miami area. Her whole family lived there, and she clearly emphasized that she had no desire to leave. Given that the South Florida area is home to only two or three major universities, finding an academic job that didn't require leaving the area would be challenging.

In academia, there is a saying, "If you want to move up, you have to move around." We all know many examples of the academic nomad—the colleague who was in California for a couple of years, then moved to Georgia, then to Massachusetts, and then to Texas. Just like many professional athletes, these scholars seem to be available to the highest bidder and to have very little attachment to their community or university. Such a nomadic existence can wreak havoc on families—children and adolescents are yanked away from their friendship networks on a moment's notice because Mom or Dad got a job offer that their current university didn't match. For academics like me who are married to non-academics, the idea of moving around the country (and sometimes around the world) looking for a better salary or more prestige is uncomfortable. In my family, we had an expression—Family Comes First— that I have always lived by. The lifestyle of the academic nomad was not consistent with my philosophy of life.

So, as I was finishing my degree at FIU, I started looking for jobs in the South Florida area. In March 2000, I came across an ad for a postdoctoral fellowship at the University of Miami. The postdoc would be housed in a research group who conducted research on family therapy for adolescent behavior problems and substance use. My combination of degrees in family/child sciences and developmental psychology seemed like a good fit—so I applied for the position. I was hired on May 1, 2000, the day after I graduated from FIU with my doctoral degree.

You might notice that I have not mentioned Dick Dunham's name much. He and I went through a nasty "divorce" at the end of my time at Florida State, and our relationship had become somewhat contentious. Dick, who had been gracious and magnanimous when I was still a lost soul and needed a great deal of guidance, had become increasingly prickly and difficult after I assumed the role of assistant lab director. The students in the lab were more likely to approach me than Dick if they had a question or concern—he could be unapproachable to people he had not "let into" his private psychological space. He seemed to be threatened by my increasing prominence within the lab, and within the identity research community generally. When I started working with Jim Côté and Al Waterman, often on papers in which Dick was not involved, he became even more upset.

Dick and I kept in touch for the first couple of years after I left Florida State and relocated to FIU, but he was never comfortable with my increasing independence from him. I brought Lisa to Tallahassee to meet Dick and Jeannie in August 1998, and we talked about some research projects we wanted to work on. However, my contact with him after that was sporadic, and we never saw each other in person again. Dick retired from academia in 1999 and moved to San Diego, and soon after that his health began to decline precipitously. He passed away in April 2002, and at the time of his death, we had not spoken in more than 2 years. When Jeannie notified me that he had died, I felt a sinking feeling in my stomach. Yes, my relationship with Dick had deteriorated considerably at the end of my time at Florida State and into my time in Miami—and yes, he had become difficult and had embarrassed me in front of his lab on several occasions because he was angry with me. But I could (and should) have been the bigger person and continued to collaborate with him. The fact that I didn't still haunts me, and—as one of my close colleagues told me when I told him the story—it will probably stay with me for the rest of my life. Dick was supportive of me when I really needed him, and he only became threatened when he thought I didn't need him anymore. He admitted to me once that he had fears of abandonment, and those fears were on display at the end of our time together. However, I remain indebted to him for the rest of my career. I would never have gotten started without him.

I had a PhD student who also had a difficult relationship with her mentor. Her story with him is very similar to my story with Dick. He was magnanimous at the beginning when she was not a threat to him, but he became increasingly territorial as she advanced in her career and as people in the lab were gravitating more toward her. Mentorship requires a wide range of skills and strengths, and not everyone will possess all of them. I have heard horror stories about mentor/mentee relationships, and my story with Dick pales in comparison with many of them.

Back to my postdoctoral position. It was a difficult group to work with. The research was wonderful, but the interpersonal dynamics were challenging. I found myself losing motivation. In early 2001, a friend of mine from my graduate-school days at FIU told me that he might be able to arrange a meeting for me with José Szapocznik, who directed another center at the University of Miami. José emailed me in late March asking me to send him my curriculum vitae. I did, and within a week I received an email from his assistant thanking me for applying for the faculty position.

What faculty position? I thought. I had not applied for anything—I had simply asked for a meeting.

On April 18, 2001, I officially interviewed for the position as José's faculty-level assistant, and on May 14, his administrative assistant emailed me and told me that José wanted to meet with me again. I met with him a few days later, and he hired me. I started with him on June 1, 2001—and I held that position for nearly 20 years. So the difficult postdoctoral position served as my point of entry into the university.

Working for (and with) José was a wonderful experience. He was one of the most visionary leaders one could imagine. He was a top-notch scientist, a community leader, and an expert clinician. He had a lot of projects going on, and I often received emails from him asking for something to be done almost immediately. Papers needed to be written, grant applications needed to be put together, and final project report deadlines were approaching. I handled everything he asked me to handle, and I was learning much in the process. José had also been one of the founders of acculturation theory and research in the 1970s, so the early work I had done on acculturation was turning into a major line of research for me. Even though some of the work José was involved in was not of direct interest to me, I found it fascinating, and it became of interest to me. Better yet, I started applying José's rigorous methods to my own personal identity work, and I was beginning to be recognized as a leader in that field. Before long, I was looking for ways to integrate acculturation theory and research into my work on personal identity.

Dick Dunham had given me sage advice at the end of my time at Florida State. He told me to collect as much data as I could during my doctoral program so that I could publish off the data during my postdoc and assistant professorship. So I gathered six or seven different college student samples at FIU during my time there—using measures that Jim Côté, Al Waterman, and others had shared with me. As Dick advised, I continued to publish off those data sets well into my faculty position at the University of Miami. If memory serves me correctly, those data supported my publishing efforts for at least 10 years after I finished graduate school—and they helped my colleagues and me launch a series of multisite college student health studies between 2007 and 2010. In turn, the multisite studies have supported more than 50 publications—many of which were led by graduate students, postdocs, or early-career faculty. So Dick's sage advice led me not only to launch my research program, but also to create major opportunities for the next generation of young scholars.

Working with José also taught me how to write grants. Grant writing can be frustrating and demoralizing because months of work appears wasted if the grant proposal is scored poorly by the review committee. But every piece of writing is an opportunity to sharpen one's skills—even if the outcome is not favorable. Receiving critical reviewer comments on my grant applications and journal manuscripts has taught me to be a better writer. Moreover, as I emphasize repeatedly in this book, many of the reasons why papers and grants get rejected have less to do with the writing itself and more to do with the study that is being proposed or reported. Even the most wonderfully written manuscript or grant proposal cannot compensate for a poorly planned or flawed study.

Of course, this does not mean that poor writing is not a reason why manuscripts and grant proposals get rejected. Of course it is! If a reviewer cannot understand what you are saying, that person is unlikely to provide a favorable recommendation regarding publication or funding. My point here—something José emphasized repeatedly during my years working closely with him—is that the quality of the writing must be considered in light of what we are writing about.

It took a few years, but the lessons I was learning—not just about writing but also about planning and carrying out rigorous research studies—led to my beginning to "break out" as a scholar. After some fairly mediocre years at the start of my faculty career, including some quite frustrating stretches where almost everything I submitted seemed to be getting rejected, the summer of 2004 served as my coming-out party. Suddenly I was publishing between 15 and 20 articles (including both lead-authored and coauthored papers) per year. My acceptance rate went from less than 25% to above 50%, where it has remained ever since. I have only had one year since 2004 when I have published fewer than 10 journal articles—and that was in 2011, when I was dealing with multiple serious family illnesses.

I also wrote, and received, my first research grant in 2004 and 2005. No exaggeration—I went through no fewer than 70 drafts of that proposal before we submitted it. I sought comments from many, many people and continually revised the proposal in response. At some points, I felt frustrated and exasperated by the prospect of having to recast the proposal over and over. Sometimes I just wanted to scream. But, as I learned through the process of writing that proposal (and many others since), moving from a first draft to a submittable draft, as well as sharpening the writing (and sharpening what we are writing about), takes patience and a great deal of work.

Since that first grant award—a Mentored Scientist award that provided me with 5 years of funding to get my career started—I have received seven additional grants. I have met many amazing colleagues along the way, most of whom have really helped me to grow my research career, sharpen my writing skills, and start new and important projects. Working with all these people has taught me how to collaborate successfully with colleagues. The primary lesson my father taught me—say what you mean and mean what you say—has been invaluable in my academic career. Also, the difficult lessons, such as the mistakes I made at the end of my relationship with Dick, have taught me how to be more patient with, and forgiving of, other people. I now work with colleagues around the world and mentor many people (both formally and informally), and I am grateful for the opportunity to serve others as well as to advance my own career.

Lessons Learned From My Academic Journey

Among the most important attributes I have maintained throughout my academic career have been resilience, humility, and a sense of humor. Bouncing back after being rejected is an essential part of being an academic. Being rejected unfairly—such as editors' rejection of your manuscripts when the reviews are favorable—is especially difficult to deal with. Allowing oneself time to be angry, and to grieve, is important. Papers that we write often become extensions of ourselves, and having them rejected can feel like a blow to our self-worth. I often allow myself two or three days to "steam" after having a paper or grant proposal rejected, and then I move on to next steps (e.g., revising the paper based on the feedback from the journal or deciding how to recast the grant proposal).

Humility is a trait that I have always valued greatly. My grandfather had a wonderful expression: "Don't ever believe your own press clippings." In other words, don't let success go to your head. As I say in my book *Reaching for Resilience*, true confidence is quiet and has no reason to brag or boast. I know that I am good at what I do, but I have no need to tell others how great I am. I prefer to give credit away to others when projects are successful. As long as you know that you are good at your work and don't need others to reassure you, you are free to share the credit.

My sense of humor keeps me grounded. There is an expression I like—if you don't laugh at life, it will make you cry. Self-deprecating humor—making lighthearted jokes about yourself as a way of getting people laughing—is especially effective because it disarms people, it isn't threatening or offensive to anyone, and it makes you seem relatable. I make jokes about myself all the time, and I love doing it. I know that what I'm saying is just a joke—I don't really think I'm stupid or oafish—but laughter really is the best medicine. Get someone laughing and they will let their guard down, so that you can really get to know them. I enjoy making other people feel good, so watching them laugh at my silly jokes helps me feel more comfortable as well. In the end, when I'm giving talks, teaching, or engaging in other interactions with my colleagues, my goal is to exchange ideas. Such exchanges are likely to be most successful when both parties are comfortable and have let their guard down.

Other lessons I have learned include the power of persistence, the importance of relationships, and being perfectionistic up to a point. Persistence is absolutely critical in academia. We know that our chances of having papers accepted in top journals are small to medium at best, so continuing to persevere even after a rejection is essential. I cover this topic in Chapters 11, 12, and 13, but some papers seem to be "cursed" and are rejected over and over. But you have to keep trying. At some point you may choose to set a paper aside after it has been rejected several times, but I would not advise doing that until you've tried at least three or four journals. I have a colleague who submitted a paper to twelve journals—each of which rejected the paper—but he tried a thirteenth journal that finally accepted the paper. Readers only know—and care about—the journal in which the paper was published. They don't know about, and are not concerned with, all of the journals that rejected the paper.

I cannot say enough about the importance of developing and maintaining relationships. Academia is a collaborative endeavor, and very few of us work alone. Collaborative relationships are often formed through conferences, through mutual colleagues, and sometimes even when one person reaches out to another and asks to collaborate. I have met close colleagues in each of these ways. I met Byron Zamboanga, one of my closest colleagues and the person with whom I have coauthored the greatest number of publications, at a conference talk in 2004. He was in the audience at my talk and introduced himself after the session had ended, and we immediately started talking about potential collaborations. We stayed in touch, followed through on some of the ideas we had discussed, and built a strong working relationship that has now been in place for 15 years. Whenever I had an idea for a project, I would tell Byron about it, and vice versa.

Sometimes people have emailed me out of nowhere and asked me to collaborate with them. I met several of my European colleagues that way. Koen Luyckx, who was then a PhD student at the Catholic University of Leuven in Belgium, emailed me in January 2005 and asked me whether I would be interested in coauthoring a paper with him. I told him I needed a couple of months to finish some other projects, and then I carefully edited his paper and sent it back to him. We wound up working together not only on that paper, but also on several more, and we also co-edited a handbook (along with another colleague of ours). Elisabetta Crocetti, who is now a professor at the University of Bologna in Italy, and Nino Skhirtladze, who is at Ilia State University in Tbilisi, Georgia, approached me in the same way. In my experience, people who approach an experienced scholar and ask to collaborate are generally hardworking, ambitious, and dedicated—and it has been more than worth my time to work with them.

Academic relationships are cultivated in much the same way as relationships in any other area of life. You treat the person with consideration and respect, you keep them in mind when thinking of new projects, and you find ways to involve them in papers that you are planning to write. You are honest with them and you don't make promises or offers unless you plan to follow through. If you say you are going to do something, you do it, even if other events get in your way. If you absolutely cannot honor your word, you let the person know as soon as possible and find a way to make things right.

Essentially, you communicate to the other person that you are trustworthy and honorable, that their well-being is important to you, and that working with them is a priority for you. Collaborative relationships are part friendships and part business partnerships, so it is important to treat close colleagues in the same way as one would treat a friend or a business partner. Remember that, in most cases, collaborators work with you because they want to, not because they have to—so you want them to keep wanting to collaborate with you.

A final point is avoiding maladaptive perfectionism. It is important to want our work to be rigorous and solid, and not to want to have our names listed on papers that are poorly written or that report erroneous results. Some degree of perfectionism may therefore be adaptive. However, maladaptive perfectionism is something to avoid. Maladaptive perfectionism is to an insistence that everything must be completely perfect, with no blemishes at all, before it can be presented. Maladaptive perfectionism freezes our progress and prevents us from submitting papers for publication because we are afraid that they are somehow not perfect enough. There is a saying that captures maladaptive perfectionism well: "The perfect is the enemy of the good." We are human, and therefore we are destined to be imperfect. Expecting absolute perfection from yourself, or from anyone else, is an exercise in frustration.

As a child, I was once afraid of tall water slides. I was terrified that they might move too fast or that I might drown. I once sat at the top of a water slide for 10 minutes until the lifeguard told me that I needed to either go down the slide or walk back down the stairs. There was a line of other kids waiting for the slide, and it wasn't fair of me to keep sitting there. Eventually I mustered the courage to go into the slide, and I loved it! All that fear had been needless.

Writing is not all that different. Especially when we are writing drafts that will be shared with colleagues so they can provide feedback, at some point we must decide that the draft is ready for our colleagues to review. The writing team as a whole decides when the paper is ready to submit for publication, as is discussed in Chapter 14. When we have done the best we can, it is time to send the draft to our colleagues. My colleague Gordon Finley taught me the law of diminishing returns, which essentially states that there is a point in the revision process where further changes are unlikely to improve the paper substantially. When we have reached that point in the process of writing drafts on our own, it's time to circulate the draft to our coauthors. Maladaptive perfectionism prevents us from doing this because we are terrified that our work is not good enough and will never be good enough. Maladaptive perfectionism is thus a trap that we should do our best to avoid.

About This Book

In this book, I offer lots of advice and tips about writing, based on what has worked for me and for my colleagues. I have written with people from all around the world, and these strategies have worked consistently in getting papers published. However, I encourage readers to add their own nuances and touches to the ideas I outline in this book. I do not expect every reader to follow everything I suggest to the letter. Writing is an idiosyncratic process, and no two people do it in exactly the same way.

This book is intended as a resource for writers at various stages of their careers, including graduate students, postdoctoral fellows, and early-career, mid-career, and senior scholars. The sequence of chapters, as described below, captures the publishing process from generating an idea all the way through acceptance of the manuscript for publication. I expect that most readers will use the book as a reference, but some people may find value in reading the chapters in sequence. I've written the book so that it can be used in either of these ways.

My assumption is that most readers have a good sense of the scientific method and of the basics of how research is conducted. Selecting a topic can be difficult—it is easy to say, "I want to study discrimination," but it is much more difficult to propose a specific set of research questions and hypotheses. One of the most difficult ideas for early-career scholars, especially students, to grasp is that it is not possible (or necessary) to do everything in one study. We have our entire careers to pursue our lines of research. Each individual study is a step along that path. We cannot traverse the entire path in one step. Chapter 1 focuses on how to narrow down a broad idea into a focused set of objectives, research questions, and hypotheses, and Chapter 2 focuses on how to design a publishable study that can provide a full test of our hypotheses.

Chapter 3 focuses on ethical issues, including ethical data analysis and avoiding conflicts of interest. I teach a course on research ethics, and when I first tell my students that there are important ethical issues involved in collecting, analyzing, and writing up data, some of them respond with a quizzical look on their faces. To put it briefly, our goal should be to conduct our research in as transparent a way as possible. Think of the last time you read a good novel where the author painted scenery and made you feel as though you were on the scene with the characters in the story. J.R.R. Tolkien, author of *The Hobbit* and *Lord of the Rings*, was a master at painting scenes in this way. Sometimes he would spend 10 pages just describing what the mountains and landscape looked like, the expressions on each character's face, the way the wind was blowing, and the sounds and smells that filled the air. We are certainly not aiming for this level of detail in writing up research articles, but we do want the reader to imagine being with us as we conceived of the idea for the project, designed the study, carried out the project, collected the data, and conducted the analyses. Concealing important information from the reader—such as the fact that the original hypotheses were not supported and that we then proceeded to develop and test a new set of hypotheses—is unethical and serves to mislead the scientific process and the field.

Several chapters focus on the scientific process. It is essential that we not start writing until we have completed data collection and analysis. We don't write until we know what we will be writing about. Further, any paper that we write is only as good as the data on which it is based. A wonderfully written manuscript cannot compensate for a flawed study. Think of it this way—would you start decorating the walls of your house if the foundation was shaky? Would you drive your new car on a road where the concrete had holes in it?

As a result, the first three chapters cover study design, conducting rigorous research, and data analysis. I provide references to more extensive treatments of these topics, but because the writing process depends on the quality of the science we are describing, I believe that chapters on the scientific process must be included in a book about scholarly writing in the social and health sciences.

I also include three chapters on the principles of good writing—specifically getting ready to write both psychologically and logistically (Chapter 5), rules of good grammar and sentence structure (Chapter 6), and how to paraphrase and cite sources correctly (Chapter 7). Individual writers will differ in terms of how useful some of this material may be to them. People whose first language is not English may find some of the mechanical and syntactical tips in Chapter 6 useful—but my experience is that many native English speakers can also benefit from a review of sentence structure, grammar, and punctuation. Especially with the advent of text-messaging lingo, which is based heavily on shorthand, the principles of good writing may have become less familiar to some writers. Some of the principles I cover, such as avoiding second person (*you, your*) and minimizing the use of contractions, may represent new ideas for some readers. Readers who are already familiar with these writing "rules" may be able to skim Chapter 6, if not skip it entirely.

Writing first drafts can also be a frustrating exercise for many people. Staring at a blank screen with the cursor flashing can be intimidating and anxiety-provoking. In Chapter 8, I offer tips on getting started—centering on transferring thoughts from one's mind onto the screen. First drafts are supposed to be poorly written. The purpose of a first draft is not to create a Shakespearean sonnet—it is to move the ideas onto the screen. *You cannot edit what is in your head!*

The anxiety that often accompanies writing for many people can freeze them in place and keep them from getting started. In this case, I recommend creating an outline and then writing within that outline—a technique that I also cover in this book. The outline can be as broad or specific as you need it to be, so long as it helps to guide your writing and to reduce your anxiety. When I use outlines, I assume that the entries I list will end up as headings in the paper. I therefore know what kind of text needs to be written within each heading. For example, if I am writing a paper about discrimination, I might include headings about structural discrimination and personal discrimination—in other words, higher-level systems (such as the justice and educational systems) that discriminate against certain groups, in contrast to specific discriminatory events (such as being ignored or called names) that occur between individuals or small groups.

Going from a first draft to a submission-quality draft can be quite a challenge for many people. Chapter 9 covers editing your own work as well as soliciting and handling feedback from colleagues. At what point do we share a draft with coauthors? How do we incorporate feedback from multiple coauthors? What happens when coauthors' recommendations conflict with one another? What about when coauthors want to take the paper in a different direction than we have in mind?

As I note several times, my experiences and perspective are just that—my experiences and perspective. Although I expect that some version of my techniques will work for most writers, I have no expectation that everyone will follow my suggestions literally. Consider my suggestions, figure out what works for you, and stick with that.

Chapters 10 (selecting journals) and 11 (thinking like a reviewer) cover material that I "learned the hard way"—how to select journals for your work and how to evaluate the contribution of your work objectively. Many authors submit manuscripts to top journals even when the result is almost certain rejection, because the paper does not represent enough of a contribution to the literature to warrant publication in a high-prestige journal. It is extremely beneficial to authors to know the journals in their field of study well enough so that they can select a set of journals that are well matched with the manuscript they have written. It is also essential to adopt sufficient scientific humility so as to be able to generate an honest evaluation of the contribution that one's work represents. There is no shame in writing a paper that represents a moderate contribution—but it is essential to be able to recognize that the paper's contribution is moderate rather than major.

I also include two chapters on the manuscript submission, review, and revision process. Chapter 12 covers the manuscript submission and review process, and Chapter 13 addresses what to do with rejected manuscripts. Even when reviewers like your paper and believe it can be published after revisions are made, they may still include harsh-sounding comments in their reviews. The first time I received a revise–resubmit decision from a journal, the reviewer comments seemed frightening. How was I ever going to make all these revisions? Fortunately, Dick Dunham guided me through the revision process, and we got that paper published. Since then, I have successfully shepherded (or helped others to shepherd) nearly 300 papers through the journal review and revision process. The response letter—where you list each reviewer comment and detail how you revised the paper in response to that comment—is extremely important in satisfying reviewers and in convincing them to recommend that your paper be published. I include chapters on dealing with editors and reviewers—as well as on what to do if a journal rejects your paper. Some papers seem to be "cursed" and are rejected by one journal after another. How do we handle those papers, and at what point do we conclude that the best course of action is to stop spending time on a paper that has been repeatedly rejected? I cover this in great detail, using my own experience as well as that of my colleagues.

The last five chapters address "special considerations" in the publication process. Chapter 14 covers working with coauthors. Coauthors are an invaluable resource in the publishing process—in the majority of cases, they provide helpful feedback, help us to spot and correct errors or omissions in our work, and offer support when we feel stuck and are not sure how to proceed with a paper. Coauthors can also be slow or difficult, and large authorship teams may be especially challenging because of the sheer volume of coauthor feedback that the lead author must sort through.

Chapter 15 covers working with public-use and proprietary data sets. writing non-empirical papers. Writers and data analysts working with large national datasets need to be aware of the unique challenges that these data sets present, such as complex sampling strategies, where results are likely to be inaccurate if the complex data structure is not modeled correctly.

Chapter 16 covers non-empirical papers. Non-empirical papers present specific challenges that empirical papers may not involve, such as laying out new theories, reviewing and summarizing extensive amounts of literature, or arguing for specific lines of research. Because these papers don't report empirical results, they are more challenging to write, and they often receive reviewer comments that are often more extensive and more difficult to address than reviewer's comments on empirical manuscripts.

Chapter 17 covers open-access and pay-to-publish journals. The open-access movement has resulted in the launching of many new journals that charge authors to publish their work. Should we submit our work to these journals, and if so, what kinds of work may be best suited for open-access journals? Writers must also know how to differentiate legitimate open-access journals from predatory open-access journals, where predatory journals should be avoided.

Chapter 18 covers how to write books and book chapters. Scholars are often asked to write book chapters, and they may also be interested in writing or editing books. There are several important considerations that should be taken into account when planning an authored or edited book (or an edited handbook). I have written and edited books in my career, and I offer guidance for planning these projects. I also offer advice for scholars who are considering whether to write a book chapter.

Each chapter begins with a set of objectives and ends with a summary, so that readers know what to expect going into the chapter and are provided with a summary of key points after finishing the chapter. The summary also makes it easier for readers to refer to points from earlier chapters without having to hunt for those points within the text of the chapter. My goal for this book was to make it as easy to read and as easy to use as I possibly could.

Now that we have finished this broad overview of the book, let's get started!

1

Getting Started and Selecting a Topic

Chapter Objectives

By the time you finish this chapter, you should feel more comfortable with:

- Conducting literature searches
- Following the latest scholarly work in a field of study
- Developing a set of research questions and hypotheses for an empirical study
- Conceptualizing a line of research as evolving from one's initial ideas
- Differentiating among association, prediction, and causation—and identifying research questions that correspond to each of these levels
- Using theory to develop and test hypotheses
- Using literature searches to ensure that your research questions have not been examined before

Most readers will be familiar with the scientific method. Broadly, the steps are as follows:

1. Observe the phenomenon (or review the literature)
2. Formulate a set of hypotheses
3. Design an empirical study to test the hypotheses
4. Analyze the study data and render a conclusion about the extent to which the hypotheses have been supported
5. Write up and publish the results

Notice where writing appears on this list. *It's the last step.*

Starting to write before we know what we're going to write about is like choosing a college for a child who hasn't been conceived yet. It's wildly premature.

First, we need to decide what it is that we want to study. Out of the vast universe of possible ideas, which ones interest us?

A close colleague of mine likes to say that "research is me-search." What he means by this is that we tend to choose topics that resonate with our own

The Savvy Academic. Seth J. Schwartz, Oxford University Press. © Oxford University Press 2022.
DOI: 10.1093/oso/9780190095918.003.0002

personal history, or with the histories of people, places, or groups we know well. For example, I became very interested in identity formation in college and graduate school because of my own acute struggles with identity earlier in my life. As a kid, I was a drifter and never really knew who I was or what my life was about. I was a below-average student despite being a math whiz, loving science and history, and having a near-photographic memory. It wasn't until I met Dick Dunham (see the Prologue) that I really started to buckle down and figure out what I was doing with my life.

However, being interested in identity is not the same thing as proposing a specific study with testable hypotheses. To be able to propose a study, we must know the literature and what the next steps are for advancing that literature. We must know what has been done before, what the "major names" in the literature have been publishing recently, and what the stakeholders (both major names and other contributors) in our chosen field believe needs to be done next. In short, we must do our homework.

When I was a postdoctoral fellow, I spent months reviewing literature. I taught myself how to write summaries of empirical articles. I would take brief notes on the introduction section, particularly on the theoretical approaches that were being used to frame the study. Eventually, I created a template that I used to summarize more than 300 journal articles during my postdoc. An example summary appears in Table 1.1. Additionally, Jaakkola (2020) provides a list of characteristics of conceptual or literature review articles that are analogous to the characteristics of empirical articles that I list in the table. For example, she substitutes "choice of theories and concepts analyzed" in place of data source and sample. I recommend consulting her article—she provides an excellent template for summarizing conceptual and literature review articles.

Not only did this template allow me to summarize articles quickly, but it also provided me with a "cheat sheet" when I was writing a paper and needed to figure out which articles to cite. It was a great way to become acquainted with the literature. Authors whose names kept showing up were clearly leaders in the field (and possible reviewers for my papers when I submitted them for publication). Journals that appeared repeatedly in my database were possible outlets for papers that I would later submit.

Searching the Literature

But how do we find sources in the first place? What do we put into the search engine so that it will "spit out" records for us to sort through?

Table 1.1 Journal Article Summary Template

Reference	Research questions	Variables/Instruments	Sample and number of data points	Analyses	Findings
Barber, Connolly, Crits-Christoph, Gladis, & Siqueland, in press (JCCP)	What is the predictive relationship between therapeutic alliance and treatment outcomes, taking into account prior treatment gains?	(1) Depression (Beck) (2) Therapeutic alliance	88 clinically referred patients (anxiety or depression disorders)—42 males, 46 females; mean age 38. Measures of alliance at sessions 2, 5, 10; measures of symptoms at intake, after every session, and at termination.	Hierarchical multiple regression—covariates (therapy type, number of sessions, and initial severity).	(1) Alliance was associated with decreased depression symptoms at termination, controlling for symptom levels at intake. (2) Alliance was associated with change in depression during the early phases of therapy, but not right away. (3) Alliance continued to predict later changes in depressive symptoms even when controlling for prior change in symptoms. (4) The relationship between alliance formation and symptom reduction is bidirectional.

Our first step is to identify the search engines we will use. Notice I am using the plural word *engines*. Although Google Scholar is quite adept at providing a comprehensive list of records, I also recommend using at least one other database—PsycInfo, Sociological Abstracts, Scopus, MedLine, and PubMed are some of the databases I have used to supplement my Google Scholar searches. Google Scholar will provide more records than most other search engines, but many of the records returned will be tangential or irrelevant to your search. The other databases are more likely to provide a narrower range of records that will be relevant to your search, but each of these databases specializes in a specific field (e.g., psychology, sociology, medicine, public health).

The next item we need is a list of keywords or search terms. Let's say we are interested in ethnic identity and substance use among Hispanic adolescents. We might enter the search terms *ethnic identity* and *substance* or *drug* or *alcohol* and *Hispanic* or *Latin** and *adolescen**.

Where each of the terms in parentheses must be present somewhere in the title, abstract, or keywords in order for a given entry to be included in the results of our search. Note that the asterisk (*) represents a wildcard character—there are multiple endings for *Latin*, and we want to make sure that *adolescent* and *adolescence* both show up in our search results.

Google Scholar uses the same algorithms that the general Google search engine uses. The most directly relevant records are returned first, and relevance decreases as we move down the list of search results. Depending on the breadth versus narrowness of our search, and of the field in which we are searching, there may be many, few, or no relevant records returned. Using more search terms narrows the range of records that will be returned, so if you are not getting any hits from a search, remove one of your keywords and try again. If you are getting too many hits, and not enough of them are relevant to what you are seeking, add a new keyword and try again. Searching the literature is an inexact science, and search engine algorithms are constantly changing. New search engines are constantly appearing as well.

Once we have a sense of who is contributing to the literature in which we are interested, we should follow those people. Many researchers maintain profiles on Google Scholar and on academic social media sites, such as ResearchGate and Academia.edu. On Google Scholar, you can simply click on someone's name to view their profile (assuming they have created one). On ResearchGate and Academia.edu, you need to create your own profile first before you can view other people's profiles. (Creating profiles on these sites is a good idea, because you will receive attention for your work as you publish and upload it.)

As you find articles through various means (search engines and academic social media), you should save PDFs of those articles on your computer so you can access them later. I often work on airplanes, in doctor's office waiting rooms, and in other places that may or may not have wireless Internet access. It is very useful to be able to access articles on my laptop even if I cannot access the Internet.

I also suggest using reference software, such as Reference Manager or EndNote. These programs allow you to save the citation information for an article directly from a search engine, so that you don't have to type the citation manually into the text and into the reference section. They also easily convert citations and references from one style to another—which saves a *lot* of time. I remember an article that was rejected from a journal that used APA style. We wanted to submit it to a journal that used Chicago style, which required several mind-numbing hours of changing every single citation and reference. Had I been using Reference Manager or EndNote, the change would have required less than a minute (and almost no effort on my part).

Keeping Up With Journals and Authors

Once you have a sense of the journals that publish articles in your field—that is, the journals that show up repeatedly in your search records—you should be sure to browse those journals regularly. You can sign up for table of contents alerts online, and you will receive an email each time a new issue is available for each journal. Some journals will also send out alerts each week with new articles that are available ahead of print (some publishers call these articles Online First). Alternatively, you can go to the journal website every couple of months and browse new content.

Google Scholar also provides an option where users can obtain a list of articles that cite a specific article. For example, let's say that we find an article by Jones and Hernandez, published in 2010. We can click the "Cited By" link within the Jones and Hernandez record, and we will be taken to a list of articles that cite the Jones and Hernandez article. Because citing articles are, by definition, more recently published than the original article, looking up citing articles is a good way to find more recent literature on the topic in which we are interested.

As already noted, it is also essential to identify major contributors to your chosen field and to keep up with their work. Academic social media sites, such as ResearchGate and Academia.edu, allow users to "follow" scholars and to view their current projects as well as published articles. Users can also communicate directly with scholars to ask about their ongoing projects, request full text of articles, and share ideas. I have found that most researchers, ranging from graduate students to senior full professors, are honored to be asked about their work and are generally responsive to requests and other communications.

Coming Up With a Testable Research Question and Hypotheses

How do we go from having a general area of interest to outlining a specific set of research questions and hypotheses? My answer to this question focuses on three general themes: science as baby steps, lines of research, and characteristics of a good hypothesis.

Science as Baby Steps

The scientific literature rarely takes huge leaps within a single study. Rather, science is advanced through coordinated steps. Each step represents a study (or a sequence of studies) and advances the literature significantly but gradually.

For example, let's say that we wanted to examine the effects of ethnic discrimination on cardiovascular functioning among ethnic minority adults. We might first conduct a correlational study examining the relationship between discrimination experiences and cardiovascular biomarkers. Assuming that we found an association between discrimination and cardiovascular functioning, we might then conduct an experimental study where we randomly assign participants to active (experiencing discrimination from a study confederate) or control (exposure to stimuli not involving discrimination) and measure cardiovascular biomarkers as study outcomes. Again assuming that the expected effects emerge, we might then conduct additional studies varying the source of discrimination (e.g., authority figure versus peer), the type of discrimination experienced (e.g., overt name-calling versus more subtle insults or invalidations), and the setting (e.g., workplace, doctor visit, casual encounter, close relationship). This series of studies, conducted in sequence, would allow us first to open a line of research examining the association between discrimination and cardiovascular health, and then to gradually explore this association with greater precision.

Notice that it would be impossible to traverse all these steps in a single study. Indeed, it would be unwise to conduct detailed experimental studies until there was evidence of a general association between our hypothesized predictor and outcome variable. Doing so would be akin to drilling for oil prior to obtaining evidence that there was indeed oil present in the location where we were planning to drill. We would run the risk of wasting valuable time and resources on an expedition that might well lead to nothing.

It might be said, then, that science takes baby steps. Yes, there are some studies that represent quantum leaps in the evolution of a scientific field, but these studies represent only a small percentage of the research that is conducted. The majority of research moves science forward incrementally, where the next steps often become apparent only after the previous step has been completed. For example, our hypothetical experimental study— conducted in a research laboratory—examining the effects of discrimination on cardiovascular biomarkers might indicate that being verbally accosted by a study confederate caused the research subjects' biomarkers to react in unhealthy ways. This finding might lead us to wonder about the conditions under which discrimination is most harmful to cardiovascular health—which would likely lead us to conduct more studies examining effects of various settings and sources of discrimination.

Lines of Research

As implied in the previous subsection, researchers tend to establish lines of work examining specific issues and phenomena. The results of one study help to generate new questions that guide the next study. Indeed, many people spend years, decades, or even whole careers investigating a specific set of phenomena. As an example, I have been studying acculturation and related issues (e.g., culturally related stressors, such as discrimination and negative context of reception) for more than 15 years. I have studied various aspects of acculturation, including its dimensional structure (e.g., how many specific components comprise it; Schwartz et al., 2011), how acculturation components are affected by the language in which the questions are asked (Schwartz et al., 2014), and how acculturation components change over time (Schwartz et al., 2015). My colleagues and I have also applied acculturation theory to specific groups of international migrants (Schwartz et al., 2018; Wang, Schwartz, & Zamboanga, 2010) and undocumented immigrants (Cobb et al., 2017). Acculturation and similar immigration-related phenomena have represented my primary line of research for the majority of my scholarly career.

Students are often zealous and ambitious about their work, particularly master's theses and doctoral dissertations. Many students want to "do everything" at once! Such youthful exuberance is to be expected, and the enthusiasm that it reflects needs to be nurtured and encouraged. However, it is important for mentors to model lines of research for their students and to help students to appreciate what can—and what cannot—be accomplished in a single study or set of studies. I tell my students that they have their whole careers to do the work that they are planning to do.

The objective of any research study is to test a specific set of research questions and hypotheses. The next subsection covers some characteristics of a good research hypothesis. For now, the point I want to emphasize is that a line of research is far more expansive than any single hypothesis (or set of hypotheses), and that many of the studies we will conduct later in our careers are dependent on those that we are conducting now. That is, the ideas and hypotheses for our future work will be generated based on the results that we—and others in our field—are obtaining now.

Characteristics of a Good Research Hypothesis

So how do we know when we have arrived at a "good" research hypothesis? My answer is that a good research hypothesis:

- Is falsifiable;
- Specifies the population that is being studied;
- Specifies the constructs and variables that need to be measured; and
- Suggests appropriate research designs that can be used.

Falsifiability is one of the most critical components of a hypothesis. That is, empirical data should be able to provide a verdict on whether the hypothesis should be supported. For example, consider the hypothesis that "exposure to substance-using peers is positively associated with alcohol consumption among adolescents." This hypothesis is falsifiable because the magnitude and significance of the correlation between substance-using peer exposure and alcohol consumption will allow us to decide whether the hypothesis should be retained or rejected. On the other hand, consider the hypothesis that "discrimination is hurtful for ethnic minority adolescents." This hypothesis is not falsifiable because we have not operationally defined what *hurtful* means.

In many cases, hypotheses are not falsifiable because they are not specific enough. If we were to modify the discrimination hypothesis to state that "exposure to discrimination is causally related to increased depressive symptomatology and cortisol secretion," it would be falsifiable because we would be able to collect data based on the hypothesis and use those data to support or reject the hypothesis.

Hypotheses should also specify the population that we will be studying. More specifically, *inclusion/exclusion criteria* will be used to screen each potential participant and determine whether that person is eligible to participate in our study. Inclusion/exclusion criteria are based on the hypotheses guiding our study. For example, if our hypothesis states that pre-migration trauma will be correlated with experiences of discrimination among Venezuelan immigrant adults in the United States, then we know that our study population is Venezuelan-born adults who currently reside in the United States. Anyone who is under age 18, was not born in Venezuela, or is not currently living in the United States is not eligible to participate. We may have additional inclusion/exclusion criteria based on the measures we are using (e.g., if we are administering survey measures, participants must be able to read and write in English or Spanish and must not currently be under acute psychiatric care). Overall, inclusion criteria tell us what characteristics someone must have if they are to be included in our study, and exclusion criteria tell us what characteristics someone cannot have if they are to be included in our study.

Hypotheses also tell us what constructs need to be included in our study. For example, let's consider the Venezuelan hypothesis listed in the previous paragraph. If our hypothesis states that "pre-migration trauma will be correlated with experiences of discrimination among Venezuelan immigrant adults in the United States," then we know we must measure pre-migration trauma and experiences of discrimination. It is essential that the study measures exactly match the constructs listed in the hypothesis. If they do not, then our study will not be able to test the hypothesis.

It is important to note that, in most cases, our hypothesis does not dictate how we should assess the variables listed in the hypothesis. For example, pre-migration trauma might be assessed using surveys, interviews, or checklists. It is up to us to select the measurement method that is most rigorous and most compatible with our study population. (It is perfectly appropriate to use multiple methods, such as both surveys and interviews.)

A good hypothesis also tells us what research designs and methods to use in our study. Hypotheses that mention associations, correlations, or relationships can usually be tested using cross-sectional designs. Hypotheses that mention prediction or temporal ordering of variables generally require longitudinal designs—where the number and spacing of assessment waves are predicated on the pace and ways in which the study phenomena change over time. Hypotheses that use causal language—words like *cause, effect, influence*, et cetera —generally call for experimental studies where participants are assigned to conditions.

Note that, in experimental studies, group assignments may or may not be random, depending on the phenomenon under study and on whether it is possible or ethical to randomly assign participants to levels of that phenomenon. For example, if we are studying the effects of child abuse on post-traumatic stress symptoms, we will not be able to randomly assign participants to abuse versus non-abuse conditions. Doing so would be highly unethical. We can use a quasi-experimental design, where the groups are already in place before the study begins. The ability to draw causal conclusions is weaker in quasi-experimental research than in designs where people are randomly assigned to conditions, because random assignment is assumed to distribute confounding variables evenly across the resulting groups. It may be advisable to recruit individuals who were abused versus not abused, for example, and randomly assign them to conditions that will expose them to varying stimuli. This way there is a random assignment component in the study, even if the primary variable (abuse) is not randomly assigned (Shadish, Cook, & Campbell, 2002). Research designs are reviewed in depth in Chapter 2.

The Role of Theory

In many fields, theories guide the research process. A *theory* is a set of postulates about "how things work." For example, the theory of planned behavior (Ajzen, 2002) holds that the likelihood that a person will engage in specific behaviors is a function of that person's attitudes, social norms (beliefs about what other people think about engagement in the behavior in question), self-efficacy (the belief that one is able to perform the behavior properly), and intentions to engage in the behavior. For example, research (e.g., Rhodes & Courneya, 2003) has indicated that the likelihood that someone will begin a physical exercise routine can be predicted by that person's attitudes toward fitness and exercise, the person's beliefs about what their friends and family members think about exercise, the person's confidence that they can engage successfully in a sustained exercise program, and the person's plans to begin an exercise program.

Theory is essential in coming up with, and justifying, specific research hypotheses. For example, social identity and self-categorization theories suggest that people organize themselves into groups—real or imagined—when confronted with a set of specific differences between "us" and "them" (Spears,

2011). These theories enumerate a number of dynamics that might occur once people have formed groups, such as allocating resources unfairly so that one's own group benefits (Brewer, 1999), developing stereotypical portrayals of people from other groups (Pettigrew & Tropp, 2011), and even attacking people from other groups (Moshman, 2007). These theoretical postulates can help to suggest research hypotheses within specific intergroup situations— such as political campaigns, sports rivalries, and wars. For example, we might expect that fans of the New York Yankees and the Boston Red Sox—two baseball teams with a rivalry that dates back more than 100 years—might characterize one another unfavorably and might want unfair advantages to benefit their respective teams. Similarly, given the animosity between their governments, Americans and Iranians might view one another with suspicion and develop negative stereotypes about one another. One could imagine any number of research hypotheses that might arise from these intergroup situations.

Without a theory to frame our hypotheses, however, we are "flying blind." Because it is unethical to analyze data prior to developing hypotheses (Kerr, 1998)—doing so is akin to cheating on a test—we have no solid basis on which to propose hypotheses. Theory tells us not only *what* hypotheses to propose, but also *why* they should be proposed and *how* they can be justified. Further, in some situations, we can compare theories—for instance, although social identity and self-categorization theories tell us what happens when people are classified into "ingroups" and "outgroups," what happens when it is not clear to which group a given person belongs? For example, are immigrants ingroup members or outgroup members? Some people see immigrants as outsiders or invaders (Murray, 2017), whereas others see them as part of the national fabric (Chavez, 2013). The specific research hypotheses suggested by social identity and self-categorization theories—namely that immigrants are likely to be marginalized from the cultural mainstream—would likely be quite different from those suggested by ingroup projection theory (Wenzel et al., 2007), which proposes that immigrants would be expected to forgo their cultural heritage and "assimilate" into the cultural mainstream. This is a clear case where two theories can be pitted against one another in developing and testing hypotheses.

I remember a manuscript I wrote once where a reviewer accused my co-author and me of "dust bowl empiricism" because we were simply describing phenomena and not invoking theory. In response, we had to consult the literature to identify theories that would have supported and given rise to the hypotheses we were proposing (and had already tested). This is not my preferred method of using theory—theory should optimally come *before* the hypotheses are generated and the study is conducted—but in a case like this, where we were admittedly sloppy and were called out for it, identifying theories after the fact was the best we could do.

Even in fields like epidemiology, where a major goal is to describe population trends and disease prevalence and incidence, theory remains essential (Krieger, 2001). For example, although documenting the spread of HIV among intravenous drug users is of extreme importance, we also need to know why and how the disease is spreading within this population. What theories account for sharing used needles and engaging in unprotected sex with people who inject drugs? Because theory specifies the mechanisms that we will study *and* that should be targeted within intervention programs, the *why* and the *how* are just as important as the *who* and the *what*. Questions of *why* and *how* are at the heart of theory.

Simply put, a project—and manuscripts that come out of it—that is not guided by theory is likely destined to fail.

Make Sure It Hasn't Been Done Before!

I have a close colleague who is at a liberal arts teaching college. He teaches two to three courses per semester, is loaded down with student advising, and is able to write only sparingly during the academic year. Most of his research and writing is done during the summer. As a result, he is less productive than other scholars at research-intensive universities where the teaching load is lower and faculty are provided with more protected time for research and writing.

On more than one occasion, my colleague has been "scooped" by other researchers who have published work on an idea he had been working on. Just as he was ready to submit a manuscript to a journal, an article would come out—written, invariably, by someone at a research-powerhouse university—on the same idea that my colleague had been pursuing.

The third time this happened, my colleague threw up his hands and sighed in frustration. What more could he have done? I was more than sympathetic, because this is an experience that many researchers will have at some point in their careers.

There is truly nothing that my colleague could have done to avoid being scooped—other than moving to an institution that would afford him more time to write so that it would take him less time to get his papers written and submitted. But there is a similar situation—one that is much easier to avoid—that can be prevented simply by keeping up with the literature.

Let's say that a doctoral student conducts a cursory literature search, using one search engine, and determines that the idea she wants to pursue is hers to take. So she starts preparing to propose her dissertation. She meets with her advisor, who calmly states, "Someone has already done this."

The project that has already been done might have appeared in some literature databases but not others, or it might be "in press"—that is, accepted for publication and posted on the journal's website but not yet assigned to a journal volume and issue. Because the student searched only one literature database, she may have missed the journal article reporting the study that was so similar to what she was planning to do.

It is worth noting that the National Institutes of Health and other funders have launched a new initiative focusing on replication. A recent international set of psychology studies (Klein et al., 2014; Nosek et al., 2015) found that only about half of the studies they attempted to replicate could be successfully redone—meaning that significant findings again emerged as significant and nonsignificant findings remained nonsignificant. So replicating prior work is becoming an increasingly worthwhile endeavor (see Goodman, Fanelli, & Ioannidis, 2016).

However, the extent to which journals are willing to dedicate space to publishing replications has not increased nearly as much as scientists have suggested that it should (Burman, Reed, & Alm, 2010; Pashler & Harris, 2012). Many replication studies consist of multiple trials conducted at different locations, to determine the conditions under which results are more versus less likely to replicate (Forsell et al., 2019). The extent to which single studies reporting replications are likely to be accepted for publication is unknown.

My contention here is that replication is not recommended as a task for beginning scholars. The scientific rigor required to determine whether a study is replicable may be higher than the rigor required to conduct an original study! Replication is not pursued accidentally (e.g., because the author didn't know that the idea had already been pursued); rather, it is pursued purposefully and under extremely stringent conditions. Additionally, establishing oneself as a serious scholar may be accomplished more effectively by publishing original theory and research. So I advise you to ensure that the work you plan to undertake has not already been done.

Think Two Steps Ahead

If you have ever played chess, you know that you have to think two or three moves ahead. What will your opponent do after you make the move you are planning to make? Will you expose your queen or king to capture? Will you gain an advantage over your opponent by making this move?

Research operates in much the same way. If our hypotheses are supported in the current project or paper, where will we seek to go next? What is the next step in this program of research? As already noted, science proceeds along lines of research that are comprised of individual studies. When planning and launching a study, we should have a good idea where that study is likely to take us.

When I plan a new research project, I generally outline at least three or four manuscripts that I plan to write using the data from that project. Of course, there is no guarantee that the results of our statistical analyses will support each of the planned papers. I have a saying: data are like children, they behave when they want to. If I outline four potential manuscripts from a project, I can pretty much guarantee that one or two of the planned papers will fall through because there won't be a story to tell. (Generally, if none of the hypotheses we are testing is supported, it's not worth trying to publish the null results. Journals generally are not inclined to publish articles that report only nonsignificant results.) Generating ideas is a wonderful exercise, but I do not suggest becoming overly invested in any idea until the analyses have yielded results that are worth publishing.

A very common question that students ask me involves the length of time they should plan to devote to a research project. My general answer is that, if you take the amount of time that you think the project will take, and then triple that amount of time, that is how much time the project will really take to complete. If we are collecting new data, there will be a whole host of delays—IRB/ethics approvals, finding and hiring staff, programming data collection software, quality assurance checks to identify and correct programming mistakes, data collection errors, scoring and merging data files, data analyses (which often require many iterations to complete), and preparing manuscripts based on the results. Unexpected snafus can occur at any point during the project, and often at multiple points. I remember one project where my colleagues and I were almost ready to submit a manuscript for publication when my statistical colleague discovered an error in the data. When he fixed the error, half of our significant results were no longer significant! Needless to say, we were quite disappointed, and the paper had to be rewritten. Whereas we had thought the results were groundbreaking, correcting the error reduced the potential impact of our findings considerably, and we had to drop down quite a bit in journal prestige. This type of occurrence is fairly common, especially with complex longitudinal and experimental studies.

An additional piece of advice I offer based on my own experience is to pursue any opportunity you can to enhance your statistical skills. You may not run all of the analyses for your manuscripts by yourself, but it is extremely advantageous if you are able to conduct at least some of them. Additionally, it is essential to be able to collaborate with statistical colleagues in writing the results section. Relying on a statistician to write the results for you is not a good idea. A manuscript needs to speak with a single voice. As a reviewer, I can usually tell when one person wrote the introduction, methods, and discussion sections, and another person wrote the results section. Reviewers often do not respond well to this approach! Writing the results section in collaboration with your statistical colleagues will help to ensure that the entire paper speaks with one voice. (Moreover, possessing advanced statistical skills can increase your marketability when you apply for positions.)

Conclusion

In summary, choosing a topic is far more complex than many beginning authors think. Moving from a general research area to a specific set of research questions and testable hypotheses can require considerable work. Especially if you are new to the field in which you plan to conduct your research, it is essential to become intimately familiar with the work being done in that field. What is the current state of knowledge? What kinds of research designs are used? Who are the leading scholars in that field, and what kind of work are they doing? What journals are publishing work in the field? What are the next logical steps that need to be pursued in the field?

Also, remember that if your research questions and hypotheses cannot be evaluated based on the results of statistical analyses, then your research questions and hypotheses are not precise enough. Statistical analyses must be able to falsify a given hypotheses. If they cannot, then the hypothesis is not sufficiently testable.

Finally—and this advice is intended for scholars at all levels of academia and related professions—your work should be part of a line of research that you are pursuing. People who publish an article or two in one field, a couple in a second field, and a couple in a third field are unlikely to attract the attention and prestige needed to secure jobs, promotions, and grants. Indeed, as someone who has reviewed many manuscripts, grant proposals, and promotion and tenure dossiers in my career, I can tell you that people who have established themselves in a specific field of study fare far better than those with scattered publications across a range of fields. Choosing a topic is not a task for a single study—rather, it is a task for the long haul.

This is not to say that people's interests cannot change over time. They do! As noted in the Prologue, I started out as a personal identity researcher and transitioned to studying acculturation (which is also an identity process) as I embraced the fascinating cultural context of Miami. People can change interests for a variety of reasons—sometimes they are exposed to new areas through collaboration, sometimes they are chasing grant money and need to align themselves with funding agency priorities, and sometimes personal experiences lead to changes in one's career path. I had a close colleague who became acutely interested in divorced fathering after his own marriage ended. He had no prior research record on divorce, but we published several articles on the topic after his divorce. Another person I know switched his research interests from ethnic identity to brain imaging so that he could compete for grant funding. And another colleague of mine became a genetics researcher after beginning a collaboration with someone who was doing work in that area.

It is worth noting, however, that all these people were senior professors and were tenured. Early in your career, you should focus on gaining expertise in a specific area and becoming known as an authority in that area. As already noted, promotion, tenure, and research grants are far more likely to be awarded to people who can easily be identified as leaders (or at least up-and-comers) in a specific field.

Summary

- We do not start writing until we know precisely what we are going to write about.
- We must know the literature in a field of study before we can come up with research questions that will contribute to that field.
- When conducting literature searches, it is imperative to use multiple search engines.
- Following major names in a field is a useful way to keep up with the literature in that field.
- Research questions must be directly testable and falsifiable.
- It is impossible to "do everything" within a single study. Many scholars spend their whole careers creating lines of research on specific topics.
- Research questions and hypotheses must be firmly rooted in established theories.

- Replication is pursued intentionally and with exceptional rigor, not because someone did not know that someone else had previously pursued the idea. Replication is generally not a task for early-career researchers (especially students) to pursue.

References

Ajzen, I. (2002). Perceived behavioral control, self-efficacy, locus of control, and the theory of planned behavior. *Journal of Applied Social Psychology, 32,* 665–683.

Brewer, M. B. (1999). The psychology of prejudice: Ingroup love and outgroup hate? *Journal of Social Issues, 55,* 429–444.

Burman, L. E., Reed, W. R., & Alm, J. (2010). A call for replication studies. *Public Finance Review, 38,* 787–793.

Chavez, L. R. (2013). *The Latino threat.* Berkeley: University of California Press.

Cobb, C. L., Xie, D., Meca, A., & Schwartz, S. J. (2017). Acculturation, discrimination, and depression among unauthorized Latino/a immigrants in the United States. *Cultural Diversity and Ethnic Minority Psychology, 23,* 258–268.

Forsell, E., Viganola, D., Pfeiffer, T., Almemberg, J., Wilson, B., Chen, Y., . . . Dreber, A. (2019). Predicting replication outcomes in the Many Labs 2 study. *Journal of Economic Psychology, 75,* Article 102117.

Goodman, S. N., Fanelli, D., & Ioannidis, J. P. A. (2016). What does research reproducibility mean? *Science Translational Medicine, 8,* Article 341ps12.

Jaakkola, E. (2020). Designing conceptual articles: Four approaches. *AMS Review, 10,* 18–26.

Kerr, N. L. (1998). HARKing: Hypothesizing after the results are known. *Personality and Social Psychology Review, 2,* 196–217.

Klein, R. A., Ratliff, K. A., Vianello, M., Adams, R. B., Jr., Bahník, Š., Bernstein, M. J., . . . Nosek, B. A. (2014). Investigating variation in replicability: A "many labs" replication project. *Social Psychology, 45*(3), 142–152.

Krieger, N. (2001). Theories for social epidemiology in the 21st century: An ecosocial perspective. *International Journal of Epidemiology, 30,* 668–677.

Moshman, D. (2007). Us and them: Identity and genocide. *Identity: An International Journal of Theory and Research, 7,* 115–135.

Murray, D. (2017). *The strange death of Europe: Immigration, identity, Islam.* London: Bloomsbury.

Nosek, B. A., Aarts, A. A., Anderson, J. E., Anderson, C. J., Attridge, P. R., Attwood, A., . . . Zuni, K. (2015). Estimating the replicability of psychological science. *Science, 349,* 943–951.

Pashler, H., & Harris, C. R. (2012). Is the replicability crisis overblown? Three arguments explained. *Perspectives on Psychological Science, 7,* 531–536.

Pettigrew, T. F., & Tropp, L. R. (2011). *When groups meet: The dynamics of intergroup contact.* Philadelphia, PA: Psychology Press.

Rhodes, R. E., & Courneya, K. S. (2003). Investigating multiple components of attitude, subjective norm, and perceived control: An examination of the theory of planned behaviour in the exercise domain. *British Journal of Social Psychology, 42,* 129–146.

Schwartz, S. J., Benet-Martínez, V., Knight, G. P., Unger, J. B., Zamboanga, B. L., Des Rosiers, S. E., . . . Szapocznik, J. (2014). Effects of language of assessment on the measurement of acculturation: Measurement equivalence and cultural frame switching. *Psychological Assessment, 26,* 100–114.

Schwartz, S. J., Salas-Wright, C. P., Pérez-Gómez, A., Mejía-Trujillo, J., Brown, E. C., Montero-Zamora, P., . . . Dickson-Gomez, J. (2018). Cultural stress and psychological symptoms in recent Venezuelan immigrants to the United States and Colombia. *International Journal of Intercultural Relations, 67*, 25–34.

Schwartz, S. J., Unger, J. B., Zamboanga, B. L., Córdova, D., Mason, C. A., Huang, S., . . . Szapocznik, J. (2015). Developmental trajectories of acculturation: Links with family functioning and mental health in recent-immigrant Hispanic adolescents. *Child Development, 86*, 726–748.

Schwartz, S. J., Weisskirch, R. S., Zamboanga, B. L., Castillo, L. G., Ham, L. S., Huynh, Q.-L., . . . Cano, M. A. (2011). Dimensions of acculturation: Associations with health risk behaviors among college students from immigrant families. *Journal of Counseling Psychology, 58*, 27–41.

Shadish, W. R., Cook, T. D., & Campbell, D. T. (2002). *Experimental and quasi-experimental designs for generalized causal inference*. Boston: Houghton-Mifflin.

Spears, R. (2011). Group identities: The social identity perspective. In S. J. Schwartz, K. Luyckx, & V. L. Vignoles (Eds.), *Handbook of identity theory and research* (pp. 201–224). New York: Springer.

Wang, S. C., Schwartz, S. J., & Zamboanga, B. L. (2010). Acculturative stress among Cuban American college students: Exploring the mediating pathways between acculturation and psychosocial functioning. *Journal of Applied Social Psychology, 40*, 2862–2887.

Wenzel, M., Mummendey, A., & Waldzus, S. (2007). Superordinate identities and intergroup conflict: The ingroup projection model. *European Review of Social Psychology, 18*, 331–372.

2
Designing a Publishable Study

Chapter Objectives

By the time you finish reading this chapter, you should be more comfortable with:

- Mapping out the steps that go into planning a study
- Using careful checks to catch errors in the study procedures, measures, and data analyses
- Selecting a study design and analytic approach
- Distinguishing among association, prediction, and causation—and identifying research hypotheses and designs associated with each of these levels of relationship
- Recruiting hard-to-reach populations
- Planning for retention in longitudinal studies
- Managing a research team
- Conducting secondary data analyses and meta-analyses
- Drawing a sample

OK, so now we have selected our topic and we are ready to get started. Easy, right?

Not exactly.

Aside from the quality of the writing—and possibly even more importantly than the written document itself—the potential for any empirical manuscript to compete successfully for publication in a peer-reviewed journal rests on the quality of the research design, measurement instruments, and data analyses presented in that manuscript. Even the most beautifully written prose cannot make up for a poorly planned, designed, conducted, or analyzed study. And once you have finished collecting your data, they are *yours*, with any and all flaws in your research design, measures, and research procedures.

The best advice I can provide is to plan carefully before carrying out the study. Choose a research design that will allow you to fully test your research hypotheses, conduct careful quality assurance checks before your study goes live, and make sure your study websites, equipment, programming, and so

The Savvy Academic. Seth J. Schwartz, Oxford University Press. © Oxford University Press 2022.
DOI: 10.1093/oso/9780190095918.003.0003

forth, work properly. If you are collecting self-report data, make sure that the questions and survey length are appropriate for your participant population. Meta-analyses of survey content and length (Rolstad, Adler, & Rydén, 2011) have found that survey completion rates decreased as survey length increased, but that participant interest in the survey content may also play an important role. Simply put, if participants lose interest in your survey—either because it's too long or because they're not interested in what you are asking—they will stop paying attention. They may even quit the survey altogether.

Several years ago, my colleagues and I carried out a 3-year longitudinal study of acculturation, culturally related stressors, family relationships, and adolescent mental health and risk behavior among recently immigrated Hispanic families in Miami and Los Angeles. Recent immigrants are notoriously difficult to retain in research studies because they often work multiple jobs, may relocate frequently, and may change phone numbers (Knight, Roosa, & Umaña-Taylor, 2009). However, we were able to retain 85% of study families through 3 years and six time points, and we did not have many problems with surveys not being completed—despite the fact that the adolescent and parent surveys each took more than 2 hours to complete.

How did we pull this off?

There are a few steps we took to ensure that we retained as many participants as possible through the study. First, we hired a dedicated tracker—a person who would be responsible for maintaining contact with participants, for reaching out to schedule and confirm appointments, and for conducting assessments when necessary. The two people we hired for the tracker position—Tatiana Clavijo in Miami and Monica Pattarroyo in Los Angeles—were so good at their jobs that many families would pick up the phone only if Tatiana or Monica was calling! Tatiana and Monica were regularly invited into families' homes for meals and to pray with the family, and even after the study ended, many families continued to stay in touch with them.

Second, we conducted quality assurance checks—"dry runs"—on all study procedures. Because some parents in our study population (recent immigrants) had low literacy levels, we voice-recorded each survey item and the associated response choices, so that the voice would read the item to respondents as the item's text appeared on the screen. The voice recording took several weeks to finish—we quickly learned that our research associates' voices would start "cracking" after an hour or two of recording, and they would have to take a break. We also listened to each recording, and if there was too much background noise, we would re-record it. On a few occasions, a recording was accompanied by a thunderclap from outside, and we had to wait out the storm before resuming the recording session.

A key task with the recording was to ensure that the item text that appeared on the screen was *exactly the same* as the words being read aloud by the recorded voice. When we conducted quality assurance checks, there were many instances where the text on the screen did not match the text from the recording. Our programming consultant was surely annoyed by the number of times we came to her with errors that needed to be fixed.

A third challenge that we have faced in many of our studies has been translation. Sireci, Yang, Harter, and Ehrlich (2006) outlined state-of-the-art procedures for translating self-report and interview measures: first, a bilingual individual translates the document from the original language into the target language, then a second bilingual individual translates the first translator's version back into the original language, and finally the two translators meet to compare the original and back-translated versions of the document in the original language. The two translators then work together to translate the final original-language version into the target language. Optimally, the final target-language version will also be reviewed by a committee of bilingual individuals to ensure acceptability. Such committee review is especially important when multiple groups with different dialects will use the translated versions—such as a French-language translated measure intended for use in France, Quebec, Switzerland, and Belgium.

We also contacted members of the Hispanic immigrant communities in Miami and Los Angeles, explained the study to them, and asked for their feedback. Although families generally liked the study and thought it resonated with their life experiences, they also suggested additional constructs for us to measure. They also gave us feedback on the wording of our items.

Simply put, these steps helped ensure that we would obtain high-quality data by identifying and eliminating potential errors from the methodology. Item wording, readability, technical issues, and other procedural issues *cannot* be corrected once the study has been conducted—and these errors will be part of the data that you obtain from the study.

Here is an example of a costly error that was caught prior to the end of the study. A close colleague and I conducted an online survey study of Venezuelan immigrant adolescents in the United States. Using a respondent-driven sampling methodology (Heckathorn, 2002), where each participant is asked to refer additional eligible people to the study, we started with a small number of participants referred to us by our community partners. When our sample size had reached 300, we performed a routine check on the data and found that many of the IP addresses were associated with Venezuelan locations. This told us that a large number of participants were not part of the study population—that is, they were not Venezuelan immigrants in the United

States, because individuals with Venezuelan IP addresses were still living in Venezuela. Because our incentives were automatically delivered after participants finished the survey, we had wasted more than $1,000 worth of incentives on participants whose data could not be used. Fortunately, however, we were able to obtain additional funding to finish data collection and reach 400 participants as we had originally planned.

Imagine if we had not discovered those Venezuelan IP addresses? We would have analyzed data from participants who were not part of our study population, and our conclusions might have wound up being incorrect as a result. Worst of all, we probably would never have known about it.

I minored in computer programming at Florida State, and one of the first lessons I learned was the difference between syntax errors and logical errors. A syntax error is an incorrect statement, such that the program will not run. You will receive an error message telling you to correct the error and run the program again. Syntax errors can be frustrating when they keep occurring, or when you cannot find the source of the error—but the good part is that we know we have made an error and that it needs to be fixed.

Logical errors, on the other hand, are far more problematic. The error does not result in an incorrect statement and the software will not flag the error for you. You will receive whatever output you requested from the software, and you may not know that an error occurred at all. For example, when I was writing code for a data collection interface a number of years ago, I mistakenly divided by 9 instead of 10. It wasn't until the program was consistently giving me strange values that I realized something had gone wrong. It took me more than 4 hours to find the error and correct it.

There are two important messages that you should take away from the syntax versus logical error example. First, most potential problems in our research procedures are more like logical errors than like syntax errors. They are not readily apparent, and we don't receive a warning that an error occurred. Indeed, in many cases we could easily finish collecting data and never know there was a problem. *This is why quality assurance checks are so important.*

Second, when we are running statistical analyses, most of the errors we make will be logical errors that won't be apparent unless we carefully review the results. Writing the wrong variable name into our input syntax, or clicking the wrong box in point-and-click software, will produce an error that is extremely difficult to identify. I like to tell my students and trainees that they must develop a "sixth sense" about statistics. If something looks wrong, it probably is!

Third, because statistical analyses can be very tedious, it is essential to have a second pair of eyes on the syntax and on the output. One misspelled variable name, one copied and pasted line of code that is not changed to include the correct variables, or even a missing command terminator (such as a semicolon or period) can lead to incorrect results. My colleagues have caught errors that I've made in my analyses, and I have caught errors that my colleagues have made. Had any of us been conducting the analyses alone with no oversight, these errors might not have been noticed and corrected.

Finally, as I cover in greater detail in the chapter on ethics in data analyses, the advent of point-and-click statistical software (such as SPSS and SAS) allows people to conduct analyses without really knowing what they're doing. All you have to do is select an analysis from the drop-down menu, put variables into each of the boxes, and click OK. The software will generate output that may wind up being meaningless!

Note that the points I am making here are not just about analyses. They refer to every stage of research—from designing the study to analyzing and writing up the results, and everywhere in between. Every decision that we make must be carefully thought out, justified, and consistent with the research questions and hypotheses guiding the study. If we make decisions that are not consistent with our study goals, our ability to properly test our hypotheses will be compromised.

So let's start with the main topic of this chapter—designing a publishable study.

Selecting a Study Design

The first step in designing a study involves choosing what type of study we are going to conduct. There are many different choices, but each design type is intended to test a specific type of hypothesis. It is essential to ensure that the design we select is properly matched with our hypothesis.

Qualitative, Quantitative, or Mixed Method?

Most broadly, we need to decide whether we are going to collect quantitative, qualitative, or mixed-method data. Qualitative methods include interviews, focus groups, narrative storytelling, and other similar methods. Broadly, the purpose of qualitative research is to obtain first-person perspectives on the phenomena we are studying. For example, a research team led by my PhD student, Saskia Vos, recently published an article (Vos et al., 2021) reporting how Hispanic youth in Miami and Los Angeles defined culturally related stress.

Saskia and her colleagues conducted a series of focus groups where they asked 10th grade adolescents to talk about various aspects of cultural stress. They then coded the discussions into themes using grounded theory methods. Briefly stated, this coding method is used to obtain a sense of general topics that emerge within an interview, group discussion, or life-story narrative. In Saskia's study, adolescents mentioned topics including discrimination from other Hispanic people, translating for parents, and laws and policies that were perceived as unfair or discriminatory.

Quantitative research can take any number of forms, but broadly it refers to studies where numeric scores are obtained for each study variable. These scores can be responses to survey items, response times when completing tasks, observational ratings of family interactions, blood pressure readings, or almost anything else. The objective is to obtain scores so that statistical analyses can be conducted on the resulting dataset.

Much of the work that my colleagues and I have conducted has used self-report surveys. In many cases, we collect data from multiple informants (generally youth and parents) to reduce the bias associated with assessing all variables from the same person (see Podsakoff, MacKenzie, & Podsakoff, 2012). Interestingly, reports on the same construct from multiple reporters often do not correlate well. For example, in one of our studies (Schwartz et al., 2016), parent and adolescent reports of family functioning correlated quite weakly ($r = .23$)—indicating that parent and youth perceptions of family relationships were quite different. Had we relied solely on parent or adolescent reports of family functioning, our conclusions might have been biased.

There are many types of both quantitative and qualitative analyses, and many books, chapters, and journal articles have been written to provide detailed information about these analyses (for example, see Kaplan, 2004, for quantitative analyses, and Denzin & Lincoln, 2018, for qualitative analyses). Different fields have their own standards for what represents acceptable scientific rigor—for example, the study of stress often includes both self-reports and biomarkers (e.g., cortisol secretion, blood pressure; Juster, Perna, Marin, Sindi, & Lupien, 2012). It is quite possible that some audiences—and reviewers—might question the scientific acceptability of stress studies that do not include biomarkers. The acceptability of self-reports without biomarkers might depend on whether the study is framed as scientific discovery (in which case biomarkers might be viewed as required) or as applied (such as evaluating interventions or characterizing a real-world setting like a workplace—in which case self-reports might be acceptable on their own).

Mixed-method research includes both quantitative and qualitative components. Bryman (2006) included a number of reasons why researchers might want to integrate these two research traditions. I explain three of these reasons here. In *triangulation*, the goal is to determine whether the qualitative and quantitative components yield the same conclusions. For example, do participants describe their experiences in a similar way when they take part in focus groups as they do when they complete surveys or engage in experimental tasks? If we administer a measure of cultural stress (e.g., discrimination, feeling shut out or unwelcome, being demonized and scapegoated for the country's problems) to a sample of immigrants and then ask them to participate in personal interviews, how well do the findings converge between the two methods?

A second use of mixed methods is *offsetting*, where one uses qualitative methods to address the weaknesses of quantitative methods, and vice versa. For example, my colleague Liliana Rodriguez wrote her doctoral dissertation using a dataset I had collected, and we and another colleague of ours (Rodriguez, Schwartz, & Whitbourne, 2010) published an article based on her dissertation research. Lili and her student colleagues coded White, Black, and Hispanic students' written responses to a series of prompts asking about what it means to be American. They coded responses both into categories (e.g., symbols, behaviors, values) and into positive versus negative valence. For example, "Americans are greedy and selfish" would have been coded into the values category (because greed and selfishness are values) and as an extremely negative response. In contrast, "Americans like to eat hot dogs and hamburgers" would have been coded into the behaviors category and as a neutral response (because no emotional description was included).

Lili then correlated the affective valence ratings with quantitative measures of personal and ethnic identity, separately for Whites, for Blacks, and for Hispanics. She found that affective ratings of participants' descriptions of Americans were correlated positively with personal identity among Whites, but negatively with ethnic identity among Blacks and Hispanics. The affective valence characterizing participants' descriptions of Americans was best captured using open-ended qualitative responses, whereas personal and ethnic identity are often assessed using quantitative scales. Administering quantitative measures of how positively or negatively participants view Americans is certainly possible, but qualitative responses provide richness (as well as the ability to identify specific categories, which would be difficult using quantitative responses). Conversely, in studies with large samples, quantitative measures of personal and ethnic identity may be more efficient than qualitative prompts.

A third way of using mixed methods research is *expansion*, when one method is used to elaborate on findings obtained using the other method. An example of this is a study that my colleague Cory Cobb conducted, along with me and some other colleagues of ours (Cobb, Meca, Xie, Schwartz, & Moise, 2017). Cory surveyed a sample of undocumented Hispanic immigrants in Houston, Texas, and Little Rock, Arkansas, regarding discrimination, negative context of reception (e.g., feeling unwelcome and barred from opportunities; Portes & Rumbaut, 2014), flourishing, and satisfaction with life. He also asked participants whether they felt that their experiences in the United States were different from those of documented Hispanic immigrants. Those who answered Yes were asked to elaborate about the differences they perceived.

Quantitative analyses indicated that undocumented immigrants who perceived their experiences as different from those of documented individuals scored significantly lower on flourishing and satisfaction with life, and significantly higher on discrimination and negative context of reception, compared to undocumented immigrants who did not perceive differences between their experiences and those of documented individuals. Responses to the qualitative prompt indicated that the vast majority of individuals who perceived differences characterized those differences in terms of fewer opportunities, less respect from others, and marginalization from society. These responses help to provide context and nuance to the quantitative results, in terms of *why* some undocumented Hispanic immigrants believed that they were treated differently than documented Hispanics are treated.

Cross-Sectional, Longitudinal, or Experimental?

We also must decide how many observation points there will be in our study, whether (or how) we will manipulate our study variables, and ultimately the types of statistical analyses we want to be able to conduct on the resulting data (see Pearl, 1999, for further discussion of the statistical implications of research designs). These decisions should be based on our research questions and hypotheses. Specifically, the philosophical and statistical distinctions among association, prediction, and causation must be considered—and the type of relationship specified in our research questions and hypotheses dictates our choice of research design.

All research questions and hypotheses refer to some sort of relationship between or among variables, or to group differences in some variable or set of variables. Note that analyses of relationships (correlation, regression, factor analysis, structural equation modeling) and analyses of group differences (*t*-tests and analyses of variance) are all housed under the general linear model family (Tabachnick & Fidell, 2007). As a result, group differences can be viewed as a special case of relationships among variables. For example, differences in work satisfaction between immigrant and native-born employees might also be thought of as relationships between nativity and work satisfaction. As a result, the points I make below regarding levels of relationship apply both to hypotheses about relationships between and among variables and to hypotheses about group differences.

Figure 2.1 illustrates the three levels of relationship that may be specified in a given research question or hypothesis. These levels are association, prediction, and causation. Consider the following three hypotheses:

Hypothesis 1: The greatest angle at which sunlight hits the ground at any given location on Earth on a given day is associated with the temperature at that location during that day.

Hypothesis 2: The greatest angle at which sunlight hits the ground at any given location on Earth on a given day predicts the temperature at that location 1 month later.

Hypothesis 3: Changes in the greatest angle at which sunlight hits the ground at any given location on Earth across months of the year cause seasonal variations in temperature at that location.

Hypothesis 1 simply states that, at a given location, the highest "sun angle" on a given day is related to the temperature at that location on that day. No assumptions are made regarding how the sun angle might predict temperatures on subsequent days, or whether changes in the sun angle across days, weeks, and months might cause seasonal changes in temperature. Such a hypothesis refers to *association* and requires only one observation for each location. Measure the greatest sun angle during a given day and the highest temperature during that day, and estimate the association between these two sets of measurements across days.

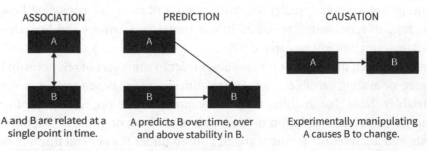

Figure 2.1 Association, prediction, and causation.

Hypothesis 2 states that, as the maximum sun angle increases across days, the highest observed temperature 1 month later will also increase—controlling for the temperatures on earlier days. For example, in the Northern Hemisphere, the high sun angles in June will predict hotter temperatures in July, and the low sun angles in December will predict colder temperatures in January. This hypothesis refers to *prediction* and requires repeated measurements of sun angles and maximum daily temperatures, as well as conducting longitudinal analyses where maximum sun angles on earlier days are allowed to predict maximum temperatures on later days.

Hypothesis 3 states that changes in maximum sun angles *cause* increases and decreases in temperature across days, and that increasing or decreasing the maximum sun angle at a given location will also increase or decrease the maximum daily temperature observed at that location. This hypothesis refers to *causation* and requires experimentally manipulating the maximum sun angle observed at a given location and observing the effect on the maximum temperature observed at that location.

Now wait a moment, you might be thinking. *How can you manipulate the sun angle? You cannot "move" the sun!*

This is certainly true—we cannot move the sun. But we can purposely vary the latitude observed (which inherently varies the maximum sun angle) and observe maximum temperatures at each latitude. For example, Cairo, Egypt, is at 30 degrees north; New York City is at 40 degrees north; and Brussels, Belgium is at 50 degrees north. The maximum sun angles on June 21 (the summer solstice) are 83° in Cairo, 73° in New York City, and 63° in Brussels. The maximum sun angles on December 21 (the winter solstice) are 36° in Cairo, 26° in New York City, and 16° in Brussels. If we measured maximum temperatures on these dates in each city across 10 successive years, we would likely find that temperatures in Cairo are warmest. But would New York City always be warmer than Brussels? (The answer is likely No, and the reason is that there are factors other than the sun angle that affect temperatures. We will come back to this example when we discuss confounding variables.)

So the type of relationship we test for depends on the level of association specified in our research questions and hypotheses. Hypotheses involving association can be tested using cross-sectional studies with only one measurement occasion; hypotheses involving prediction can be tested using longitudinal[1] studies with multiple measurement occasions; and hypotheses

---

[1] Note that the term *longitudinal* includes cross-sequential designs and other types of studies that examine change over time but do not intervene with, or deliberately change, any of the study variables.

involving causation can be tested using experimental studies where an independent variable is manipulated and changes in one or more dependent variables are observed (see Table 2.1).

An important reason why many journal manuscripts are rejected is because the research design used does not allow the hypotheses to be tested properly.

One example of this phenomenon involves cross-sectional tests of mediation. By definition, mediation is a longitudinal or causal process where variable A predicts or causes variable C *through* variable B (MacKinnon, 2008). For example, psychoneuroimmunology research indicates that chronic stress causes illness by taxing the body's stress response system (Chrousos, 2009). Testing this proposition requires examining (or experimentally manipulating) stressful events, measuring stress hormones like cortisol, and observing the number of colds, sick days, or other indicators of illness. The measurements would also need to be staggered, so that the stressor occurs or is measured first, the cortisol secretion is measured later, and the illness is measured last. (In studies where experimental manipulation does not occur, all variables should be measured at all time points, so that we can conduct analyses to determine the most likely sequence.)

Now what happens if we try to test a mediational hypothesis using a cross-sectional design? To answer this question, let's consider two potential mediational hypotheses—one predictive and one causal.

Table 2.1 roperties of Cross-Sectional, Longitudinal, and Experimental Studies

Design	Primary Purpose	Key Advantages	Key Disadvantages
Cross-Sectional	To characterize a population at one point in time	• Easy to collect • No concerns about retention	• Developmental, directional, or causal conclusions cannot be drawn
Longitudinal	To follow a cohort over time	• Allows drawing developmental or directional conclusions	• Retention can be challenging • Causal conclusions cannot be drawn (unless specific statistical methods are used)
Experimental	To test effects of an intervention or manipulation on dependent variables	• Allows drawing causal conclusions • Provides strongest test of theory	• Same exact procedures must be used with each participant • Data cannot be analyzed until the study is finished (for randomized clinical trials)

Hypothesis 1: Discrimination experiences will predict heightened rejection sensitivity, which in turn will predict greater depressive symptoms. (Predictive)

Hypothesis 2: A coping skills intervention will decrease depressive thoughts, which in turn will decrease the likelihood of suicide attempts. (Causal)

First, let's consider the most appropriate research designs for testing each of these hypotheses. Hypothesis 1, which proposes a predictive mediational sequence, might best be tested within the context of a longitudinal study with at least three waves (see Figure 2.2). Discrimination experiences and rejection sensitivity should both be measured and entered into our analytic model at Time 1, rejection sensitivity and depressive symptoms should both be measured and entered into our analytic model at Time 2, and depressive symptoms should be measured and entered into our analytic model at Time 3. Controlling for prior levels of our mediating (rejection sensitivity) and outcome (depressive symptoms) variables allows us to draw strong directional inferences, which are essential for assuming mediation (Cole & Maxwell, 2003).

Hypothesis 2, which proposes a causal mediational sequence, should be tested using a randomized experimental design (see Figure 2.3). That is, randomly assigning participants to intervention and control conditions allows us to conclude that experimentally manipulating coping skills causes decreases in depressive thoughts, which in turn leads to decreases in suicide attempts.

When conducted carefully and rigorously, randomized experimental manipulation allows us to assume causality for at least two reasons (see Ong-Dean, Hofstetter, & Strick, 2011, for further review and discussion). First, because assignment to conditions is random, no other study variables can predict this assignment—and therefore the directionality must proceed from

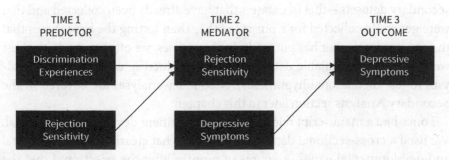

Figure 2.2 Predictive mediational design.

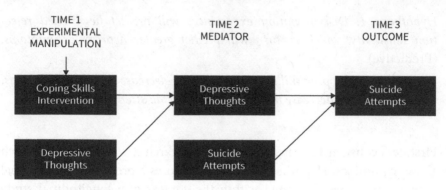

Figure 2.3 Causal mediational design.

the experimental manipulation (and the variable that is manipulated in the experiment) to the mediating and outcome variables, and not vice versa. Second, random assignment is intended to distribute confounding variables evenly among the study conditions. Both of these assumptions must be evaluated statistically, however—the intervention may affect the mediating and outcome variables through mechanisms other than the one suggested by the researchers, and some confounding variables may not be evenly distributed. Montgomery (2017) and Schneider et al. (2007) provide additional details on analyzing experimental data.

The point here, however, is that cross-sectional data cannot satisfy the assumptions needed to demonstrate mediation. No variables are experimentally manipulated, and prior levels of mediating and outcome variables cannot be statistically controlled (Maxwell & Cole, 2007; O'Laughlin, Martin, & Ferrer, 2018). This is not to say that mediation analyses absolutely cannot be conducted with cross-sectional data—rather, my point is that when we are planning a study, we should do so using the research design that will provide the strongest tests of our hypotheses.

Of course, not everyone designs their own studies. Many researchers use secondary datasets—that is, datasets that have already been collected and that were generally collected for a purpose other than testing the hypotheses that the current researcher has put forth. In these cases, we often must do the best we can with the available data (including conducting cross-sectional analyses to test mediational hypotheses). Secondary analyses are covered in the Secondary Analysis section later in this chapter.

I once had a manuscript rejected from a prominent developmental journal. We used a cross-sectional dataset to examine what clearly were longitudinal and developmental issues. A couple of months after the rejection, I met the editor of the journal at a conference. I took him aside, thanked him for his time and effort in evaluating our manuscript, and asked him what we could have done better. "When you have a longitudinal question, you need longitudinal data," he responded.

Simply put, you need a dataset that allows you to test your hypotheses as fully as possible. By "longitudinal question," the editor meant that we were advancing hypotheses about predictive relationships between variables. Cross-sectional datasets are not equipped to test these kinds of hypotheses. We were eventually able to publish that paper, but in a less prominent journal and with lots of caveats and cautions regarding the use of cross-sectional data to test longitudinal hypotheses.

Cross-Sectional Studies

So what are cross-sectional studies good for? What are their advantages? Are there ways to reduce some of their limitations if we do not have the resources to conduct a longitudinal or experimental study?

First, let's enumerate some of the "proper" uses of cross-sectional studies and data. We can estimate prevalence rates using cross-sectional data, as long as our sample is representative of the population about which we wish to make inferences. Polling, for example, generally uses cross-sectional samples that are described as representative of "likely voters" (see Brick, 2011, for an extended discussion). An important assumption in this type of polling, of course, is that the key demographics of the sample are similar to the key demographics of the population (in this case, the population refers to all likely voters within the given country, state, province, city, etc.). Such an assumption is critical to satisfy, given that many news outlets often rely on poll results during their coverage (Rosenstiel, 2005).

In 2004, the progressive website MoveOn.org held an informal poll of visitors to the site, asking for whom they would vote in the upcoming election between Republican George W. Bush and Democrat John Kerry. Not surprisingly, the poll results indicated that more than 90% of respondents would vote for Kerry. However, Bush won the election. How could this poll have been so far off base?

The simple answer is that the MoveOn.org visitor base is not representative of the American voting public. The site promotes itself as a tool supporting the progressive movement, suggesting that most people who visit the site are affiliated with the Democratic Party. The number of Republicans who visit MoveOn.org is likely quite small. As a result, a poll conducted by the site is liable to oversample Democratic voters and to undersample Republican voters. (Similarly, a poll conducted by Republican-leaning Breitbart News would almost certainly have predicted Bush as the overwhelming favorite.)

Cross-sectional studies are also useful for estimating prevalence rates. The Centers for Disease Control and Prevention, for example, conducts surveillance studies to estimate the prevalence of various diseases, such as cancer, diabetes, heart disease, and HIV (see www.cdc.gov). The University of Michigan Institute for Social Research conducts an annual Monitoring the Future study (see Miech et al., 2019, for a recent report) on adolescent substance use. These studies are cross-sectional because their primary purpose is to estimate the percentage of the population who have been diagnosed with a given illness or who have engaged in a given set of behaviors. To paraphrase the editor I met at that conference and who had rejected my paper, a cross-sectional question can be addressed using a cross-sectional design.

Because they are limited to examining associations, prevalence rates, and other similar descriptive information, cross-sectional studies are often difficult to publish unless the sampling strategy is purposeful and rigorous. Some journals explicitly refuse to publish cross-sectional studies with convenience samples, especially those using self-report survey measures. For example, the *Journal of Research in Personality*'s guide for authors states that "Cross-sectional, self-report studies conducted among convenience samples . . . are relatively easy to conduct and have some important limitations. Papers that rely solely on cross-sectional designs and self-report questionnaire methods among convenience samples are often rejected without review." Indeed, in many cases it is not clear what information can be gleaned from this type of study. For example, I could survey a college class—or a set of classes—about attitudes toward financial planning, but the generalizability of this information is questionable. Let's say that we surveyed a set of psychology classes at a major public university. Psychology students are not representative of the young adult population—and they are not even representative of the overall college student population. Students in the social sciences are overwhelmingly female (American Psychological Association, 2015)—many of my college student samples have been 75% to 80% women. Further, depending on the demographics of the specific university where the data are collected, different ethnic groups may be overrepresented or underrepresented. My colleagues and I once collected a large dataset from 30 colleges and universities around the United States, and the demographics of the various institutions were vastly different from one another (Corker, Donnellan, Kim, Schwartz, & Zamboanga, 2017). So it is difficult to argue that the results from these samples—especially in cross-sectional studies where prediction and causation cannot be tested—are sufficiently informative to warrant publication.

Longitudinal Studies

Longitudinal studies are generally conducted to test predictive relationships, as well as to map the developmental course of one or more phenomena. For example, longitudinal studies are useful in generating an understanding of how children learn to read (see Verhoeven & van Leeuwe, 2008), predictors of school dropout (see Fortin, Marcotte, Diallo, Potvin, & Royer, 2013), and mental health patterns among adult children from divorced families (see Uphold-Carrier & Utz, 2012).

Longitudinal studies are labor intensive. Aside from recruitment and sampling strategies, which apply to most types of research and are discussed in the Sampling section later in this chapter, the primary challenge in longitudinal studies is retaining participants across time. Indeed, attrition (dropout) is among the greatest threats to the validity of longitudinal studies and the data they produce. Nonrandom attrition—where specific participant, setting, or time characteristics predict who drops out of the study and who remains engaged—requires a sophisticated set of analyses that are likely not necessary otherwise (Little, 2013). Further, high attrition levels threaten our ability to draw firm conclusions from the study results. For example, if we conducted a 2-year longitudinal study but 75% of participants dropped out before the final assessment point, how much trust would you place in the data from this study?

The specific strategies needed to prevent or reduce attrition depend on the specific study design and population (see Cotter, Burke, Stouthamer-Loeber, & Loeber, 2005, for an example). Intensive follow-up and contact procedures may be needed for participants who are highly residentially mobile, whose lives are unstable, and who engage in high-risk behavior (e.g., sex workers, drug users). Participants whose cultural backgrounds are different from those of the researchers, or who are vulnerable for cultural reasons (e.g., recent immigrants, unaccompanied and undocumented minors, refugees), may require culturally syntonic recruitment and engagement strategies (see Knight, Roosa, & Umaña-Taylor, 2009, for a compilation of such strategies).

In our work, we have followed many of Knight et al.'s (2009) suggestions. In our study with recent-immigrant Hispanic families in Miami and Los Angeles (Schwartz et al., 2015, 2016), our recruiters were all fluent Spanish speakers who understood the local cultural contexts. For each family, we obtained information for three "contact persons" who would know where the family members were if we could not reach them to schedule a follow-up assessment. We sent holiday and birthday cards to each family, and we called each family at least once between assessment points to ask whether they needed anything. When President Barack Obama signed an executive order authorizing Deferred Action for Childhood Arrivals (DACA)—a program that provided undocumented immigrants brought to the United States as children with work permits and relief from deportation—our research team provided letters of reference for adolescents who were applying for DACA status. Finally, as mentioned earlier, we designated two team members—who were especially adept at bonding with families and gaining their trust—as our trackers. The trackers were responsible for all contacts with families—and our 85% retention rate through 3 years and six assessment points was largely attributable to the trackers.

Retention strategies may be somewhat different in short-term, intensive longitudinal studies. The term *intensive longitudinal design* refers to studies where participants are assessed one or more times per day (see Bolger, Davis, & Rafaeli, 2003, for a review of these methods). Intensive longitudinal studies include daily diaries, where participants are asked to complete a battery of assessments every day, as well as ecological momentary assessments, where participants are paged at random times and asked to answer questions about their activities, whereabouts, or mental and emotional states.

In some cases, intensive longitudinal studies are conducted by themselves, such that participants are asked to take part for only a few days (see Schwartz et al., 2019, for an example). In other cases, an intensive longitudinal component (sometimes referred to as a "diary burst") is embedded within a larger longitudinal study (Becht et al., 2016). For intensive longitudinal studies where participation is required for only a few days, email or text reminders might be provided each day (along with reminder calls for participants who have not completed study activities on a given day). In some cases, especially where additional tasks are required—such as providing saliva samples at home and storing them until an assessor comes to retrieve them—mobile apps may be used to remind the participant to complete the task. Some of my colleagues have developed such an app and are currently testing its efficacy.

Retention in longer longitudinal studies, including those that incorporate diary bursts within the structure of the larger study, requires a set of intense strategies (Knight et al., 2009). In cases where assessments occur across long periods of time, such as once or twice per year, it is often necessary to contact participants between assessment points to update contact information. In the past, such contacts generally took the form of phone calls, but with advances in technology, researchers can text participants or contact them on social media. (It is probably a better idea to message someone on Facebook, Twitter, or Instagram than to "friend" or "follow" them; researchers do not need to have access to participants' personal social media posts.) I recommend setting up a study phone number and providing mobile phones to staff members who will be calling, texting, or otherwise contacting participants. Staff members should generally not be expected to use their personal phone plans for research activities, and having an official study phone number can help to lend credibility to the study and to people reaching out to participants on behalf of the study. Having business cards printed (as well as e-cards created) for study staff may also be reassuring to participants.

There may be times, however, when explicitly affiliating a study with a university or other formal institution may create more problems than it solves. When my colleagues in Los Angeles were recruiting families for our longitudinal acculturation study, they encountered a considerable amount of difficulty—far more than we were encountering in Miami. They gave brief presentations in classrooms where interested youth provided their parents' contact information, but many parents did not answer the study team's phone calls. In many cases, adolescents had provided their families' home addresses, but when the assessment team knocked on the door, no one would answer. Our team members became very frustrated and concerned that we would not be able to recruit our Los Angeles sample.

After some struggles, my colleague and friend Daniel Soto, who was the project director for the Los Angeles site and is one of the smartest and hardest-working people I know, suggested that we ask some of the people we had already recruited to serve as ambassadors for the study. Many undocumented people know one another, and perhaps asking participants to "vouch" for us would help with recruitment. Daniel's approach helped to overcome some of the obstacles we had faced with recruitment, and we recruited the number of participants we needed. So, in this case, and likely in many others, a more informal approach—relying on participants' connections with one another rather than on the prestige of the researchers' university—was far more efficacious.

Retention efforts in our acculturation study were facilitated largely by our two trackers. The trackers forged relationships with many of the study families, and when they called a family, they were often asked to share a meal with them. *Retention in longitudinal studies is all about relationships.* If the tracker (or whoever else is making calls to participants) is leaving the study, it is essential for the tracker to contact each family and to introduce the new person who will be taking over. Especially with all of the phone scams that are now so prevalent, many people will simply not answer calls from a number they do not recognize. Text messages may be more likely to be answered, but as Knight et al. (2009) noted, participants are most likely to respond to someone with whom they have an existing relationship.

Sending birthday and holiday cards is also a nice touch that participants are likely to appreciate. Social media sites like Facebook, Twitter, and Instagram allow users to send birthday, holiday, and other messages to others—and social media has been shown to help with retention in longitudinal studies (Mychasiuk & Benzies, 2012). I know that I always appreciate receiving birthday cards from doctor's offices and car dealers—and I may be more likely to continue to engage with someone who remembers my birthday.

In his classic book *How to Win Friends and Influence People*, Dale Carnegie notes that a person's name and other details are extremely important to that person. A woman who worked on the same floor I worked on in my previous position told me in passing one day that she was a breast cancer survivor. Several months later, I ran into her and asked how she was feeling. I said I had been thinking about her because of her battles with cancer. Tears welled up in her eyes and she hugged me. Few other people had asked her about her health, and she told me that my asking had really touched her.

What does this have to do with retention in longitudinal studies? The answer is *everything*. If you know something personal about someone—perhaps their son is in college, or maybe their mother has been ill—you can use that information to form a bond with that person. For example, in one intervention study that my colleagues conducted, they were able to engage and retain a Chilean immigrant father in their parenting intervention because the intervention facilitator was married to a Chilean man (Pantin, Schwartz, Coatsworth, Briones, & Szapocznik, 2007). The father had been reluctant to participate until the facilitator started talking about how much she loved Chile. Less than 30 minutes later, the father had agreed to participate. Any commonalities that study personnel have with participants can be used to form a bond, and other information—such as birthdays, health information, family members' activities, and so forth—can be used to show participants that you care about them. Of course, you can't just say that you care about them—you have to mean it.

Experimental Studies

Some experimental studies, such as those conducted in social psychology, involve only one or two participation sessions. Others, such as randomized clinical trials, often involve repeated contacts with participants, sometimes over a span of months or years. Retention in long-term experimental studies (such as randomized clinical trials) is similar to retention in longitudinal studies—and retention is generally not an issue for single-session studies like those often conducted in social psychology. I therefore do not discuss retention issues in this subsection on experimental studies.

Because they are used to infer causality, experimental studies must be carried out with airtight methods (see Baltes, Reese, & Nesselroade, 2014, for a collection of reviews). By "airtight," I mean that the experiment is conducted in exactly the same way for each participant (or that sources of variability in implementation are measured so they can be covaried in analysis), that the experimental and control groups differ only in the experiment and its components (and that any demographic differences between groups are controlled in analysis), and that control and experimental group participants not interact with one another during the course of the study. Each of these potential problems can bias the results of the experiment. Differences in how the experiment is delivered across participants can introduce error variability that cannot be statistically controlled (unless the source of the error is measured). Demographic differences between the experimental and control groups can weaken the study conclusions by providing an alternative explanation for the findings (i.e., that the group differences, and not the experiment, are responsible for the effects observed). Contamination between experimental and control condition participants—especially in randomized clinical trials of behavioral interventions—can decrease differences between groups when control group participants learn about what is being covered in intervention sessions (Moerbeek, 2005).

Where possible, random assignment is the "gold standard" in experimental studies (Charness, Gneezy, & Kuhn, 2012). Because assignment to experimental and control conditions is random, the group assignment has no predictors—and therefore it can be regarded as causal as long as the experiment is carried out properly. In some cases, however, randomization is not practical or ethical. If we are studying abused versus non-abused children, for example, we cannot randomly assign children to be abused. If we are examining differences in cultural orientations between German and Chinese people, we cannot randomly assign people to be German or Chinese. In cases like these, we would use a quasi-experimental design (see Reichart, 2009, for an in-depth review). In a quasi-experimental design, the groups exist prior to the beginning of the study—and as a result, causal inferences are more difficult to draw. Indeed, whereas no variables can predict a random condition assignment, there may be many predictors of naturally occurring groups. For example, abused and non-abused children, or German and Chinese people, likely differ on a wide range of characteristics.

A number of statistical methods can be used to draw stronger inferences from quasi-experimental data than can be drawn using standard inferential statistics like analyses of variance. One such method is propensity score matching (Guo & Fraser, 2014). Propensity score matching can be used to statistically equate participants in cases where randomization is not possible or did not occur. Propensity scores are generally utilized to evaluate the effects of treatments, policies, or other interventions over time. Other methods include matched controls, where each participant from Group A is matched with a participant from Group B on several key variables (such as gender, educational attainment, or income level). Hancock (2004) also outlined the Multiple Indicators, Multiple Causes (MIMIC) method of controlling for confounding variables, as well as some other analytic strategies for quasi-experimental data.

A Note on Planning

As noted throughout this chapter, regardless of the research design used, it is of the utmost importance that the study be carefully planned, adequately staffed, and carried out as cautiously as possible. Any errors in measurement, execution, or any other part of the study will quite likely compromise the study results, and by extension, impair the ability of the study to properly test the hypotheses that it was designed to test.

I cannot say enough about planning. Knowing who will do what, exactly what order the study activities will follow, and precisely what will be done with each participant is essential. It is also important to establish an organizational chart for the study indicating who is responsible for what, and who reports to whom. Figure 2.4 displays the organizational chart that my colleagues and I are using for our ongoing study of Puerto Rican Hurricane Maria survivors who relocated to the Orlando and Miami areas after the storm. (Credit goes to my colleague Chris Salas-Wright for creating this chart.) Notice that each of the three principal investigators—myself, Chris, and Mildred Maldonado-Molina—is responsible for supervising a group of staff members. Chris provided job descriptions for each person on the team (including the principal investigators) so that it would be *abundantly* clear who is responsible for whom and for what.

Anyone who has worked on any kind of project team has experienced diffusion of responsibility—the phenomenon where something doesn't get done but everyone says it was someone else's job to do it. Without a clear organizational chart, the likelihood of diffusion of responsibility occurring in your project is high. With a clear description of who is responsible for what, rigorous training sessions for each staff member, and regular lab meetings to update everyone on the team's progress, people are much more likely to know which tasks fall within their job description.

In almost every major grant I have ever written—and I have now received four major grant awards from the National Institutes of Health and other funders—the first year of the study is dedicated to planning. The planning phase includes:

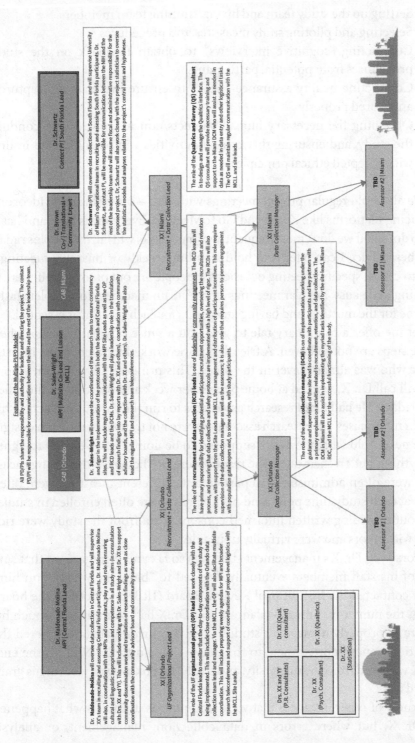

Figure 2.4 Sample organizational chart.

Features of the Multiple PI/PO Model:
All PD/PIs share the responsibility and authority for leading and directing the project. The contact PD/PI will be responsible for communication between the NIH and the rest of the leadership team.

Dr. Maldonado Molina
MPI | Central Florida Lead

Dr. **Maldonado-Molina** will oversee data collection in Central Florida and will supervise XX's team in recruiting and assessing Central Florida participants. Dr. Maldonado Molina will also, in coordination with the MPIs and consultants, play a lead role in ensuring cultural and linguistic appropriateness and competence in all study aims (in consultation with Drs. XX and YY). This will include working with Dr. Sales-Wright and XX to support community dissemination work and translation of research findings as well as close coordination with the community advisory board and community partners.

Dr. Sales-Wright
MPI | Multisite Co-Lead and Liaison (MCLL)

CAB | Orlando

Dr. **Sales-Wright** will oversee the coordination of the research sites to ensure consistency and rigor in the implementation of the protocols in both the South and Central Florida sites. This will include regular communication with the MPI Site Leads as well as the OP and RCD leads and the DCMs. Dr. Sales-Wright will play a leadership role in the translation of research findings into lay reports with Drs. XX and others), coordination with community advisory boards, and the collection (with Dr. XX and others). Dr. Sales-Wright will also lead the regular MPI and research team teleconferences.

CAB | Miami

Dr. Brown
Co+/ | Translational + Community Expert

Dr. Schwartz
Contact PI | South Florida Lead

Dr. **Schwartz** (PI) will oversee data collection in South Florida and will supervise University of Miami's operational team in recruiting and assessing South Florida participants. Dr. Schwartz, as contact PI, will be responsible for communication between the NIH and the rest of the leadership team and will assume fiscal and administrative responsibility for the proposed project. Dr, Schwartz will also work closely with the project statistician to oversee the statistical models and analyses related to the project's central aims and hypotheses.

XX | Orlando
Recruitment + Data Collection Lead

XX | Miami
Recruitment + Data Collection Lead

The role of the **recruitment and data collection (RCD) leads** is one of leadership + community engagement. The RCD leads will have primary responsibility for identifying potential participant recruitment opportunities, overseeing the recruitment and retention process, and ensuring that data collection and safety protocols are implemented with a high level of rigor. The RCDs will also oversee, with support from the Site Leads and MCLL, the management and distribution of participant incentives. This role requires supervision of the data collection manager as well as the assessors; it is also a role that requires person-to-person engagement with population gatekeepers and, to some degree, with study participants.

The role of the **Quatrics and Survey (QS) Consultant** is to design and manage the Qualtrics interface. The QS consultant will provide necessary training and support to the Miami DCM who will assist as needed in data entry and other logistical tasks. The QS will maintain regular communication with the MCLL and site leads.

XX | Orlando
UF Organizational/Project Lead

The role of the UF **organizational project (OP) lead** is to work closely with the Central Florida lead to monitor that the day-to-day components of the study are being implemented. This will include close coordination with the Orlando data collection team lead and manager. Via the MCLL, the OP will also facilitate multisite coordination. This will include preparing weekly agendas for MPI and broader research teleconferences and support of coordination of project-level logistics with the MCLL Site Leads.

XX | Orlando
Data Collection Manager

XX | Miami
Data Collection Manager

The role of the **data collection managers (DCM)** is on of implementation, working under the guidance and supervision of the site lead to coordinate with participants and key partners with a primary emphasis on activities related to recruitment, retention, and data collection. The DCM in Miami will also assist in implementing the myriad tasks identified by the site lead, Miami RDC, and the MCLL for the successful functioning of the study.

TBD
Assessor #1 | Orlando

TBD
Assessor #2 | Orlando

TBD
Assessor #1 | Miami

TBD
Assessor #2 | Miami

Drs. XX and YY
(P.R. Consultants)

Dr. XX (Qual. consultant)

Dr. XX
(Psych. Consultant)

Dr. XX, XX (Qualtrics)

Dr. XX
(Statistician)

- Setting up the study team and hiring/training team members
- Selecting and piloting study measures and procedures
- Conducting "cognitive interviews" to obtain feedback on the study procedures from potential participants
- Conducting quality assurance checks to ensure that data are captured and stored properly
- Obtaining the necessary human subjects/ethical approvals to conduct the study, and ensuring that project activities will be conducted in line with accepted ethical principles

We also hold regular project meetings with staff—often through videoconferencing platforms like Zoom and GoToMeeting. Everyone is busy and has a lot to do, and if we don't meet frequently, project tasks will fall off people's radar. The best advice I can offer is to hold standing weekly or biweekly meetings, and to cancel specific meeting occasions if people are out of town or if there is nothing to discuss. Regular meetings "force" team members to complete tasks in time for the meeting, and having an agenda for each meeting is essential.

Let me offer a cautionary tale to give you a sense of what happens when these steps are not followed. A friend of mine worked for a principal investigator who was almost never in the office. This principal investigator, whom we will call Dr. X, worked at home 6 days per week and was only in the office on Fridays. He had hired research associates to run the various projects in his lab. In many cases, the research associates were not trained in research design, were never told what they were supposed to be doing, and were left to figure everything out on their own. The results were predictable—the wrong measures were often administered to participants, different measures were often used at each study time point, and participants were often enrolled in studies without providing written informed consent. Data from the study were riddled with errors and were virtually unusable.

Worse yet, Dr. X's management style was so lax and disorganized that several of his staff members eventually decided to "blow the whistle" on him. They contacted the Institutional Review Board (IRB) and notified the board about the numerous ethical violations that Dr. X had committed through his failure to properly manage his studies. The IRB investigated, discovered the violations, and reported them to the university and to the NIH. In the end, Dr. X was fired from the university, and the NIH took away several of his grant awards.

I know of other instances that were not quite as drastic as what happened to Dr. X, but where errors in data collection, management, or analysis compromised the study findings. In most of these instances, the errors were a result of lack of adequate planning. In one case, some colleagues of mine were studying the ability of an intervention to increase social support among HIV-positive women. The social support measure required participants to write in the names of people from whom they sought or received support, and for each support source, they were asked a series of questions. Over time, participants discovered that listing fewer support sources would lead to fewer questions being asked, which in turn would help them complete the measure more quickly. The end result was that participants in both the intervention and control conditions appeared to be receiving less support over time, even though participants in the intervention condition reported more effective coping strategies across time. Had my colleagues gone through their measurement battery carefully and conducted cognitive interviews with participants (see Beatty & Willis, 2007, for a detailed review of cognitive interviewing procedures), their cognitive interviewing participants would have alerted them to the problems with the social support measure.

Here is another example. In our study of Puerto Rican Hurricane Maria survivors in Florida, we considered including a measure of the extent to which participants perceived conflict between their Puerto Rican and U.S. identities. Our community partner, who is well connected and established in the Hurricane Maria survivor community in Florida, told us that this measure would not work well with this population. Although their homeland is a U.S. territory, Puerto Ricans have a complicated relationship with the United States (Acosta-Belén & Santiago, 2018). For example, Puerto Ricans are U.S. citizens at birth and can travel anywhere on the U.S. mainland without a passport—but Puerto Rico competes as a separate nation in the Olympics and other international tournaments. The issue of potentially becoming a U.S. state has been extremely controversial among Puerto Ricans, some of whom support statehood and others of whom would rather become an independent country (Torres, 2017). As a result, asking Puerto Ricans about their identity as Americans is akin to stepping into a minefield, as our community partner suggested.

Had we decided to include the identity-conflict measure in our assessment battery, not only would the resulting data likely have been biased, but also we would have risked losing participants from our sample. In longitudinal research—including randomized trials, which also involve repeated assessments—any measure or procedure that is likely to upset or alienate participants should be avoided.

Secondary Analyses and Meta-Analyses

Thus far, the discussion has focused on issues involved in primary data collection—that is, where the study involves collecting new data. However, many research projects involve analyzing existing datasets or empirically summarizing results across a set of studies. Although the challenges involved in planning a study and supervising data collection and other study procedures are generally not present, other challenges do need to be addressed (see Trzesniewski, Donnellan, & Lucas, 2010, for a collection of reviews). This section first discusses secondary data analyses and then discusses meta-analyses.

Secondary Data Analyses

Among the primary challenges involved in secondary data analysis is not having control over the dataset. If you are designing a study and collecting data, you and your colleagues get to decide what the study population will be, which measures to include, and how and when the assessments will be conducted, among other decisions. You have full control over the dataset that will be generated as a result of the study.

With secondary data, you are using a dataset that someone else collected. As a result, you may have to use data from measures that you would not have chosen had you conducted the study yourself. There may be errors in the dataset that you would have caught had you been in charge of the study. The team who conducted the study may have made decisions along the way that affected the data but that may never have been disclosed to anyone outside the study. The documentation for the dataset may be unclear, and you may have to do some detective work to figure out how to use the dataset.

Several years ago, one of my PhD students wanted to study predictors of adolescent sexual behavior. Because she was an epidemiologist, my student wanted to use a national, population-based dataset. We found a dataset for her to use, but the documentation was so complex that learning the dataset took her more than a year. The study team had used sampling weights to ensure that the sample would be representative of the U.S. adolescent population. (I discuss sampling weights later in this section.)

My student diligently learned the dataset and conducted a rigorous set of analyses, which we published (Shneyderman & Schwartz, 2013). Honestly, as someone who has almost always collected my own data, I am not sure whether I would have had the patience that she had. However, as I discuss in detail in Chapter 15, she was able to make much more authoritative statements using a population-based dataset than we could have made had we collected our own data.

Thus, secondary data analyses may take several forms. One such form involves analysis of large, population-based datasets. Disciplines like sociology, political science, demography, and public health often dictate—either implicitly or explicitly—that these kinds of datasets are necessary to make statements about whole populations. Indeed, the "mission statements" of these disciplines involve studying and drawing inferences about populations (Franco, Malhotra, Simonovits, & Zigerell, 2017). Although some people, such as my colleague Deborah Schildkraut (2014) at Tufts University, collect their own population-based datasets, most researchers who use population-based datasets use datasets collected by others. Population-based datasets are discussed in greater detail in Chapter 15.

A second form of secondary data analysis involves using data that one's colleagues have collected. Many graduate students, for example, use their mentors' datasets for their master's theses and doctoral dissertations. In many cases, datasets generated by large grants are collected to test specific hypotheses, but the data can then be used for other purposes.

Several years ago, some of my Dutch colleagues allowed me to use some of their data to conduct longitudinal analyses of personal identity exploration and commitment processes. (At that time, I had never collected my own longitudinal data and had to rely on my colleagues' generosity.) The datasets were easy to learn because the data managers had clearly labeled the variables in the dataset—though I did need some help because the labels were in Dutch. Although only a few of my colleagues provided comments on drafts of the papers we wrote, all of the "owners" of the dataset were listed as authors.

Listing the data's owners as authors is common practice when the dataset belongs to colleagues, but it is not generally done with large national datasets. Rather, the study team is sometimes acknowledged in a footnote. The National Longitudinal Study of Adolescent Health (Add Health), for example, requires that authors using the Add Health dataset insert a specific paragraph in their acknowledgments section listing the primary members of the Add Health research team.

National or regional datasets are often explicitly collected to serve as repositories for researchers. For example, the United States Centers for Disease Control and Prevention collects the Youth Risk Behavior Surveillance Survey (YRBSS; see https://www.cdc.gov/healthyyouth/data/yrbs/index.htm). The YRBSS dataset is used to provide prevalence rates for a range of adolescent risk behaviors, such as risky alcohol use, illicit drug use, and impaired driving—as well as to examine predictors of, and trends in, youth risk behavior. For example, Choo et al. (2014) used the YRBSS dataset to study the effects of state medical marijuana laws on adolescent marijuana use. Such an analysis would be difficult to conduct using anything other than a national probability sample.

A third type of secondary dataset is the *proprietary* dataset. Proprietary datasets are similar to national probability datasets, except that the dataset's owners carefully control access to the data and often insist on approving all analyses and manuscripts that use the dataset. Proprietary datasets are discussed further in Chapter 15—but a key decision to be made when considering whether to use such a dataset is whether one is willing to expend the time and effort needed to gain access to the dataset and to "jump through all the hoops" necessary to publish using the dataset.

Sampling Weights

Researchers collecting national or regional probability samples use *sampling weights* to ensure that smaller groups are properly represented in the sample and that each group's contribution to the study results is proportional to that group's share of the population. For example, if Group A comprises 20% of a population and Group B represents 30% of that population, patterns from Group A should contribute 20%, and patterns from Group B should contribute 30%, to the overall pattern of results obtained from the dataset. This proportional representation should hold even if, for example, Group A makes up 40% of the sample and Group B makes up 10% of the sample.

Broadly, a sampling weight is computed as , where %P represents a given group's share of the population and %S represents that group's share of the sample. In the example in the previous paragraph, where Group A represents 20% of the population but 40% of our sample, the patterns for Group A will be weighted half as much (20% divided by 40%) as they would be using an unweighted analysis. Asparouhov (2005) provides a more technical and detailed treatment of how to analyze data with sampling weights.

Sampling weights allow us to oversample smaller groups so that the statistical estimates for these groups are stable. For example, let's say that we are sampling five groups from a population (see Figure 2.5). Our plan is to gather a sample of 500 people in total. Because the aqua group represents only 5% of the population, if we sampled each group exactly in proportion to its representation in the population, we would sample only 25 people from the aqua group. But a sample of 25 cases is likely to yield unstable estimates, especially for more complex statistical models (Asparouhov, 2005). We might decide

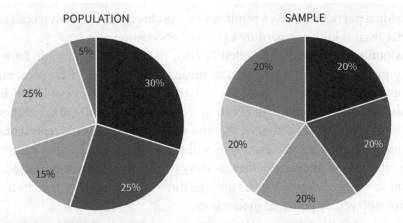

Figure 2.5 Hypothetical population and sample.

instead to sample evenly across the five groups—that is, 100 people from each group—and weight the resulting data so that results from our analyses would represent the population.

In this case, we have oversampled the aqua group (because they comprise 20% of the sample but only 5% of the population) and undersampled the blue group (because they comprise 20% of the sample but 30% of the population). To correct for this oversampling and undersampling, we use sampling weights. The weight for the aqua group would be 0.25 (5% divided by 20%), and the weight for the blue group would be 1.5 (30% divided by 20%). The yellow, gray, and orange groups would be weighted in a similar fashion, using their representations within the population and in the sample.

As an example, Morgan et al. (2009) collected a population-based sample of healthy adults in the United Kingdom and surveyed experiences of psychosis. Because relatively few Black Caribbean adults resided in the study's catchment area, the researchers oversampled this group by taking longer to recruit them than they took to recruit the other ethnic groups in the sample. Morgan et al. then used sampling weights to ensure that Black Caribbean participants contributed to the study results in proportion to their representation in the communities from which the sample was drawn.

Meta-Analysis

Meta-analysis is a form of "empirical literature review" in which results from a series of studies are statistically synthesized and reported as a single set of findings. In a meta-analysis, the unit of analysis is studies rather than individual participants. As a result, a well-conducted meta-analysis can summarize what is known regarding a given phenomenon.

As outlined by Field and Gillett (2010), meta-analyses provide four primary pieces of information: (1) the mean association or difference within a population, (2) the variance around that mean at the population level, (3) the extent of variability in effects across studies, and (4) effects of moderator variables. That is, provided that the researchers include a representative sample of studies, the meta-analysis will tell us the average effect within the population, how much this effect is likely to vary within the population, the extent to which different studies provide differing estimates of the effect, and the roles played by potential moderators.

As an example, Olatunji, Davis, Powers, and Smits (2013) conducted a meta-analysis of the outcomes of randomized trials evaluating cognitive-behavioral therapy for obsessive-compulsive disorder. They first conducted a literature search using multiple databases and identified abstracts that matched the search terms (e.g., *obsessive-compulsive*, *cognitive-behavioral*, *randomized trial*). Abstracts that did not mention randomized trials for obsessive-compulsive disorder were omitted from consideration, and the authors proceeded to obtain full-text versions of the remaining articles. They then carefully reviewed each of these articles to ensure that the studies reported had compared an active cognitive-behavioral treatment against a comparison or waitlist control condition. Effects reported within each of the qualifying articles were then entered into the meta-analysis.

Olatunji et al.'s meta-analysis included a number of summary statistics. First, the Hedges' *g* statistic (a measure of effect size) reflects the average change in symptoms during treatment, in standard deviation units (Rosenthal, 1991). That is, Hedges' *g* tells us by how many standard deviations the average patient's obsessive-compulsive disorder symptoms decreased as a result of treatment—compared to a control condition that did not receive treatment. Second, a 95% confidence interval is provided for the Hedges' *g* statistic. This confidence interval provides an index of variability around this average effect size. A larger confidence interval tells us that the average effect size is less precise. Third, the Q statistic (Bowden, Tierney, Copas, & Burdett, 2011) provides an estimate of heterogeneity across studies, where a significant Q value suggests that effects of moderator variables should be examined. Fourth, the effects of potential moderators were examined using meta-regression analysis (Stanley & Jarrell, 1989), where the results of individual studies—rather than data from individual people—are used as the input. Finally, a set of statistics, such as the trim-and-fill-method (Rücker, Carpenter, & Schwarzer, 2011), are used to estimate the effect of publication bias (i.e., manuscripts reporting nonsignificant results not being submitted or accepted for publication). Effects of interest can be reported with maximal confidence if they remain significant even with potential effects of publication bias taken into account.

When conducting meta-analyses, it is essential to include theses, dissertations, and other student outputs that may not have been subsequently published. It is also a good idea to contact researchers working in the subject area of the meta-analysis and ask them whether they have new findings that can be included in the meta-analysis. If the information needed for a meta-analysis is not included in published articles, you should contact the author of the article and ask for that information. I have often been contacted by people and asked for means and correlations among a set of study variables—which serve as the input matrix for meta-analyses of associations among variables (Field & Gillett, 2010).

Meta-analytic articles often also include a flow chart indicating how many abstracts were originally included, how many full-text articles were reviewed, and how many studies were ultimately included in the meta-analysis. Olatunji et al. (2013), for example, initially identified 234 abstracts, downloaded 39 articles for review, and included 16 articles in their meta-analysis. The search terms, databases, and range of dates used in the literature review should be specified, so that a reader could replicate the search.

Students and colleagues often ask me how far back literature searches should go. My response is often that, aside from classic citations (e.g., founders of a field of inquiry, developers of statistical techniques), citations should generally be restricted to the last 10 to 15 years. Science accelerates at such a pace that much of the literature from the 1990s, and even the early 2000s, is now outdated. As I write this chapter in December 2019, I very rarely cite anything published prior to 2000. I am even hesitant to cite anything published prior to 2005.

Some types of citations must be extremely current. Prevalence rates, for example, *must* be based on extremely recent sources. I have reviewed manuscripts and seen authors claiming that the prevalence rate for a given condition is high—but then cite a 20-year-old source. Prevalence rates change constantly, so what was prevalent in 2001 may not be prevalent in 2021 (and vice versa). Citations to current events should also be very recent.

So what do these principles mean for meta-analyses? Unless there is a compelling reason to do otherwise, studies included in a meta-analysis should be as recent as possible. This guideline is especially important in fields where measurement has evolved, and where older studies used measures that were less precise or rigorous than those used in more recent studies. Alternatively, year of publication might be used as a moderator, such that findings from earlier studies might be statistically different from those of more current studies.

In their meta-analysis, Olatunji et al. (2013) noted that the practice of cognitive-behavioral psychotherapy had remained largely consistent and stable, such that older studies were also important to include. It should be noted that 10 of the 16 studies (63% of the studies) they included were published in 2000 or later. Smith and Silva (2010), in their meta-analysis of ethnic identity and well-being, included 184 studies, of which 118 (64%) were published in 2000 or later. As time continues to pass and more studies are added to the literature, the share of pre-2000 articles included in meta-analyses will continue to decrease.

An essential rule to follow in meta-analysis is that, within a single meta-analysis, only one entry can be included for a given dataset (Field & Gillett, 2010). Most datasets produce multiple publications, but the means, variances, and correlations for a given set of variables will be the same for each publication. Including more than one publication for the same dataset would unfairly weight that dataset more heavily than other datasets are weighted.

Sampling

The final topic to be considered in this chapter is sampling. There are many excellent sources that provide in-depth information and recommendations for selecting and implementing a sampling strategy (e.g., Lohr, 2019; Thompson, 2013), so I provide only a fairly brief overview of sampling considerations. My coverage here focuses primarily on general sampling considerations and far less on specific types of samples. I should note, however, that sampling is absolutely critical to our ability to draw accurate inferences from our results. We draw a sample from our population of interest, conduct our study with this sample, and then infer or generalize our results back to the population.

Figure 2.6 displays this process. What is essential to understand is that *the quality of the inferences we can draw regarding our population is dependent on the quality of our sampling procedures*. Polling is an example of an activity where sampling is of the utmost importance. To be able to say that Candidate A is ahead of Candidate B by 6 percentage points among likely voters, we must have polled a sample that is representative of people who are likely to vote in the upcoming election. Similarly, if we want to publish a report on the prevalence of unprotected sexual behavior among adolescents, we must recruit a population-based sample from this age group—or at least identify and recruit from all of the subgroups that comprise the adolescent population, and then

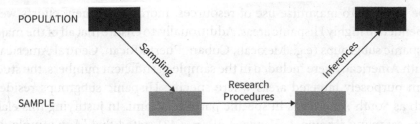

Figure 2.6 The importance of sampling.

use sampling weights to correct for underrepresentation or overrepresentation of each subgroup within the sample versus the population.

The "best" type of sample to be recruited depends on the population under study, the goals of the project, and the available resources. Stratified random sampling, where each segment of the population is identified and participants are recruited at random from each segment, is generally regarded as a sound strategy for epidemiologic and public health research (see LaVange et al., 2010, for an example from the Hispanic Community Health Study). However, in social psychology, convenience samples like Amazon's Mechanical Turk are often considered adequate (Buhrmester, Kwang, & Gosling, 2011). Indeed, in epidemiology and public health, the goal is generally to make statements about whole populations—such as rates, predictors, and consequences of risk factors and disease outcomes among groups. Social psychology, on the other hand, is more concerned with testing theoretical propositions about intergroup relations and processes, with the hope of generalizing the findings to real-world situations. The types of samples gathered to achieve these goals are clearly different.

As examples, let's consider studies designed to estimate predictors and prevalence of cardiovascular disease among Hispanic adults in the United States and studies designed to test ingroup projection theory (Wenzel, Mummendey, & Waldzus, 2007), a social psychological perspective positing that the majority group in a given country or region is likely to equate itself with the country or region itself (such as White Americans implicitly assuming that Whites are "more American" than other ethnic groups are; Devos & Heng, 2009). These two examples are quite different and require vastly different sampling approaches.

The Hispanic Community Health Study set up field sites in four major U.S. cities—New York City, Miami, Chicago, and San Diego—and used a two-stage sampling process within each city (see LaVange et al., 2010). First, they used U.S. Census data to identify areas that were more-versus-less heavily Hispanic, and then they randomly selected households to visit within each type of area. To maximize use of resources, more recruitment efforts were expended in highly Hispanic areas. Additionally, to ensure that all of the major Hispanic subgroups (e.g., Mexican, Cuban, Puerto Rican, Central American, South American) were included in the sample in sufficient numbers, the study team purposely targeted areas where specific Hispanic subgroups resided, such as South Americans in specific parts of Miami. In justifying this elaborate sampling scheme, LaVange et al. (p. 643) stated that "Any sample design that uses nonrandom selection (e.g., a convenience sample) produces a nonprobability sample. . . . Accompanying the simplicity and lower cost associated with nonprobability sampling is [the problem that] there is no direct theoretical basis for making estimates of population characteristics from the sample."

In contrast, Bianchi, Mummendey, Steffens, and Yzerbyt (2010) conducted a series of social-psychological experiments in Germany and Italy to test ingroup projection theory. The samples for all three experiments consisted exclusively of university students, and no attempts were made to recruit outside of one Italian university and one German university. An implicit assumption within such a design is that the effects of social-psychological experiments on the intergroup processes taking place among university students are universal, and that, in effect, the sample doesn't matter. A social-psychological colleague of mine once told me directly that all samples are basically equivalent. At least at the time these studies were conducted, the views on sampling between epidemiology and social psychology could not possibly have been more divergent.

So, in cases where representing and making statements about the population is among the study goals, convenience sampling is likely not a good choice. Peterson and Merunka (2014) compared 42 U.S. university student samples in terms of gender differences in mean endorsement of capitalist values. They found that gender differences in capitalism scores favored men in some samples, favored women in other samples, and were nonsignificant in still other samples. In other words, convenience samples may not provide much generalizable information.

Among the reasons why convenience samples may not provide generalizable information is that certain subgroups of the population are likely to be underrepresented or omitted. For example, Schwartz (2016) reviewed differences in identity processes and substance use rates between college students and non-college-attending young adults. Compared to their similarly aged peers who do not attend institutions of higher education, college students were less likely to endorse identity commitments, more likely to be confused or uncertain about their future, more likely to engage in binge drinking, and less likely to use illicit drugs or engage in unprotected sexual intercourse. Using student samples to examine any of these outcomes—and especially to generalize findings to the young adult population as a whole—is likely to result in inaccurate conclusions.

In some cases, the goal is to make statements or inferences about hidden or difficult-to-reach populations. In these cases, random sampling is generally not possible. For example, in our work with Hurricane Maria survivors in Florida (Scaramutti, Salas-Wright, Vos, & Schwartz, 2019) and with Venezuelan immigrants in Miami and Bogotá, Colombia (Schwartz et al., 2018), my colleagues and I have used respondent-driven sampling (Wejnert & Heckathorn, 2008). Respondent-driven sampling is similar to snowball sampling in that a small group of "seed" participants are recruited and are asked to refer other people who also meet the study's inclusion criteria. Each of the referred participants is then asked to refer additional people, and the chain continues until the desired sample size is reached. Unlike snowball sampling, which is a convenience approach, respondent-driven sampling requires that referral chains be carefully documented and controlled for in analysis (Heckathorn, 2012). Heckathorn (2002) outlined procedures for using respondent-driven samples to provide prevalence rates and other information about a population.

Qualitative studies may use entirely different sampling strategies than quantitative studies use (see Koerber & McMichael, 2008, for a review of qualitative sampling strategies). In general, the goal of most qualitative sampling strategies is not to produce a representative sample, but to provide a range of participant characteristics as a way of maximizing the richness of the resulting data. At the same time, qualitative work must remain rigorous, and it is essential to ensure that the sample includes representation from all of the subgroups about whom inferences will be drawn.

Indeed, purposive qualitative sampling represents an attempt to capture a population of interest for qualitative inquiry (Onwuegbuzie & Leech, 2007). Onwuegbuzie and Leech reviewed a number of qualitative sampling strategies and noted that the goal of qualitative sampling is to provide saturation—that is, to capture all of the themes or constructs of interest. It is therefore important to select a sample that is both diverse and inclusive enough to provide the full range of response categories that would be expected to emerge from the population. For example, if we were asking immigrants to describe their experiences in their new countries of residence, we would want to purposively sample both recent and longer-term immigrants, immigrants from a variety of source countries and ethnic groups, and immigrants from a range of socioeconomic brackets. It is quite plausible that a given immigrant's experience in the new country of residence would vary as a function of time since migration, country of origin, and socioeconomic status.

Sampling strategies for randomized trials have been discussed less frequently than have sampling strategies for descriptive and epidemiological studies, because the primary goal of a randomized trial is to evaluate the efficacy or effectiveness of an intervention. Given that random assignment to experimental versus control conditions allows for causal conclusions to be drawn, sampling concerns may be regarded as somewhat less important. However, a commonly endorsed approach to randomized trials research (Rounsaville, Carroll, & Onken, 2001) holds that a behavioral intervention should be tested for efficacy in at least two trials, with two different populations, before it can be tested for effectiveness. (Note that testing for *efficacy* refers to evaluating an intervention under controlled laboratory conditions, whereas testing for *effectiveness* refers to evaluating the intervention in community settings.) As a result, sampling *does* matter for randomized clinical trials—we can conclude that an intervention is efficacious or effective only for the participant populations or groups with whom it has been tested.

For example, Muir, Schwartz, and Szapocznik (2004) described a randomized trial of a parent-centered substance use preventive intervention with Hispanic and African American families in Miami. The intervention was designed to provide support and community connections for immigrant families. Results indicated that the intervention was efficacious for Hispanic families, but that it had iatrogenic (hurtful) effects for African American families. When interviewed later, several of the African American parents indicated that the intervention did not meet their needs—they were already well connected in their communities and had plenty of support from neighbors and friends. They indicated that what they needed was access to resources for their children, such as tutors, newer textbooks, and mental health treatment. These findings suggest that the content and structure of parenting interventions must match the expressed needs of the population the intervention is designed for.

As another example, Multisystemic Therapy (Henggeler, Schoenwald, Borduin, Rowland, & Cunningham, 2009) is an intervention designed to reduce antisocial behavior among children and adolescents. As outlined by Henggeler et al., this intervention has been tested in several efficacy and effectiveness studies with different populations (e.g., serious juvenile offenders, youth in psychiatric crisis) and has since been implemented in standard clinical care in the United States, Canada, and Norway, among other countries (Schoenwald, Heiblum, Saldaña, & Henggeler, 2008). Each time

Multisystemic Therapy was tested on a different population, a sample had to be recruited from that population.

However, no attempt was made to ensure that the samples of delinquent or psychiatrically impaired youth were randomly selected or otherwise representative of their respective national populations. Indeed, such an endeavor would likely have been impossible—no national registries exist for delinquent or psychiatrically impaired youth, and it is not clear whether respondent-driven sampling (where psychiatrically impaired youth refer other psychiatrically impaired youth, for example) would have produced a representative national sample either. The fact that Multisystemic Therapy significantly outperformed control conditions in several randomized trials provides evidence that the intervention is efficacious and effective.

In conclusion, the sample collected for a given study should match the objectives, discipline, and scope of that study. Studies that aim to support statements about a population must sample representatively from that population—whether by sampling randomly from across the population, by specifically targeting subpopulations and sampling randomly within them, or by using respondent-driven methods to capture hidden populations. Studies whose primary aim is to test theory should sample within the population of interest, but representativeness may be less of a priority. My social-psychological colleague's statement that "samples don't matter" may be challenged by the current replication crisis in psychology and other social sciences, where up to half of previously published results cannot be replicated with new samples. Although there may be other explanations for the inability to replicate prior findings (Open Science Collaboration, 2015), the use of convenience samples may limit generalizability, and perhaps reproducibility as well (Pruchno et al., 2008).

At the same time, convenience samples may have some utility. For example, they may be useful in exploring new phenomena or populations and in providing guidance about how to investigate these phenomena or populations in subsequent studies. My colleague Chris Salas-Wright and I, along with several other collaborators, recruited a convenience sample of Venezuelan immigrant adolescents in Florida and surveyed them with regard to alcohol use, pre-migration trauma, family relationships, and other dimensions of adjustment and social functioning. The articles we have published so far using this dataset—indicating that Venezuelan youth who experienced food insecurity prior to migration were likely to report symptoms of depression following migration (Salas-Wright, Vaughn, Cohen, & Schwartz, 2020a), and that Venezuelan immigrant youth were more likely than other youth to report problematic alcohol use (Salas-Wright et al., 2020b)—will serve as preliminary findings for an upcoming grant application to recruit a population-based sample of Venezuelan immigrant families and study them longitudinally.

Conclusion

This chapter discusses the importance of study design, measurement, sampling, and other considerations (see Table 2.2 for a study design checklist). Although the writing process itself is mentioned only occasionally in this chapter, the decisions made regarding how the study will be carried out will ultimately dictate what can, and cannot, be included in the written document. Causal language can be used only if a randomized experiment has been carried out—or if causality can be established statistically. (Readers are referred to Judea Pearl's Causality Blog [http://causality.cs.ucla.edu/blog/] for an in-depth treatment of how causality can be tested in the absence of an experimental design.) Predictive language can only be used with longitudinal

Table 2.2 Study Design Checklist

Sampling	Measures	Retention
• Have you defined the population to which you want to generalize your findings? • Have you decided how to draw your sample? • Have you defined inclusion/exclusion criteria to determine whether a given individual can be enrolled in your study?	• Have you identified how you will measure each construct? • Do you know exactly how to administer and score/ code each measure? • Is each measure appropriate for your study population? Are there any reasons why any measure would not work with your population?	• For longitudinal studies, how will you stay in touch with participants to limit dropout from your study? • Will specific retention methods be used for certain types of populations (such as highly mobile individuals)?
Design	**Recruitment**	**Procedures**
• Will you use a crass-sectional, longitudinal, or experimental design? • Does your chosen design match your study hypotheses? • Have you identified potential confounding variables and ways to account for them?	• How will you obtain your sample? How will you gain access to them, and how will you enroll them in your study? • Will your sample represent the population? Why or why not? Are there biases in your sampling and recruitment that will oversample or undersample certain groups?	• What will each participant have to do during each study visit? • How will you ensure that these procedures are as consistent as possible across participants and visits? • How will research staff be monitored to prevent "drift" from study protocols?

data where prior levels of mediating and outcome variables can be statistically controlled. The research design used in a study should match the research questions guiding the study, so that the proper level of association can be discussed in papers based on the study. The type of data to be collected—quantitative, qualitative, or mixed method—should also be based on the research questions underlying the study.

I also emphasized the importance of planning. Once the study has been conducted, the data are ours—including any errors that occurred along the way. Unplanned variations in study implementation, covariates that were not measured, and questions that were not asked essentially become error variance in the analyses that we conduct. When participants drop out of a study in large numbers, the validity of the results may be threatened. When study staff are not properly trained and commit errors, the resulting data will be compromised. As the old saying goes, failure to plan is planning to fail. And in most cases, even the most sophisticated statistical analyses cannot make up for mistakes made during the study or in data collection. In science, there are few things that are as useless as a heavily flawed dataset. Planning properly can help to head off many potential errors and to maximize the validity of the data we collect.

Summary

- Using a rigorous research design is an essential prerequisite to being able to publish high-quality articles in top journals.
- Planning is essential if we are to eliminate as many errors as possible from our study.
- Once we have completed our study, the data are ours—including any problems or errors.
- The types of statements that we can include in our manuscripts—such as association, prediction, and causation—are directly tied to the type of research design that we used to collect the data.
- The research design that we choose for our study must allow us to test our hypotheses fully.
- Regular research team meetings are crucial to ensure the progress and success of a study.
- Secondary data analyses allow us to access data without having to collect our own dataset—but we do not have control over the variables in the dataset, and the data collection may have included errors that we are not aware of.

- Sampling weights can be used to correct for overrepresentation or under-representation of certain groups in our sample relative to the population to which we wish to generalize.
- Meta-analysis is essentially an empirical method for reviewing and summarizing a body of literature.
- The quality of statistical inferences is dependent on how well we have sampled from our target population. Different fields of study maintain different standards regarding the "ideal" types of samples.

References

Acosta-Belén, E., & Santiago, C. E. (2018). *Puerto Ricans in the United States: A contemporary portrait* (2nd ed.). Boulder, CO: Lynne Rienner.

American Psychological Association (2015). 2005–2013: Demographics of the U.S. psychology workforce. Retrieved May 3, 2018 from http://www.apa.org/workforce/publications/13-demographics/index.aspx

Asparouhov, T. (2005). Sampling weights in latent variable modeling. *Structural Equation Modeling, 12*, 411–434.

Baltes, P. B., Reese, H. W., & Nesselroade, J. R. (2014). *Life-span developmental psychology: Introduction to research methods.* New York: Psychology Press.

Beatty, P. C., & Willis, G. B. (2007). Research synthesis: The practice of cognitive interviewing. *Public Opinion Quarterly, 71*, 287–311.

Becht, A. I., Nelemans, S. A., Branje, S. J. T., Vollebergh, W. A. M., Koot, H. M., Dennisen, J. J. A., & Meeus, W. H. J. (2016). The quest for identity in adolescence: Heterogeneity in daily identity formation and psychosocial adjustment across 5 years. *Developmental Psychology, 52*, 2010–2021.

Bianchi, M., Mummendey, A., Steffens, M. C., & Yzerbyt, V. (2010). What do you mean by "European"? Evidence of spontaneous ingroup projection. *Personality and Social Psychology Bulletin, 36*, 960–974.

Bolger, N., Davis, A., & Rafaeli, E. (2003). Diary methods: Capturing life as it is lived. *Annual Review of Psychology, 54*, 579–616.

Bowden, J., Tierney, J. F., Copas, A. J., & Burdett, S. (2011). Quantifying, displaying and accounting for heterogeneity in the meta-analysis of RCTs using standard and generalised Q statistics. *MBC Medical Research Methodology, 11*, Article 41.

Brick, J. M. (2011). The future of survey sampling. *Public Opinion Quarterly, 75*, 872–888.

Bryman, A. (2006). Integrating quantitative and qualitative research: How is it done? *Qualitative Research, 6*, 97–113.

Buhrmester, M., Kwang, T., & Gosling, S. D. (2011). Amazon's Mechanical Turk: A new source of inexpensive, yet high quality, data? *Perspectives on Psychological Science, 6*, 3–5.

Charness, G., Gneezy, U., & Kuhn, M. A. (2012). Experimental methods: Between-subject and within-subject design. *Journal of Economic Behavior and Organization, 81*, 1–8.

Choo, E. K., Benz, M., Zaller, N., Warren, O., Rising, K. L., & McConnell, K. J. (2014). The impact of state medical marijuana legislation on adolescent marijuana use. *Journal of Adolescent Health, 55*, 160–166.

Chrousos, G. P. (2009). Stress and disorders of the stress system. *Nature Reviews Endocrinology, 5*, 374–381.

Cobb, C. L., Meca, A., Xie, D., Schwartz, S. J., & Moise, R. K. (2017). Perceptions of legal status: Associations with psychosocial experiences among undocumented Latino/a immigrants. *Journal of Counseling Psychology, 64*, 167–178.

Cole, D. A., & Maxwell, S. E. (2003). Testing mediational models with longitudinal data: Questions and tips in the use of structural equation modeling. *Journal of Abnormal Psychology, 112*, 558–577.

Corker, K. S., Donnellan, M. B., Kim, S. Y., Schwartz, S. J., & Zamboanga, B. L. (2017). College student samples are not always equivalent: The magnitude of personality differences across colleges and universities. *Journal of Personality, 85*, 123–135.

Cotter, R. B., Burke, J. D., Stouthamer-Loeber, M., & Loeber, R. (2005). Contacting participants for follow-up: How much effort is required to retain participants in longitudinal studies? *Evaluation and Program Planning, 28*, 15–21.

Denzin, N. K., & Lincoln, Y. S. (Eds.). (2018). *The SAGE handbook of qualitative research* (5th ed.). Thousand Oaks, CA: SAGE.

Devos, T., & Heng, L. (2009). Whites are granted the American identity more swiftly than Asians: Disentangling the role of automatic and controlled processes. *Social Psychology, 40*, 192–201.

Field, A., & Gillett, R. (2010). Expert tutorial: How to do a meta-analysis. *British Journal of Mathematical and Statistical Psychology, 63*, 665–694.

Fortin, L., Marcotte, M., Diallo, T., Potvin, P., & Royer, E. (2013). A multidimensional model of school dropout from an 8-year longitudinal study in a general high school population. *European Journal for the Psychology of Education, 28*, 563–583.

Franco, A., Malhotra, N., Simonovits, G., & Zigerell, L. J. (2017). Developing standards for post-hoc weighting in population-based survey experiments. *Journal of Experimental Political Science, 4*, 161–172.

Guo, S., & Fraser, M. W. (2014). *Propensity score analysis: Statistical methods and applications* (2nd ed.). Newbury Park, CA: SAGE.

Hancock, G. R. (2004). Experimental, quasi-experimental, and nonexperimental design and analysis with latent variables. In D. Kaplan (Ed.), *The SAGE handbook of quantitative methodology for the social sciences* (pp. 317–344). Newbury Park, CA: SAGE.

Heckathorn, D. B. (2002). Respondent-driven sampling II: Deriving valid population estimates from chain-referral samples of hidden populations. *Social Problems, 49*, 11–34.

Heckathorn, D. B. (2012). Comment: Snowball versus respondent-driven sampling. *Sociological Methodology, 41*, 355–366.

Henggeler, S. W., Schoenwald, S. J., Borduin, C. M., Rowland, M. L., & Cunningham, P. B. (2009). *Multisystemic Therapy for antisocial behavior in children and adolescents* (2nd ed). New York: Guilford.

Juster, R.-P., Perna, A., Marin, M.-F., Sindi, S., & Lupien, S. J. (2012). Timing is everything: Anticipatory stress dynamics among cortisol and blood pressure reactivity and recovery in healthy adults. *Stress, 15*, 569–577.

Kaplan, D. (Ed.). (2004). *The SAGE handbook of quantitative methodology for the social sciences.* Thousand Oaks, CA: SAGE.

Knight, G. P., Roosa, M. W., & Umaña-Taylor, A. J. (2009). *Studying ethnic minority and economically disadvantaged populations: Methodological challenges and best practices.* Washington, DC: American Psychological Association.

Koerber, A., & McMichael, L. (2008). Qualitative sampling methods: A primer for technical communicators. *Journal of Business and Technical Communication, 22*, 454–473.

LaVange, L. M., Kalsbeek, W. D., Sorlie, P. D., Avilés-Santa, L. M., Kaplan, R. C., Barnhart, J., . . . Elder, J. P. (2010). Sample design and cohort selection in the Hispanic Community Health Study/Study of Latinos. *Annals of Epidemiology, 20*, 642–649.

Little, T. D. (2013). *Longitudinal structural equation modeling.* New York: Guilford.

Lohr, S. L. (2019). *Sampling, design, and analysis* (2nd ed.). Boca Raton, FL: Taylor and Francis.

MacKinnon, D. P. (2008). *Introduction to statistical mediation analysis.* New York: Guilford.

Maxwell, S. E., & Cole, D. A. (2007). Bias in cross-sectional analyses of longitudinal mediation. *Psychological Methods, 12,* 23–44.

Miech, R. A., Johnston, L. A., O'Malley, P. M., Bachman, J. G., Schulenberg, J. E., & Patrick, M. (2019). *Monitoring the Future national survey results on drug use, 1975–2018: Volume I, Secondary school students.* Ann Arbor: Institute for Social Research, The University of Michigan.

Moerbeek, M. (2005). Randomization of clusters versus randomization of persons within clusters: Which is preferable? *The American Statistician, 59,* 173–179.

Montgomery, D. C. (2017). *Design and analysis of experiments* (9th ed.). New York: Wiley.

Morgan, C., Fisher, H., Hutchinson, G., Kirkbride, J., Craig, T. K., Morgan, K., . . . Fearon, P. (2009). Ethnicity, social disadvantage, and psychotic-like experiences in a healthy population based sample. *Acta Psychiatrica Scandinavica, 119,* 226–235.

Muir, J. A., Schwartz, S. J., & Szapocznik, J. (2004). A program of research with Hispanic and African American families: Three decades of intervention development and testing influenced by the changing cultural context of Miami. *Journal of Marital and Family Therapy, 30,* 285–303.

Mychasiuk, R., & Benzies, K. (2012). Facebook: An effective tool for participant retention in longitudinal research. *Child: Care, Health, and Development, 38,* 753–756.

Olatunji, B. O., Davis, M. L., Powers, M. B., & Smits, J. A. J. (2013). Cognitive-behavioral therapy for obsessive-compulsive disorder: A meta-analysis of treatment outcome and moderators. *Journal of Psychiatric Research, 47,* 33–41.

O'Laughlin, K. D., Martin, M. J., & Ferrer, E. (2018). Cross-sectional analysis of longitudinal mediation processes. *Multivariate Behavioral Research, 53,* 375–402.

Ong-Dean, C., Hofstetter, C. H., & Strick, B. R. (2011). Challenges and dilemmas in implementing random assignment in educational research. *American Journal of Evaluation, 32,* 29–49.

Onwuegbuzie A. J., & Leech, N. L. (2007). A call for qualitative power analyses. *Quality and Quantity, 41,* 105–121.

Open Science Collaboration. (2015). Estimating the reproducibility of psychological science. *Science, 349,* Article aac4716.

Pantin, H., Schwartz, S. J., Coatsworth, J. D., Briones, E., & Szapocznik, J. (2007). Familias Unidas: A systemic, parent-centered approach to preventing problem behavior in Hispanic adolescents. In P. H. Tolan, J. Szapocznik, & S. Sambrano (Eds.), *Preventing youth substance abuse: Science-based programs for children and adolescents* (pp. 211–238). Washington, DC: American Psychological Association.

Pearl, J. (1999). Causal inference in statistics: An overview. *Statistics Surveys, 3,* 96–146.

Peterson, R. A., & Merunka, D. R. (2014). Convenience samples of college students and research reproducibility. *Journal of Business Research, 67,* 1035–1041.

Podsakoff, P. M., MacKenzie, S. B., & Podsakoff, N. P. (2012). Sources of method bias in social science research and recommendations on how to control it. *Annual Review of Psychology, 63,* 539–569.

Portes, A., & Rumbaut, R. G. (2014). *Immigrant America: A portrait* (4th ed.). Berkeley: University of California Press.

Pruchno, R. A., Brill, J. E., Shands, Y., Gordon, J. R., Genderson, M. W., Rose, M., & Cartwright, F. (2008). Convenience sampling and caregiving research: How generalizable are the findings? *Gerontologist, 48,* 820–827.

Reichart, C. (2009). Quasi-experimental design. In R. E. Millsap & A. Maydeu-Olivares (Eds.), *The SAGE handbook of quantitative methods in psychology* (pp. 46–71). Newbury Park, CA: SAGE.

Rodriguez, L., Schwartz, S. J., & Whitbourne, S. K. (2010). American identity revisited: The relation between national, ethnic, and personal identity in a multiethnic sample of emerging adults. *Journal of Adolescent Research, 25*, 324–349.

Rolstad, S., Adler, J., & Rydén, A. (2011). Response burden and questionnaire length: Is shorter better? A review and meta-analysis. *Value in Health, 14*, 1101–1108.

Rosensteil, T. (2005). Political polling and the new media culture: A case of more being less. *Public Opinion Quarterly, 69*, 698–715.

Rosenthal, R. (1991). *Meta-analytic procedures for social research* (revised edition). Thousand Oaks, CA: SAGE.

Rounsaville, B. J., Carroll, K. M., & Onken, L. S. (2001). A stage model of behavioral therapies research: Getting started and moving on from Phase I. *Clinical Psychology: Science and Practice, 8*, 133–142.

Rücker, G., Carpenter, J. R., & Schwarzer, G. (2011). Detecting and adjusting for small-study effects in meta-analysis. *Biometrical Journal, 53*, 351–368.

Salas-Wright, C. P., Vaughn, M. G., Clark Goings, T., Oh, S., Marsiglia, F. F., Cohen, M., . . . Schwartz, S. J. (2020b). Disconcerting levels of alcohol use among Venezuelan immigrant adolescents in the United States. *Addictive Behaviors, 104*, Article 106269.

Salas-Wright, C. P., Vaughn, M. G., Cohen, M., & Schwartz, S. J. (2020a). The sequelae of pre-migration hunger among Venezuelan immigrant children in the United States. *American Journal of Preventive Medicine, 58*, 467–469.

Scaramutti, C., Salas-Wright, C. P., Vos, S. R., & Schwartz, S. J. (2019). The mental health impact of Hurricane Maria on Puerto Ricans in Puerto Rico and Florida. *Disaster Medicine and Public Health Preparedness, 13*, 24–27.

Schildkraut, D. J. (2014). Boundaries of American identity: Evolving understandings of "us." *Annual Review of Political Science, 17*, 4.1–4.20.

Schneider, B., Carnoy, M., Kilpatrick, J., Schmidt, W. H., & Shavelson, R. J. (2007). *Estimating causal effects using experimental and observational designs* (report from the Governing Board of the American Educational Research Association Grants Program). Washington, DC: American Educational Research Association.

Schoenwald, S. K., Heiblum, N., Saldaña, L., & Henggeler, S. W. (2008). International implementation of Multisystemic Therapy. *Evaluation and the Health Professions, 31*, 211–225.

Schwartz, S. J. (2016). Turning point for a turning point: Advancing emerging adulthood theory and research. *Emerging Adulthood, 4*, 307–317.

Schwartz, S. J., Meca, A., Ward, C., Szabó, A., Benet–Martínez, V., Lorenzo-Blanco, E. I., . . . Zamboanga, B. L. (2019). Biculturalism dynamics: A daily diary study of bicultural identity and psychosocial functioning. *Journal of Applied Developmental Psychology, 62*, 26–37.

Schwartz, S. J., Salas-Wright, C. P., Pérez-Gómez, A., Mejía-Trujillo, J., Brown, E. C., Montero-Zamora, P., . . . Dickson-Gomez, J. (2018). Cultural stress and psychological symptoms in recent Venezuelan immigrants to the United States and Colombia. *International Journal of Intercultural Relations, 67*, 25–34.

Schwartz, S. J., Unger, J. B., Baezconde-Garbanati, L., Zamboanga, B. L., Córdova, D., Lorenzo-Blanco, E. I., . . . Szapocznik, J. (2016). Testing the parent-adolescent acculturation discrepancy hypothesis: A five-wave longitudinal study. *Journal of Research on Adolescence, 26*, 567–586.

Schwartz, S. J., Unger, J. B., Zamboanga, B. L., Córdova, D., Mason, C. A., Huang, S., . . . Szapocznik, J. (2015). Developmental trajectories of acculturation: Links with family functioning and mental health in recent-immigrant Hispanic adolescents. *Child Development, 86*, 726–748.

Shneyderman, Y., & Schwartz, S. J. (2013). Contextual and intrapersonal predictors of adolescent risky sexual behavior and outcomes. *Health Education and Behavior, 40*, 400–414.

Sireci, S. G., Yang, Y., Harter, J., & Ehrlich, E. J. (2006). Evaluating guidelines for test adaptations: A methodological analysis of translation quality. *Journal of Cross-Cultural Psychology, 37*, 557–567.

Smith, T. B., & Silva, L. (2010). Ethnic identity and personal well-being of people of color: A meta-analysis. *Journal of Counseling Psychology, 58*, 42–60.

Stanley, T. D., & Jarrell, S. B. (1989). Meta-regression analysis: A quantitative method of literature surveys. *Journal of Economic Surveys, 19*, 299–308.

Tabachnick, B. G., & Fidell, L. S. (2007). *Using multivariate statistics.* Boston, MA: Allyn & Bacon.

Thompson, S. K. (2013). *Sampling* (3rd ed.). New York: Wiley.

Torres, K. M. (2017). Puerto Rico, the 51st state: The implications of statehood on culture and language. *Canadian Journal of Latin American and Caribbean Studies, 42*, 165–180.

Trzeskiewski, K. H., Donnellan, M. B., & Lucas, R. E. (Eds.). (2010). *Secondary data analysis: An introduction for psychologists.* Washington, DC: American Psychological Association.

Uphold-Carrier, H., & Utz, R. (2012). Parental divorce among young and adult children: A long-term quantitative analysis of mental health and family solidarity. *Journal of Divorce and Remarriage, 53*, 247–266.

Verhouven, L., & van Leeuwe, J. (2008). Prediction of the development of reading comprehension: A longitudinal study. *Applied Cognitive Psychology, 22*, 407–423.

Vos, S. R., Shrader, C. H., Alvarez, V. C., Meca, A., Unger, J. B., Brown, E. C., . . . Schwartz, S. J. (2021). Cultural stress in the age of mass xenophobia: Perspectives from Latina/o adolescents. *International Journal of Intercultural Relations, 80*, 217–230.

Wejnert, C., & Heckathorn, D. D. (2008). Web-based network sampling: Efficiency and efficacy of respondent-driven sampling for online research. *Sociological Methods and Research, 37*, 105–134.

Wenzel, M., Mummendey, A., & Waldzus, S. (2007). Superordinate identities and intergroup conflict: The ingroup projection model. *European Review of Social Psychology, 18*, 331–372.

3

Key Principles in Ethical Data Analysis and Handling Conflicts of Interest

Chapter Objectives

By the time you finish reading this chapter, you should feel more comfortable with:

- The role of researcher degrees of freedom in research results
- Avoiding questionable research practices
- The concept of statistical power
- Identifying financial and other types of conflicts of interest
- How "publish or perish" can compromise research procedures and results
- Using collaborative relationships to increase one's publication count
- Identifying and avoiding p-hacking and hypothesizing after the results are known
- Using registered reports to specify research questions and hypotheses
- Considering pressures to bring in grant money as potential conflicts of interest

Let's say that we have designed and carried out our study, and now we have our dataset. The rest is easy, right? All we have to do is sit down and analyze the data, and poof—we have our results. Isn't it that easy?

The short, medium-length, and long answers are all the same. *No.*

I teach a course on research ethics, and one of the lectures I give is on ethics in data analyses. Every time I introduce students to the class and tell them that we will discuss ethical issues in data analyses, some of them recoil in shock. What? Ethical issues in analyzing data? Aren't data analyses straightforward? You just run the analyses—what could possibly be unethical about that?

The answer is embedded in John P. A. Ioannidis's (2005) article titled "Why most published research findings are false." Ioannidis reviews a number of factors that contribute to non-replicability of scientific findings. Although many of these factors have to do with study design, such as small samples that do not provide sufficient statistical power, some of the reasons also involve

The Savvy Academic. Seth J. Schwartz, Oxford University Press. © Oxford University Press 2022.
DOI: 10.1093/oso/9780190095918.003.0004

what are sometimes called "researcher degrees of freedom" (Simmons, Nelson, & Simonsohn, 2011). Researcher degrees of freedom refer to decisions made by a given researcher or research group that may be made differently by other researchers or research groups. Often, the decisions are not reported in journal articles; therefore, readers cannot tell why different research groups report different findings for similar research questions.

Weicherts et al. (2016) enumerated 34 different decision points that could represent researcher degrees of freedom. Almost half (15) of these involved data analysis, and several others were methodological but were closely related to the analytic plan (e.g., conducting power analyses, selecting and specifying covariates, specifying the independent and dependent variables). In many cases, researchers go into the analytic plan with the best of intentions, but when the original results do not come out as planned, the researchers adjust the analytic plan in an iterative fashion until a significant result emerges. Worse yet, the final set of analyses is then presented in the journal article as though it were the only set of analyses that was conducted—so that readers are not informed about all the other analytic attempts that did not produce significant results (Ioannidis, 2008).

Some of the blame for this sleight of hand can be attributed to journal editors and reviewers as well as to authors. Many journals have strict word or page limits that preclude detailed reporting of results. Public health and medical journals are known for having extremely short page limits—for example, the *Journal of Adolescent Health* limits authors to 3500 words, the *American Journal of Preventive Medicine* limits authors to 3000 words, and the *American Journal of Epidemiology* limits authors to 3500 words. Social-science (especially psychology) journals are usually more generous, although psychology studies are often more complex and include original data collection (whereas public health studies often use large secondary datasets and medical studies often utilize very straightforward methods).

In my experience at least, reviewers often ask authors to remove what they view as superfluous details from papers that they review. I remember a paper that my colleagues and I submitted to a journal in 2007 or 2008. We were reporting the results of a four-site study of identity and personality, and due to a programming error in the study website, one of the sites had more missing data than the others. We conducted the analyses both with and without this site to ensure that the missing data did not affect the study results. In the manuscript, we reported the results both with and without that site—but one reviewer asked us to remove this "extraneous" information from the paper. As I discuss in Chapters 11, 12, and 13, authors are in a "one down" (subservient) position during the review process—reviewers often must recommend acceptance before the editor will accept the paper for publication—so the best strategy is generally to make the changes that reviewers recommend. So, we removed the information about the programming error and missing data from the paper, and this information does not appear in the published article.

Questionable Research Practices

Let's get back to arguments by Ioannidis (2005, 2008) and others regarding why many published findings may not be reliable. Among the key reasons are lack of statistical power, conflicts of interest, p-hacking (massaging data until they generate a significant result), and presenting exploratory or post hoc results as though they had been hypothesized in advance. This last practice is known as hypothesizing after the results are known (HARKing; Kerr, 1998). Each of these topics is covered immediately below.

Statistical Power

In the Neyman-Pearson approach to statistical tests—that is, the approach that is generally taught in introductory psychology courses (see Table 3.1)— statistical significance is often used as the most important barometer for judging the extent to which research findings are worthy of dissemination and publication (see Anderson, 2020, for a review and critique of this approach). Here, I steer clear of the controversy regarding whether p-values should be used at all (see Kline, 2013, for an extended treatment of this controversy), and I instead focus on how significance testing can be used effectively and in the way it was originally intended.

In the Neyman-Pearson approach to statistical hypothesis testing, there are four key parameters that contribute to determining whether a given effect

Table 3.1 Neyman-Pearson Approach to Hypothesis Testing

Population Truth	Researcher's Decision	
	Retain H_0	Reject H_0
H_0 is true (no effect present)	Correct	Type I error (α)
H_0 is false (effect is present)	Type II error (β)	Correct

Note: H_0 refers to the null hypothesis that there is no relationship or effect in the population.

will emerge as statistically significant (Cohen, 1988). These parameters are the Type I error rate (α), the Type II error rate (β), the observed or expected effect size (*ES*), and the sample size (*N*). Briefly, α represents the likelihood that a true null hypothesis will be incorrectly rejected; β represents the likelihood that a false null hypothesis will be incorrectly retained; *ES* represents the magnitude of the observed finding—generally expressed as the percentage of variability in the dependent variable explained by the finding (for tests of relationships) or as the size of the difference between or among means in standard deviation units (for tests of group differences); and *N* is the number of cases in the sample. (For some multilevel analytic methods, the sample size may be determined by both the number of clusters and the numbers of cases within each cluster; Scherbaum & Ferreter, 2009.)

Statistical power is computed as $1 - \beta$. That is, power represents the likelihood of obtaining a significant finding that will allow us to reject the null hypothesis when it is false. Generally, 80% power is regarded as the gold standard in the social sciences (Kraemer & Blasey, 2015). This power rate means that, if the null hypothesis is false in the population, we will obtain a statistically significant result in our sample 80% of the time.

The first question that popped into my mind when I first heard this statement in a statistics course was "Why not have 100% power? Then we could reject the null hypothesis *every time* it's false!"

The answer to this question involves the difference between statistical significance and practical importance. If our null hypothesis states that the correlation between vehicle speed and likelihood of a crash is zero, *how false* would this null hypothesis need to be for us to advocate for speed limits on highways? If the correlation was .02, meaning that 0.04% of variability in likelihood of a car crash was accounted for by the speed of the vehicle, would we want to set and enforce speed limits—which would require time and effort from police officers and would potentially inconvenience drivers? What if that correlation was .50, meaning that 25% of variability in likelihood of car crashes was accounted for by vehicle speed? Would we be willing to implement speed limits then?

Because *p*-values are a function of both sample size and effect size—that is, we can make any nonzero effect statistically significant if we sample enough cases—having too much power is a waste of resources. Obtaining enough cases just so that minuscule effects reach significance is effectively pointless. Seeking 100% power would lead us to collect so much data that virtually everything would be significant. Because most research requires resources—financial, human, or otherwise—resources must be allocated judiciously. *We do not collect any more data than we absolutely need to.*

Look at it this way: suppose an experimenter were asking adults to read a fictitious newspaper article and to respond to a set of questions afterward. In this scenario, 80 participants are required to reach 80% power, but the experimenter wants 100% power. So you are the 125th participant in this study. Your data are unnecessary and will allow trivial and unimportant effects to be detected as statistically significant.

Is this a good use of your time? Probably not.

There is also a mathematical reason for restricting the desired power to 80% rather than 100%. When we increase the amount of power we are seeking, each of the other quantities—Type I error risk, the effect size that can be detected as statistically significant, and the required sample size—also increase. Raising our desired amount of power beyond what we really need will require us to recruit more cases, increase our risk of incorrectly rejecting a true null hypothesis, and/or prevent us from detecting smaller effects as statistically significant.

So, assuming that we have settled on 80% as our desired level of power, we can conduct a power analysis to determine how many cases we need to recruit. An a priori power analysis—which is the kind we conduct when planning a study—requires us to specify the highest Type I error risk we would be willing to take (this is what α represents, and we usually set α to .05), our desired amount of power, and the effect size that we expect to find in our study. Specifying an effect size can be tricky, especially in emerging literatures where there isn't much prior information to go on. If we are planning a randomized trial in a field where several such trials have already been conducted, we can refer to these previous trials and use the effect sizes that they reported. When it is not clear exactly what effect size to specify, I have a "trick" that I use. I cannot take credit for this technique—I learned it from José when I was writing grants for him (and later writing grants with him). This technique requires us to have a "ballpark" range of sample sizes that we might be able to recruit, so that we can identify the smallest effect size that we want to be able to detect.

Let me provide an example. When my colleagues and I were planning our study of Hurricane Maria survivors in Florida, our first task was to create a draft budget and "cost out" all of the expenses that we knew we would need to include. The National Institutes of Health (NIH) stipulate that a research project grant—often referred to as an R01—can request a maximum of $500,000 in direct project costs per year, and the majority of most research budgets goes toward paying investigator and staff salaries. So we knew that we needed to stay under the budget limit, and the number of participants we could potentially recruit and compensate was clearly not infinite. With a sample size of

500, which was the largest we could afford in our budget and that we could reasonably recruit within the study time frame, we would be able to detect a cross-lagged path coefficient of .19 or greater as statistically significant. So, in this case, we determined the smallest effect size that we would be able to detect by working backward from our largest possible sample size.

Power analyses are fairly easy to conduct—several software programs are available, some of them for free. However, many studies are still underpowered. Button et al. (2013) found that the average post hoc statistical power of human neuroscience studies was 18%, and that the average post hoc power of neuroimaging studies was 8%. Both of these numbers are well below the 80% power recommended by Cohen (1988).

I taught introductory biostatistics in the biomedical PhD program at the University of Miami from 2010 to 2014. When I talked about power analysis, students often raised their hands and indicated that what I was saying didn't apply to them. I would ask why not, and students often responded that they generally used two or three cases in their research. One student in my class told me that she used *one mouse* in her doctoral work, and that she used the left eye as the "treatment eye" and the right eye as the "control eye." My thoughts immediately shifted to how a quantitative methodologist would react to this kind of research (not well, I suspect).

The relationship between statistical power and the other parameters (α, *ES*, *N*) suggests that underpowered studies should not yield any significant findings. Although this is often true, it is not always the case. Significant findings sometimes do emerge from underpowered studies—but these findings often cannot be replicated. This phenomenon is called the "winner's curse" (Button et al., 2013) and is a likely reason why many significant findings cannot be replicated with other samples (Ioannidis, 2005, 2008). Ioannidis notes that studies in the biomedical sciences—and especially those involving animal research—are least likely to replicate, and that small sample sizes and lack of statistical power may be to blame. My student's research with the two mouse eyes may have been a prime example.

Maxwell (2004) illustrated the winner's curse concept by contrasting the power to detect a *specific* effect against the power to detect *at least one* effect from among a series of tests. In a 2-way analysis of variance with two levels of each category, three dependent variables, and 20 cases within each cell, entering a series of dependent variables yields 59% power to detect a single prespecified (hypothesized) effect as statistically significant, but 93% power to detect at least one of the three effects as statistically significant. Similarly, in a multiple regression model with five predictor variables and $N = 100$, we would have 26% power to detect a specific hypothesized predictor as significant, but 84% power to detect at least one of the five predictors as significant.

To avoid p-hacking and HARKing, the scientific method requires that we specify in advance what effects we hope to find and that we test *only* for those effects. We do not "fish" for results—casting a line into a crowd of fish, catching one randomly, and then claiming that the fish we caught was the one we had planned to catch all along. Such an approach is disingenuous because the next person will not likely be able to catch that same fish and will then wonder why they could not replicate our catch. Indeed, the concept of statistical power is *meaningless* when applied outside of the framework for which it was intended. Power refers to the likelihood of detecting an effect that we hypothesized a priori if that effect is indeed present in the population. Power does not refer to the likelihood of "something" coming out significant from a set of analyses that we conduct—or from a set of predictors or outcomes included in a single analysis.

Indeed, Anderson (2020) suggested that multiple testing—conducting more than one analysis to test a single hypothesis, or accepting any significant result, even if it was not specifically hypothesized, as support for one's hypothesis—is largely responsible for the replication crisis and for the misuse of *p*-values. My first statistics instructor taught us a wonderful expression about avoiding multiple testing: *One Hypothesis, One Test*. If multiple tests are to be used to evaluate a single hypothesis, the Type I error risk (α) needs to be lowered to compensate for the multiple testing. This adjustment is necessary because of family-wise error—the inflated Type I error risk that accompanies conducting multiple tests for a single hypothesis. The family-wise Type I error risk (α_{FW}) can be computed as , where t represents the number of tests conducted. For example, with a standard $\alpha = .05$, if we conduct four tests for a single hypothesis, the family-wise Type I error risk is .19. This means that our likelihood of committing a Type I error by rejecting the null hypothesis for any of the four tests is 19%—far higher than the 5% that we specified in advance.

Back to the subject of statistical power: I argue that underpowered studies are unethical. The ethical concept of *beneficence* holds that participants will benefit from, or at least not be harmed by, research studies and procedures (Sims, 2010). Asking someone to participate in a study that is unlikely to produce reproducible results is, in effect, wasting that person's time. Although I am not likely to be "harmed" when my time is wasted, there are surely other things I might prefer to have done with that time. The informed consent form, which specifies that the study's objective is to produce generalizable knowledge, may be viewed as misleading when the study is underpowered and generalizable knowledge is unlikely to be produced.

So am I saying that research studies are useless unless they meet the standards of a formal power analysis? Of course not. Many studies are conducted for reasons other than testing pre-specified hypotheses. When I served on the University of Miami Institutional Review Board from 2008 to 2010, the majority of the studies I reviewed were small pilot projects that were designed to generate effect sizes for power analyses, to identify side effects of new medications, or to solicit feasibility and acceptability ratings for new behavioral interventions. Some agencies within NIH offer intervention development (R34) awards, whose purpose is to create and pilot-test new interventions. There is no expectation that these studies will generate sample sizes large enough to provide 80% statistical power.

The point for which I am advocating here is *truth in advertising*. If your study is exploratory, *say so*. If you did not propose specific hypotheses going into the study, *say so*. Do not "fish" for significant results and then write your introduction as though these results were hypothesized in advance. Last, even if no a priori power analysis was conducted for your study, you can still conduct a post hoc power analysis to determine how much power you had. It is never a bad idea to report post hoc power in a journal article, especially if a priori power analyses were not conducted.

Conflicts of Interest

A conflict of interest (COI) is any influence, whether internal or external, that compromises one's objectivity in conducting research, analyzing data, or reporting results (Brody, 2011). Many of the most prominent COIs are financial—such as among physicians who receive research funding from pharmaceutical companies to evaluate the company's products (Krimsky, 2012). Not surprisingly, financial COIs can bias study results—for example, there is some evidence that studies where one or more authors report COIs may be more likely to report positive results than are studies where no authors report COIs (Friedman & Richter, 2004). Clearly, having a financial incentive to produce significant results can bias researchers' objectivity.

Let me use a prominent example to illustrate this point. A number of years ago, a well-known psychiatric researcher was receiving speaking fees to endorse pharmaceutical companies while he was also conducting NIH-funded clinical trials of these companies' drugs. Clearly, the two activities taken together represent a COI—how can someone objectively evaluate products marketed by a company that is also paying the person to promote their products? When this COI was discovered, the researcher was fired from his university position and the NIH barred him from applying for grants for 3 years.

However, the concept of COI extends well beyond financial interests (see Maj, 2008, for an example). We are all invested in our work—otherwise we would not be doing it—but some researchers are so strongly invested in their research agenda (or in their own personal reputation) that they may be willing to "push the envelope" to see their work published and cited. Perhaps the most prominent such case in psychology is Diederik Stapel, a Dutch social psychologist who fabricated or falsified data for 24 scholarly publications (see Markowitz & Hancock, 2014, for an in-depth review of Stapel's case). Stapel was already a tenured full professor when he began engaging in scientific misconduct, and he stated in his own account (Stapel & Brown, 2014) that "publish or perish" did not figure into his activities. Rather, he noted that "I became impatient, overambitious, reckless. . . . I wanted to go faster and better and higher and smarter, all the time" (p. iii). Stapel's egotism, rather than external pressures, led him to commit multiple egregious incidents of scientific misconduct—to the extent that many of his articles have been formally retracted by the journals in which they had been published.

Where is the COI in Stapel's case? Well, his self-interest took priority over his allegiance to scientific discovery, and, as a result, he misled and deceived his field of study. Although the COI in this case was not financial, the end result was extremely similar to the results of many financial COIs. Research results were distorted or, in some cases, completely made up. I argue that the personality traits associated with research misconduct (Tijdink et al., 2016)— such as Machiavellianism (unemotional detachment from conventional moral standards, tendency to manipulate others, and prioritizing one's own achievements over collaborative success)—represent a form of COI.

Another important form of COI is the publish-or-perish pressures that many universities and departments place on academic researchers. Pressures to publish as many articles as possible can lead to duplicate or piecemeal publication (publishing multiple papers that are very similar to one another; van Dalen & Henkens, 2012), scientific misconduct (intentional or otherwise; Grimes, Bauch, & Ioannidis, 2018), and other questionable research practices. We know that most people make more mistakes when they are rushing to complete a task than when they are able to take their time. The research process is painstakingly slow—planning a study can take months, many longitudinal studies and randomized trials can take years to complete, the process of putting together a publishable manuscript (including incorporating comments from coauthors) can take several months, and the journal review and revision process can take more than a year. So, in many cases, academic output can be slow in coming.

When I was first hired at the University of Miami in 2000, I was told that I needed to publish 30 articles to be promoted to the rank of associate professor, and that I would need 50 published articles to be promoted to the rank of full professor. Those hard-and-fast standards can be easy to achieve for some people and in some fields, and difficult for other people and in other fields. This kind of "bean counting" can be detrimental to science, because not all publications are of the same impact and quality. Publishing in top journals often requires more time and effort than publishing in lower journals, because top journals reject the overwhelming majority of manuscripts submitted for consideration, and only manuscripts reporting the most rigorous and groundbreaking studies have a realistic chance at publication. So, as José used to tell me, one publication in *Science* or *Nature* may be worth 10 publications in more field-specific journals.

Bean counting has unfortunately made its way into our mentoring relationships with our students. When a student approaches me for advice on landing a postdoctoral fellowship or a tenure-track academic position, my first question is usually "How many publications do you have?" I may then ask where those articles are published, but the first question is almost always about the number of publications (both total and first-authored). Further, even though some of my students have published in highly ranked journals, the emphasis is always "More! Publish more!" Like a college football coach who is back on the recruiting trail the week after his team wins the national championship, many of us take only a short time to celebrate a long-awaited acceptance letter before we move on to the next paper.

Publish-or-perish pressures are a form of COI because they often induce desperation—and as the saying goes, desperate people do desperate things. In my former department, assistant and associate professors were reviewed every year for reappointment (and progress toward tenure for those people who are on the tenure track). Each year, at least one or two faculty members would receive the feedback that they were not publishing enough. On one occasion, we reviewed someone who averaged only one or two publications per year—although this person's publications were in outstanding journals and were heavily cited. This person was warned to "pick up the pace" because the publication count was too low. José's advice about major publications being worth more than other publications was not being heeded.

At many major universities—and at most medical schools—faculty are also under great pressure to bring in grants as a way of generating revenue for the university (Lilienfeld, 2017; Lowenstein, Fernandez, & Crane, 2007). In the journal *Social Work Research*, Thyer (2011) titled his guest editorial "Harmful Effects of Federal Research Grants." Among the harms he enumerated were wasted time on grant applications that were not funded, federal research priorities directing departmental hiring practices and the work that faculty members are encouraged (or allowed) to conduct, and the anxiety that faculty members experience regarding needing to secure enough funding to cover their salaries or their students' stipends. Indeed, my colleagues and I have experienced or witnessed all of these detrimental effects of pressures to bring in grant money. I have lain awake at night worrying about how my salary would be covered during the next fiscal year, and I have spent weeks or months on a grant application that was not funded (and therefore I wasted much of that time). Colleagues of mine have switched their entire research portfolios to align with NIH funding priorities—one colleague switched his interests from ethnic identity to brain imaging, and another moved away from his original interests in child maltreatment to focus on developmental neuroscience. In both cases, these people told me that the switches occurred because they needed to bring in grant money, and because many NIH agencies have emphasized neuroscience, genetics, and biomarkers in their funding priorities. As Thyer (2011) observed several years ago, the increasing emphasis on biological processes and outcomes in psychology and other social sciences has served to de-emphasize traditional psychosocial research (see also Schwartz, Lilienfeld, Meca, & Sauvigné, 2016). The shifts in funding agency priorities have important consequences for the future of psychology as a field (Eisenberg, 2014; Lilienfeld, 2017)—and they also may lead researchers to move to fields that they don't know very well, which may compromise the quality of the research.

Publish-or-perish and bring-in-money pressures can also lead to questionable research practices. Van Dalen and Henkens (2012) use the term *salami slicing* (another term for piecemeal publication) to refer to the practice of publishing small pieces of research as separate publications, rather than publishing larger articles with greater impact. In their survey of faculty in management sciences, Bedeian, Taylor, and Miller (2010) found that 86% of respondents knew someone who published the same data in two or more journal articles. Clearly, this kind of piecemeal publication is intended to artificially increase the authors' publication count—without really adding much to the scientific record. A couple of years ago, I reviewed a manuscript for a prominent journal, and the findings struck me as extremely similar to those reported in a previous article in a different journal, ostensibly written by the same author group. I alerted the journal editor about my suspicions and sent him a copy of the previous article. He promptly rejected the manuscript and admonished the authors for attempting to publish results in his journal that had already been published elsewhere.

Publications are also a prerequisite to securing grant funding. Applicants for NIH research project (R01) grants, for example, are required to present preliminary data—which is expected to have been published. Applicants for NIH fellowship (F series) and career development (K series) grants must document a publication record to support their application. Simply stated, NIH reviewers and agencies will not award grants to people who do not have a reliable track record of publication.

Investigators are also expected to publish from the data they collect as part of their funded projects. Indeed, in the NIH review panel on which I was a standing member, applicants were often scored less favorably if they did not publish enough off their current or prior grants. In my experience, most of the articles published off a grant come at the end of the project period or after the project has ended—for many types of projects, such as longitudinal cohort studies and randomized clinical trials, it is difficult (and sometimes unethical) to publish the data before the study is completed. For most randomized trials, except for planned interim analyses (which are generally conducted by people not affiliated with the trial), investigators are not supposed to look at efficacy or effectiveness data before the trial is finished (Schulz & Grimes, 2005). So, in many cases, investigators may have active grants that have generated few or no publications.

In some cases, funders will expect—or investigators will perceive that funders expect—positive results from a current project in order to secure funding for future projects. Many years ago, I worked with a researcher who was funded by a major government agency. He sat with me to review the data for his current trial (which I was helping to manage), and he instructed me to delete cases that were "performing at chance levels." In other words, he was seeking to ensure that the data would support his hypothesis. I later learned that he had had a conversation with the funding agency, and that they were interested in awarding him another grant provided that the results of the current project were favorable.

In my opinion, all of these scenarios represent COIs. The primary mission of science—to objectively test hypotheses and to advance knowledge—is compromised whenever outside influences prompt scientists to engage in unethical or questionable practices. I certainly recognize that some of the pressures I've described here are endemic to academia and are not going away anytime soon. Following the Great Recession of 2008–2009, many state legislatures slashed their higher education budgets, prompting universities to place greater demands on faculty to bring in grant money to make up some of the shortfall (Barr & Turner, 2013). One university I know of closed programs and departments that were not generating grant money and warned the surviving programs and departments that they needed to increase their grant submission activity. Several years ago, when I was serving on my university's Medical School Appointment, Promotion, and Tenure Review Committee, I was assigned to review a faculty member who was in the final year of her tenure clock. She would either receive tenure or be asked to leave the university. This faculty member had experienced some health challenges, and her department chair was asking for an additional year for her to publish more articles and improve her curriculum vitae. This person had been at the university for several years and had averaged fewer than two publications per year. The additional year (which was not granted by the university) would have forced her to publish quickly—and as I noted above, the publication process is extremely slow. Asking her to suddenly come up with five or six publications in 1 year would have been unreasonable and might have pressured her to engage in questionable research practices. (This possibility was part of the university's rationale for denying the request for an additional year.)

I would be remiss if I did not mention the new metrics that have been introduced to evaluate the quality of people's publications. Among these are the journal impact factor (Garfield, 1999; *PLOS Medicine*, 2006) and the h-index (Bornmann & Daniel, 2007). The impact factor is a property of journals and is calculated by dividing the total number of citations of a journal in a given year by the number of articles published in that journal during that same year. For example, a journal that published 150 articles in a year, but that received 300 citations in that year, would have an impact factor of 2. You can usually find a journal's impact factor on the journal's website. Be mindful that some journals don't have an impact factor.

A major weakness of the impact factor is that it is field-specific (Althouse, West, Bergstrom, & Bergstrom, 2009). For example, within the behavioral sciences, *American Psychologist*, the flagship journal of the American Psychological Association, had a 2018 impact factor of 4.9. In contrast, the top medical journals—the *Journal of the American Medical Association* and the *New England Journal of Medicine*—had 2018 impact factors of 51 and 70, respectively. Surely top medical journals are more prestigious than top psychological journals—but likely not 10 to 15 times more prestigious. The top medical journals are read and cited by authors in fields as diverse as public health, cardiology, genetics, neuroscience, and hematology. In contrast, the top psychological journals are cited primarily by psychologists. So the number of citations—the numerator in the impact factor formula—is much larger for top medical journals than for top psychological journals.

Impact factors can also vary wildly over time. When I published my first article in the *American Psychologist* (Schwartz, Unger, Zamboanga, & Szapocznik, 2010), the journal's impact factor was above 7. It has since decreased to below 5. Therefore, an author publishing in this journal in 2021 will receive fewer "prestige points" when requesting promotion or tenure than I received when I went up for tenure in 2011. Furthermore, because I was a behavioral scientist working in a medical school, the promotion and tenure committee was probably far less impressed with the *American Psychologist* impact factor than they would have been with the impact factor of the *Journal of the American Medical Association*, which publishes primarily medical articles. Finally, the impact factor is a property of the journal for a specific year. It cannot fairly be used to evaluate authors or individual articles—because the index is silent regarding which articles in the journal are being cited. A poorly cited article in a top journal and a well-cited article in a mediocre journal will be evaluated solely based on the journals in which they appear. Of course, more rigorous research is more likely to appear in top journals, but this is not always the case.

The h-index was developed to measure the impact of scholars themselves. My h-index reflects how well regarded my work is among my peers. If my h-index is 30, that means that 30 of my articles have been cited at least 30 times. Within a given career stage, researchers with higher h-index scores are publishing work that is being cited at a greater rate. You can look up someone's h-index (including your own) on Google Scholar, Scopus, and other search engines.

One key problem with the h-index is that it is biased toward senior researchers. For me to have an h-index of 80, I must have published at least 80 papers, and these papers must have been available in the literature for a long enough period of time to be cited 80 times. According to Google Scholar, as of December 2019, my 2001 article in *Identity* had been cited 833 times, and my 2010 article in the *American Psychologist* had been cited 1,676 times. Does this mean that the 2010 article was twice as popular as the 2001 article? My answer would be "not really," because the 2001 article had been in the literature for twice as long. Similarly, an assistant professor with an h-index of 15 cannot be compared to a full professor with an h-index of 80. Such a comparison would be akin to saying that a 35-year-old professional basketball player who has been in the league for 15 years has had a better career than a 17-year-old high school player.

Although the impact factor and the h-index have their flaws, they have been among the key elements used in deciding whether to award tenure and promotion, how to evaluate a grant applicant team, and which candidate to hire for an open position (Browman & Stergiou, 2009). As part of our yearly faculty evaluation in my former department, faculty were asked to list impact factors next to each of their publications. When I served on the promotion and tenure committee at my former university, impact factors and h-index values regularly came up in discussions about candidates. When he was considering whether to put me up for tenure in 2009, José implored me to publish in higher-impact journals. It wasn't until the 2010 *American Psychologist* article came out that he was convinced I was ready to be evaluated for tenure.

Short of retiring or leaving academia, I do not imagine a scenario where faculty can exempt themselves from the publish-or-perish and bring-in-money pressures that can represent conflicts of interest in science. Rather, we must learn to manage these pressures without resorting to questionable practices. Some of the ways in which I have done this in my career are maintaining a large collaborative network, adopting an assembly-line approach, and partnering with younger colleagues (or with older colleagues earlier in my career). I briefly review each of these strategies here.

Maintaining a Large Collaborative Network

When I was a boy, my father, who was a costume jeweler, maintained what was once known as a Rolodex—a circular binder full of index cards, each of which displayed the name and phone number of a sales contact. My father was extremely proud of his Rolodex and all of the contact information that it contained. Once I started my academic career, my father's advice to me was to always keep expanding my Rolodex. That is, keep adding colleagues to my network and not subtract anyone from my network.

I have taken that advice seriously throughout my career, and I maintain a virtual Rolodex (now a Microsoft Outlook contact list) of colleagues around the world. In my career I have published with hundreds of people, and I have done my best to maintain these collaborative relationships. On only a few occasions have I lost people from my network—usually because they retire, leave academia, or shift their research interests. Falling-outs or conflicts have been rare in my career; I've learned that academia is a very small world. For example, in April 2019, I was visiting some colleagues in New Zealand, more than halfway around the world. During that trip, I was introduced to someone who turned out to be close friends with one of my closest colleagues in the United States. So, I travel to the other side of the world and I still cannot get away from the smallness of the academic world.

Many of my colleagues invite me to collaborate on their papers, and I invite them to collaborate on mine. Even in years when I was extremely busy writing grants, running a PhD program, and now editing an academic journal, I was still able to publish with my colleagues by providing detailed feedback on their papers. In 2019, for example, I published 17 journal articles, and only two of them were first-authored. The pressure on me to "publish or perish" is virtually nonexistent because of the large network that I maintain.

So how did I assemble this network? Early in my career, I stayed in touch with my graduate school classmates, I attended many academic conferences, and I presented as many talks and posters as I could. I also followed Dick Dunham's advice and collected as much data as I could while I was in graduate school—and as I included more and more people within my network, I would invite them to collaborate with me on papers based on the data I had collected. In November 2003, I presented a poster on identity at the inaugural meeting of the Society for the Study of Emerging Adulthood. I knew that I wanted to invite both Jim Côté from the University of Western Ontario and Jeff Arnett from the University of Maryland to coauthor an article with me based on the poster. As each of them walked by the poster, I asked them whether they wanted to coauthor, and each of them agreed. I then started working on the paper almost immediately and sent them drafts within a month after the conference. The result of that collaboration was an article that has now been cited nearly 1,000 times (Schwartz, Côté, & Arnett, 2005).

After publishing a number of articles with me, my collaborators naturally began to reach out to one another (often independently of me) and start projects together. Sometimes I would be invited to join in on those projects, and these collaborative endeavors have served as a constant source of publications. I always smile when I see an article come out with several of my collaborators as authors, even if my name isn't included in the authorship.

Adopting an Assembly-Line Approach

A common complaint I have heard from early-career colleagues is that the excitement of an acceptance letter is followed by a long lag until the next manuscript is submitted. Working on one paper at a time will, by definition, lead to a very slow publication rate. Although many graduate students are first learning to publish and may have a difficult time working on multiple papers at once, doing so is an invaluable skill in academia.

Imagine a juggler throwing one ball up in the air, waiting for it to come down, and then throwing it back up again. Would that be challenging to do or exciting to watch? Probably not. The juggler would have nothing to do while the ball was in the air, and the process would not be terribly efficient.

Now imagine that same juggler managing five balls at once. Four are in the air while the juggler catches the fifth one and quickly throws it back up into the air. The juggler must have quick reflexes, because the next ball is coming down quickly.

This juggling analogy is extremely similar to how I approach working on publications, and how I manage to publish between 15 and 25 articles per year. I am actively writing or editing one paper while my coauthors are working on the others. Emails are constantly coming in with drafts for me to edit, and I edit them one at a time and send them back to the lead author. As I am able, I work on my own first-authored papers and send them to my coauthors to review and edit.

My usual practice is to have at least one first-authored or coauthored manuscript in each of the stages of preparation, review, and revision—one paper in the conceptualization and analysis phase, one in the writing and editing phase, one under review, and one under revision. Of course, this doesn't mean that I personally am doing all of these things at once—rather, it means that I am involved in at least one paper (as lead author or as coauthor) in each of these phases. Doing so maximizes the likelihood that I will maintain a steady flow of publications.

One important point on unreasonable ambition as a conflict of interest: not every paper has to be groundbreaking. Every successful academic writer will publish some "smaller" articles. Expecting every article to be a field-changer is like a basketball player expecting to score 50 points every game. This kind of unreasonable ambition was the crux of Diederik Stapel's undoing, as he noted in his book detailing the scientific misconduct in which he engaged. It is just fine to publish some articles that represent smaller advances, and others that represent larger advances.

It is also difficult to anticipate which papers will garner the greatest readership. One of my most widely read articles on ResearchGate is one that was rejected by three general psychology journals before being accepted by a more highly specialized journal. The article proposes a theory of the role of personal and cultural identity in terrorism and terrorist ideologies (Schwartz, Dunkel, & Waterman, 2009). I honestly didn't think it would attract a lot of attention, but apparently it has. Conversely, some other articles that I thought would be highly read and cited have not been. So the bottom line is that we must do our best within the context, resources, and limitations in which we find ourselves. Make the most of your situation—for example, I spent the first 4 years of my academic career as José's faculty assistant, so much of my time was dedicated to doing his work rather than my own. However, I strategically found time to do my own work whenever I had finished something for José and he hadn't yet asked me to do anything else. I also took note of the methodological rigor José applied to his own research and started applying it to my own work. Now I have my own mentees who are adopting a similar approach—modeling their working approaches after mine.

One piece of wisdom I have learned both from mentoring and from parenting: you are being watched and copied, even when you don't realize it. Your children and mentees will copy what you do far more than they will listen to what you say. If your children see you littering and treating people badly, they may follow suit. If your mentees see you cutting corners in your work, they may think it's acceptable for them to do so as well. José did me the hugest favor he could possibly have done by modeling exceptional rigor and care in his research. I hope I have done the same for my mentees.

Partnering with Senior and Junior Colleagues

In October 2018, I was invited to present my approach to mentoring at a workshop organized by the National Institute on Alcohol Abuse and Alcoholism. The crux of my approach, I explained, was that senior researchers have a lot data but not a lot of time, whereas junior researchers have a lot of time but not a lot of data. The result is a marriage made in heaven—senior researchers can allow junior researchers to use their data to analyze and write, and the senior researcher becomes a de facto mentor to the junior researcher.

Early in my career, I was the junior person who had a great deal of enthusiasm, but most of the data I had collected was from convenience samples. If I was going to publish in top journals, as José was urging me to do, I needed to have access to longitudinal datasets. So I reached out to some senior researchers I had met at conferences, and I asked whether they would allow me to analyze their data to answer some of my research questions. The answer was generally Yes, and people knew that I follow through and keep my promises. These secondary data analyses I conducted helped me to publish in highly ranked journals, successfully apply for tenure, and receive an R01 award from the NIH.

As my career progressed, younger scholars started reaching out to me and inviting me to collaborate with them. Several European researchers—usually graduate students, postdocs, and beginning assistant professors—have asked me to write with them, and the answer has always been Yes. In many cases they wanted to work with an experienced researcher who was also a native English speaker—and I was happy to oblige. These individuals generally had their own data and had ideas for how to analyze it, but they needed help writing for English-language journals. I viewed such collaborations as a chance for me to "pay forward" what José had taught me.

A second group of individuals have contacted me and asked to use *my* data. These individuals were also generally students, postdocs, or early-career faculty members, but they either did not have an attentive mentor or were working in a different field of study than their mentor was pursuing. One person had recently switched advisors in her graduate program, and her new advisor didn't have access to a dataset with variables that were of interest to her. So her advisor recommended that she reach out to me. A second person had a conflictual relationship with her advisor and was not receiving the support that she needed, so she reached out to José (having read his work) and he referred her to me. A third person didn't have access to the type of data he needed and reached out to me (we knew each other from conferences). As senior colleagues had done for me early in my career, I happily shared my datasets with these people. All of them have become close colleagues. As is noted at the beginning of this subsection, when senior researchers share datasets with early-career colleagues, the result is a win–win situation for everyone involved. Younger people, who are not yet weighed down with administrative responsibilities, can collaborate with senior scholars and receive mentoring in the process. Furthermore, the publish-or-perish pressure on both younger and senior scholars is reduced because publications are being generated from the senior scholar's datasets. (For senior scholars who have active grants, funding agencies are also pleased when the work they are supporting is being published.)

P-Hacking

When we read a journal article, we generally assume that the research process was conducted exactly as described in the article (with some details omitted for brevity, of course). This assumption also applies to the statistical analyses, which readers usually assume were conducted exactly as stated in the results section. If the text in the results section says that a multivariate analysis of variance (MANOVA) was conducted, then we assume that the MANOVA was performed with the categories, dependent variables, and covariates specified in the article. If the text states that the analyses were conducted on a sample of 400 participants, then we assume that the plan for the study was to collect data from 400 cases and stop. Simply put, truth in advertising is a key principle in reporting research results.

P-hacking violates the truth in advertising principle. As Lakens (2015) outlined, p-hacking involves "massaging" data until significant results emerge. Such massaging can include inserting or removing covariates, changing the type of analysis conducted (e.g., analysis of variance versus multiple regression), removing outliers from analysis, collecting more data to increase statistical power and decrease p-values, or stopping a study prematurely as soon as significant results emerge. Simply put, p-hacking involves playing with the data until one sees p-values just under .05 in one's output, and then stopping and pretending that the results one produced through the massaging process were really from the first set of analyses that one conducted.

The p-value is among the most misused statistical concepts. As Kline (2013) noted in his book on reforming significance testing in the behavioral sciences, our obsession with "$p < .05$" often clouds our better judgment in conducting and reporting statistical analyses and results. As taught in introductory statistics classes, there are only two possible decisions we can make regarding a null hypothesis—reject it or retain it. If our p-value is less than or equal to .05, we reject the null hypothesis and conclude that there is an effect to be reported. If our p-value is above .05, we conclude that there is nothing worth reporting.

Compounding this issue are journals' inclinations toward publishing significant effects and against publishing effects that do not reach significance. I once received a rejection letter from a journal that cited the lack of support for our study hypotheses as the primary reason for the rejection. Pautasso (2010) reviewed this "file drawer problem" in various fields, where the published literature is biased toward significant findings and overestimates effect sizes (because nonsignificant effects are generally not published). So, as long as our p-values narrowly scrape below .05, we can publish our results and they are added to the knowledge base in our field. If our p-values are above .05, the study is set aside and forgotten.

When we combine this kind of dichotomous thinking with publish-or-perish pressures in academia and related disciplines, it is no surprise that researchers engage in questionable practices to obtain significant findings (see McShane, Gal, Gelman, Robert, & Tackett, 2019, for an extended discussion). Publications are the currency in academia, and statistical significance is a prerequisite for being able to publish one's findings; therefore, logic suggests that many people will do whatever they must so that they can accumulate publications.

As is true of statistical power, any statistical value is valid to the extent to which its use meets the assumptions on which it is based. One key assumption of p-values is that the "p-curve"—the sampling distribution of p-values—should be fairly smooth (Bruns & Ioannidis, 2016). Instead, as Bruns and Ioannidis report, there is a considerable "bulge" just below .05, meaning that p-values between .04 and .05 are far more common than would be expected given the statistical distribution of p-values. P-hacking distorts the p-curve and undermines the statistical assumptions on which p-values are based.

Head, Holman, Lanfear, Kahn, and Jennions (2015) also note that the p-curve drops off precipitously just above .05—suggesting the presence of publication bias (where findings that don't reach significance are not submitted or accepted for publication), as well as p-hacking, where p-values above .05 are "massaged" so that they drop below .05. So, by being largely unwilling to accept papers that report nonsignificant results, journals are complicit in distorting the use and meaning of p-values—both through the file drawer problem and by inadvertently encouraging p-hacking.

Perhaps the greatest problem with p-hacking is that it reifies the existing data and treats it as truth (Schmidt, 2010). Indeed, the central limit theorem tells us that, if we were to sample infinitely from a population, the sample means would be normally distributed around the population mean. This theorem also states that variability between and among the sample means would be due to *sampling error*—imprecision caused by selecting certain cases, but not other cases, from the population. Indeed, if you were to randomly choose people from your city or town, and then randomly choose another group of people from the same city or town, the characteristics of your two random samples would not be identical. Survey responses, experimental data, and other information would differ across the two samples as well. So neither of your two samples would exactly represent the "truth" about the population from which the samples were drawn. Schmidt (2010) referred to this imprecision as the "lies that data tell."

With this imprecision in mind, *p-hacking is similar to post hoc model modification in structural equation modeling*, where we attempt to improve the model fit indices by adding or deleting parameters after we have initially assessed the fit of the model (Kline, 2012). P-hacking is essentially modifying our statistical model by adding or deleting predictors, covariates, or cases—or changing the type of analysis—and in doing so, it treats the data as the absolute truth that we must fit as perfectly as possible (or must massage until it provides significant results).

So what do we do about this problem? Various solutions have been proposed. Probably the most extreme has been the new editorial policy at *Basic and Applied Social Psychology*, which in 2015 banned reporting of p-values and related significance testing information (including confidence intervals; see Fricker, Burke, Han, & Woodall, 2019). Thompson (2007) suggests reporting effect sizes and their associated confidence intervals along with (or in place of) null hypothesis tests. More than 20 years ago, Harlow, Mulaik, and Steiger (1997) published an edited book called *What If There Were No*

Significance Tests? Later, Kline (2013) titled his book *Beyond Significance Testing: Statistics Reform in the Behavioral Sciences.* These authors have provided a range of suggestions for moving away from sole reliance on $p < .05$ as the criterion by which statistical results are judged as worthy (or not) of publication and addition to the research literature.

My personal practice is as follows—I report a statistical test and a p-value, but I also report an effect size (and a confidence interval for that effect size if one is available). I also report p-values between .05 and .10 as "approaching significance." Although there has been some controversy surrounding reporting findings as "approaching significance" (Daniel, 1998), it is essential to avoid the dichotomous decision-making (reject versus retain the null hypothesis) that leads to p-hacking and to the "bulge" in the p-curve just below .05. When accompanied by a potentially practically important effect size, a marginal p-value can signify an important finding.

How I Avoid P-Hacking in My Work

I avoid p-hacking in my work in several ways. First, by using an assembly-line approach and having enough "irons in the fire" at any one time, I am able to avoid placing so much emphasis on one paper or set of analyses that I need to "bend the rules" to find significance. For example, as part of my NIH Mentored Scientist (K01) award, my colleague Craig Mason and I conducted a series of analyses on two secondary datasets that José and his colleagues had collected. One of Craig's visits to Miami was especially frustrating—we spent 2 days conducting analyses (some hypothesis-driven and some exploratory), but nothing was anywhere close to significance. The data simply weren't behaving as we wanted them to. At the end of the trip, we laughed at our misfortunes. But we still published four other articles from that project. In other words, we didn't pin our hopes on any one set of analyses producing significant findings.

Second, each article that I write tests multiple hypotheses, so that failing to find significant results for one or two of these hypotheses generally doesn't doom the paper. For example, in an article that my colleagues and I published a few years ago (Schwartz et al., 2015), we explored the developmental trajectories of heritage and U.S. cultural practices, values, and identifications among a sample of Hispanic immigrant adolescents. We also examined the predictive effects of these trajectories on outcomes such as self-esteem, prosocial behavior, and family relationships. Because the developmental trajectories of multiple acculturation components had not previously been examined within a recent-immigrant sample, our findings would have been important regardless of how they came out. Further, whether or not the trajectories predicted the outcome variables, these predictive relationships would have shed light on important developmental processes and outcomes among this population. Even a finding that acculturation trajectories didn't predict outcomes still would have been valuable. So there was no need to p-hack the results.

Of course, people conducting experimental studies have more of a stake in the results emerging as statistically significant. No one wants to spend years designing, conducting, and analyzing data from a randomized clinical trial only to find that the intervention did not produce significant changes in the mediating and outcome variables. In these cases, my suggestions would be to use multiple mediating and outcome variables (as specified by the theory of change undergirding the intervention; Rogers, 2008); to carefully document every step and component of the study methods, including intervention delivery and adherence monitoring, to ensure that methodological errors or slippages can be ruled out as explanations for lack of significant findings; and to include, to the extent possible, additional assessment points after the end of the intervention so that "sleeper effects" can be detected (see White, Mun, Pugh, & Morgan, 2007). In this way, we can increase the odds of finding a significant effect—and, if a significant effect does not emerge, we may still be able to publish an article (likely a brief report) on a rigorously controlled study where the intervention did not exert significant effects.

For example, José and his colleagues designed a "one-person" version of their Brief Strategic Family Therapy intervention for adolescent substance use. More or less, the intervention would be delivered to a single family member but would address the family dynamics that are linked with substance use among youth. José and his collaborators conducted a randomized controlled trial comparing the one-person version of the intervention to the version delivered to the entire family (Szapocznik, Kurtines, Foote, Perez-Vidal, & Hervis, 1986). Results indicated no significant differences between the two versions of the intervention. However, the carefully documented methodological rigor of the study reassured the editor and reviewers that the nonsignificant differences were not due to methodological sloppiness or errors. As a result, the results were published as a brief report in a top-ranked clinical psychology journal.

Third, I tend to pursue topics and studies where whatever we find is interesting and potentially important. Of course, because most of my research is etiological rather than clinical or experimental, I am less strongly invested in observing specific results. However, as noted in the previous paragraph, carefully documenting the study methods can vastly decrease the odds that failure to find significant results is due to errors or inconsistencies in executing the study. If we were to find no significant differences in learning outcomes among several instructional approaches, this result would be just as important for teachers and school administrators as would a finding that one method was superior or inferior to the others. Such findings would offer much-needed guidance for educators regarding what types of teaching styles and practices work best for facilitating children's learning.

HARKing

I once worked with a research group who conducted a clinical trial but did not find significant results. They tried conducting the analyses several different ways (i.e., they engaged in p-hacking), but no significant findings emerged. So they conducted a series of fishing expeditions to see whether *anything* would come out significant. They finally created a set of composite variables and found that their intervention changed these composite variables significantly more than the control condition did. They then wrote an article around the composite variables, including organizing the entire introduction around these constructs—which were not the original primary outcome variables.

Kerr (1998) labeled this practice as hypothesizing after the results are known (HARKing). HARKing is akin to driving on a random set of roads, liking the destination, and drawing a map as though this had been the route you had planned to take all along. Simply put, HARKing misinforms the scientific literature—and it also reifies the existing data (cf. Schmidt, 2010, who emphasizes that results from a single sample do not tell us the "truth" about the phenomena we are studying). There is a good chance that the fishing expedition that produced the HARKed results would have generated a different set of findings with a different sample from the same population.

Ioannidis (2005, 2008) identified p-hacking and HARKing as among the primary reasons why so much published scientific research cannot be replicated and may be false. I know I keep repeating myself, but statistical analyses are based on a set of assumptions—a major one of which is that the scientific method has been followed. That is, the researcher's hypotheses need to be formulated before the study is conducted or the data are analyzed. (This principle applies to secondary analyses as well as to original data collection.) When we HARK, we are misusing statistical tools. Imagine trying to use a screwdriver to cut a piece of wood and wondering why it doesn't work—that is what HARKing is like, except that we often don't know that what we are doing is "not working."

Recall what I said in Chapter 2 about point-and-click statistical packages, such as SPSS and SAS. Someone can open a dataset, select analyses from the drop-down menus, and place variable names in the various boxes—and the results will likely be meaningless. HARKing follows the same principle, but to a far lesser and more nuanced degree. Patterns observed in a dataset may be statistically reliable, or they may be based on chance variability that will almost certainly not be present in a new sample gathered from the same population. When we HARK, we cannot be sure which kind of variability we are tapping into.

Classical test theory (see Petrillo, Cano, McLeod, & Coon, 2015, for a brief review) postulates that any observed score is comprised of two components—the true score and error (see Figure 3.1). Because any construct is measured with error or imprecision, the score that we have in our dataset is *not* the "true" value of the corresponding construct for the case in question. Self-report variables are affected by many sources of error, some of which can be minimized through survey design (Dillman, Smyth, & Christian, 2014). Even biological variables are measured with error—cortisol and brain-derived neurotropic factor, for example, fluctuate throughout the day and can be affected by events like menstruation and menopause (Pluchino et al., 2009).

Per the scientific method, when we hypothesize an effect in advance and design our study specifically to investigate that effect, we are most likely to capitalize on true-score variability. When we search for effects that our study was *not* designed to detect, we run a much larger risk of capitalizing on error variability. Imagine aiming a bow and arrow directly toward the target and shooting the arrow at the center of the target. Then imagine closing your eyes and aiming the same bow and arrow without looking at the target. Which method do you think maximizes your chances of hitting the target?

When we HARK, we write the article as though we aimed directly at the target, even if we really just closed our eyes and shot.

At its essence, HARKing is a reproducibility problem. We found an effect that is likely to capitalize on chance variability and that is unlikely to emerge again with a new sample. As an analogy, the rules of billiards (also known as "pool") dictate that players must name the ball that they are seeking to sink and the pocket in which they seek to sink the ball. If I sink a ball that I didn't specify in advance, then I lose my turn. Quite simply, only shots that other players are likely to be able to replicate are counted. "Scratch" shots—where a ball goes into a pocket by chance—do not count because they were not planned. It is not a coincidence that unskilled players are more likely to sink balls through scratch shots and less likely to sink balls through planned shots. In this respect, billiards has a great deal in common with the scientific method.

To continue with the billiards analogy, when we HARK, we sink a ball through a scratch shot—only we don't tell others that we didn't call the shot in advance. Then, when other players try to repeat the shot that we executed by chance, they will likely not be able to do so. The result is a failure to replicate, which is troublesome for science because we do not know which study capitalized on error variability—the original study, the replication attempt, or both (Open Science Collaboration, 2015).

Avoiding Questionable Research Practices

Preventing P-Hacking and HARKing Through Registered Reports

Recently, some scientists (e.g., Nosek & Lakens, 2015) have suggested *pre-registration* as a way of preventing p-hacking and HARKing. Simply put, a preregistered report is like a billiards player calling the ball and the pocket— the researcher specifies the research design, sample size, and exact analytic plan and then executes the specified plan. Any post hoc modifications or deviations are described in the article where the results of the study are reported. The Center for Open Science (https://cos.io/prereg/) provides more information on how to create and submit a preregistered report.

Thus far, the registered report format has been used primarily for replication studies, where the methodology and analytic plan used in the original study serve as guides for the replication. Registered reports have also been used for "adversarial collaborations" (see Matzke et al., 2015), where an adversarial collaboration is a project in which investigators with competing hypotheses or research programs each contribute hypotheses, measures, and procedures (see Kahneman, 2003, for a further description of adversarial collaboration). In a preregistered adversarial collaboration, each investigator or group submits a set of analyses that they would want conducted. In some cases, a neutral third party conducts all of the analyses to ensure objectivity. As Kahneman observed, adversarial collaborations are an empirical alternative to the more traditional "rejoinder" format, where scholars comment on one another's work but empirical data are not brought directly to bear on the dialogue between opposing viewpoints.

Although registered reports have rarely been used for original research, there is no reason why they could not be used for this purpose. A registered report for original research would, in effect, "call the ball and the pocket" before the study was conducted—to assure the scientific community that the work was performed with the highest ethical integrity and that p-hacking and HARKing did not occur. Registered reports would also help to address Ioannidis's (2005, 2008) concerns regarding "researcher degrees of freedom" and statistical machinations (p-hacking) that were, in effect, conducted behind the scenes and not reported in the scientific literature.

Registered reports would also ensure that the scientific method is followed appropriately. Specifically, registering one's hypotheses and analyses in advance would eliminate the possibility of HARKing, where the researchers develop hypotheses to accompany a set of analyses they have conducted. With covariates, sample size, and independent and dependent variables specified in advance, there is no "wiggle room" to deviate from the "ball and pocket" that have been declared ahead of time.

Of course, investigators are always free to conduct post hoc or exploratory analyses to investigate significant (or nonsignificant) findings, or to look for other potential stories if the original analyses do not produce significant results. However, following the truth-in-advertising principle (which underlies the registered report concept), exploratory and post hoc analyses should be declared as such. There is nothing wrong with conducting additional analyses to identify the effects of an intervention or associations among a set of variables, but the authors should be clear that additional work is necessary to examine these findings more definitively. Following classical test theory, it is essential to design a new study whose explicit purpose is to investigate the phenomena that were "discovered by chance." Chance findings that capitalize on error variance are unlikely to replicate—so designating them as exploratory will help inform the scientific community about which findings may be most likely to replicate and which findings may more likely be due to chance.

Being transparent involves some sacrifices and scientific humility. Findings that were not hypothesized in advance and that emerged through exploratory analyses may not be seriously considered for publication in top journals. It may therefore be necessary to have multiple publications underway at any one time to maximize the likelihood that at least some of them will produce results that can be published in the most highly ranked journals.

Scientific humility on the part of authors must be accompanied by similar humility on the part of journals' reviewers and editors. Penalizing authors for not having their results come out exactly as they expected is unfair and unreasonable. Such a policy is akin to parents' punishing their children for telling the truth. If we want to encourage truth-telling, honesty, and humility among authors, then we should not penalize them for complying. Encouraging authors to publish nonsignificant results from well-controlled studies as brief reports would be an extremely positive step among journal editors. The focus on replication (Open Science Collaboration, 2015) must be accompanied by a willingness among journal editors to publish replication studies, as well as a willingness among funding agencies to de-emphasize innovation as a criterion for reviewing applications and selecting projects for funding. By definition, replication studies are not innovative, but they are much needed, given the reproducibility crisis in many scientific fields (Begley & Ioannidis, 2015). As Nosek and Lakens (2015) noted, even failures to replicate are important, because they help us identify potential moderating variables that may contribute to the strength of observed effects. Replication studies are also important in estimating the sample-specificity of results, in keeping with the concept of sampling error from the central limit theorem (Schmidt, 2010). In short, replication—and registered-report studies that replicate prior work— are an essential component of the scientific enterprise.

Addressing Conflicts of Interest in Research

As said repeatedly in this book, it is unreasonable to expect scholars' behavior to change unless the culture of academia changes as well. As a result, this subsection is directed as much at departmental and university administrators, funding agencies, and other "controllers" of academic advancement as it is toward individual scholars. As a parent, I know that my children are most likely to change their behavior if I change the way I relate to them and provide rewards for "appropriate" behavior. A similar principle applies to the individuals who reward (or do not reward) academic work.

As already noted, by definition, COIs occur in any situation that compromises researchers' objectivity or increases the likelihood of unethical behavior. COI disclosure policies have been put in place to address financial COIs (Loewenstein, Sah, & Cain, 2012). Other forms of COI, such as ideological biases toward or against specific types of work, unreasonable ambition, and publish-or-perish and bring-in-money pressures applied by departmental and university administrators, must be addressed separately. Here I propose some ideas for administrators, journal editors, and funding agencies to consider so that the incentive system in academia can be reworked to encourage and reward ethical research and analysis practices. I also propose strategies for researchers to conduct themselves as ethically as possible within the current reward systems in most academic institutions and similarly structured research enterprises.

Recommendations for Departmental and University Administrators

In many medical school departments, and increasingly in "hard money" departments where faculty salaries are guaranteed for most of the year, the focus is on securing grant money. Although administrators in many departments give lip service to being interested in the subject matter and scientific objectives of funded projects, often what they really care about is how much money—especially for indirect costs like staff, equipment, and other operating expenses—the grant is providing. Faculty are effectively viewed as commissioned salespeople who are hired to bring in grant money.

In many medical schools and schools of public health, faculty are also expected to cover some portion of their salaries with grant money. Some departments provide a percentage of "hard salary" for faculty members, whereas other departments provide nothing. Faculty are on their own to secure enough grant funding to cover their salaries, and if they are unable to do so, they will likely lose a portion of their salary. Medical school and public health salaries are often higher than those in hard money departments, but the increased pay comes at a cost. When I was in a medical school, my colleagues and I were constantly submitting grant applications to make sure that our salaries and those of our team members and students were covered. A friend of mine in my former department likes to say that we were "on a treadmill," and that we often felt guilty when we were doing anything other than working on a grant application.

When I was in graduate school, many of the faculty members I worked with did not write grants. Their salaries were covered from September to May, and they had the summer to do as they pleased (although they were not paid for the summer). Faculty who did have grants or who taught classes during the summer were paid "summer salary," but otherwise there were no pressures to bring in grant money.

As Barr and Turner (2013) noted, the Great Recession of 2008–2009 changed all of that. University administrators had their budgets slashed by state legislatures, and private universities lost some of their donors. Faculty members were asked to write grants to make up the shortfall. A few years ago, when I was co-editing a handbook, I asked a colleague to contribute a chapter. She reluctantly declined, saying that "although I would love to write beautiful chapters for books like yours, my university is pushing me to write grants." Candidates for positions in hard-money departments are routinely asked about their grant funding portfolio and about what grants they plan to write in the near future.

As long as faculty members are beholden to funding agencies to support their livelihood, the incentive to "cut corners" or otherwise gain unfair advantages persists. Grant funding is extremely competitive, and review committees are very difficult to please. I have reviewed grants for NIH since 2009—and I served on a standing NIH review committee for 4 years—and no more than 10% of the grants we reviewed had a realistic chance of being funded. Further, even receiving a good score from a review committee is not a guarantee of receiving a grant. The funding agency must then consider the application in light of their research priorities, and at times, even grants with excellent scores are not selected for funding.

So what does any of this have to with writing for publication?

The answer is *everything*.

Review committees evaluate applicants based, in part, on their publication record in the subject area of the application, and preliminary data—often in the form of published articles by the research team—are viewed favorably. So scholars must publish if they want to apply successfully for grants (and if they want to keep their jobs—I discuss publish-or-perish pressures later in this subsection). The impact factors and prestige of the journals in which applicants have published often serve as criteria for receiving a good score from a grant review committee. So all of the pressures described earlier in this chapter—obtaining significant results and having the majority of one's hypotheses supported—are part of competing successfully for grants.

In short, p-hacking and HARKing are often rewarded in the form of grants. If publishing often and in the best journals is a prerequisite for receiving grant funding, and if obtaining significant results is a prerequisite for publishing in top journals, then are we not encouraging people to massage their data to ensure that their hypotheses are supported?

Is this the kind of reward system that creates the problems that Ioannidis (2005, 2008) and others have cited as contributing to the replication crisis in psychology and other sciences? Thyer (2011) seemed to think so, and I am inclined to agree.

There is yet another problem that universities' reliance on funding agencies has created. The NIH has appointed neuroscientists and geneticists to the directorships of many of the NIH institutes that have traditionally funded behavioral and psychosocial research—such as the National Institute of Child Health and Human Development, the National Institute of Mental Health (NIMH), the National Institute on Drug Abuse, and the National Institute on Alcohol Abuse and Alcoholism. As a consequence, the funding priorities within these institutes have shifted away from traditional psychological research and toward biomedical research (see Schwartz, Lilienfeld, Meca, & Sauvigné, 2016, for an extended discussion). Schwartz et al. reviewed 3 years of psychology department hiring practices and found that neuroscientists are in high demand—in 2013, half of all tenure-track job advertisements published in the *Monitor of the American Psychological Association* required or preferred neuroscience expertise. In an editorial for the Association for Psychological Science, Eisenberg (2014) explicitly tied these hiring practices to funding agency priorities and cautioned that we may be becoming too narrowly focused and are in danger of not providing students (and other constituents, such as counselors and educators) with the information that they need.

Consider this example: I have a colleague who is a cultural identity researcher in a psychology department at a public university. The majority of the faculty her developmental psychology program has hired over the past several years have been neuroscientists—but the graduate students who come into the program want to work with her! They are far less interested in brain imaging and other neuroscience-related work.

The point here is not that neuroscience research is not valuable. Of course it is. The point is that, when departmental and university administrators attach themselves to funding agencies and indirect costs as a way of supporting their operations, a conflict of interest arises. Faculty may be pressured to conduct research in areas that don't especially interest them because "that's where the money is," and they may be pressured to publish groundbreaking findings as often as possible. Although everyone wants to publish groundbreaking findings, expecting everything you publish to be revolutionary simply isn't reasonable. Sometimes the data don't behave as we would like them to behave—and although no one dataset can tell us what is true, I can say with certainty that manipulating the data (or the analyses) to get the story we want will very likely produce results that are *not* true.

A word to administrators: placing immense pressure on faculty members to publish or perish and to submit one grant application after another is not a great way to incentivize ethical research and data analytic procedures. We need to see the forest first and the trees second. If we want our universities' reputations to be enhanced by solid, rigorous, and honest work, we need to incentivize that kind of work directly. Take some of the pressure off faculty members and you will see their best work. (Notice I didn't say to take *all* the pressure off—some people work well under pressure—but the kind of pressure that many academics face is not healthy for anyone and actually rewards unethical behavior in some cases.)

Recommendations for Journal Editors

My colleague Byron Zamboanga and I (Schwartz & Zamboanga, 2009) published an article more than 10 years ago where we provided some recommendations for how journal editors should conduct themselves. Here, I will add a few items to that list that are directly related to encouraging honest and transparent research and data analytic practices. (I am now a journal editor myself, so I am practicing what I preach.) First, it is important for journals to seriously consider and to publish carefully conducted replication studies—including preregistered reports. I once had a paper rejected from a prominent journal despite positive and enthusiastic reviews. The editor stated in his letter that our paper did not make a strong enough contribution to warrant publication in that journal. In my estimation, this criterion should be loosened considerably to accommodate studies that replicate (or fail to replicate) prior work. Just as I would recommend to funding agencies that innovation should be de-emphasized as a criterion for reviewing grant applications, I would similarly recommend that the "it doesn't advance the field enough" criterion should be de-emphasized as a reason for rejecting journal manuscripts. Stating that a study does or does not advance the field considerably carries the assumption that the field's current foundation is solid and secure—an assumption that the current replication crisis in psychology and other sciences is leading us to question. A study that solidifies a field's current knowledge base is at least as important as one that represents a considerable step forward from what is currently known. As Ioannidis (2005) noted in his article explaining why most published findings are false, studies in "hot" fields (where there is a great deal of competition to create major breakthroughs) may be especially likely to involve questionable research practices. Instead of expecting authors to submit the most *revolutionary* papers, it may be a better idea to encourage authors to submit the most *solid* papers.

Further, the tendency for journals to accept articles with significant results, and to reject those with null results, leads us to overestimate the effect sizes within a given field of study (Ioannidis, 2008). The math here is simple: if we have a set of six numbers—say 1, 3, 5, 7, 9, and 11—but we decide to count only the three largest numbers and take the average of those, then our computed average (9.0) will be far greater than the true average among the set of numbers (6.0). In this case, the three largest numbers can represent the effect sizes that were large enough to reach significance and warrant publication, whereas the three smallest numbers represent effect sizes that were too small to reach significance and that were not published.

A key assumption that editors and reviewers make when they choose to consider and accept papers with significant effects, but not papers with nonsignificant effects, is that the studies that produced nonsignificant effects may have included flaws that prevented the findings from reaching significance, but that the studies reporting significant results did not include flaws that may have distorted the effects reported. In other words, the assumption is that nonsignificant findings are a warning that something may have gone wrong with the study to prevent significant results from emerging, but such caution is not necessary for significant findings. (Ironically, Ioannidis, 2005, 2008, reached almost the opposite conclusion.)

I recommend that, for all studies reporting statistical tests, authors be required to provide a "methodological rigor" section detailing how the study procedures were implemented as identically as possible across participants, how the study measures were selected and administered in the most rigorous way possible, and how the analyses were conducted specifically to test the study hypotheses. (Even for journals that do not require this information, I suggest that authors provide as much such information as possible.) Especially given that most journals are now published online and printing costs have been vastly reduced, the emphasis on word and page limits should be relaxed to allow for replicability information to be provided.

For qualitative studies, the primary problem is subjectivity (Bott, 2010). Although the researcher's personal position is important in qualitative studies and analyses, analytic rigor remains a priority. "Cherry-picking" cases or quotes to fit one's preexisting theoretical perspective or hypotheses is akin to HARKing in quantitative research. Just as authors of quantitative papers need to convince reviewers and editors that their work is sufficiently rigorous, so do authors of qualitative papers. Where possible, coders should be blind to the study hypotheses so that they do not inadvertently code in a way that supports the hypotheses. In cases where study authors are among the coders and cannot be blind to the hypotheses, the coding process should be conducted with, and described in, exquisite detail so that the roles of bias and subjectivity are reduced as much as possible (Syed & Nelson, 2015). It is essential that editors allot space for such descriptions, and that reviewers are counseled not to ask authors to remove information about methodological and analytic rigor.

Recommendations for Funding Agencies

Having served as an NIH reviewer for more than 10 years, and having held seven NIH grants as principal investigator, I have a fairly good idea of how the world's largest funding agency operates. Other U.S. federal agencies, such as the National Science Foundation, the Institute for Education Sciences, the National Institute of Justice, and the Department of Defense, deviate from the NIH model to varying extents, but the process is fairly similar across agencies.

(Private foundations are different—they are not taxpayer-funded and are far more idiosyncratic in the ways they operate.)

Within most federal funding agencies, applicants must deal with two sets of preferences—(1) reviewers' own interests and opinions and (2) the agency's own priorities. Whereas the journal review process places the editor in the role of arbiter and decider and the reviewers in the role of advisors, grant review committees are not similarly accountable to an arbiter. With some limitations (e.g., reviewers are not allowed to include budgetary concerns in their review scores), reviewers can pretty much say whatever they want, and applicants do not have any recourse. The NIH rarely considers appeals of peer review, and differences of scientific opinion between applicants and reviewers are not considered to be grounds for appeal. Even if a reviewer misreads your application, and even if you can document that the error was the reviewer's and not yours, the odds of a successful appeal are extremely low.

Reviewers' biases sometimes make it into their reviews. Two examples stand out in my mind from my own experiences as a reviewer. On one occasion, a reviewer criticized an application for proposing an attention-control condition to account for participants' meeting as a group with a facilitator. Without an attention control, we would be comparing an active group intervention condition to an inert control condition where participants receive no intervention at all—and we would not be able to rule out the possibility that simply meeting with other participants and a facilitator accounts for the gains observed in the intervention condition (see Freedland, Mohr, Davidson, & Schwartz, 2011, for a review). Many studies have successfully used attention-control conditions, including some that my colleagues have conducted. However, this reviewer scored an application poorly because of the attention-control condition. When the application was discussed, I challenged this reviewer, and he adjusted his score somewhat. Had I (or someone else with a similar mindset) not been there to challenge him, his poor score might have prevented that application from receiving serious funding consideration.

The second example occurred several years later and involved a reviewer with a strong bias toward including biomarkers in research studies. On several occasions this reviewer said "psycho-phys, psycho-phys" (psychophysiology) over and over again during the discussion, to the point that I remarked that not every study needs to have a biomarker component. I sent an email to the scientific review officer for that committee about this reviewer's biases, and the reviewer was not invited back to serve on the committee again.

The point is that these kinds of biases occur in almost every review committee. *Everyone* has biases, and if someone else in the room doesn't challenge us when we express them, they may have an effect on the funding decision for the application in question. Although funding agencies have priorities and preferences, an application with a less-than-stellar score will rarely be funded, even if it is perfectly matched with the agency's priorities. The way the NIH review process is constructed dictates that the reviewers will seldom be overruled (as they sometimes are in the journal review process).

My suggestion to the NIH and other agencies would be to urge reviewers to separate their assessment of the *rigor* of a study from how much they *like* or *agree with* the methods proposed. I personally have given excellent scores to applications where I personally disagreed with the theories and methods underlying the application. If the science is solid, give it a good score—and factor out your bias. For such a scenario to occur successfully, someone would have to oversee the reviewers, read their reviews, and make an independent decision on each application (rather than simply averaging reviewer scores and rank-ordering applications, as many NIH agencies do).

For the agencies themselves, the agency director's ideology often leads to the agency's being reorganized so that the director's top priorities receive a disproportionate share of the money that the agency is assigned. For example, NIMH once funded a wide range of psychological research on mental health. However, the appointment of Thomas Insel as director signaled a major change in the agency's priorities. Insel (see Insel & Cuthbert, 2015) has consistently framed mental problems as brain disorders, and he reorganized the agency to focus on the biological underpinnings of psychopathology. Psychological research on mental health was largely excluded from consideration. So, following Insel's appointment as agency director, NIMH addressed only specific aspects of mental health.

In 2018, when my colleagues and I were preparing to submit our proposal to study mental health among Puerto Rican Hurricane Maria survivors in Florida, I mentioned NIMH as a possible agency for the application. One of my colleagues, who has had many years of NIH funding and knows the NIH as well as anyone I know, quickly nixed the idea. She told me that she and her colleagues had discussed a similar proposal (focusing on hurricane survivors still living in Puerto Rico) with project officers at NIMH, and they told her that they would be interested only if she was planning to include neuroscience or biomarker measures in her study. We quickly decided to send the application to a different agency.

Because grant funding is a prerequisite to being able to conduct large-scale research, the NIH directors' ideologies effectively dictate the course of science. In my opinion, this kind of ideology should not dictate which science is able to be conducted and which science is not. If our goal for the study was to gather information on hurricane survivors who had relocated to Florida so that we could then develop interventions to address their experiences and needs, then whether this information is gathered via rigorous self-reports, interviews, brain scans, or blood draws may be immaterial. The NIH's motto—"Turning Discovery into Health"—should take precedence over ideological biases in one direction or another.

Recommendations for Scholars

So what about people doing research? What do we do? My answer is that we simply must do our best. When you take a job, be clear what the expectations are. Will you be expected to cover a portion (or all) of your salary through grants? What are the expectations regarding publications? How heavily are impact factors and h-indices weighted in tenure and promotion decisions? (Note: administrative changes, especially when a new dean or provost is brought in, will change many of the rules by which faculty are evaluated—so whatever is promised to you needs to be in writing before you accept an offer.)

For me, the assembly-line and "expanding my Rolodex" approaches have shielded me from many of the publish-or-perish pressures that my colleagues face. The various research teams of which I am part are productive enough that we are able to publish enough without p-hacking or HARKing. With regard to grants, I have submitted many applications, and I have been fortunate enough to receive seven from the NIH as principal investigator and another (also as principal investigator) from the US–Israel Binational Science Foundation. I have not changed my research portfolio to align with NIH institute priorities—indeed, I have never measured a biomarker—yet I have been continuously funded by the NIH since 2005 and was able to survive in a soft-money position (including some coverage for teaching and administrative work) for more than 20 years before I finally moved into hard money. I have no idea how representative my story and experiences are vis-à-vis the general population of scholars, but I suspect that I am far from the only person who has had success without changing one's professional identity to align with funding agency priorities.

Let me say this—everyone will go through dry spells where grants are not being scored well and manuscripts are being rejected. No one is immune from the ups and downs of academic life. If your institution expects you to bring in grant money, you should lean on your collaborative network to come up with ideas and submit applications. My various NIH grants have involved several different research teams, such that I am often submitting applications with three or four different groups. NIH grants are a numbers game—as a friend of mine at one of the agencies likes to say, the best predictor of getting a grant is submitting applications. The more you submit, the better your chances are of being funded (as long as the grants are solid—I have a colleague who once submitted 20 grants in a year and none came close to being funded).

Some hard-money departments expect faculty to *submit* grant applications on a regular basis, with less expectation that the grants will be awarded. Other hard-money departments, and almost all soft-money departments, expect faculty to bring in grant money (with varying extents of penalties for faculty who do not bring in enough grant money). If you are uncomfortable with the expectations placed on you regarding grant funding, you may wish to consider relocating to a different institution with different expectations. However, as the old saying goes, the grass is not always greener on the other side. Your new department may have other expectations—such as an increased teaching load or additional administrative responsibilities.

In terms of writing articles, be as rigorous as you possibly can in explaining your methods and analyses. Many journals allow supplemental material (such as tables and figures) to be placed online if this material would otherwise cause the paper to exceed the journal's word or page limit. Do not omit details that would make your study "look bad"—reviewers will likely ask for this material anyway. In the event that your paper makes it through the review process without some important details being disclosed, readers may email you and ask for the information. As I tell my students, you can never "de-publish" anything—once your article is published, it's out there for everyone to read.

An important consideration for researchers is what to do if they are involved in a study as a coauthor and suspicions of p-hacking, HARKing, or outright fraud occur. That is, the lead author (or whoever is responsible for the analyses) may engage in behaviors that you, as a coauthor, do not want associated with your name. The first step I suggest is to contact that person and express your concerns. If the person is evasive or otherwise unwilling to address your concerns, I would notify the other authors as well as your department chair. If the paper is under review, contact the journal editor and indicate that you would like your name removed from the authorship of the paper. If the paper is already published, notify the journal editor.

We place a great deal of trust in our colleagues when we agree to participate in articles they are leading. Plagiarizing, falsifying, fabricating, HARKing, or p-hacking threatens or destroys that trust. Finding out that your colleague engaged in questionable or fraudulent behavior on a paper you were involved with is probably similar to finding out that your friend has been stealing from you. It's a form of betrayal.

In relation to how authors should handle potential nonfinancial COIs, such as strong ambition or investment in one's own work, my practice is to have a dedicated statistician (or statistically oriented colleague) conduct or review the analyses for papers I am leading. I have enough experience with analyses to be able to conduct and write them up myself, but I prefer to have a second pair of eyes on my input and output to ensure that everything is done correctly. Often, I don't have enough time to conduct the analyses myself—it is a good idea to budget a statistical person on your grants and to delegate the analyses to that person. For papers where I am lead author, I review the analyses and output with that person before writing up the results section. For papers where someone else is lead author, I encourage that person to meet with the study statistician to review the analyses and output.

Having an independent person conduct the analyses (or at least asking that person to review the analyses) helps to avoid COIs where we are overly invested in obtaining positive results. Questionable analytic decisions—such as removing outliers—are made by multiple research team members rather than solely by the person who is most invested in finding significant effects. (Hint: a common practice with outliers is to conduct the analyses both with them and without them to determine their effects on the results; see Stanimirova, Daszykowski, & Walczak, 2007, for an illustration.)

Finally, most questionable research practices are not malicious, and many are not intentional. Most researchers do not set out to falsify or to mislead the scientific record. People who engage in HARKing, p-hacking, or other questionable practices are usually not "bad" people. The pressures of academia and related disciplines are such that some people believe that they must cut corners and bend the rules in order to survive. To some extent, p-hacking and HARKing are as much symptoms of a larger systemic problem as they are personal faults of the individuals engaging in these practices. Although financial conflicts of interest that result in questionable research practices tend to be egregious and clear violations of professional ethics, other types of COIs are far less well understood. I am certainly not saying that people should be excused for engaging in questionable or unethical behavior; rather, I am saying that this behavior must be understood within the context in which it occurs. Understanding that "desperate people do desperate things" is essential in ensuring that *you* don't become desperate enough to engage in these behaviors.

Conclusion

This chapter reviews the principles of ethical data analysis. It discusses the many pitfalls involved in analyzing data—many of which present themselves when one's original analyses do not produce significant results. These pitfalls include p-hacking, HARKing (which usually follows fishing for significant results without strong hypotheses to guide the analyses), and COIs. The chapter describes ways to prevent the type of desperation or unreasonable ambition that increases the likelihood of these practices, as well as "checks" to ensure that COIs do not bias research results. The discussion includes the many pressures that academic scholars experience and suggestions for the systems that apply the pressures. I include some of my own strategies for ensuring that I do not face publish-or-perish situations and for maximizing the odds that my grant submissions (which support my research projects and manuscripts) will be successful.

This chapter also reviews some of the problems with underpowered studies and the ways in which underpowered studies can be unethical. I also emphasize that statistical concepts such as power and p-values carry their intended meanings only when the underlying assumptions are met—such as hypotheses being specified in advance and testing only for these pre-specified effects. In the majority of cases, honesty and transparency are the best policies—it's better to tell readers that you didn't find anything in your primary analyses and that you have shifted to exploratory analyses, rather than reporting exploratory findings as though they had been hypothesized in advance.

The primary point of this chapter is that we, as scientists, are entrusted by the public to engage in rigorous hypothesis generation and testing, and that our primary responsibility is to provide the public with an honest accounting of what we have done and what we have found. Ethical data analysis and reporting are about honesty and truth in advertising. Our ability to replicate prior work is likely to increase when more details from that prior work are made available. Ultimately, ethical scientific practice will contribute to advancing the public interest. Our work is not just about us—it is also about the populations we study and serve.

Summary

- Data analyses may be conducted differently by some research groups than by other research groups. These differences are referred to as "researcher degrees of freedom" and are a major source of replication failures.
- Ensuring adequate statistical power is an essential component of ethical data analysis.
- The "winner's curse" refers to statistically significant findings that emerge from underpowered studies and that are unlikely to replicate in other samples.

- P-hacking—which refers to "playing" with data until findings become significant—is unethical and distorts the meaning and interpretation of *p*-values.
- HARKing (hypothesizing after the results are known) is likely to capitalize on chance variability and violates the spirit of the scientific method.
- Conflicts of interest are conditions that compromise researchers' objectivity and that may potentially lead researchers to engage in questionable research practices. Although many conflicts of interest are financial, some personality characteristics—and some university, journal, and funder expectations—can also create conflicts of interest.
- Publications are essential to securing grant funding.
- Researchers should monitor the impact factors of the journals in which they are publishing, as well as their own personal h-index values.
- An "assembly-line" approach to publishing helps to increase one's publication count and to decrease publish-or-perish pressures.
- Truth in advertising is essential when reporting analyses and results.
- Registered reports represent a way to specify hypotheses and analyses prior to conducting a study. Registered reports help one to avoid p-hacking and HARKing.

References

Althouse, B. M., West, J. D., Bergstrom, C. T., & Bergstrom, T. (2009). Differences in impact factor across fields and over time. *Journal of the American Society for Information Science and Technology, 60*, 27–34.

Anderson, S. F. (2020). Misinterpreting p: The discrepancy between p values and the probability the null hypothesis is true, the influence of multiple testing, and implications for the replication crisis. *Psychological Methods, 25*, 596–609.

Barr, A., & Turner, S. E. (2013). Expanding enrollments and contracting state budgets: The effect of the Great Recession on higher education. *Annals of the American Academy of Political and Social Science, 650*, 168–193.

Bedeian, A. G., Taylor, S. G., & Miller, A. N. (2010). Management science on the credibility bubble: Cardinal sins and various misdemeanors. *Academy of Management Learning and Education, 9*, 715–725.

Begley, C. G., & Ioannidis, J. P. A. (2015). Reproducibility in science: Improving the standard for basic and preclinical research. *Circulation Research, 116*, 116–125.

Bornmann, L., & Daniel, H.-D. (2007). What do we know about the h-index? *Journal of the American Society for Information Science and Technology, 58*, 1381–1385.

Bott, E. (2010). Favourites and others: Reflexivity and the shaping of subjectivities and data in qualitative research. *Qualitative Research, 10*, 159–173.

Brody, H. (2011). Clarifying conflict of interest. *American Journal of Bioethics, 11*, 23–28.

Browman, H. I., & Stergiou, K. I. (2009). Factors and indices are one thing, deciding who is scholarly, why they are scholarly, and the relative value of their scholarship is something else entirely. *Ethics in Science and Environmental Politics, 8*, 1–3.

Bruns, S. B., & Ioannidis, J. P. A. (2016). P-curve and p-hacking in observational research. *PLOS One*, *11*, Article e0149144.

Button, K. S., Ioannidis, J. P., Mokrysz, C., Nosek, B. A., Flint, J., Robinson, E. S., & Munafò, M. R. (2013). Power failure: Why small sample size undermines the reliability of neuroscience. *Nature Reviews: Neuroscience, 14*, 365–376.

Cohen, J. (1988). *Statistical power analysis for the behavioral sciences* (2nd ed.). Hillsdale, NJ: Lawrence Erlbaum.

Daniel, L. G. (1998). Statistical significance testing: A historical overview of misuse and misinterpretation with implications for the editorial policies of educational journals. *Research in the Schools, 5*(2), 23–32.

Dillman, D. A., Smyth, J. D., & Christian, L. M. (2014). *Internet, mail, and mixed-mode surveys: The tailored design method* (4th ed.). New York: Wiley.

Eisenberg, N. (2014). Is our focus becoming overly narrow? Retrieved September 7, 2014 from http://www.psychologicalscience.org/index.php/publications/observer/2014/september-14/is-our-focus-becoming-overlynarrow.html

Freedland, K. E., Mohr, D. C., Davidson, K. W., & Schwartz, J. E. (2011). Usual and unusual care: Existing practice control groups in randomized controlled trials of behavioral interventions. *Psychosomatic Medicine, 73*, 323–335.

Fricker, R. D., Jr., Burke, K., Han, X., & Woodall, W. H. (2019). Assessing the statistical analyses used in *Basic and Applied Social Psychology* after their p-value ban. *The American Statistician, 73*, 374–384.

Friedman, L. S., & Richter, E. G. (2004). Relationship between conflicts of interest and research results. *Journal of General Internal Medicine, 19*, 51–56.

Garfield, E. (1999). The impact factor: A brief review. *Canadian Medical Association Journal, 161*, 979–980.

Grimes, D. R., Bauch, C. T., & Ioannidis, J. P. A. (2018). Modelling science trustworthiness under publish or perish pressure. *Royal Society Open Science, 5*, Article 171511.

Harlow, L. L., Mulaik, S. A., & Steiger, J. H. (Eds.). (1997). *What if there were no significance tests?* Philadelphia, PA: Psychology Press.

Head, M. L., Holman, L., Lanfear, R., Kahn, A., & Jennions, M. D. (2015). The extent and consequences of p-hacking in science. *PLOS Biology, 13*, Article e1002106.

Insel, T. R., & Cuthbert, B. N. (2015). Brain disorders? Precisely. *Science, 348*, 499–500.

Ioannidis, J. P. A. (2005). Why most published research findings are false. *PLOS Medicine, 2*, Article e124.

Ioannidis, J. P. A. (2008). Why most discovered true associations are inflated. *Epidemiology, 19*, 640–648.

Kahneman, D. (2003). Experiences of collaborative research. *American Psychologist, 58*, 723–730.

Kerr, N. L. (1998). HARKing: Hypothesizing after the results are known. *Personality and Social Psychology Review, 2*, 196–217.

Kline, R. B. (2012). *Principles and practices of structural equation modeling* (3rd ed.). New York: Guilford.

Kline, R. B. (2013). *Beyond significance testing: Statistics reform in the behavioral sciences* (2nd ed.). New York: Guilford.

Kraemer, H. C., & Blasey, C. (2015). *How many subjects? Statistical power analysis in research.* Newbury Park, CA: SAGE.

Krimsky, S. (2012). Do financial conflicts of interest bias research? An inquiry into the "funding effect" hypothesis. *Science, Technology, and Human Values, 38*, 566–587.

Lakens, D. (2015). What p-hacking really looks like: A comment on Masicampo and LaLande (2012). *Quarterly Journal of Experimental Psychology, 68*, 829–832.

Lilienfeld, S. O. (2017). Psychology's replication crisis and the grant culture: Righting the ship. *Perspectives on Psychological Science, 12,* 660–664.

Loewenstein, G., Sah, S., & Cain, D. M. (2012). The unintended consequences of conflict of interest disclosure. *Journal of the American Medical Association, 307,* 669–670.

Lowenstein, S. R., Fernandez, G., & Crane, L. A. (2007). Medical school faculty discontent: Prevalence and predictors of intent to leave academic careers. *BMC Medical Education, 7,* Article 37.

Maj, M. (2008). Non-financial conflicts of interest in psychiatric research and practice. *British Journal of Psychiatry, 193,* 91–92.

Markowitz, D. M., & Hancock, J. T. (2014). Linguistic traces of a scientific fraud: The case of Diederik Stapel. *PLOS One, 9,* Article e105937.

Matzke, D., Niewenhuis, S., van Rijn, H., Slagter, H. A., van der Molen, M. W., & Wagenmakers, E.-J. (2015). The effect of horizontal eye movements on free recall: A preregistered adversarial collaboration. *Journal of Experimental Psychology: General, 144,* e1–e15.

Maxwell, S. E. (2004). The persistence of underpowered studies in psychological research: Causes, consequences, and remedies. *Psychological Methods, 9,* 147–163.

McShane, B. B., Gal, D., Gelman, A., Robert, C., & Tackett, J. L. (2019). Abandon statistical significance. *The American Statistician, 73,* 235–245.

Nosek, B. A., & Lakens, D. (2015). Registered reports: A method to imcrease the credibility of published results. *Social Psychology, 45,* 137–141.

Pautasso, M. (2010). Worsening file-drawer problem in the abstracts of natural, medical and social science databases. *Scientometrics, 85,* 193–202.

Petrillo, J., Cano, S. J., McLeod, L. D., & Coon, C. D. (2015). Using classical test theory, item response theory, and Rasch measurement theory to evaluate patient-reported outcome measures: A comparison of worked examples. *Value in Health, 18,* 25–34.

PLOS Medicine. (2006). The impact factor game. *PLOS Medicine, 3,* Article e291.

Pluchino, N., Cubeddu, A., Begliuomini, S., Merlini, S., Giannini, A., Bucci, F., . . . Genazzani, A. R. (2009). Daily variation of brain-derived neurotrophic factor and cortisol in women with normal menstrual cycles, undergoing oral contraception and in postmenopause. *Human Reproduction, 24,* 2303–2309.

Rogers. P. J. (2008). Using programme theory to evaluate complicated and complex aspects of interventions. *Evaluation, 14,* 29–48.

Scherbaum, C. A., & Ferreter, J. M. (2009). Estimating statistical power and required sample sizes for organizational research using multilevel modeling. *Organizational Research Methods, 12,* 347–367.

Schmidt, F. (2010). Detecting and correcting the lies that data tell. *Perspectives on Psychological Science, 5,* 233–242.

Schulz, K. F., & Grimes, D. A. (2005). Multiplicity in randomised trials II: Subgroup and interim analyses. *Lancet, 365,* 1657–1661.

Schwartz, S. J., Côté, J. E., & Arnett, J. J. (2005). Identity and agency in emerging adulthood: Two developmental routes in the individualization process. *Youth and Society, 37,* 201–229.

Schwartz, S. J., Dunkel, C. S., & Waterman, A. S. (2009). Terrorism: An identity theory perspective. *Studies in Conflict and Terrorism, 32,* 537–559.

Schwartz, S. J., Lilienfeld, S. O., Meca, A., & Sauvigné, K. C. (2016). The role of neuroscience within psychology: A call for inclusiveness over exclusiveness. *American Psychologist, 71,* 52–70.

Schwartz, S. J., Unger, J. B., Zamboanga, B. L., Córdova, D., Mason, C. A., Huang, S., . . . Szapocznik, J. (2015). Developmental trajectories of acculturation: Links with family functioning and mental health in recent-immigrant Hispanic adolescents. *Child Development, 86,* 726–748.

Schwartz, S. J., Unger, J. B., Zamboanga, B. L., & Szapocznik, J. (2010). Rethinking the concept of acculturation: Implications for theory and research. *American Psychologist, 65*, 237–251.

Schwartz, S. J., & Zamboanga, B. L. (2009). The peer-review and editorial system: Ways to fix something that might be broken. *Perspectives on Psychological Science, 4*, 54–61.

Simmons, J. P., Nelson, L. D., & Simonsohn, U. (2011). False-positive psychology: Undisclosed flexibility in data collection and analysis allows presenting anything as significant. *Psychological Science, 22*, 1359–1366.

Sims, J. M. (2010). A brief review of the *Belmont Report*. *Dimensions of Critical Care Nursing, 29*, 173–174.

Stanimirova, I., Daszykowski, M., & Walczak, B. (2007). Dealing with missing values and outliers in principal component analysis. *Talanta, 72*, 172–178.

Stapel, D., & Brown, N. J. L. (2014). Faking science: A true story of academic fraud. Available at https://errorstatistics.files.wordpress.com/2014/12/fakingscience-20141214.pdf

Syed, M., & Nelson, S. C. (2015). Guidelines for establishing reliability when coding narrative data. *Emerging Adulthood, 3*, 375–387.

Szapocznik, J., Kurtines, W. M., Foote, F., Perez-Vidal, A., & Hervis, O. (1986). Conjoint versus one-person family therapy: Further evidence for the effectiveness of conducting family therapy through one person with drug-abusing adolescents. *Journal of Consulting and Clinical Psychology, 54*, 395–397.

Thompson, B. (2007). Effect sizes, confidence intervals, and confidence intervals for effect sizes. *Psychology in the Schools, 44*, 423–432.

Thyer, B. A. (2011). Harmful effects of federal research grants. *Social Work Research, 35*, 1–7.

Tijdink, J. K., Bouter, L. M., Veldkamp, C. L. S., van de Ven, P. M., Wicherts, J. M., & Smulders, Y. M. (2016). Personality traits are associated with research misbehavior in Dutch scientists: A cross-sectional study. *PLOS One, 11*, Article e0163251.

van Dalen, H. P., & Henkens, K. (2012). Intended and unintended consequences of a publish-or-perish culture: A worldwide survey. *Journal of the American Society for Information Science and Technology, 63*, 1282–1293.

Weicherts, J. M., Veldkamp, C. L. S., Augusteijn, H. E. M., Bakker, M., van Aert, R. C. M., & van Assen, M. A. L. M. (2016). Degrees of freedom in planning, running, analyzing, and reporting psychological studies: A checklist to avoid p-hacking. *Frontiers in Psychology, 7*, Article 1832.

White, H. R., Mun, E. Y., Pugh, L., & Morgan, T. J. (2007). Long-term effects of brief substance use interventions for mandated college students: Sleeper effects of an in-person personal feedback intervention. *Alcoholism: Clinical and Experimental Research, 31*, 1380–1391.

4

Developing an Outline

Chapter Objectives

By the time you finish this chapter, you should be comfortable with:

- Using outlines to keep oneself on message and to avoid distractions
- How to turn one's initial ideas into an outline
- The purpose and structure of each section of an empirical manuscript
- How to outline theoretical, review, and position papers
- Agreeing with your coauthors on an outline

Now that our study has been designed and conducted and we have our results, it's time to write! Some people may find this idea enticing—after all, they have been ready to write for quite a while. Other people, however, may be scared to start writing: *What if I don't write well enough? What if I don't really have enough to say? How do I get started anyway?*

My postdoctoral supervisor taught me the value of creating outlines. An outline allows us to map out what we want to say, and the order in which we want to say it, before we get started. Writing an outline is like creating a map before you set out on a road trip. You know which roads to take, and where to turn or get off the highway. You can even decide on places to stop during your trip. When you create a map like this, the trip is planned and you don't have to worry whether you are going in the correct direction. It has already been mapped out for you.

When I was a graduate student, I had a difficult time writing a complete introductory section. I would start writing ideas, but then I would get stuck. I knew I hadn't said enough, but I didn't know what else to say! I once tried to write an introductory section but I had covered everything within a single paragraph! That can't be possible, can it?

When my postdoctoral supervisor taught me to create outlines, I became a much better writer. I could list the major points I wanted to cover, and then I could write around those. Even though I might still not always finish my

The Savvy Academic. Seth J. Schwartz, Oxford University Press. © Oxford University Press 2022.
DOI: 10.1093/oso/9780190095918.003.0005

thoughts as well as I needed to (more on that in Chapters 6 and 10), I knew I would not miss key points—and I knew that I would not include superfluous information that wasn't needed to understand the study I was setting up.

Headlines and Tangents

Have you ever had a course instructor who always goes off on tangents while lecturing? The person starts out with a thought, stumbles on something interesting, and is suddenly talking about something that has little or nothing to do with the substance of the lecture. A speaker like this is difficult to follow and listen to, because it's not clear what point they are trying to make.

I have reviewed many manuscripts that have this same problem.

A colleague of mine had this same problem when I started working with her several years ago. She knew what she wanted to say, but when I read her drafts, she was here, there, and everywhere. Each sentence was making a different point. Trying to follow her line of logic was like trying to follow a blind snake. First, this way! Then that way! Now another way! My head would wind up spinning before I finished the introduction. Then I started suggesting that she create outlines before she started writing, and her drafts improved dramatically.

Many writers have ideas in their head that they want to cover, but without an outline, they often think of these points randomly—so the writing meanders from one point to the next, and often back to the original point. I have reviewed papers like this, and it is almost impossible to judge the value of the work reported when the line of logic is so difficult to follow. Trying to read a poorly organized paper is like trying to figure out what a puzzle is supposed to look like when the pieces are strewn across the floor. When I edit papers like this, I have to stop and rewrite much of the text so I can understand what the authors are saying.

I've come up with a term for this kind of disorganized writing—*all over the place* (AOTP). As is covered in Chapter 8, first drafts are often AOTP unless an outline is used (and even then there may be some AOTP writing). An outline does, however, prevent tangents from distracting from the points you are trying to make. Points that are not part of your outline generally are not addressed in your paper.

Creating an Outline

In a research report (a manuscript reporting the results of an empirical study), the introduction and discussion are the sections that are most likely to require outlines. The method and results sections are formulaic and are less likely to require outlines—although, for beginning writers, outlining these sections is never a bad idea. Note that you may wish to design your outlines based on the outlines I provide here, and you might even create a blank outline template that you can use for each new paper you are getting ready to write.

So let's start by going over what an outline of an introductory section might look like. But before we outline the introduction, we need to review what the purpose of the introductory section is.

Outlining the Introductory Section

The purpose of the introductory section is to orient the reader toward your study. Nothing more, nothing less. Simply put, the reader needs to understand the populations, constructs, methods (if you are using a new or unfamiliar method), settings, and other key components of your study. For example, a recent paper of mine (Schwartz et al., 2019) reported a daily diary study of biculturalism, and its effects on well-being and internalizing symptoms (anxiety and depression), among Hispanic college students in Miami. For the reader to understand the basis for the study, we needed to review the following:

- The U.S. Hispanic population, including its size and growth rate as well as overrepresentation of young people in this population;
- Miami as a context for Hispanic immigration and the city's diverse Hispanic population;
- Hispanic college attendance rates and the unique cultural needs and traits of Hispanic college students;
- Acculturation and biculturalism; and
- Well-being and internalizing problems.

These bullet points represented subsection headings in our introduction, to ensure that all of our "bases" were covered in introducing the reader to our study. By the time the reader reaches the method section heading, it should be clear what the study will be about, what gap in the literature is being filled, and why filling this gap is important and advances the literature. If the reader is not clear on all of these things by the end of the introduction, then something is missing.

So let's go through my outline for the introductory section of this paper. Most people learn more by doing than they do by passively reading or listening, so I would like you to create your own outline as you read through mine. Note that I use traditional Roman numerals and letters when I create outlines—but you can use whatever format you are most comfortable with.

I. The U.S. Hispanic Population
  A. Size and Growth Rate
  B. Overrepresentation of Adolescents and Young Adults
  C. Concerns regarding Youth are Especially Relevant to Hispanics
II. Miami as a Context for Hispanic Immigration
  A. Original Cuban Migration (1960s and 1970s)
  B. Other Hispanic Groups (Nicaraguans, Colombians, Venezuelans, Argentinians, Peruvians, etc.)
  C. Much of the City's Political and Economic Power is Held by Hispanics
  D. Miami as a Highly Bicultural City
III. Hispanic College Students
  A. Increased Hispanic High School Graduation Rates
  B. Increased College Enrollment
  C. However, Hispanics Lag Behind Whites in Degree Completion
  D. Barriers to Degree Completion among Hispanic Students
    i. Cultural Barriers (e.g., individualistic expectations for a more collectivistic population)
    ii. Dissonant Expectations from Family and from University
    iii. Poor Well-Being
    iv. Internalizing Symptoms (anxiety and depression)
IV. Acculturation and Biculturalism
  A. Acculturation as a Bidimensional Process (U.S. and Heritage Acculturation as Separate Dimensions)
  B. Biculturalism as Endorsement of Both Cultural Systems
  C. Types of Biculturalism
    i. Integrated/Hybridized
    ii. Alternating/Conflicted
    iii. Key Differences Between Types
    iv. Biculturalism as Most Adaptive in Bicultural Contexts
V. Well-Being and Internalizing
  A. Dimensions of Well-Being

    i. Self-Esteem
   ii. Subjective Well-Being/Life Satisfaction
   iii. Psychological Well-Being (mastery, competence)
   iv. Eudaemonic Well-Being (self-discovery, challenging activities)
   v. How Well-Being Promotes Academic and Social Success
  B. Internalizing Symptoms
   i. Anxiety
   ii. Depression
   iii. How Internalizing Symptoms Interfere with Academic and Social Success

Thus, this outline provides me with a structure for my writing. The first-level headings (capital Roman numerals) become first-level headings; the second-level headings (capital letters) become second-level headings or themes; and the third-level headings represent topics that must be discussed within each of the second-level headings. Again, topics not listed in my outline will not appear in the introduction—ensuring that tangents are unlikely to be a problem. I also largely avoid the AOTP problem because I specify what is to be written in each subsection. (As noted, I can still be AOTP within a paragraph, but I will probably not be AOTP within the section as a whole.)

Outlining the Method Section

As noted, the method section generally does not need an outline, but I will take this opportunity to review what the method section generally looks like. In general, for an empirical manuscript, the method section provides the following information:

- Who participated in the study (number of participants, as well as their characteristics);
- How the sample was recruited or otherwise accessed;
- Number of times participants were contacted or provided data;
- What study procedures were carried out, and in what order;
- What interventions or experimental procedures were applied, and whether (and how) participants were randomized to conditions; and
- How each study construct was measured (self-report, interview, experimental task, biomarker assay, etc.)—including reliability and validity information for each measure.

So let's return to the biculturalism daily diary study to which I referred earlier, and outline the method section.

I. Sample
   A. 824 Hispanic college students
      i. 76% female
      ii. Mean age 20.86 years ($SD = 2.80$, range 18–29)
      iii. 34.5% of participants born outside the United States; 45% U.S.-born with both parents born outside the States; 20.5% U.S.-born with one U.S.-born parent
      iv. 41.0% Cuban, 13.2% Colombian, 7.5% Nicaraguan, 7.2% Venezuelan, 6.5% Dominican, 24.6% other nationality
      v. 27.7% freshmen, 14.6% sophomores, 30% juniors, 27.8% seniors
   B. Recruited from psychology courses through a research participation system
   C. Received course credit for their participation
II. Procedures
   A. 12-day diary study
   B. Started on a Thursday, ended on a Monday
   C. Full surveys completed on Days 1 and 12; single items completed on Days 2–11
   D. Completion rates on each study day were between 80% and 90%
III. Measures
   A. Biculturalism
      i. Bicultural blendedness and harmony
      ii. Bicultural hybridizing and blendedness
   B. Well-Being
      i. Self-esteem
      ii. Life satisfaction
      iii. Psychological well-being
      iv. Eudaemonic well-being
   C. Internalizing Symptoms
      i. Anxiety
      ii. Depressive symptoms

Notice that the outline for the method section is extremely brief. This brevity is one reason why the method section does not normally need to be outlined. Method sections are formulaic, in that the same general subsections (sample, procedure, measures) appear in most method sections. Additional subsections, such as those describing interventions, interventionist training, adherence monitoring, and assaying of biological measures, may also appear where applicable.

Outlining the Results Section

Results sections do not have a set structure. Rather, the results section reports descriptive statistics and other essential descriptive information (e.g., bivariate correlations for papers reporting structural equation models), followed by tests of each of the study hypotheses. Results sections also include tables and figures as necessary—in general, a table is used whenever more than four numbers of the same type (e.g., means, correlations, percentages) are reported, and a figure is used in situations where "a picture is worth a thousand words." In some cases, tables and figures can be anticipated and written into an outline, whereas in other cases, the need for a table or figure doesn't become apparent until you are have started drafting the text (or until a coauthor suggests including a table or figure).

Here I provide the outline for the results section from the biculturalism daily diary paper. As I noted, however, the structure of the results section for another paper might deviate somewhat from the results presented here. Results sections from qualitative or mixed-method papers will also look different from those from quantitative papers—quotations will be interspersed within the text, and the results section will present themes in place of (or as well as) statistical analyses.

I. Analytic Plan
   A. Bivariate Correlations to Examine Relationships between the Two Sets of Biculturalism Constructs (Research Question-Hypothesis 1)
   B. Cross-Lagged Panel Modeling to Examine Directionality between Sets of Biculturalism Constructs (Research Question-Hypothesis 2)
   C. Examining Overlap in Daily Fluctuations among Biculturalism Constructs (Research Question-Hypothesis 3)
      i. Computation of fluctuation scores (standard deviation of a series of repeated measurements for the same variable) for Days 2–11
      ii. Correlations among fluctuation scores
   D. Fluctuation Scores Predicting Outcome Variables (Research Question-Hypothesis 4)
      i. Creating latent variables for well-being and for internalizing symptoms at Days 1 and 12

ii. Regressing Day 12 latent outcome variables on biculturalism fluctuation scores, controlling for latent outcome variables on Day 1

II. Bivariate Correlations on Day 1 (for Research Question-Hypothesis 1)
   A. Table Needed
III. Random Intercept Cross-Lagged Panel Models (for Research Question-Hypothesis 2)
   A. Table Needed
IV. Correlations Among Fluctuation Scores (for Research Question-Hypothesis 3)
   A. Table Needed
V. Structural Equation Models (for Research Question-Hypothesis 4)

It is essential to note that the results section can be outlined prior to knowing what the results are—but clearly the results section cannot be written until we know what the findings are. The discussion section, however, cannot be outlined until we know the results.

Outlining the Discussion Section

Discussion sections have several overall goals, and the structure of the discussion section is largely consistent across papers. Broadly, the discussion should accomplish six objectives. First, it is important to restate the purpose of the study. After reading the method and results sections—which are very detail-oriented—the reader may need to be reoriented to the larger "story" underlying the study. Restating the research questions and hypothesis may be helpful as well.

Second, the findings are restated in words. Results sections can sometimes be opaque and difficult to read, so the discussion needs to lay out the findings in plain language. Importantly, the discussion needs not only to restate the findings, but also to interpret what they mean. That is, not only *what* was found, but also *why* the findings came out as they did. In particular, unexpected findings need to be explained.

Let me provide an example. A few years ago, my colleagues and I (Schwartz et al., 2018) conducted a cross-national study of cultural stress and internalizing problems (depressive and anxiety symptoms) among Venezuelan immigrant adults in South Florida and Bogotá, Colombia. The United States generally does not recognize medical and other degrees from many foreign universities (Public Radio International, 2018)—so many Venezuelan doctors, engineers, and scientists have taken jobs as ride-share drivers, restaurant servers, and pizza deliverers in Florida (Newkirk & Crooks, 2017). Further, many Venezuelans have applied for asylum in the United States (U.S. Customs and Immigration Services, 2019), although the outcome of these asylum applications is highly uncertain. The Trump administration attempted to crack down on unauthorized immigration and asylum seeking (Woods & Arthur, 2017). In contrast, Venezuela and Colombia share a common language and culture, and the Colombian government has been largely receptive to Venezuelans seeking safety and security (Baddour, 2019). So we hypothesized that Venezuelan immigrants in the United States would report more discrimination and a worse context of reception compared to Venezuelan immigrants in Colombia.

The results actually supported an opposite conclusion—Venezuelans in Colombia reported more discrimination, and a worse context of reception, compared to those in Florida. Anecdotal evidence from our community partners in the two locations suggested that many Colombians were displeased with the influx of Venezuelans, many of whom were homeless. In contrast, South Florida has been home to a cohort of wealthy Venezuelans since the mid-1990s (Robles & Jordan, 2019), and many Venezuelans in the United States are highly educated. In fact, in our sample, nearly half of the Venezuelans in Florida—compared to 25% in Colombia—had completed college degrees. It is possible that the greater educational attainment within the U.S. sample—in contrast to the largely negative perception of Venezuelans in Colombia (at least among the Colombian public)—accounts for the more favorable reception among Venezuelans in the United States.

Third, a discussion section should state the "verdict" regarding each of the study hypotheses. That is, was each hypothesis fully supported, partially supported, or refuted? Some of the verdicts may be stated when the results are summarized in words, but it should be clear in the discussion how much support each of the study hypotheses received.

Fourth, the findings should be integrated into the literature that was reviewed in the introduction. What contribution does the present study make to the field? Do the present findings affirm, extend, or refute prior work? If the findings are not consistent with prior work, why might that be the case? Might there be methodological or theoretical differences (e.g., different measures, different types of samples, different conceptual approaches) that might explain the divergence in findings? Do we need additional research to resolve the inconsistency between the present study and prior work?

Fifth, discussion sections should list limitations and future directions. No one study can do everything, and every study has shortcomings that can be addressed in future research. So we need to provide a roadmap for future work by listing the ways in which our study was "flawed" (while still remaining positive about our own work) and ways in which these limitations can be overcome in subsequent studies. In Chapters 9 and 10, I provide concrete tips for writing a limitations subsection that eloquently lists shortcomings without undermining the contributions of the study.

Finally, the discussion section ends by stating the "take-home points" from the paper. What should the reader take away from your study? What key messages do you want to communicate? Are there specific implications for future research, for intervention, or for policy that should be stated? The conclusion section is the place to make hard-hitting statements about what your study has contributed and what its practical and applied value might be.

With these components in mind, let's outline the discussion section from the biculturalism daily diary article.

I. Restate Purpose of Study
   A. Examine Overlap among Biculturalism Dimensions
   B. Examine Directionality between Biculturalism Models
   C. Daily Biculturalism Fluctuations as Predictors of Mental Health
II. Summarize Findings
   A. Bicultural Blendedness and Harmony Predict Bicultural Hybridizing
   B. Bicultural Alternation as a Situational Process
   C. Fluctuations in Blendedness Predict Well-Being and Internalizing Symptoms
III. Interpreting Findings
   A. What Is Biculturalism?
      i. Blended and harmonious mixture of heritage and destination cultural systems
      ii. Hybridizing emerges as a consequence of such blending and harmony
      iii. Alternating represents a separate phenomenon and may be situationally determined rather than characterological
   B. Biculturalism as Facilitated by Bicultural Contexts
      i. Unclear whether findings would have been similar in a more monocultural context
      ii. Miami as a unique cultural context (majority-minority and much of the political and economic power in the hands of immigrants)

IV. Limitations
    A. Short Time Span (12 Days)
    B. College Sample Cannot be Generalized to Non-College Young Adults
    C. Overrepresentation of Women—Findings May Not be Generalizable to Men
    D. Focus on Process Does Not Speak to Content of Bicultural Identities
V. Conclusion
    A. Take-Home Points
    B. Implications for Counseling
    C. Implications for Higher Education

So we can write the discussion section around this outline.

Outlining Theoretical Articles, Literature Reviews, and Position Papers

As is discussed in Chapter 16, theoretical, review, and position papers are far more difficult to write than empirical articles are. There is no set structure, and we don't have data and empirical results to lean on. The entire paper is "fair game" for criticism from reviewers—and because the whole article is based on our arguments rather than on data—our theoretical and conceptual background needs to be even stronger than it does for an empirical article. As my colleague Al Waterman used to say, "It is very, very hard to publish theory." His statement has been quite true in my experience, though I have been fairly successful in publishing theoretical papers (30 in my career as of November 2020). In my experience, reviewer comments for theoretical, review, and position papers have often been more extensive and more difficult to address compared to reviewer comments for empirical articles.

As a result, for theoretical, review, and position papers, *the entire article needs to be outlined at once*. It is essential to stay as "close" to existing theory and research as possible—you are likely to be penalized for logical leaps or for statements that cannot be readily defended and justified. I suggest starting with a clear problem statement, a review of the gap in the literature that the paper is addressing, and the rationale for the paper. The potential value of the contribution that the paper represents needs to be stated early in the paper, and the contribution should be restated toward the end.

I had a colleague in graduate school who summarized the art of giving conference presentations in one sentence: "Tell them what you're going to tell them, then tell them, and then tell them what you told them." Theoretical, review, and position papers follow much the same principle. At the beginning, you tell readers what your purpose is, then you lay out your arguments, and then at the end of you summarize what your arguments were.

So let's go over the outline for a theoretical paper. We'll use an article that my colleagues and I published in the *American Psychologist* (Schwartz et al., 2010). In that article, we introduced a new model of acculturation that extended and expanded upon John Berry's (1980) classic theorizing on cultural adaptation. Reviewer comments on this paper were quite challenging—one reviewer characterized the paper as a "badly written dissertation literature review"—but fortunately the associate editor liked the paper. (Editors have varying amounts of power in the review process, depending on the style they adopt; see Chapter 12.)

I. Rates of International Migration
II. Purpose of the Paper
    A. Expanding Acculturation Theory
    B. Considering Contexts of Reception
    C. Considering the Role of Ethnicity
    D. Considering Types of Migrants
    E. Reinterpreting the Immigrant Paradox
    F. Introducing a New Model of Acculturation
III. Existing Acculturation Theory
    A. Berry's Four-Category Model
        i. Widely used and applied to many cultural contexts
        ii. Somewhat simplistic
        iii. Not clear which specific cultural domains Berry's model refers to (e.g., practices, values, identifications)
        iv. Assumes that all categories exist and are equally valid
        v. Marginalization category (rejects both heritage and destination cultures) may not be valid
        vi. Multiple types of biculturalism (endorses both heritage and destination cultures) may exist
IV. Rethinking Acculturation Theory and Research
    A. Migrant Type, Ethnicity, and Cultural Similarity
        i. Acculturation may be "easiest" for migrants who are phenotypically similar to the dominant ethnic group in the destination country
        ii. Acculturation may be "easiest" for migrants who already speak one or more of the destination country's languages
        iii. Acculturation may be most difficult for refugees and asylum seekers, many of whom experienced severe trauma in their homelands

    iv. Migrants of color may need to explore how they fit into the destination society's ethnic hierarchy

  B. To Whom Does Acculturation Apply?

    i. May not apply to individuals who migrated as young children *if* they can "pass" as members of the dominant ethnic group

    ii. People who migrate as adults may have difficulty adjusting, or they may settle in ethnic enclaves where they are largely insulated from the destination culture

    iii. Acculturation applies to some second-generation migrants—primarily those from visible-minority groups

    iv. Acculturation applies to later-generation individuals living in ethnic enclaves and bicultural areas—because they must balance multiple cultures

  C. Immigrant Paradox and Measurement of Acculturation

    i. Simplistic, unidimensional measures of acculturation are used in many public health studies

    ii. Bidimensional measures (separating destination-culture acquisition from heritage-culture retention) are needed to examine how acculturation is related to health outcomes

    iii. Biculturalism is often associated with the most favorable outcomes, but the models used in public health studies do not acknowledge biculturalism

  D. Domains of Acculturation

    i. Practices (language use, media, food, friends)

    ii. Values (individualism, collectivism)

    iii. Identifications (ethnic and national identity)

    iv. An Integrative Perspective

V. Context of Reception

  A. Unfavorable Contexts of Reception Create Acculturative Stress

  B. Contexts of Reception as Changing Over Time and Across Locations Within a Country

  C. Context of Reception Interacts with Acculturation to Predict Health Outcomes

VI. Conclusions and Future Directions

I can say with great confidence that I could never have written that article without a detailed outline. We covered so many topics that writing without an outline would have easily led me to be AOTP—and, in fact, one reviewer essentially accused us of being AOTP when they referred to our original submission as a "poorly written dissertation literature review."

In fact, I wrote the outline and shared it with my coauthors before I started drafting the paper. In the next section, I discuss how to use outlines to reach agreement with coauthors on the direction and content that the paper will cover.

Outlines as Agreements Among Coauthors

An outline can also be used as an agreement among coauthors in terms of the structure of the paper or section. That is, you can create an outline, circulate it to your coauthors for feedback, and come to an agreement regarding what will be covered. In this way, the authorship team is deciding in advance what will be covered. Coauthors will have comments and edits, of course, but disagreements regarding the overall structure or mission of the paper or section will (hopefully) be less likely to occur once everyone on the team has settled on an outline.

Chapter 14 covers more about working with coauthors, but for now I will say this: the working style among the writing team should be settled and agreed upon in advance. The strategy I use, which I learned from José, is: First Author Makes the Call. That is, the first author, who is doing the majority of the "heavy lifting" on the paper—drafting each section, integrating coauthors' feedback, and undertaking most of the editing and revising—is the final arbiter regarding the direction of the paper. Coauthors provide input, but the first author reserves the right to incorporate whichever comments seem most germane to the direction and goals for the paper.

Note, however, that the fact that a coauthor has signed off on the outline does not prevent that coauthor from providing comments—or even changing their mind completely once they have seen the fully drafted section or paper—later on. Think of it this way: you might have seen an artist's rendition of your new house, but your thoughts once you walk into the completed structure might be quite different from what you thought when you looked at the illustration. So my guidance here is to *be reasonable*. In most cases, coauthors' goals for the paper are the same as yours—get the paper published so that its impact on the field is as strong as possible—so I suggest viewing their comments with this shared goal in mind.

Therefore, I view outlines as a starting point for the writing process. Sharing an outline with coauthors decreases the likelihood of major disagreements regarding the direction and content of the paper, but sharing the outline does not guarantee that conflicts will not occur. Providing coauthors with the opportunity to provide input early on does, however, engage them more fully in the writing process.

Conclusion

This chapter presents outlines as a way of starting the writing process, organizing your thoughts, and laying out the content of the paper. The introduction and discussion, in particular, should be outlined to ensure that we avoid the AOTP problem. Papers that are poorly organized are extremely difficult to read and to understand.

For beginning writers, it may also be helpful to outline the method and results sections. Although these sections are generally formulaic, an outline can help to ensure that all of the subsections and information are included. As I write this, I have just desk-rejected a manuscript from the journal that I edit, in part because many of the subsections in the method and results sections were either missing or extremely substandard. The authors would have benefited from outlining these sections prior to initiating the writing process. (For example, there was no description of the sample in the method section.)

Outlines may also be used as a way to engage coauthors in the writing process and to come to a preliminary agreement on what should be included in the paper. Outlines can help the writing team to map out the paper—although team members are free to change their minds or to provide additional input once the sections have been drafted.

In closing, outlines are an important tool for both beginning and experienced writers. As is mentioned in other chapters, first drafts are unlikely to be polished—we often write our thoughts down as they come to mind—so an outline will help to structure our ideas. Even the most experienced authors can be AOTP if they do not plan their ideas in advance.

Summary

- Outlines are helpful in structuring a manuscript and ensuring that the line of logic remains consistent throughout.
- Outlines help to avoid tangents when we are writing a first draft.
- The introduction and discussion are the most important sections to outline prior to drafting them.
- When we are writing theoretical, review, and position papers, we outline the entire paper at once.
- Outlines can be used to propose a structure for a planned paper and receive feedback from coauthors.

References

Baddour, D. (2019, January 20). Colombia's radical plan to welcome millions of Venezuelan migrants. *The Atlantic.* Retrieved from https://www.theatlantic.com/international/archive/2019/01/colombia-welcomes-millions-venezuelans-maduro-guaido/581647/

Berry, J. W. (1980). Acculturation as varieties of adaptation. In A. M. Padilla (Ed.), *Acculturation: Theory, models, and some new findings* (pp. 9–25). Boulder, CO: Westview.

Newkirk, M., & Crooks, N. (2017, May). Venezuela's crisis has professionals scrubbing toilets in Miami. Retrieved from https://www.bloomberg.com/news/articles/2017-05-11/venezuela-s-crisis-has-professionals-scrubbing-toilets-in-miami

Public Radio International. (2018, March 28). Highly trained and educated, some foreign-born doctors still can't practice medicine in the US. Retrieved from https://www.pri.org/stories/2018-03-26/highly-trained-and-educated-some-foreign-born-doctors-still-can-t-practice

Robles, F., & Jordan, M. (2019, January 24). Venezuelans living in America watch crisis back home with hope and caution. *New York Times.* Retrieved from https://www.nytimes.com/2019/01/24/us/venezuelans-florida-noticias-news.html

Schwartz, S. J., Meca, A., Ward, C., Szabó, A., Benet-Martínez, V., Lorenzo-Blanco, E. I., Zamboanga, B. L. (2019). Biculturalism dynamics: A daily diary study of bicultural identity and psychosocial functioning. *Journal of Applied Developmental Psychology, 62,* 26–37.

Schwartz, S. J., Salas-Wright, C. P., Pérez-Gómez, A., Mejía-Trujillo, J., Brown, E. C., Montero-Zamora, P., Dickson-Gomez, J. (2018). Cultural stress and psychological symptoms in recent Venezuelan immigrants to the United States and Colombia. *International Journal of Intercultural Relations, 67,* 25–34.

Schwartz, S. J., Unger, J. B., Zamboanga, B. L., & Szapocznik, J. (2010). Rethinking the concept of acculturation: Implications for theory and research. *American Psychologist, 65,* 237–251.

United States Customs and Immigration Services. (2019). Asylum. Retrieved from https://www.uscis.gov/humanitarian/refugees-asylum/asylum

Woods, J., & Arthur, C. D. (2017). *Debating immigration in the age of terrorism, polarization, and Trump.* Lanham, MD: Lexington.

5

Getting Ready to Write

Chapter Objectives

When you finish reading this chapter, you should feel comfortable with the following:

- Putting yourself into a mental state that will facilitate writing
- Prioritizing writing time on a regular basis
- Allowing thoughts to flow from your mind onto the screen
- Recognizing ideal, and less than ideal, times to write
- Realizing the value of taking breaks and recharging yourself, and of knowing your limits
- Dealing with writing-related anxiety
- The role of mentors and coauthors in the writing process
- Dos and Don'ts of Academic Writing
- When to cite sources
- Use of first- and second-person pronouns in scholarly writing

So, once the outline is completed, we are all ready to get started writing. This is what we have been waiting for, correct?

Sitting at the computer and looking at the blank screen, with the cursor flashing, can be very anxiety-provoking for many people. Thoughts run through your mind, but you are not sure what to write—so you may not write anything. A saying I like is: *The hardest word to write is the first one.*

Even as an experienced writer, I experience this feeling often. I fumble with my fingers, start typing words and then delete them, and after 30 minutes I have written only one or two lines. Sometimes I have to get up and do something else for a few minutes to reset my mind—mental blocks are more likely to go away once we stop focusing on them.

The Savvy Academic. Seth J. Schwartz, Oxford University Press. © Oxford University Press 2022.
DOI: 10.1093/oso/9780190095918.003.0006

Carving Out Time to Write

My friend Al Waterman used to say that he could only really write "when the muse was on his shoulder." That is, he would write when he felt inspired to write. Often, that would be in the middle of the night, when the house was quiet and he was able to focus. I am naturally a night owl—unless I have to wake up early in the morning, I generally do my best work in the late evening and shortly after midnight. During the summer, when my children are out of school, I like to start writing around 8 or 9 p.m. and stop around 1 or 2 a.m. That's my "sweet spot" in terms of prime writing time. I know other people who prefer to wake up before sunrise and who do their best writing at 5 or 6 a.m.

It is essential to carve out time for writing. Other tasks can easily eat into your writing time if you allow them to. I reserve Friday as my writing day, and I don't allow meetings to be scheduled on that day. Even before the coronavirus pandemic, on Fridays, I almost always worked at home, where no one could knock on my door and disturb me just as I was settling into a writing groove.

I'm sure you have had the experience of waking up in the night to use the bathroom, and then once you crawl back into bed, it takes a while to fall asleep again. That same delay often occurs after your writing groove is interrupted by meetings, teaching, or other tasks. You have to dedicate large blocks of time to writing so that you can give yourself time to get into the groove and stay there.

Some people don't have large blocks of time available. They have lots of administrative responsibilities, or they have a heavy teaching load, or they have many students whom they are responsible for advising. When I was at the University of Miami, I directed a PhD program, I was the Institutional Review Board (IRB) approver for my department, and I was a member of a standing NIH review committee. During many weeks, I literally had no time to write. *This is OK. Trust me, it is.*

Administrative loads are not the same every week—and neither is student mentoring or advising. Some weeks will be lighter than others—and when you have a lighter week, that's when you need to make sure to carve out some writing time. Remember that, unless someone is defending their dissertation next week, or unless there is a grant deadline coming up, or unless there is a fire that absolutely must be put out right now, most meeting requests (aside from standing meetings) can be pushed back a week. You are the best judge of what is urgent and what is not, but as I have learned in my career, we must set boundaries with other people. It is often tempting to give up writing time when your calendar is filling up, but if you don't make time for writing, then the weeks will go by and the writing will not progress.

Evenings and weekends may sometimes be good writing time, depending on your family responsibilities. When I had young children, I would write after they went to bed—but as they grew older and started staying up later, that writing time began to disappear. When my daughters were in elementary and middle school and were bringing home lots of homework, I usually helped them with it—which took away some of my writing time. (Now that they are in high school, they complete most of their work without needing my assistance, so some of my evening writing time has returned.)

Some of my colleagues say that academia and parenting don't fit well together, and I can see why that may be true in some cases. I've been an extremely involved parent ever since my daughters were born, and I have rarely missed one of their performances or events. My wife and I share the childcare responsibilities fairly evenly, and I handle most of the homework, almost all the parent–teacher meetings, and many of the doctor's appointments. However, I can also say that my productivity increased dramatically after I became a parent. Parenting forced me to manage my time extremely well and to fit in writing whenever I could.

So the point here is that the quality of your writing will depend heavily on how much time you dedicate to it. You cannot just sit down and expect to be in the groove immediately—you need to carve out regular writing time and to train yourself to tune out distractions. As a distance runner, I would never try to run a half marathon if I hadn't been running regularly. I wouldn't try to lift heavy weights if I wasn't in good enough shape to handle it. So why would writing be any different?

Here I use the term *good writing habits* to refer to ways in which you can keep your writing skills sharp. Think about when you first learned how to ride a bicycle or to drive a car. Chances are you made lots of mistakes at the beginning, but riding or driving became easier and easier as you practiced and as the motor skills became second nature. Writing is similar. We learn to write by writing and receiving feedback from others. My mentors taught me to write by giving me critical, constructive feedback on my drafts. As I spent more time writing, their comments became more positive and less critical—and I became more comfortable as a writer.

So, good writing habits involve protecting your writing time, writing frequently, and seeking critical feedback on your drafts. I cannot overemphasize the need to identify the correct people to read your work—you don't need "yes people" who will just read and tell you how terrific your writing is. You need people who will read every word, correct every mistake they see, point out anything that looks even potentially questionable, and challenge you to be-come a better writer. José provided that for me, and I provide it for the people I mentor and with whom I collaborate.

Another important principle is that the best way to learn something is to teach it to someone else. Reviewing journal manuscripts and grant proposals, as well as commenting on other people's drafts, has helped me to identify my own writing mistakes. As soon as you pick up skills from people who read and comment on your work, pass those skills on to others by reading and commenting on their work. Take whatever opportunities you have to help others with their writing—and doing so will help you with your own writing as well.

It is worth reinforcing that writing time should not be sacrificed. I know it's tempting to do something else instead of working on that dreaded manuscript—but doing so will not help that paper get written. My wife uses the term *creative avoidance* to refer to the art of doing almost anything other than the task that needs to be done. If I have a paper I need to finish, but I re-ally don't want to work on it, I might run analyses for another paper, revise my curriculum vitae, or look over my lecture notes again. I once had a postdoc-toral fellow who was absolutely brilliant but didn't like to write. She always said that writing scared her and that she didn't believe she was very good at it. So she finished her post-doc with only one first-authored publication. She spent much of her time organizing data files and completing other tasks that were helpful for me and for our lab, but that didn't advance her career. Creative avoidance involves working on other tasks that are important, but preventing yourself from getting to the primary tasks that you really don't want to work on. It is essential to identify when you are engaging in creative avoidance and to "call yourself out" for it.

Again, even though I am an experienced writer, I still fall prey to creative avoidance. I've had plenty of manuscripts and grants that I avoided working on for weeks, months, or even years. Eventually, though, I had to complete these tasks. Other people were counting on me—my coauthors, students, and mentors. Ultimately, I had to force myself to sit there and write, and eventually I was able to find my writing groove and finish the work.

For people whose first language is not English, but who want to publish in English-language journals, good writing habits are especially important. English is one of the most difficult European languages to learn, and as my Colombian colleague likes to say, English grammar can be "devilish." There are many different words that sound the same, or are even spelled the same, but that have completely different meanings (I cover some of these in greater detail in Chapter 6). If English is not your native language, learning how to write well in English takes a great deal of practice, as well as feedback from native English speakers.

I work with several colleagues from other countries, as well as many people who are immigrants to the United States or to other English-speaking countries. Several of them have told me that their English writing has improved through writing with me and receiving my detailed edits and feedback on their drafts. It is an honor to hear this—of course—but I consider it to be a service to the profession.

So, for those readers who are not native English speakers, practice is key. Sit down at your laptop (or desktop computer) and work on a paper. Even if the words don't come out as smoothly as you would like—or if you are afraid of making mistakes—just let your thoughts come out. Importantly, force yourself to write in English, rather than writing in your native language and translating into English. The point is that you need to teach yourself to think in English so that you can become a better writer in English.

Allow Thoughts to Flow From Your Mind Onto the Screen

As is discussed in greater detail in other chapters, the purpose of a first draft is to move your thoughts from your mind to the computer screen. It is essential that you not try to censor or to perfect your thoughts while they are still in your mind. You *cannot* edit what is in your head—and I don't suggest that you should attempt to. Once the ideas are on the screen, you can change them, add to them, and move them around—preferably after the first draft has been completely written. Especially for novice writers, writing and editing should be done during different writing sessions—so you don't cut off the creative process until it's finished. Attempts to edit, censor, or cut off one's thoughts are counterproductive until the thoughts have been transferred to the screen. The point of a first draft is to ensure that your ideas are written down—you can worry about organizing them later.

Note that I am not inviting you to be AOTP. As I suggest in the next section, you might want to paste the relevant parts of your outline under each section heading and write within the structure that the outline provides. If you are AOTP within a subsection of your outline, that is far easier to fix compared to the whole section or paper being AOTP.

Chapter 1 describes the dangers of maladaptive perfectionism—the insistence that every word must be perfect before you can write it (or before you can leave it alone and continue writing). If you have maladaptive perfectionist tendencies, I strongly suggest that you do your best to put them aside before you start writing your first draft. As noted above, first drafts are supposed to have problems and are not supposed to be perfect. The editing phase, which begins after the first draft is completed, is your opportunity to identify and to correct the problems in your first draft. The advice provided before bears repeating: *Do not attempt to edit your ideas while they are still in your head, or while you are still in the process of transferring them to the screen.* I generally do not start editing until my first draft is completed and after I have set it aside for a few days. (There is much more detail on editing in Chapter 9.)

Some people get anxious when they sit down to write. If this happens to you, I recommend that you take some time to practice mindfulness techniques, meditation, centering, or whatever other exercises will help to calm your anxiety. I am an anxious person myself, and I can tell you that my performance in almost anything I'm trying to do is adversely affected by anxiety. If I can't calm myself down at a given point in time, then I cannot write well at that time—so I don't even try.

I've always said that I do my best writing when I allow the words to flow through me and when I don't stop and think too much about what I'm writing. Csikszentmihalyi (1990) introduced the concept of flow, which he defined as a cognitive-affective state where we are extremely involved in the activity, we forget about our personal problems, and we stop thinking and worrying about whether we are "doing it right." In other words, we are too engrossed in the activity to analyze ourselves to death. We just do what we know we need to do.

Athletes, actors, and other performers generally perform best when they are in a flow state. When a baseball player is striking out too much, or a basketball player is not shooting the ball well, the explanation they often provide for their struggles involves overthinking. Imagine a stage actor stopping, looking at the audience, and wondering whether their performance is good enough for that audience. How well do you think that stage actor would perform under those circumstances?

When you try to edit your words while they are in your head, while they are being transferred onto the screen, or before you are finished putting your thoughts into your first draft, you are making the same mistake as the baseball player who is overthinking and striking out, or the stage actor who is overthinking and forgetting lines. In other words, you are being a maladaptive perfectionist—and most of the time, maladaptive perfectionism will compromise the quality of the work you are producing. Let the words flow out of you like water out of a faucet. You will have lots of time to think about those words later on, after they have been written.

People often ask me how I'm able to write so well: *What's your secret?* I've been asked that question many times, and my answer is usually some variation of what I wrote in the previous paragraph. The words just flow out of me, almost as though they're not even mine. I feel them coming through me, but it doesn't feel as though I am the source of the words. They are coming from a divine source, passing through my mind and my fingers, and settling onto the screen.

I have just described how the concept of flow can be applied to writing—*any* type of writing. If you have to think too much, it won't work. Overthinking will shut off the flow state. Flow and mindfulness have a great deal in common, which is why I recommend mindfulness training and meditation as a way to calm your anxiety and to place yourself into a flow state. It can take a while to get into the flow state, and distractions will pull you out of it very quickly— which is why I recommend setting aside long, undisturbed blocks of time to write.

Stephen King, the horror novelist, once said in an interview that people often ask him where he gets his ideas—and he laughs at the question. The ideas come to him when he isn't expecting them to. I have had the same experiences with manuscript, grant, or project ideas—they often occur to me in dreams, while I'm running, or even while I'm in the shower. One of my best paper ideas came to me while I was rocking my baby daughter to sleep at 3:00 a.m. A common assumption is that writers come up with their ideas like a witch brewing a stew. A little bit of this, a little bit of that, and *voilà*—here's my idea! This assumption is generally false. The best ideas are often those that we don't come up with on purpose.

Let me summarize this section briefly. When we are writing a first draft, we need to place ourselves into a flow state and avoid overthinking. Trust yourself, let go, and allow the words to flow out of you. Don't try to edit or censor the words as they are coming out—just act as though you are dispassionately observing the words as they are appearing on the screen. Paste your outline for each section of the paper into that section and write within each heading. Don't worry about being AOTP—just let the words come out. You can—and will—edit them later.

Know When Is a Good Time to Write, and When Is Not

Just as there are some days you don't feel up to running, swimming, talking on the phone, or whatever else you might have planned to do, there are some days that are not especially conducive to writing. If you just had an argument with someone close to you, or you're not feeling well, or other events are occurring that are interfering with your ability to focus and concentrate, then I would advise putting the writing aside for a short while and sorting out the issues you're facing.

Although I said that we need to preserve our writing time, now I'm saying that sometimes we need to accept that the present moment is not the best time to write. Some readers might see a contradiction here and be confused about what I am suggesting. So let me clarify. If there are specific circumstances that are interfering with your concentration, then try to resolve these problems (if they can be resolved—some issues, such as family illnesses, cannot be re-solved, and you must learn to live with them and try to put them out of your mind when you're trying to write) and come back to writing when you are less distracted. If you are trying to creatively avoid a writing task, try to force your-self to sit down and write even though you don't really want to. Trust yourself to know the difference between "today is just not a good time to write because of circumstances that are beyond my control" and "I just don't feel like writing right now."

Anyone who is old enough to remember the events of September 11, 2001, probably remembers exactly where they were and what they were doing when they first found out about the attacks. I was driving to work and listening to sports talk radio when an announcement came over the radio that a plane had hit the World Trade Center in New York City. I arrived at the office just in time to watch the second plane hit, and to watch both towers collapse. I am a native New Yorker, and the September 11th attacks hit me especially hard. I tried to write later that day, but I just couldn't. My brain just couldn't do it. So I put the writing off—it was several days before I was able to concentrate well enough to do any writing at all.

September 11th is an extreme example, but there are other events that will make it difficult to devote the mental energy needed to write well. If I have a nasty argument with my wife one day, that would probably not be a good day for writing. Sometimes I am just exhausted or burned out and need some time away from writing. In my experience, mental exertion is often more ex-hausting than physical exertion—I have more energy after finishing a half marathon than I do after writing nonstop for several days—so if you need a break, take one. I almost never work on Sundays, and if I am especially ex-hausted and I can afford to take Saturday off as well, then I will. You are un-likely to write well when you are burned out or exhausted.

It's OK to push yourself to a point, but you also must know your limits. Know when you are too tired or distracted to work effectively. Breaks are essential for your mental health, and your mental health is essential for doing your best writing. Sometimes a weekend off is what you need to recharge. As I tell my students, vacations are a *must*. I take off 2 weeks during the winter holidays and 2 weeks during the summer. Working through the holidays is not a good idea if you want to be fresh and energetic in March and April. José was one of the hardest workers I've ever met, but he regularly took 2- and 3-week vacations to recharge himself. He needed to—if not, he could never have kept up the 7-day workweeks for which he was famous.

There is an important parallel between writing and distance running—both of which I do regularly. *You must conserve your energy.* If I sprint through the first mile of a half marathon, I will probably be way ahead of most other people my age at the end of that mile, but I will be gasping for air by the eighth or ninth mile. Similarly, I can write for a few hours, but then I need a break—or I need to do something else that is less mentally draining. I have learned what my limits are, and I have learned to respect and honor them.

A Word on Anticipatory Anxiety

In my experience, one of the most troublesome types of anxiety is the type you experience when you are thinking—and worrying—about future events that have not yet happened, or when you are dreading doing something that you have a lot of fears about doing. In many cases, I have lain awake at night worrying about how I'm going to support my family next year after one of my grants runs out, or how I'm going to get through a talk I have to give in front of a large audience, or about how I'm going to deal with a difficult colleague who has requested a meeting with me—a meeting I know will be uncomfortable and aversive.

The term *anticipatory anxiety* refers to this kind of worrying. When we are worrying about future events that have not happened yet, this kind of worrying is usually pointless (unless it leads us to take action to prevent an undesirable outcome). When anticipatory anxiety is attached to a specific activity that we cannot avoid, it can interfere with our performance in that activity. If we are afraid of writing—and some people are—we need to work on overcoming that fear so that we can accomplish what we need to get done.

As I note several times in this chapter, mindfulness can help us to center ourselves and calm down. However, some concrete strategies may be needed to overcome the anxiety that you may experience while you are performing the activity. Mindfulness can take away anticipatory anxiety, but we don't want the anxiety to come back when we sit down to write.

For many people, staring at a blank screen is especially anxiety-provoking. The hardest word to write is the first one! Many writers find themselves writing a couple of words, deleting them, writing a few more, deleting those, and not accomplishing very much. I was once one of those writers.

José taught me a trick for getting around the "blank screen" anxiety. This strategy is covered more in Chapter 8, but I will provide a quick preview here. José taught me that, when I'm writing an empirical research paper, I should start with the method section rather than with the introduction. Remember that the method section is extremely mechanical and formulaic. It is by far the easiest section of the paper to write. There is relatively little complexity in telling the reader who participated in your study, how participants were recruited, what measures were used, and what procedures were carried out. José's advice was a stroke of brilliance—I went from being scared of looking at a blank screen to being able to start almost any paper without having to worry.

Once the method section is written, then we write the results (how to write a results section is reviewed in Chapter 8). The results are not quite as mechanical as the method is, but the layout of the results section is fairly formulaic once we know what the hypotheses were and how we tested them. A quick word about writing results sections: the results section is not about statistics, and it's not about impressing your audience with fancy statistical symbols and flashy numbers. The results section is essentially a story—the story of how the hypotheses were tested and what the outcomes of the statistical tests were. Outlining the results section and writing the story within that outline is an important strategy for beginning writers (and for many experienced writers as well).

Only *after* we have written the methods and results sections do we go back and write the introduction. This way, the introduction has a clear destination and endpoint where it needs to leave off (the structure of the introduction section is discussed further in Chapter 8). After the introduction is finished, we write the discussion, which is also covered in Chapter 8. José's method allows us to write the most formulaic sections of the paper first; therefore, it allows us to "warm up" and reduce the anxiety associated with not knowing where to start.

Many of my colleagues have talked about "writer's block" preventing them from writing. In my opinion, writer's block is just another word for the anxiety (both anticipatory anxiety and the anxiety that one feels when one is trying to write) that sometimes accompanies someone's writing attempts. Anxiety clouds the mind and closes off the flow of words onto the screen. It also interferes with the "third-person observer" perspective that people often experience when they are in a state of flow—the feeling that the words are coming *through* me, but not *from* me. Anxiety makes us self-conscious and often causes us to judge our own performance, where such judgment is the antithesis of flow. So calming and managing writing anxiety will, in many cases, help to alleviate writer's block.

Finally: whatever you are experiencing when you sit down to write is real and true for you. Please don't judge or criticize yourself for what you are thinking or feeling. Condemning yourself for being anxious while writing only compounds the problem. Accept whatever you are thinking or feeling and consider it a starting point. If you're anxious and scared, or you have writer's block, or you just can't find the words to write, that's okay. You will find them eventually. Allow yourself to fully own the thoughts and feelings. There is a great line in Neale Donald Walsch's (1996) book *Conversations with God*: What you resist persists, and what you look at disappears. If you try to pretend that you are not anxious or scared, but you really are, that feeling will become even more difficult to overcome. Accept the feeling, own it, and have faith that you will get past it. Trust me—I have been there many times.

Writing as a Collaborative Endeavor

Many beginning writers make the mistake of thinking that they must do everything themselves. They must make the paper perfect on their own—and only once it's perfect can they share it with anyone else. This kind of unrealistic expectation often leads to writer's block and creates a lot of the anxiety that beginning writers experience. Like Atlas, the Greek god condemned to hold up the entire Earth on his own, many novice writers take on far more burden than they really need to.

The reality is that very few papers are single-authored. Most papers have multiple authors—and the number of authors on the average scholarly article has increased over time (Mallapaty, 2018). Coauthors are a resource for the primary author to lean on and to ask for input and assistance (I discuss working with coauthors in greater detail in Chapter 14). The point here is you don't have to do it all yourself—just get the paper into good enough shape for your coauthors to work with, and then let them provide feedback to help you improve the paper.

Most people learn to write scholarly papers by working with mentors. I learned most of what I know about scholarly writing from Dick and José. Mentors read our drafts, make detailed edits and comments, and meet with us to discuss their feedback. I learned from my mentors, and my mentees learn from me, by incorporating the mentor's feedback and understanding the writing principles that the feedback conveys. There is no shame in writing with mentors, or in leaning on mentors as you polish your writing skills.

In some cases, scholars are expected to demonstrate increased "independence" from their mentors. Such an expectation is often applied to assistant professors—they are supposed to start writing papers "on their own," without their mentors to lean on, before they will be seriously considered for tenure and promotion. In these cases, it is essential for young scholars to "pick and choose" which papers will involve their mentors and which ones will not. A former post-doc of mine has capitalized on the many connections I helped him to establish, and he has started projects with other colleagues of ours (and I fully support him in doing so). He has written many papers on which I am not a coauthor, as well as many on which I am a coauthor—and we discussed this arrangement in detail when he learned that his department expected him to establish independence.

Note, however, that when my former post-doc was still working in my lab, I worked closely with him to help him develop his writing skills, and I gave him careful feedback on everything he wrote. I also invited him to collaborate on papers that I was writing, so that he could learn the art of team writing. These kinds of activities are what a mentor should be doing with mentees, so that the mentees are able to establish independence later on. Mentoring is a lot like being a good parent—allow your mentees and children to develop as much independence as they can handle, but still make sure they know that they can come to you if they need help or support. Eventually, they will need you less and less—and that is how the process should work. Establishing independence is natural for children and mentees—they will only remain dependent on you long-term if they have not developed sufficient life or career skills or you have convinced them that you need them to remain at your side. In other words, independence is a natural outcome of healthy mentoring relationships. My former mentees still work with me, but they are not dependent on me—and nor would I want them to be. If they need anything from me, I am always here for them. If they invite me to write with them, I provide detailed feedback on their papers or grant applications. In some cases, I lean on them for help and support with my own work.

Back to the issue of leaning on coauthors when you are starting out as a writer: coauthors (especially experienced writers) know that novice writers need detailed feedback and that novice writers may need more help with writing style and organization. However, not all coauthors are equally patient and responsive. It is essential that you choose coauthors who will go through your drafts thoroughly and provide extensive feedback and editing. Someone who gives your paper the "summer vacation treatment" (to quote my friend

Jeff Arnett) and just tells you that it looks terrific probably is not an ideal co-author for a novice writer. As you continue writing with various coauthors, you may want to identify the coauthors with whom you want to continue collaborating—as well as those who are less responsive and helpful.

In sum, the point here is that, when working with coauthors, your goal should be to advance the paper as far as you can and then send it to your coauthors for review. If you feel "stuck" in your writing and are not sure how to proceed, it is often a good idea to request a meeting with one or more coauthors (or to send them your current draft) and to ask for help. You can call on coauthors as many times as you need to, so it is important not to feel that you have to perfect the paper on your own. Call on your coauthors as frequently (or infrequently) as necessary during the writing process. (I discuss working with coauthors in much greater detail in Chapter 14.)

Dos and Don'ts of Academic Writing

Academic writing is very different from other types of writing. Many people who have written novels, newspaper articles, blog posts, or opinion editorials (op-eds) find academic writing to be surprisingly difficult. Students have complained to me that academic writing is boring, ponderous, and uninteresting. My response is generally that I understand their point of view, but that academic writing becomes increasingly interesting as we spend more time reading and producing it. It is a style to which one must become accustomed, but that becomes "second nature" after engaging in it for a long enough time. In this section, I list some characteristics of academic writing, as well as some Dos and Don'ts of writing scholarly articles, chapters, and books. Specifically, I cover issues of neutrality, highlighting the study purpose without denigrating prior work, when to cite sources, abbreviations and acronyms, use of first- and second-person pronouns, and use of contractions. Additional writing principles are covered in Chapter 6.

Neutrality

Academic writers strive to be neutral and not to express their own opinions in their papers. Even if we are writing about topics that are very important to us, we must strive to be objective in our treatment of the topic.

For example, compare the following two paragraphs. The first is written with the author's opinions clearly expressed, and the second is written neutrally.

First: Drug users cause a lot of problems in our society. They contribute nothing to society and just hurt people. They should be in jail so that they do not harm anyone else. They need to take responsibility for their actions and stop relapsing.

Second: Drug use is a considerable societal problem. Costs associated with treatment, incarceration, and crime exceed $1 billion in the United States alone. Research indicates that providing access to clean needles and to safe rehabilitation services can increase the likelihood of recovery among drug-addicted individuals.

In a neutral writing stance, we should avoid strong and opinionated words—words like *horrible*, *terrific*, *wonderful*, and *awful*. Although it is not possible to separate scholars' personal values from their work (Kurtines, Azmitia, & Gewirtz, 1992)—our values guide the topics that we decide to study and the methods that we use to study the topics—we should nonetheless strive to be as neutral as possible. Readers should not be able to discern our personal values, beliefs, and political orientations simply by reading our work.

Academic writing should also be modest. We should discuss our results tentatively, even if we think they are extremely strong. Remember Schmidt's (2010) caution about the lies that data tell—what we find with one sample may not emerge with a different sample drawn from the same population, or with a sample drawn from a different population. So words like *demonstrate* should probably be avoided, unless we have conducted a series of studies (as is common in social psychology) and have increased confidence in our results. Even if we do have more confidence, it is better to be modest about our study's contribution.

The word *prove* should never be used in scientific writing. We can never prove anything in science.

When discussing results, we should be tentative rather than definitive. We should say "Our results may suggest support for our hypotheses" rather than "Our results confirm our hypotheses." Patterns from one study, even if they appear to strongly support the a priori hypotheses, do not produce a definitive finding. Remember the findings from the Open Science Collaboration (2015), where less than half of all research findings in psychology were able to be replicated in new samples. Our writing style must leave open the possibility that our results could fail to replicate in the future—or someone else may come up with a more effective methodological approach and report different findings than we reported.

Take a look at the following two paragraphs. The first paragraph includes some strong statements, whereas the second paragraph is more tentative and modest.

First: Our results demonstrate that pro-diversity attitudes cause companies to increase in profits. These findings confirm that including members of various demographic groups in the workforce is always good for business. These findings provide proof of a principle that has been advanced in the industrial/organizational psychology literature for decades.

Second: Our results suggest that pro-diversity attitudes may be beneficial vis-à-vis corporate profits. It is possible that the intergroup contact that accompanies diversity-based hiring helps companies to appeal to a wider range of customers. The present findings may help to support the diversity principle within industrial/organizational psychology.

Notice how the first paragraph is very strident and forceful, whereas the second is more modest and tentative. Given the incremental progress of science, each step should be taken carefully and with full knowledge that replication is essential before we can consider any set of results to be reliable. Even results with large effect sizes should be discussed carefully and with scientific reservation.

There are two additional principles of scientific modesty. The first is that we can only cite sources as saying what they actually say, and empirical sources (including meta-analyses) are more authoritative than claims that are made without direct support from data. José was a major proponent of this principle—if I cited a statement that someone made in an article as though it were fact, he would push back and advise me to find an empirically based source. Sometimes we are looking for a citation to support a statement we want to include in an article we are writing, and we cannot find a direct citation— but we do find something that's "close." For example, suppose we want to say that perceptions of discrimination may influence e-cigarette use among immigrant adolescents, but we cannot find a source that has studied that. However, we do find a source (Unger, Schwartz, Huh, Soto, & Baezconde-Garbanati, 2014) indicating that discrimination predicts use of regular cigarettes (not e-cigarettes) among a sample of U.S. Hispanic adolescents, some of whom were immigrants. Can we "stretch" the Unger et al. citation to cover the claim we want to include in our paper?

The answer depends on what we mean by "stretching," and whether the stretch renders our use of the citation dishonest. We may need to change the statement to match the source, such as:

There is evidence that perceived discrimination may predict use of tobacco products among adolescents from immigrant or minority backgrounds (Unger et al., 2014).

This statement is consistent with what Unger et al. (2014) found, and we may be able to use it to support our argument that discrimination appears to predict use of a specific type of substance (in this case tobacco products) within a specific population (in this case a minority group whose members are primarily first- and second-generation immigrants). In this way, we are "finessing" the argument without citing the source as saying something that it does not actually say.

The second principle of scientific modesty comes into play when we are discussing our own results in an empirical manuscript. Our statements should not go beyond what our research design and results can reasonably support. If we found a negative correlation between physical activity and depressive symptoms, then all we can discuss is an association between the two variables. We cannot talk about prediction or causation, because our research design was not longitudinal or experimental. Our statements also should not go beyond the sample that we used in our study—for example, if we surveyed a sample of college students from a psychology course, we cannot generalize our findings to the population of young adults as a whole.

Let's say that we surveyed a sample of college students and found that physical activity is negatively related to depressive symptoms. Assume that the study was cross-sectional, that we did not attempt to recruit anyone who was not attending a college or university, and that our measure of depressive symptoms allows us to assess the person's extent of depressive thoughts and feelings—but does not provide a clinical diagnosis of major depression. As before, I will present two paragraphs—one "wrong" paragraph that goes beyond our research design and results, and one "right" paragraph that accurately summarizes our findings:

First: Our results demonstrate that engaging in physical activity protects against depression among young adults. Specifically, young adults who are physically active are unlikely to be depressed. Our results indicate that programs designed to prevent depression among young adults should promote physical activity.

Second: Our results suggest that engaging in physical activity is inversely related to college students' reports of depressive symptoms. Students who are physically active may report fewer depressive symptoms compared to individuals who are more sedentary. If replicated longitudinally, these results may suggest that interventions to prevent or decrease depressive symptoms among college students might include activities to promote physical activity.

Notice that the first paragraph uses the term *protects against*, which implies a negative predictive association (Mustanski & Liu, 2013). The first paragraph also references young adults in general, even though the sample is comprised only of college students. The first paragraph also uses the words *depression* and *depressed*, terms that refer to clinical diagnoses. All these statements go beyond what our study can support.

In contrast, the second paragraph is more faithful to the research design and sample used in the study we are reporting. The text refers to an inverse relationship, to a college population, and to depressive symptoms. In this way, someone who skipped the method and results sections and only read the discussion (which I would not advise, of course) would have a good idea of what the study findings were and how they might be used to inform intervention efforts.

It is important to note that academics are not the only people who will read your work. Practitioners, policymakers, and other non-academic audiences may also read what you write. These people may not be able to fully understand the results section, so they will depend on the discussion to be faithful to your sample, measures, research procedures, statistical analyses, and findings.

A few years ago, I received a call from a divorce attorney. She was representing a father who was seeking shared custody of his infant daughter. A number of years earlier, my colleague Gordon Finley and I had published a series of articles on college students' recollections of their relationships with their fathers (Finley & Schwartz, 2007, 2010; Schwartz & Finley, 2009). Our core message across these articles was that college students from divorced families—particularly those whose mothers were awarded sole physical custody—reported significantly lower levels of involvement from their fathers than did college students from intact families. The divorce attorney had found our papers and emailed me, asking whether I would be willing to serve as an expert witness on behalf of her client.

When I spoke to this attorney on the phone, she expressed her gratitude for the work we had conducted, and she confessed that she was not well versed in statistics and had only read our discussion sections. I agreed to serve as an expert witness, and the family court judge also read our articles. He, too, only read the discussion sections. Had we overstated our results, the consequences for the father (who ultimately won his case) might have been quite negative once the attorney and judge discovered that we had misled them about our findings and their implications.

Standing on the Shoulders of Others

In the introduction to a research article, we need to justify the gap in the literature that we are seeking to fill. In doing so, we trace prior literature and note where the prior work has left off and why the advance that we are proposing is necessary and important. In essence, we are indicating how our work will extend the literature beyond prior work.

As a beginning writer, my style was often to disparage prior studies for what they had not done. I might have said something like "Prior studies have failed to consider," and then state all of the limitations and shortcomings of prior work. In making the case for the study I was reporting, I would often "slam" prior work for not having already done what my colleagues and I were writing about.

In his statesmanlike and eloquent way, José suggested that I might consider standing on the shoulders of prior studies rather than criticizing them for not having already done what we had done. In other words, review prior work respectfully, and then neutrally state where the field needs to go next. For example, we might say that "Prior studies have suggested that family therapy may be efficacious in decreasing adolescent behavior problems. A next possible step might be to examine the mediating mechanisms that drive this effect."

There are three main advantages to José's statesmanlike approach compared to criticizing prior studies for what they did not do. First, as Al Waterman—who spent more than 20 years of his life as a journal editor or associate editor—told me many years ago, editors often choose reviewers for a manuscript based on who is cited in the reference list. So if you cite my work and disparage it, I may be asked to review your manuscript—and I will likely not take kindly to having my work criticized. The statesmanlike approach, in contrast, praises and honors prior work and credits it for having brought the field to the place where our current study is picking up. Reviewers are more likely to support publication of a paper that praises their work compared to a paper that disparages their work.

Second, the statesmanlike approach reflects the evolution of the scientific literature, in which the prior studies we cite represented advances at the time they were published—just as our study represents an advance now. Imagine if each step of the scientific process criticized prior work for not taking the current step earlier? This kind of criticism is akin to having a thought right now and then criticizing yourself for not having had that thought 3 years ago. It places an unreasonable burden on prior researchers and creates an adversarial atmosphere for scientific progress. In short, each step of scientific progress is important and should not be disparaged for not also taking the next step.

Third, readers may be more likely to accept and endorse your justification for why your work is necessary if you frame your justification respectfully and positively. Think of how most people react to negative political campaign advertisements. When I watch negative campaign ads, my first reaction is, "Don't tell me why I shouldn't vote for the other person— tell me why I *should* vote for *you!*" Similarly, when you are writing an introduction to a journal article, don't tell me what others have not done. Tell me what you are doing and why it is important for the field.

So let's contrast two paragraphs—one that is critical of prior work and one that is respectful (I have omitted citations for brevity, but if we were to write these paragraphs for publication, we would need to cite sources):

First: Prior work testing the hypothesis that parent–adolescent acculturation discrepancies predict compromised family functioning has been limited in at least three ways. First, many prior studies in this area have been cross-sectional and have not permitted analyses of predictive relationships between acculturation discrepancies and family functioning. Second, other studies have failed to include youth or parent outcomes—as a result, we do not know whether parent–adolescent acculturation discrepancies predict parent or youth adjustment *through* family functioning. Third, parent–youth acculturation discrepancies have been measured at only one point in time, which is a limitation because we do not know how these discrepancies may evolve over time.

Second: Prior work has suggested that parent–adolescent acculturation discrepancies may be associated with compromised family functioning. This prior work has been important in opening a line of research on the consequences of acculturation discrepancies in immigrant families. Building on this prior research, a number of important research directions may be important to follow, including (a) examining the link between acculturation discrepancies and family functioning longitudinally, (b) examining the extent to which acculturation discrepancies predict youth and parent outcomes indirectly through family functioning, and (c) examining trajectories of, as well as individual scores on, acculturation discrepancies.

Notice how the second paragraph pays tribute to prior research and uses it as a starting point for the present work. José referred to this approach as "standing on the shoulders" of prior research. When José developed his Brief Strategic Family Therapy intervention, he stood on the shoulders of pioneering family therapists and researchers like Minuchin (1974) and Madanes (1981)—and among his primary innovations was integrating the structural (e.g., focusing on family hierarchy and healthy family roles) and strategic (e.g., intervening at specific points in time and to correct specific family dynamics that may be related to the family's presenting problem) family therapy traditions (see Szapocznik, Schwartz, Muir, & Brown, 2012, for a review of this integration). I can distinctly remember José telling me that he never criticized Minuchin, Madanes, and others for not proposing the integration that he later proposed—rather, he stood on their shoulders and integrated the pioneering lines of work that they had conducted. Indeed, whenever we conduct research, review literature, or propose theory, we are always standing on the shoulders of those whose work came before ours. It is important to acknowledge and pay tribute to this prior work so that our contribution can be properly situated within the literature and so that others can stand on our shoulders when they extend and build upon our work.

Citing Sources

When I have taught workshops on writing for publication, many attendees have told me that they are confused about when to cite sources and when not to cite sources. Novice writers (as well as experienced writers) are often unsure about when citations are needed and what kinds of citations are needed. For example, what happens if we are working with a new population about which very little has been published in the literature? There may be many sources in the popular media—is it okay to cite those? What about Census reports and other similar population estimates and profiles? Which sources may be trustworthy and which sources may not be trustworthy? Do specific recruitment strategies and measurement instruments need citations? When we describe statistical analyses, do we need to cite sources? If we are integrating our findings into the literature in the discussion, do we need to cite sources?

Let's take these questions one at a time. First, regarding when to cite a source, I will proceed section by section, starting with the introduction. Second, regarding which sources to cite, I provide some specific guidance as I discuss each of the sections.

Introduction Section

In the introduction, we need to cite a source for prevalence rates and population estimates. For example, if we are providing the number of Asian immigrants in the United States, or the number of people who contracted HIV in 2019, or the number of people who lost their jobs in the last 5 years, we need to cite a source for these estimates. Government sources are generally the most authoritative—such as the U.S. Census Bureau for population figures, the Centers for Disease Control for disease prevalence and incidence rates, the Department of Education for statistics on school enrollment and completion, and the Department of Defense for military enrollment and spending. (Most other countries have similar ministries and bureaus that publish reports on a regular basis.) Some nongovernmental organizations, such as the Pew Research Center, RAND Corporation, and Research Triangle International, also publish trustworthy facts and figures.

As a general rule, popular-media sources are less preferable compared to official government sources and nongovernmental organizations. Newspapers, television channels, and radio stations likely vary in terms of the research that they conduct and the sources on which they depend for their information. If you can avoid doing so, do not rely on a popular-media report for information that can be obtained from a more trustworthy source. I remember finding a story in the *Miami Herald* once about Cuban immigration to South Florida. I considered citing that story, but instead I used Google to find a more authoritative source (in this case the American Community Survey, which is conducted by the U.S. Census Bureau).

We also need to cite a source for factual-sounding statements that appear anywhere in our manuscript, unless they are taken directly from our own findings. Even if we are citing our own prior work, we must include a formal citation. As already noted, the sources that we cite for factual-sounding statements must actually say what we are citing them as saying, and empirically based sources are preferable to theoretical or speculative statements.

Method Section

In the method section, citations are generally not needed for commonly used sampling and recruitment strategies. However, new or uncommonly used strategies, such as respondent-driven sampling (Goel & Salganik, 2010), should be accompanied by citations. Self-report measures should be cited, using the original authors (if the original version of the measure was used) or the authors who adapted the measure (if an adapted version is used). If you are using a version that you adapted, then cite the original version and indicate what adaptations you made (e.g., inserting or deleting items, changing the response scale, simplifying item wording).

If you are using a functional magnetic resonance imaging machine, genotyping procedure, biological assay, or other similar equipment, the customary citation involves listing the name of the company that manufactures or administers the equipment and the location where the company is based. For example, Alexander et al. (2009, p. 1529) cited one of their biological measures as follows: "A topical anesthetic (EMLA cream; AstraZeneca, Wilmington, DE) was applied to the antecubital area of both arms and an hour later a flexible intravenous catheter was inserted into both of the arms." No corresponding entry in the reference section is needed.

Research procedures generally do not require citations unless they are proprietary. A number of cognitive and social tasks have been developed to measure executive functioning, social ostracism, authoritarianism, and other constructs that may be difficult to assess validly through self-report. For example, Williams and Jarvis (2006) developed the Cyberball task to assess social ostracism. Other players (who are actually computerized avatars) throw a ball back and forth to the person playing the game, but eventually they exclude the person and throw the ball only between each other. The assumption is that participants will feel excluded, and that social and biological processes related to exclusion will be activated after playing the game—thereby allowing for administration of self-report measures or collection of biological samples that are assumed to be associated with ostracism. As another example, the Trier Social Stress Test (Kirschbaum, Pirke, & Hellhammer, 1993) was developed to induce stress that can then be assessed via cortisol secretion and other biomarkers. Participants are asked to deliver a speech on a predetermined topic, and audience members (who are actually the experimenters' confederates) jeer and laugh at the participant. Biological samples are then collected following the task.

Results Section
Most standard analytic procedures do not require a citation. In my estimation, any analysis that is taught in an introductory or intermediate statistics course can be considered standard and does not need a citation. Examples include t-tests, analyses of variance, chi-square tests of independence or association, most regression techniques (e.g., linear, logistic, Poisson, negative binomial), factor analyses, discriminant function analyses, cluster and latent class analysis, and tests of proportions. Structural equation modeling, survival analysis, and multilevel modeling have become mainstream enough that these techniques no longer require citations.

Some newer analytic techniques, such as some types of mixture modeling (e.g., factor mixture modeling; Lubke & Muthén, 2007) are not well known or commonly used, and I recommend citing references for these techniques. Bayesian analytic techniques (see Gelman & Shalizi, 2013, for a review) are likely less well known to many nonstatistical audiences than are frequentist analyses like general linear models (e.g., *t*-tests, analyses of variance, and multiple regression)—and citations can help link readers with sources where they can learn more about the analyses used in a given study. Especially with regard to statistical analyses (but also with regard to methodological techniques), citations are used both to ground one's methods in existing literature and to provide resources where readers can obtain additional information about the methods. Indeed, on many occasions, I have become aware of new recruitment methods, experimental tasks, or statistical analyses by reading or reviewing journal articles, and then I have looked up the sources cited in the articles. Some of the techniques later became part of my own research repertoire.

Discussion Section

The discussion generally contains fewer citations than the introduction does, and citations are used most often to compare the present findings to prior literature, to offer reasons why the present study's hypotheses may not have been fully supported, or to suggest the present study's implications for further research, intervention, or policy. Although discussion sections do need citations, remember that the focus of the discussion is on the present study's findings and contributions to the literature. The discussion is not the place to introduce new concepts unless they are being related directly to the present findings. With some rare exceptions, the discussion is also not the place to introduce new results. Indeed, the purpose of the discussion is to present the "bottom line" regarding the study's contribution, provide a verdict on the study hypotheses, integrate the present results with prior literature, and suggest limitations and future directions. The discussion is where the study "comes together" and where the take-home messages are presented—and citations should be provided for these purposes.

Abbreviations and Acronyms

Abbreviations and acronyms are a major pet peeve of mine. On more occasions than I can remember, I would be reading or reviewing a paper or grant application, and the authors would introduce a series of abbreviations or acronyms. Invariably, as I continued reading, I would forget what the abbreviation or acronym meant, and I would have to go back and look it up. This experience was frustrating, and when José told me his view on abbreviations and acronyms, I agreed with it immediately. He said that abbreviations and acronyms should be avoided unless they will be used "50 times" in the paper. He was exaggerating, of course, but his point was well taken. If you are going to use an abbreviation or acronym only a few times, just spell it out. It is much easier for readers to follow your argument when they don't have to constantly go back and remind themselves what an abbreviation or acronym means.

Of course, some abbreviations and acronyms are common knowledge and don't even need to be defined. Acronyms like HIV, FBI, and USA are used so frequently that some readers may not even know (or care) what they stand for. Some acronyms, such as fMRI (functional magnetic resonance imaging), may or may not need to be defined, depending on the readership to whom the paper is aimed. Neuroscientists will likely know what fMRI means, whereas sociologists may or may not know. The bottom line with acronyms is "when in doubt, spell it out"—unless the acronym will be used over and over again in your paper.

First- and Second-Person Pronouns

Some professional societies and writing styles discourage the use of first-person pronouns (*I*, *we*). The line of thinking behind this aversion to first-person pronouns is that the writing should be focused on the science rather than on the individuals conducting or reporting the science. In more recent years, as the role of researchers and their own value systems within the scientific enterprise has been increasingly recognized, first-person pronouns have become increasingly accepted in some fields (*Nature*, 2016). Although there is little agreement among writing styles regarding the acceptability of first-person pronouns (Bennett, 2009), I have had many reviewers tell me that first-person pronouns are preferable to passive-voice sentences. Look at the following two sentences, for example:

First person: We recruited participants using snowball sampling techniques.
Passive voice: Participants were recruited using snowball sampling techniques.

Passive-voice sentences are often clumsy and difficult to read, and the typical subject–predicate sentence structure (discussed in greater detail in

Chapter 6) is often out of order. On many occasions, reviewers have asked me to reword passive-voice sentences into active-voice form. When describing study methods or analyses, the subject of the sentence is generally a first-person pronoun, and passive voice represents a way to remove these first-person pronouns from scientific writing. So there is a trade-off between avoiding first-person pronouns and using passive-voice sentence structures that can be clumsy to read.

Earlier in my career, I actively avoided using *I* or *we* in my writing. In my undergraduate and graduate training in the 1990s, I was taught that first-person pronouns are not appropriate for use in scientific writing. However, as reviewers have pointed out, active-voice sentences are more intuitive and easier to understand, and the American Psychological Association (2020) has loosened its rules regarding the use of personal pronouns. I encourage you to use active voice whenever possible and to include first-person pronouns as needed.

Second-person pronouns (*you*, *your*), however, should not be used in scientific writing. Although I use second-person pronouns in this book because I am speaking directly to the reader, in scientific writing we are reporting research, reviewing literature, or proposing theory or policy—and therefore we are not speaking directly to the reader.

Sometimes we use *you* in informal speaking and writing to refer to the general or hypothetical case—for example, "When you conduct research, you have to be careful to document all of your results." In formal writing, we use *one* to refer to the general or hypothetical case—such as "When one conducts research, one must be careful to document all of one's results." So there is never a reason to use second person in formal academic writing.

Contractions

The English language includes a number of contractions, most of which use apostrophes to replace the omitted letters. For example, the second *o* in *do not* is replaced with an apostrophe in *don't*. Similarly, the *h* and *a* in *I have* are replaced with an apostrophe in *I've*. Contractions serve as a form of shorthand, and they are a hallmark of informal writing.

In formal academic writing, however, we generally avoid contractions. Formal writing is just that—formal—and contractions convey a sense of informality. As a reviewer, if I spot contractions in a manuscript, not only do I ask the author to correct them, but also I may take the author (and the manuscript) less seriously. More or less, reviewers expect authors to know not to use contractions in scientific writing.

Conclusion

This chapter addresses issues that writers should know as they prepare to convert their outlines into manuscript drafts. It covers good writing habits, in which writing skills are similar to other types of skills—that is, they must be continually practiced, maintained, and improved. Active scholars need to carve out time for writing so that their skills remain sharp. Active scholars also should seek feedback on their work and must learn to welcome, rather than shy away from, critical and challenging comments from colleagues. The "yes person" who just tells you that your work is terrific is not helping you to grow and develop as a writer.

I also describe the process of allowing ideas to flow from your mind onto the screen and the ways in which self-doubts and anxiety can disrupt this flow. The flow state—characterized by engrossment in an activity and a lack of concern with one's personal problems—is most conducive to writing, and many people do their best writing when they are in a state of flow. The flow state also requires that we try not to criticize or edit our thoughts as they are transferred from our mind onto the screen. Editing is often best done after the draft has been completed.

Another key point in this chapter is the difference between recognizing the ideal times to write and creatively avoiding the writing process. Sometimes external events create distractions and difficulties that interfere with our ability to enter the flow state, and writing might best be saved for another time. However, it is essential to recognize when we are just putting off the writing task and to force ourselves to sit down and complete the writing that we have been creatively avoiding.

Finally, this chapter emphasizes the role of coauthors in the writing process and lays out some Dos and Don'ts of academic writing. Coauthors are a resource that can—and should—be leveraged to help you improve your manuscripts. One way to work effectively with coauthors is to do as much as you can with the paper and then to seek feedback and help from your coauthors. Choose your coauthors carefully—people who don't provide good feedback or who don't respond to your requests for comments are probably not the best choices as coauthors for beginning writers (or for more experienced writers, either). Coauthors who are overly combative are also not good choices. (More coverage of working with coauthors appears in Chapter 13.)

In terms of Dos and Don'ts, there are "unwritten rules" that can help ensure that our work is taken as seriously as possible. Academic writing is neutral (we do not express our personal opinions or use overly biased language) and modest (we do not overstate our results). We stand on the shoulders of those who came before us, rather than criticizing prior work for what it did not do. We cite sources for our claims, statements, and any methods and analyses that are not commonly known. We should avoid abbreviations and acronyms in most cases, and contractions should not be used in formal academic writing. The use of first-person pronouns may be preferable to passive voice, where the subject of the sentence may be difficult to identify. Again, following these guidelines may help to ensure that your writing receives the attention and respect that it deserves—both from reviewers and from readers.

Summary

- Creating time to write is an essential part of becoming a successful writer.
- It is important to write frequently as a way of building one's writing skills and confidence.
- Be sure to seek out critical feedback on your writing from coauthors.
- People whose first language is not English should write in English as often as they can, rather than writing in their native language and translating to English.
- A key writing principle involves allowing thoughts to flow from one's mind onto the screen.
- It is important not to edit thoughts and ideas until after you have finished writing.
- The concept of flow refers to being completely engrossed in an activity and not worrying about making a mistake—and writing is often best accomplished when one is in a state of flow.
- Sometimes writing is more difficult to accomplish when one is distracted or bothered—and writers need to know when they are, and are not, in a "good writing place."
- For empirical manuscripts, starting with the method section can help to decrease writing-related anxiety and facilitate more productive writing sessions.
- Early-career writers should consult their mentors frequently as they are learning how to write scholarly manuscripts.

- Academic writing should be neutral, modest, and accurate, and should stand on the shoulders of prior work (rather than criticizing prior work for what it did not do).
- Sources should be cited for factual-sounding statements, for measurement instruments, and for analyses that are more advanced than those taught in introductory statistics.

References

Alexander, K. E., Ventura, E. E., Spruijt-Metz, D., Weigensberg, M. J., Goran, M. I., & Davis, J. N. (2009). Association of breakfast skipping with visceral fat and insulin indices in overweight Latino youth. *Obesity, 17*, 1528–1533.

American Psychological Association. (2020). *Publication manual of the American Psychological Association* (7th ed.). Washington, DC: Author.

Bennett, K. (2009). English academic style manuals: A survey. *Journal of English for Academic Purposes, 8*, 43–54.

Csikszentmihalyi, M. (1990). *Flow: The psychology of optimal experience*. New York: Harper & Row.

Finley, G. E., & Schwartz, S. J. (2007). Father involvement and long-term young adult outcomes: The differential contributions of divorce and gender. *Family Court Review, 45*, 573–587.

Finley, G. E., & Schwartz, S. J. (2010). The divided world of the child: Divorce and long-term psychosocial adjustment. *Family Court Review, 48*, 516–527.

Gelman, A., & Shalizi, C. R. (2013). Philosophy and the practice of Bayesian statistics. *British Journal of Mathematical and Statistical Psychology, 66*, 8–38.

Goel, S., & Salganik, M. J. (2010). Assessing respondent–driven sampling. *Proceedings of the National Academy of Sciences, 107*, 6743–6747.

Kirschbaum, C., Pirke, K.-H., & Hellhammer, D. H. (1993). The "Trier Social Stress Test": A tool for investigating psychobiological stress processes in a laboratory setting. *Neuropsychobiology, 28*, 76–81.

Kurtines, W. M., Azmitia, M., & Gewirtz, J. L. (Eds.). (1992). *The role of values in psychology and human development*. New York: Wiley.

Lubke, G., & Muthén, B. O. (2007). Performance of factor mixture models as a function of model size, covariate effects, and class-specific parameters. *Structural Equation Modeling, 14*, 26–47.

Madanes, C. (1981). *Strategic family therapy*. San Francisco, CA: Jossey-Bass.

Mallapaty, S. (2018, January 30). Paper authorship goes hyper. *Nature Index*. Retrieved from https://www.natureindex.com/news-blog/paper-authorship-goes-hyper

Minuchin, S. (1974). *Families and family therapy*. Cambridge, MA: Harvard University Press.

Mustanski, B., & Liu, R. T. (2013). A longitudinal study of predictors of suicide attempts among lesbian, gay, bisexual, and transgender youth. *Archives of Sexual Behavior, 42*, 437–448.

Nature. (2016). Write on: Biologists are using more informal language in their papers. *Nature, 539*, 140.

Open Science Collaboration. (2015). Estimating the reproducibility of psychological science. *Science, 349*, Article aac4716.

Schmidt, F. (2010). Detecting and correcting the lies that data tell. *Perspectives on Psychological Science, 5*, 233–242.

Schwartz, S. J., & Finley, G. E. (2009). Mothering, fathering, and divorce: The influence of divorce on reports of and desires for maternal and paternal involvement. *Family Court Review, 47*, 506–522.

Szapocznik, J., Schwartz, S. J., Muir, J. A., & Brown, C. H. (2012). Brief strategic family therapy: An intervention to reduce adolescent risk behavior. *Couple and Family Psychology: Research and Practice, 1*, 134–145.

Unger, J. B., Schwartz, S. J., Huh, J., Soto, D. W., & Baezconde-Garbanati, L. (2014). Acculturation and perceived discrimination: Predictors of substance use trajectories from adolescence to emerging adulthood among Hispanics. *Addictive Behaviors, 39*, 1293–1296.

Walsch, N. D. (1996). *Conversations with God: An uncommon dialogue*. New York: Putnam.

Williams, K. D., & Jarvis, B. (2006). Cyberball: A program for use in research on social ostracism and acceptance. *Behavior Research Methods, 38*, 174–180.

6
Principles of Good Writing

Chapter Objectives

When you finish reading this chapter, you should feel comfortable with:

- Levels of writing (grammar and sentence structure, flow within a paragraph, flow within a section, and flow across sections)
- Rules of good grammar and punctuation
- Improving flow within a paragraph
- Improving flow between paragraphs

This chapter covers some additional principles of writing clearly and effectively, building on the Dos and Don'ts presented in Chapter 5. I cover grammatical structure, punctuation, avoiding overused words, flow within and between paragraphs and sections, parenthetical phrases, and how to craft a strong opening paragraph to draw readers' attention.

Figure 6.1 illustrates the levels of the writing process—starting with grammar and punctuation and continuing to sentence structure, flow between sentences and paragraphs, flow between sections, and the strength and coherence of the overall argument. The principles of outlining covered in Chapter 4 help to address some of the flow issues between sections, but if the more fine-grained syntax and structure are not in place, the paper will be very difficult to read.

A word of caution about the "micro" levels of writing, such as grammar and punctuation: readers will often stop trying to read your paper if it is poorly written. Imagine trying to drive on a road that is full of potholes and bumps—you probably won't be able to drive very fast. That's what it's like trying to read a paper with poor grammar, punctuation, and sentence structure. As José told me once about his experiences editing poorly written papers, readers often become frustrated with the paper (and with the person who wrote it).

The Savvy Academic. Seth J. Schwartz, Oxford University Press. © Oxford University Press 2022.
DOI: 10.1093/oso/9780190095918.003.0007

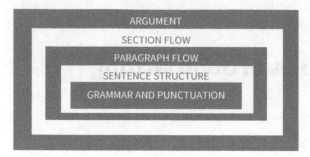

Figure 6.1 Levels of Writing.

(When I review papers—either for colleagues or for journals—I have to stop and correct grammatical and punctuation errors so that I can read the paper properly.)

I have written many papers with colleagues who are not native English speakers, and often part of my role is to correct grammatical mistakes so that the writing is easier to read. I have great respect for anyone who can write in a second language—something I cannot do—but my advice to people who are learning to write in English is to find a native English speaker to edit their drafts and help them improve their grammar. I remember reviewing a manuscript once for a very prominent journal. The paper was written by an author group whose native language was not English. The writing was very choppy, and many words were misused. The authors found a number of significant interaction effects, and they described how they "entangled" those interactions (the word they meant to use was *explored*). Another reviewer slammed the authors for their poor English and used the writing problems as part of their reasoning for recommending rejection. I felt bad for the authors, who were writing in a second language, but I also understood the reviewer's point. It's difficult to grasp the larger message of a paper when the writing is choppy, clumsy, or full of grammatical and syntactical errors.

So let's start with the basics of English sentence structure. Readers whose native language is English may wish to skip this section, although I have encountered many native English speakers whose grammar needs some improvement. In my experience, immigrants and international students are sometimes better writers than people born in the United States, because they don't take English grammar and syntax for granted.

Grammar and Punctuation

Grammar

In terms of grammar, writers must attend to several common issues, such as subject and predicate, subject–verb agreement, noun–pronoun agreement, subject–object pronoun agreement, prepositional phrases, essential and non-essential clauses, and conjunctions (this list is not exhaustive).

Subject and Predicate

In English, every sentence must have a subject and a verb. That is, we must know who or what we are talking about, as well as what that person, place, or thing is doing (or how it is being described). The subject of the sentence is the noun or pronoun that denotes who or what we are referring to, and the predicate is the part of the sentence that contains the verb and tells us what the subject is doing or how the subject is being described.

There are two general types of sentences—action sentences and descriptive sentences. In an action sentence, the subject is doing something. For example, anyone who learned to type probably knows the sentence "The quick brown fox jumped over the lazy dog." (That sentence is used to teach typing because it uses every letter in the alphabet.) In this sentence, "the quick brown fox" is the subject—the fox is what we are referring to in the sentence, along with adjectives that describe the fox. "Jumped over the lazy dog" is the predicate, because it tells us what the fox is doing, has already done, or will do.

Descriptive sentences often use forms of the verb *to be*. In these sentences, the predicate is used to describe the subject. For example, in the sentence "Your mother is very nice," your mother is the subject of the sentence, and the predicate tells us that she is very nice. Descriptive sentences can also use verbs like *seem*, *look*, or *appear*—for example, "The sun looks larger when it is rising or setting than at other times during the day." (Notice that *seems* or *appears* could have been used in this sentence as well.)

In simple sentences, it's easy to ensure that both the subject and the predicate are present—but in more complex sentences, it can be somewhat more difficult to ensure that all of the components appear in the correct places. Sometimes we can mistake a clause for the predicate, and the result is a sentence fragment (where either the subject or the predicate is missing).

In some romance languages, such as Spanish and Italian, the subject of the sentence is sometimes omitted because the form of the verb tells us what the subject is (e.g., verbs are conjugated differently for first, second, and third person, and differently for singular versus plural subjects). In English, verbs often have only two forms within a given tense—for example, in the present tense, the verb *think* has only two forms, namely *think* for first-person, second-person, and third-person plural subjects, and *thinks* for third-person singular subjects. As a result, the subject must always be written out. (The only exception is command sentences, where *you* is assumed—for example, "Take this to the kitchen" means "You take this to the kitchen.")

Subject–Verb Agreement

The form (singular or plural) of the subject of a sentence must agree with the form of the verb. For example, we say "the man assumes" and "the men assume." Subject–verb agreement also applies to pronouns—in general, third-person singular pronouns (*he, she, it*) are accompanied by singular verbs, and most other pronouns are accompanied by plural verbs. As already stated, these rules are easy to follow in simple sentences, and easier to violate in more complex sentences.

Clauses are discussed later in this section, but when there is a clause in a sentence, subject–verb agreement should be evaluated as though the clause was not present. For example, let's consider the following sentence:

My friends, who live down the street, are from another country.

The clause "who live down the street" is not included when we select the correct form of the verb.

Noun–Pronoun Agreement

When we replace a noun with a pronoun, the form of the pronoun needs to match the form of the noun it is replacing. For example, when we are referring to multiple people, places, or things who are neither the speaker nor the audience, we use *they*—and in most cases, when we are referring to a single person who is not the speaker or the audience, we use *he* or *she*. The word *it* is used only to refer to places, things, and nonhuman animals—we do not use *it* to refer to people. (I have seen newborn babies referred to as *it*, but this usage does not comport with any writing style that I know of.)

When we are referring to a general case, pronoun use becomes tricky. Technically, if we are referring to a single hypothetical person, the rules of English grammar dictate that we must use *she* or *he* as the pronoun. In recent years, *they* has become acceptable in this situation. For example, traditionally a sentence would have been written like this:

When a person comes to see you, she or he must come to your desk, give you her or his name, and start filling out the forms that you give her or him.

Some people have begun to write this sentence like this:

When a person comes to see you, they must come to your desk, give you their name, and start filling out the forms that you give them.

My solution has generally been to pluralize the sentence:

When people come to see you, they must come to your desk, give you their names, and start filling out the forms that you give them.

Pluralizing sentences allows us to avoid having to decide whether to use singular or plural pronouns to refer to a single hypothetical person. Because English does not have a third-person singular pronoun that is appropriate for use with people, the singular form of the sentence often either reads clumsily or appears to be grammatically incorrect. Pluralizing has been my solution to this problem.

Subject–Object Pronoun Agreement

Except within phrases and clauses, pronouns serving as the subject of the sentence should be subject pronouns (*I*, *he*, *she*, *we*, *they*), and pronouns appearing in the predicate should be object pronouns (*me*, *him*, *her*, *us*, *them*). (An exception is descriptive sentences, where subject pronouns in used in the predicate—such as "It is I.") Confusion sometimes occurs when multiple pronouns are used in a sentence. Take a look at the two sentences below, both of which use pronouns incorrectly:

Him and I are going to the store together.
Between you and I, he will never get this job.

The first sentence uses an object pronoun and a subject pronoun together in the subject of the sentence. The correct form is "He and I are going to the store together." The second sentence uses a subject pronoun in a prepositional phrase (object pronouns should generally follow a preposition). The correct form is "Between you and me, he will never get this job."

Prepositional Phrases

A prepositional phrase is a group of words that starts with a preposition (such as *with*, *between*, *from*, *through*, or *without*) and ends with a noun or pronoun. The purpose of a prepositional phrase is to clarify the meaning of the subject or predicate. To illustrate the importance of prepositional phrases, let's look at a hypothetical sentence both with and without prepositional phrases in the subject and predicate (prepositional phrases are underlined).

With: The man <u>from human resources</u> came to see you <u>with some forms</u>.
Without: The man came to see you.

Without the prepositional phrases, we don't know who the man is or why he came to see us. Prepositional phrases become problematic when several of them appear in a row. Sentences can quickly become confusing:

We need to visit the post office <u>with the letter from the lady from the place with the building under the tree around the corner from the library</u>.

This sentence contains seven prepositional phrases in a row! Yes, we need to know what we need to bring to the post office, but by the time we finish reading the sentence, we may be more confused than when we started.

My recommendation is that no more than three prepositional phrases appear consecutively. The reader needs time to take a breath and digest the sentence. If more information is needed, we can add another sentence.

We can take the above sentence—with the seven prepositional phrases—and make it clearer by breaking the sentence up into multiple sentences:

We need to visit the post office <u>with the letter from the lady</u> we met earlier. She was <u>from a company with an office in a tall building</u>. The building is <u>under the tree near the library</u>.

Notice that we are using more words, but the meaning is clearer.

Clauses

A clause is a group of words, usually starting with *that, which, who,* or *where,* that describes the noun, pronoun, adjective, or adverb that the clause follows. Clauses can appear in the subject of a sentence, or in the predicate, or in both.

There are two types of clauses—essential and nonessential. An essential clause would change the meaning of the sentence if it were removed:

With: We are standing in the place where your father was born.
Without: We are standing in the place.

When the clause is not included, we have no idea what place is being referenced. So the clause is essential. Essential clauses generally begin with *that* if they refer to inanimate objects, *who* or *whom* if they refer to people, *when* if they refer to time, and *where* if they refer to specific locations. Essential clauses generally do not begin with *which* unless we are trying to avoid ending a sentence with a preposition. (There is more below about how to avoid ending a sentence with a preposition.)

In contrast, a nonessential clause is one that does not change the meaning of the sentence if it is removed:

With: My aunt, whom you met last year, invited us over for dinner.
Without: My aunt invited us over for dinner.

In this case, even when the clause is removed, we still know that my aunt is inviting us for dinner. So the clause is nonessential. Nonessential clauses generally begin with *which* when referring to inanimate objects, *who* or *whom* when referring to people, *when* when referring to time, and *where* when referring to locations. Nonessential clauses do not begin with *that*.

Importantly, nonessential clauses are set off from the rest of the sentence with commas. Essential clauses are not set off with commas. (Proper use of commas is covered later in this chapter.)

It is also possible to combine clauses with prepositional phrases—and when we do this in formal writing, we must ensure that the clause or sentence does not end with a preposition. We can do this by moving the preposition to the beginning of the clause. For example:

Incorrect: She is the one who you went to the game with.
Correct: She is the one with whom you went to the game.

Keep in mind that, when we use this kind of structure, *who* becomes *whom*. (*Whom* is the object reference, and *who* is the subject reference, when we are referring to people.) Additionally, when we move a preposition to the beginning of a clause, *that* becomes *which*. For example:

Incorrect: This is the book *that* you were referring to.
Correct: This is the book to *which* you were referring.

Also, remember that clauses should not be considered when evaluating subject–verb and noun–pronoun agreement. For example:
The coach for whom they played is one of the best in the state.
In this example, notice that *the coach*—not *they*—is the subject of the sentence, so the verb needs to be singular. The principle would be the same if the clause were nonessential and set off with commas.

Clauses should appear as close as possible to the word that they are describing. When the clause is further away from the word it is describing, the meaning can be unclear. For example, read the following two sentences:

- The participant, who was recruited from a clinic, came to our office.
- The participant came to our office, who was recruited from a clinic.

In the first sentence, it is clear that the participant was recruited from a clinic. However, in the second sentence, it appears that our office may have been recruited from a clinic—which is probably impossible. When a clause appears at the end of a sentence but it is not clear what it is describing, the result is a *dangling participle*. Dangling participles should be corrected.

Articles
One of the most confusing features of the English language, especially for speakers of non-Romance and non-Germanic languages, is the use of articles (*a*, *an*, and *the*). Colleagues of mine from Russia, Georgia, China, Korea, and other parts of the world have expressed their puzzlement over when they should use articles and when they should not.

In general, for singular nouns, articles are needed provided that the noun can be pluralized. For example, if we are referring to a singular lion, we would use *the lion* or *a lion*—because there can be more than one lion. However, if we are referring to outer space, we would not need an article because there is only one "outer space." Similarly, if we are referring to "science" in general, we do not need an article; but if we are using "science" to refer to an individual scientific discipline such as chemistry or physics, we would need an article. Take a look at these two sentences:

- Science is the empirical study of natural phenomena.
- A science is defined by the specific phenomena on which it focuses.

Plural nouns do not need an article unless we are referring to a specific set of items. For example:

General: Sports are an enjoyable distraction and a way to stay fit.
Specific: The sports I enjoy most are baseball and basketball.

So when do we use *a* or *an*, and when do we use *the*? If we are referring to a general case, we use *a* or *an*. If we are referring to a specific item, we use *the*. For example:

General: A star is needed to provide light and heat to planets.
Specific: Our Sun is the star that provides Earth with light and heat.

Split Infinitives

Unlike many other languages, in English the infinitive (i.e., root or stem) of a verb consists of two words (e.g., *to be*, *to want*). However, for grammatical purposes, the infinitive is viewed as a single word. As a result, it is grammatically incorrect to place another word in the middle of the infinitive. When such an additional word is included in the middle of an infinitive, the result is called a *split infinitive*. Split infinitives should not appear in formal writing. Here is an example:

Incorrect: We want to definitely bring this study to a close.
Correct: We definitely want to bring this study to a close.

Conjunctions

The words *and*, *or*, and *but* are often used to connect two sentences within a complex sentence. For example:

- We are waiting for you, and if you don't come soon, we are going to leave.
- You should hand in your homework, or you will fail the course.
- She was happy with her new car, but she really wanted a manual transmission.

Note that we use a comma before the conjunction when the conjunction is used to separate two sentences.

In formal writing, we do not start a sentence with a conjunction. Use *further* or *also* in place of *and*, use *alternatively* or *on the other hand* in place of *or*, and use *however* or *nonetheless* in place of *but*. For example:

Incorrect: He called me to say that he was not coming. And he was not happy that he was not able to make it.
Correct: He called me to say that he was not coming. Further, he was not happy that he was not able to make it.
Incorrect: We thought of going to the restaurant. Or we could just order something to go.
Correct: We thought of going to the restaurant. Alternatively, we could just order something to go.
Incorrect: Her mother was always very nice. But this time she was angry.
Correct: Her mother was always very nice. However, this time she was angry.

Note that *like* is not a conjunction. In fact, I discourage use of *like* unless it is used as a verb (e.g., "participants were asked whether they liked the task"). For other uses of *like*, use *such as* instead. For example:

Incorrect: I have been to many Asian countries, like Korea and Japan.
Correct: I have been to many Asian countries, such as Korea and Japan.

If and *Whether*

Both *if* and *whether* are conditional words—that is, they reference a situation where something is possible but not definite. In general, *if* is used in the subject of a sentence, whereas *whether* is used in the predicate. There are some important exceptions that I note below. Meanwhile, here are common examples of how *if* and *whether* can be used correctly:

Subject: If the participant decided to take part in the study, we would ask for signed consent.
Predicate: Participants were asked to decide whether they wanted to take part in the study.

In general, *if* should not appear in the predicate. However, look at the following two sentences, and note that the meaning is quite different depending on whether we use *if* or *whether* in the predicate:

- Let us know *whether* you need our help.
- Let us know *if* you need our help.

In the first sentence, we are asking the other person to answer a Yes or No question—Do you need our help? The second sentence is more tentative—we are asking the person to reach out to us only if our help is needed. So sometimes we can use *if* in the predicate to denote a more tentative situation, or that we will not do anything unless the other person indicates that we are needed.

We can also use *whether* as the first word in an essential clause—and in this case, the clause serves as the subject or predicate of the sentence. For example:

Subject: Whether or not you need our help should be something that you decide on your own.
Predicate: You need to decide whether you need our help.

Note that *if* should not be used as the first word in a clause. In cases where you may want to use *if* as the first word in a clause, use *whether* instead.

Further, sometimes *whether* can be used on its own, and in other cases it may make more sense to use *whether or not*.

Of and *From*

As my Colombian colleague often says, English grammar can be devilish. A primary example of this confusion is the use of the prepositions *of* and *from*. In many languages, *of* and *from* are the same word—and in English, *of* and *from* can sometimes be used interchangeably. *Of* can sometimes be used as a synonym for *among*, especially as the first word in a sentence. However, *of* often reads clumsily when it appears as the first word in a sentence. I suggest *among* instead. For example:

> *Clumsy*: Of the 100 participants in our study, 76 were born outside the United States.
> *Clearer*: Among the 100 participants in our study, 76 were born outside the United States.

I suggest using *from* rather than *of* when you are describing something that was requested from someone:

> *Clumsy*: Nothing further was asked of the participants in our study.
> *Clearer*: Nothing further was requested from the participants in our study.

Reveal and *Show*

Reveal and *show* are two of my "pet peeve" words when they are used in describing or interpreting results. The word *reveal* means to uncover something that was previously hidden, and the word *show* is overused and has many different meanings. I almost always delete or replace these words when I edit manuscript or grant proposal drafts. I don't like these words because they do not accurately explain what the results have done. Results can indicate, suggest, or illustrate something—but they cannot reveal anything. If I move the curtains covering my window to reveal the daylight outside, then what is happening? The light was previously blocked from view, but once the curtains are moved, the light becomes visible. However, when I conduct a set of analyses and interpret the results, is anything uncovered that was previously blocked from view?

Although *show* has many meanings, we can explore what may be the closest meaning to what our results are doing for us. When a real estate agent shows you a house, the agent is guiding you around the house and explaining its features. Results don't do anything analogous to this—the results emerge, and we interpret them. Results can suggest or indicate something, but they cannot show anything. For example:

Clumsy: Results revealed that brain activity was related to anxiety.
Clumsy: Results showed that brain activity was related to anxiety.
Clearer: Results indicated that brain activity was related to anxiety.

While and *Since*

Two words that are often misused in scientific writing are *while* and *since*. The word *while* denotes multiple events that are occurring, occurred, or will occur at the same time. Here are two examples (with *while* italicized):

- *While* I was cleaning the stove, she was mopping the floor.
- We conducted our study *while* they were collecting their data.

While is often used as a synonym for *although* or *whereas*—but this usage of *while* is incorrect. Take a look at these two sentences in which *while* is used incorrectly:

- While discrimination has been widely studied, context of reception has been largely overlooked as a cultural stressor.
- The study of free will often focuses on how people make choices, while the study of determinism focuses on how biological or environmental factors influence people's behavior.

Below, these two sentences are rewritten with *although* or *whereas* in place of *while*.

- Although discrimination has been widely studied, context of reception has been largely overlooked as a cultural stressor.
- The study of free will often focuses on how people make choices, whereas the study of determinism focuses on how biological or environmental factors influence people's behavior.

The word *since* is used to refer to events that have occurred following the event that is referenced in the sentence. For example:

Since my father moved out, everyone has been depressed.

The word *since* is sometimes used as a synonym for *because*, but this usage is not correct. For example:

Incorrect: Since discrimination is not synonymous with context of reception, the two terms should not be used interchangeably.

Correct: Because discrimination is not synonymous with context of reception, the two terms should not be used interchangeably.

So, *while* and *since* should only be used with reference to time. If the reference is to something other than time, use *whereas* or *although* in place of *while*, and use *because* or *given that* in place of *since*.

Than Versus *Compared to*

The word *than* is used to indicate a comparison between or among items. However, in some cases, the comparison becomes ambiguous. For example:

Men are more skilled at this game than women.

Does this sentence mean that men are more skilled than women at the game, or does it mean that they are more skilled at the game than they are at women?

My solution in this case is to replace *than* with *compared to*:

Men are more skilled at this game compared to women.

Or, alternatively:

Compared to women, men are more skilled at this game.

This and *That* as Indefinite References

Using *this* or *that* (as well as their respective plurals, *these* and *those*) without a descriptor can be confusing because it is often unclear what the word is referencing. For example:

This is a problem.

Reading this sentence does not tell us what precisely the problem is. Even if the problem was specified in the previous sentence, we should not assume that the reader will know what *this* means. The solution is often simply to replace *this* or *that* with a more precise descriptor. For example:

Our lack of communication is a problem.

There Is Sentence Structure

In sentences that start with "There is . . . ," it is often unclear what the subject and predicate are. In my opinion, *there is* sentences should be rephrased with a clearer subject and predicate. For example:

- *Less Clear*: There is another way to solve this problem.
- *Clearer*: This problem can be solved another way.

Avoiding Too Many Ands

Sometimes it is difficult to follow a sentence where the word *and* appears too many times. Here are two examples:

- We were interested in the relationship between brain functioning and behavior and perception.
- Our study investigated acculturation and cultural stress and was focused on first-generation immigrants.

In the first sentence, the word *between* is used, suggesting that two items would follow—but instead three items appear. So we don't know what the *between* is referencing. Are we comparing brain functioning to behavior and perception, or are we comparing brain functioning and behavior to perception?

I use the *of . . . with* structure to resolve this confusion. The *between* is replaced with *of*, and one of the *and*s is replaced by *with*. For example, if we are comparing brain functioning to both behavior and perception, we might say:

We were interested in the relationship of brain functioning with behavior and perception.

Notice how the *of . . . with* structure clarifies the meaning of the sentence.

In the second example, we would use a comma and a multiple-sentence structure to resolve the confusion. We want to make clear that the study examined acculturation and cultural stress, as well as that it was conducted among first-generation immigrants. We might rewrite as follows:

Our study investigated acculturation and cultural stress, and the study was focused on first-generation immigrants.

So the comma makes clear what each *and* is connecting.

Anthropomorphisms

An anthropomorphism is a scenario where an inanimate object is framed as doing something that only a person or group of people can do. For example:

> The current study sought to examine the link between anxiety and depression.

This sentence needs to be reworded because a study cannot seek to do anything. It needs to be clear that we, the investigators, are the ones who sought to examine this link:

> In the current study, we sought to examine the link between anxiety and depression.

We need to be sure that a human (or group of humans) is the subject to which human actions are attributed.

Run-On Sentences

A general principle is that, if a sentence takes up more than two full lines of text (not including citations), it is too long and should be broken up. For example, consider the following sentence:

> Immigrants are often confronted with discrimination, and they need to become resilient, and they can lean on their families, and they must learn to navigate the destination country's systems of work, housing, banking, and other critical domains of functioning.

We could easily break this single sentence up into three or four sentences.

> Immigrants are often confronted with discrimination. They need to become resilient, and they can lean on their families. They must also learn to navigate the destination country's systems of work, housing, banking, and other critical domains of functioning.

If a sentence seems overly complex, it probably is. It never hurts to break up a longer, more complex sentence into two or more simpler sentences.

Use of *e.g.* and *i.e.*

When items are listed in parentheses, we may not want to (or may not be able to) list all of the items. This is where the abbreviation *e.g.* (short for *exempli gratia*, which means "for example") is used. We list examples of items, but the list is not exhaustive. For example:

> Some European countries (e.g., France, Germany, Italy, the United Kingdom) have fast and efficient rail systems that reduce the need to drive.

Notice that, with *e.g.*, we do not use *and* before the last item—because the list is not exhaustive.

When we are listing all possible items, or when we are using a parenthetical note to clarify what we mean, we use *i.e.* (short for *id est*, which means "that is"). With *i.e.*, the word *and* is included before the final item because the list is exhaustive. For example:

> The three North American countries (i.e., Canada, the United States, and Mexico) entered into their first trade agreement in 1993.

Use of *et cetera*

Sometimes we are writing out a list, and we don't want to list all of the items. When we think that the reader will know what we mean even if we stop listing more items, we can use *et cetera*. Sometimes, *et cetera* is abbreviated as *etc.*, but I do not generally use this abbreviation. I don't use *etc.* because the *et cetera* often appears at the end of a sentence, and using *etc.* at the end of a sentence either would require two consecutive periods (which looks strange) or would create confusion regarding whether the *etc.* is the end of the sentence. Look at this example:

> Graduate students must engage in a lot of mundane tasks, including literature reviews, compiling references, creating grant budgets for their advisors, etc. These tasks can take quite a bit of patience.

Because *etc.* ends with a period and the sentence is also supposed to end with a period, we don't know whether the *etc.* is the last word in the sentence. We therefore do not know whether the next word should be capitalized. It would be clearer to write:

> Graduate students must engage in a lot of mundane tasks, including literature reviews, compiling references, creating grant budgets for their advisors, et cetera. These tasks can take quite a bit of patience.

Numbers

The final grammatical issue involves how numbers are written in journal manuscripts. In general, numbers below 10 should be written as words (e.g., three, six), whereas numbers 10 or greater should be written as numbers (e.g., 20, 517). Numbers below 10 can be written as numbers if they are written along with larger numbers. For example:

- *Comparison or Enumeration*: Participants included 6 men and 15 women.
- *No Comparison or Enumeration*: The sample was comprised of seven participants.

Additionally, if a number is the first word in a sentence, it must be written as a word rather than as a number. When a more complex number (especially numbers above 100) would be the first word in a sentence, I advise inserting additional words in front of the number so that the complex number doesn't have to be written as a word. For example:

Clumsy: Six hundred forty-three people were recruited for the study.
Clearer: A total of 643 people were recruited for the study.

Punctuation

With regard to punctuation, the discussion here covers commas, periods, apostrophes, colons, semicolons, question marks, and exclamation points.

Commas

Commas are used for the following reasons:

- To separate nonessential clauses or appositive phrases from the rest of the sentence
- To separate items within a list
- To separate sentences that are joined with a conjunction
- Following prepositional phrases that appear at the beginning of a sentence (e.g., "From start to finish, this was the best race I have ever run")
- After introductory words like *However*, *Nevertheless*, and the like (e.g., "Nevertheless, the study was a success."). When *however* falls at the end of a sentence, a comma should placed before the word (e.g., "The study did appear to succeed, however.").

Importantly, commas should not appear following a verb unless the verb is part of a list (e.g., "I wrote, edited, and submitted the paper myself"). We would not say "He biked, to the office." Generally, a comma is used whenever we would pause if we were reading the sentence aloud.

An important note involving commas relates to the *Oxford (serial) comma*. The Oxford comma is a comma inserted before the final item in a list. Some writers use the Oxford comma, but others do not. Here is how sentences look with and without the Oxford comma:

With: We drove, ran, and biked in the park.
Without: We drove, ran and biked in the park.

In simple sentences, it does not appear to matter whether the Oxford comma is used. However, in some more complex sentences, using the Oxford comma can help to clarify the meaning:

With: Participants wrote, spoke, and typed and then proceeded to read what they had typed.
Without: Participants wrote, spoke and typed and then proceeded to read what they had typed.

Without the Oxford comma, we appear to encounter the "too many *ands*" problem. My preference is always to use the Oxford comma. Note, however, that different forms of English differ in terms of whether the Oxford comma is acceptable or common. For example, American English sometimes uses the Oxford comma, but British English almost never uses it, except when the sentence would be ambiguous without it.

Periods

Generally, a period appears at the end of each sentence. The period tells us that the thought has been completed and that we can "take a breath" before moving on to the next sentence. (Important: A comma cannot be used to mark the end of a sentence.)

In American English (but not British English), periods are used at the end of some abbreviations, such as *Mr.* (Mister), *Mrs.* (Missus), *Prof.* (Professor), and *St.* (Street). Importantly, these abbreviations are only used when referring to a specific person, road, or other item by name. For example, we might say "I am going to see Dr. Lopez," but "I am going to see the doctor." In the first example, we are naming the specific doctor, but in the second example, we are not naming the doctor (and therefore we do not use the abbreviation).

Also in American English—but not in British English—periods are sometimes used in degree designations, such as *Ph.D.*, *M.D.*, and *M.S.W.* These degree designations can be used with or without the periods—so both *PhD* and *Ph.D.* are correct.

Apostrophes

Apostrophes are used for three general reasons—to denote possession, to replace letters within a contraction, and, as single quotation marks, to place a quotation within another quotation. Each use is reviewed here.

To denote possession, for a singular noun (including nouns that end in *s*), simply add *'s* to the end of the noun. So *fox* becomes *fox's*, *person* becomes *person's*, and *fuss* becomes *fuss's*. For plural nouns that end in *s*, place an apostrophe after the *s* at the end of the word. So, *snakes* becomes *snakes'*. For plural nouns that do not end in *s*, add *'s* to the end of the word. So, *people* becomes *people's*, and *children* becomes *children's*.

For contractions, replace the missing letters with an apostrophe. The most commonly contracted words are *not* (e.g., *do not* becomes *don't*), *have* (e.g., *would have* becomes *would've*), *had* (e.g., *I had* becomes *I'd*), and *are* (e.g., *you are* becomes *you're*). Importantly, there is no contraction for "am not."

Finally, single quotation marks (apostrophes) are used with a quotation inside of another quotation. For example:

> My father said "I don't want you coming home and telling me 'Dad, I forgot about my curfew.' I don't believe that."

In this case, the father's quote is embedded within the speaker's larger quote. Remember that apostrophes are not used to signify plurals. For example:

> *Incorrect*: We made sure to visit all the house's.
> *Correct*: We made sure to visit all the houses.

Quotation Marks

Quotation marks are used to separate a direct quote from the rest of the sentence. Quotation marks are generally used for quotes that are less than one full sentence long. For example (this quote is fictitious):

> Waterman (2008, p. 154) noted that "happiness is inherently subjective, and its measurement must reflect that subjectivity."

When material quoted directly from a source appears in a manuscript, we must provide the page number where the quoted material appears in the source.

Longer quotations (more than a full sentence) should appear as *block quotes*—moved to a separate line, presented in smaller font, and with all lines of the block quote indented. No quotation marks are used when a block quote is presented.

For example (this quote is also fictitious):

Smith (2013, pp. 204–205) has expanded on this topic in greater depth:
When groups come into contact with one another, there is often an inherent suspicion that decreases as individual group members come into contact with one another. It is this personal contact that allows for intergroup anxiety to be overcome.

It is also possible to include only parts of the source material in a quotation. In this case, ellipses (three spaced ellipsis points) are used to indicate that some text has been omitted from the quotation. For example (this quote is fictitious):

Hong (2018, p. 528) observed that "biomedical treatments for anxiety are often ineffective . . . without co-occurring counseling or therapy."

Notice that, when a clause or sentence ends with a quotation mark, the period or comma should be placed inside the closing quotation mark. Question marks and exclamation points should appear outside the quotation mark unless they are part of the material being quoted.

Colons and Semicolons

Colons (:) and semicolons (;) are used for very specific purposes. Colons are used to signify that a list is coming (e.g., "The attendees were:"). Colons are also used in a dialogue to indicate who is speaking. For example, consider this fictitious dialogue between a mother and daughter:

MOTHER: I have been worrying about you.
DAUGHTER: Why?
MOTHER: You have been coming home very late, and I never know where you are.
DAUGHTER: My friend has been very depressed, and I've gone to help her. I'm sorry for not telling you.
MOTHER: From now on, can we please communicate better?
DAUGHTER: Yes.

Semicolons are used to separate sentences that have been joined together without a conjunction, to separate items in a list when one or more of the items has a comma embedded in it, or to signify the end of each item within a list (where each item is listed on a separate line). Here are examples of using semicolons to join sentences and to separate items in an enumerated list:

> *Joining Sentences*: We usually go away during the summer; this year, we are going to Hong Kong.
> *Separating Items in a List*: The rules prohibit running; smoking, chewing, or vaping tobacco products; skateboarding; and using foul language.

A note on using semicolons to join sentences: I suggest not doing this very often. In academic writing, individual sentences tend to be long, so joined sentences are often especially long. I would also never join more than two sentences together using semicolons.

Question Marks and Exclamation Points

Question marks (?) and exclamation points (!) are used very infrequently in formal writing. In some cases, research questions are written out in question form (in which case each item ends with a question mark). Writers may also pose hypothetical or rhetorical questions in their writing, although this occurs infrequently.

Exclamation points are almost never used in formal writing. They may appear in qualitative excerpts where direct quotes from participants are included. On rare occasions, an exclamation point may be used in the title of a manuscript to convey emphasis.

Other Word-Usage Issues

Three additional word-usage issues should receive attention: avoiding overused words, distinguishing between or among homonyms, and varying your language. These issues are important because, although text that violates the principles described here may not be technically incorrect, it may appear clumsier than text that follows the principles. The goal in any type of writing is to communicate as well as possible and to have the writing taken as seriously as possible. Elegant writing—as long as it is understandable and not overly complex—is generally preferable to clumsy writing.

Overused Words

Some words have been used so often that they have lost much of their meaning. These words also tend to have general and broad meanings—if you look up the words *do* or *make* in the dictionary, you will find several different definitions. These words are not precise, and there are often much more appropriate words that can be used to convey the meaning that the authors wish to communicate.

Here is a list—which is by no means exhaustive—of words that I try to avoid using in formal writing because they are overused and imprecise:

- Very
- Good
- Bad
- Better
- Do
- Make
- Get
- Thing

Whenever we think of using one of these words, we should identify the precise meaning we want to communicate and then look for a synonym that conveys that precise meaning. For example, consider the word *better*. This word can be used to convey several meanings—here are some examples with the intended meanings in parentheses:

- Your team is *better* than my team. (More skilled)
- Highways are a *better* way to commute than are surface roads. (More efficient)
- Biomarkers are a *better* way to measure stress than are self-reports. (More accurate)
- Are you feeling *better* now than you were before? (Healthier)

We could create similar lists of uses for the other overused words as well. Therefore, I recommend replacing *better* (or any of the other overused words) with a more precise synonym—and I generally avoid using *better* in formal writing.

Distinguishing Between and Among Homonyms

Homonyms are words that sound alike or are spelled the same but have different meanings. For example, if we were walking down the street and we saw a store with a sign that read "POLISH," we would not know whether the store specialized in polishing nails or in serving food from Poland.

Other sets of words are often mistaken for one another but have completely different meanings. One such pair of words is *compliment* and *complement*. If I give someone a *compliment*, I am saying something positive about that person. On the other hand, if two measures *complement* one another, they fit together and compensate for one another's weaknesses. Similarly, *accept* and *except* are pronounced the same, but the former is a verb and the latter is a preposition, a conjunction, and a verb. If I *accept* a paper for publication, I am happy with it and regard it as finalized. On the other hand, if I say that every-thing was satisfactory *except* the kitchen, then I am saying that the kitchen was the only item about which I am complaining.

Another pair of words that are often confused are *effect* and *affect*. In most cases, *effect* is a noun that refers to the impact of something on something else. *Affect* has two primary meanings: (a) as a verb meaning "to influence or change something," and (b) as a synonym for emotion or emotional valence. The most general meanings of *effect* and *affect* are quite similar—if variable A *affects* variable B, then variable A has an *effect* on variable B. In this example, *affect* is a verb and *effect* is a noun.

There are several other homonym pairs whose meanings are quite dif-ferent: (a) *censor* is a verb meaning "to cut off" and *sensor* is a noun referring to a device that detects something; (b) *principal* is either a noun referring to the director of a school or an adjective meaning "primary" or "most im-portant," and *principle* is a noun referring to a value, rule, or ideal; (c) *dis-crete* is an adjective meaning "bounded" or "sectioned off from something else," and *discreet* is an adjective meaning "not emphasized" or "communi-cated carefully"; (d) *your* is the possessive form of *you*, and *you're* is a con-traction for *you are*; (e) *its* is the possessive form of *it*, and *it's* is a contraction for *it is*; (f) *allusion* is a noun meaning "reference" or "indirect statement," and *illusion* is a noun referring to a visual effect that does not actually exist; (g) *personal* is an adjective referring to something private or that belongs to someone, and *personnel* is a noun referring to employees or members of a group; and (h) *precede* is a verb meaning "to come before," and *proceed* is a verb meaning "to go ahead." Finally, be aware of three words that sound the same—*their* (the possessive form of *they*), *there* (referring to a location), and *they're* (a contraction of *they are*).

Varying Language

One of the first pointers that Dick Dunham gave me about writing was that I should vary my language. That is, if I refer to the same concept twice in the same paragraph, I should use a synonym rather than repeating the word. For example:

> *Word Repeated*: Participants took part in an experiment involving random assignment to one of two conditions. When participants arrived, the experiment began with a set of instructions for them to follow. At the conclusion of the experiment, participants were debriefed regarding the objectives and hypotheses.

> *Varying Language*: Participants took part in research involving random assignment to one of two conditions. When participants arrived, the experiment began with a set of instructions for them to follow. At the conclusion of the study, participants were debriefed regarding the objectives and hypotheses.

Dick's point was that varying our language makes the paper more interesting to read. If we use the word *experiment* four or five times in a paragraph, readers may find this usage repetitious. However, as José taught me later in my career, when we are using terms for specific study constructs, the terms must be used consistently (i.e., not varied) throughout the paper. For example, one of my interests is in adolescent engagement in sexual behaviors that may have harmful long-term consequences, such as HIV and other sexually transmitted diseases. In one paper I wrote, I referred to this construct in various places as "risky sexual behavior," "unsafe sexual behavior," and "sexual risk taking." In his comments on my draft, José asked me whether I was referring to three different constructs. The lesson he was teaching me was that study constructs and other technical items should be referred to using the same term throughout the manuscript. The point is to avoid confusing reviewers and readers unnecessarily.

I think that both Dick and José are right. With regard to ordinary language, we should aim to avoid being repetitive by varying our language. With technical or scientific terms, the same term needs to be used for the same construct throughout the paper. We want our work to be easily readable and not confusing.

Flow Within a Paragraph

So far, the discussion in this chapter has been focused on the building blocks of sentences—grammar, punctuation, and word choices. Now we move on to examine flow between sentences and within a paragraph.

Generally, paragraphs should consist of three to five sentences. Roger Levesque, editor of the *Journal of Youth and Adolescence*, says it best when he advises authors that each paragraph needs an opening sentence that sets up the point of the paragraph, one to three supporting sentences, and a strong concluding sentence to wrap up the paragraph. (Roger has provided this guidance each time I submitted a manuscript to his journal, and the guidance is definitely worth sharing.) In short, each paragraph should have a clear message that is being communicated, and each of the sentences should help to communicate that message.

Sentences within a paragraph should flow together such that there are no "logical leaps" within a sentence. For example, look at these two sentences:

Anxiety is a debilitating psychological condition. We therefore must conduct functional neuroimaging to identify the brain regions that are activated when someone is experiencing a severe anxiety attack.

There is clearly a "piece missing" between these sentences. If we state that anxiety is a debilitating condition, does that necessarily mean that we need to identify the parts of the brain that are implicated in an anxiety attack? We may need to insert an additional sentence between the two sentences to explain why targeting brain functioning may help to alleviate anxiety. Let's take a look at how these sentences might look with the additional sentence inserted (underlined):

Anxiety is a debilitating psychological condition. Brain-based treatments may represent a promising method for reducing anxiety. We therefore must conduct functional neuroimaging to identify the brain regions that are activated when someone is experiencing a severe anxiety attack.

Logical leaps are one problem that can appear within a paragraph—and if there are too many leaps within the paragraph, then the paragraph will be AOTP (all over the place). Clearly, AOTP writing is extremely difficult to read. Imagine trying to follow a bird or insect that is flying all over the place, almost faster than your eyes can track. You would probably get a headache!

I sometimes develop a major headache trying to follow a paper that is full of AOTP writing.

Developing an outline for each paragraph may not be worth the effort unless you are prone to AOTP writing. If you know that you tend to be AOTP when you write, then it may be a good idea to outline each paragraph. What is the point of each sentence? How can we be sure that the point is made fully and completely? For example, let's consider the paragraph on anxiety and brain functioning, and let's quickly outline the themes for five sentences within that paragraph.

1. Anxiety as a debilitating condition
2. Many treatments have been attempted
3. Possibility of brain-based treatments
4. Need to identify the brain regions associated with anxiety
5. Then treatments can target these brain regions

Notice that the final sentence in a paragraph needs to finish the thought so that we can start a new thought in the next paragraph. When I was in graduate school, I had a lot of trouble finishing my thoughts. My wife was a huge help in solving that problem—she offered to edit one of my drafts for me, and she spent almost a month marking it up with her red pen. By far, her most common comment was "Finish this thought! Where is this idea going?" The first time I looked at her marked copy of my paper, I shook my head in amazement. She was 100% correct—and her comments helped me to overcome a huge obstacle I had been facing as a writer.

So I will pass this lesson on to you. When you finish each paragraph, ask yourself whether the thought has been completely expressed. In Roger Levesque's words, do you have a strong concluding sentence to wrap up the thought? If not, add a wrap-up sentence to your paragraph.

Let me show you an example of a paragraph with lots of unfinished thoughts, and with bracketed, italicized notes for why the thoughts are unfinished:

The ways in which people develop a sense of identity carry important implications for adult functioning. {*Why? What are the implications?*} Adulthood is a time of life when people must make a series of decisions that will dictate the life course. {*What are these decisions? Give examples.*} It is therefore essential to provide resources to help young people to develop a coherent and workable sense of identity. {*OK, but what would these resources look like? Some examples or parameters are needed here.*}

In this paragraph, we don't have an AOTP problem—but we have an unfinished thought problem. If we say that identity has important implications for adult functioning, then we need to tell the reader what we mean. What kinds of implications are we suggesting? If we mention that resources are needed, we need to be specific and provide examples. Unfinished thoughts are a common problem among young writers—so learning to recognize unfinished thoughts and to fill in the gaps is essential to improving the quality of your writing.

In addition, logical leaps are emblematic of both AOTP and unfinished-thought writing. The primary difference is that, in the AOTP case, the logic spins off in different directions unexpectedly without sentences to complete the connection—whereas in the unfinished thought case, the line of logic ends prematurely. Another common writing problem within a paragraph is distractions, where extraneous text appears and diverts the reader's attention away from the main point of the paragraph. Two primary types of distractions are covered here—interesting tidbits and sidebars.

An *interesting tidbit* is a piece of factual information that is not necessary to include. For example, in an article about epidemiology, saying that "John Snow founded the discipline of epidemiology in the 19th century" is interesting, but it is unnecessary. Readers do not need to know about John Snow to be able to understand the message of your paper. Indeed, the note about John Snow may be distracting for readers, and it should be removed.

Some interesting tidbits involve references to classic thinkers, whereas others can be statements supported by citations. What makes a statement an interesting tidbit is that it is out of place and "sticks out like a sore thumb." In most cases, the solution is simply to remove the interesting tidbit from the paragraph. Some minor rewriting may be necessary so that the paragraph flows well after the tidbit sentence is removed.

A *sidebar* is a longer string of text—perhaps an entire paragraph—that is out of place in the paper and that distracts from the flow of ideas. For example, in an introductory section focused on behavioral treatments for anxiety, a paragraph on brain imaging would be a sidebar. If a paragraph starts out in one direction but then changes direction in the middle, then the sentences at the end of the paragraph are probably a sidebar. For example:

Immigrants have been coming to North America since before the American Revolution. The first major wave of immigrants was the Irish in the 18th century. Scandinavian and German immigrants followed in the early to mid 19th century. A large wave of Southern and Eastern Europeans arrived in the United States and

Canada during the late 19th and early 20th centuries. It is noteworthy that these waves of immigration largely bypassed the U.S. South. Indeed, the South has been largely ethnically homogenous since it was originally colonized in the 17th century. Many Southerners can trace their ancestry directly to the British Isles.

This paragraph is about immigration, but then it switches to focus on the U.S. South. Assuming that the paper is about immigration (and not about the South), the information about the South is a sidebar and can be removed. If the paper is about recent immigration to the South, then information about the South should appear in a different paragraph—and perhaps under a different heading—from the information about earlier waves of immigration.

Similar to sidebars are "sharp turns," where the topic of the paper switches suddenly and without warning. Sharp turns may be the result of sidebars that are carried over into the subsequent text, such that the writer forgets about the original intent of the paper and starts writing about something else. Fixing a sharp turn often involves rewriting whole paragraphs, because sidebar text is not related to the purpose and theme of the paper. For example, let's say that we continued writing about the U.S. South in the next paragraph, even though the paper is about immigration (and not about the South). The topic of the South would represent a sharp turn and would have to be removed and rewritten.

Flow Between Paragraphs

Assuming that we are able to organize each paragraph so that the text flows well and so that each paragraph presents a coherent argument, we still must address the issue of flow between paragraphs. That is, the argument needs to progress in a continuous, linear fashion. If paragraphs don't fit well together, we may be AOTP.

Writing within an outline will likely help to maximize flow between paragraphs. Knowing where we are planning to go in each section of the paper will suggest what content needs to appear in what order. Nonetheless, we still need to be sure to avoid the AOTP and logical-leap issues. Sometimes, a piece is missing between two paragraphs. To solve this problem, we need to follow one of three steps: (1) insert text at the end of the first paragraph so that it sets up the second paragraph more clearly, (2) insert text at the beginning of the second paragraph so that it connects more clearly to the first paragraph, or (3) write a new paragraph between the first and second paragraphs so that the logical leap is filled in. We can also use a combination of two or more of these possibilities.

Let's look at an example where we have a logical leap between two paragraphs, and we will experiment with ways to fill in the leap:

> Gun violence is a major public health problem in the United States. Each year, nearly 40,000 people die from gun-related injuries. Although the majority of these deaths are suicides, homicides comprise 37% of gun-related deaths in the United States—or nearly 15,000 gun-related homicides per year. It is therefore urgent that policies be enacted to protect people from gun violence.
>
> The National Rifle Association (NRA) is funded largely by gun owners and gun-rights activists. The NRA has been advised to consider the impact of its policies on the welfare and lives of U.S. residents, but it has declined to do so. Indeed, the NRA has remained silent as people have been shot to death in schools, houses of worship, shopping malls, and elsewhere. Through its silence and refusal to advocate for stricter gun laws, the NRA's positions on gun violence have contributed to this epidemic.

In this case, the first paragraph is about rates of gun violence, and the second paragraph is about the NRA. There is clearly a piece missing between the two paragraphs. So we need to decide how to fill in that missing piece. The first step here is to determine what the missing piece is, and then we can decide whether it warrants a full paragraph versus one or two connecting sentences attached to one of the existing paragraphs.

As an exercise, let's try all three strategies. First, let's try adding two sentences at the end of the first paragraph (the new sentences are underlined):

> Gun violence is a major public health problem in the United States. Each year, nearly 40,000 people die from gun-related injuries. Although the majority of these deaths are suicides, homicides comprise 37% of gun-related deaths in the United States—or nearly 15,000 gun-related homicides per year. It is therefore urgent that policies be enacted to protect people from gun violence. These policies require buy-in and endorsement not only from gun-control activists, but also from law-abiding gun owners and gun-rights activists. Buy-in from gun owners and gun-rights activists would help to assure law-abiding gun owners that their Second Amendment rights are not under threat.
>
> The National Rifle Association (NRA) is funded largely by gun owners and gun-rights activists. The NRA has been advised to consider the impact of its policies on the welfare and lives of U.S. residents, but it has declined to do so. Indeed, the NRA

has remained silent as people have been shot to death in schools, houses of worship, shopping malls, and elsewhere. Through its silence and refusal to advocate for stricter gun laws, the NRA's positions on gun violence have contributed to this epidemic.

Does adding these two sentences solve the problem? It appears that adding these sentences now introduces a contradiction between the paragraphs, as we are arguing for buy-in from gun owners and activists in the first paragraph but blaming these same people for the gun-violence epidemic in the second paragraph.

So let's try keeping the two new sentences in the first paragraph and then adding some new sentences in the second paragraph. Some rewriting may be necessary in the second paragraph to remove contradictions and improve flow, but we will hold off on that for now:

Gun violence is a major public health problem in the United States. Each year, nearly 40,000 people die from gun-related injuries. Although the majority of these deaths are suicides, homicides comprise 37% of gun-related deaths in the United States— or nearly 15,000 gun-related homicides per year. It is therefore urgent that policies be enacted to protect people from gun violence. These policies require buy-in and endorsement not only from gun-control activists, but also from law-abiding gun owners and gun-rights activists. Buy-in from gun owners and gun-rights activists would help to assure law-abiding gun owners that their Second Amendment rights are not under threat.

Obtaining buy-in from law-abiding gun owners and gun-rights activists may best be accomplished by engaging organizations to which these individuals belong. A key organization to engage in such efforts is the National Rifle Association (NRA), which is funded largely by gun owners and gun-rights activists. The NRA has been advised to consider the impact of its policies on the welfare and lives of U.S. residents, but it has declined to do so. Indeed, the NRA has remained silent as people have been shot to death in schools, houses of worship, shopping malls, and elsewhere. Through its silence and refusal to advocate for stricter gun laws, the NRA's positions on gun violence have contributed to this epidemic.

Now the logical leap has been filled in, but there are some contradictions between the new text and the existing text. We are now saying that we need to engage the NRA, but we are still criticizing them for their inaction. We need to soften and temper these criticisms. Below is an attempt to do so. The revised text is underlined:

> Gun violence is a major public health problem in the United States. Each year, nearly 40,000 people die from gun-related injuries. Although the majority of these deaths are suicides, homicides comprise 37% of gun-related deaths in the United States—or nearly 15,000 gun-related homicides per year. It is therefore urgent that policies be enacted to protect people from gun violence. These policies require buy-in and endorsement not only from gun-control activists, but also from law-abiding gun owners and gun-rights activists. Buy-in from gun owners and gun-rights activists would help to assure law-abiding gun owners that their Second Amendment rights are not under threat.
>
> Obtaining buy-in from law-abiding gun owners and gun-rights activists may best be accomplished by engaging organizations to which these individuals belong. A key organization to engage in such efforts is the National Rifle Association (NRA), which is funded largely by gun owners and gun-rights activists. The NRA has been advised to consider the impact of its policies on the welfare and lives of U.S. residents, but _they might be more likely to do so if they are approached collaboratively rather than adversarially. The NRA has a key role to play in reducing the number of_ people _who are_ shot to death in schools, houses of worship, shopping malls, and elsewhere. _By engaging law-abiding gun owners and gun-rights activists in efforts to reduce gun violence, we may be most able to fight back against gun violence._

It appears that this combination of strategies has filled in the logical leap. Additionally, we are now able to express our position without being critical of the NRA. Remember José's advice about standing on the shoulders of others and not criticizing them? Although we are not "standing on the shoulders" of the NRA, our argument is more likely to be received well if we are positive and encouraging rather than critical and negating. We are also suggesting a way forward rather than simply criticizing the NRA and blaming them for the gun-violence epidemic.

This example exemplifies another principle (discussed further in Chapter 9)—spotting and correcting contradictions in your writing. José once told me that a paper needs to follow a straight line from start to finish, with no internal contradictions. The logic needs to be crisp and clear, without distractions or logical leaps. The reader should be able to focus on your argument without being distracted or confused.

As noted in Chapter 5 and covered in more detail in Chapter 8, writers should not worry about any of these issues when they are putting together a first draft. The purpose of a first draft is to transfer your ideas from your mind onto the screen. Don't worry about logical leaps, contradictions, or distractions. (However, I suggest using outlines, including outlining each paragraph if necessary, to prevent being AOTP. AOTP writing requires a great deal of effort to fix.) More or less, turn off your "internal editor" and just let the words flow through your fingers and onto the screen.

More is said about this issue in Chapter 8, but first drafts are supposed to be messy. Writing is a stream-of-consciousness process, and attempting to edit your words as they are coming to you is likely to stifle the creativity that you need in order to write well. Further, in most cases, you will write your first draft across several sessions, and you may not remember what you have already written during earlier writing sessions. This is OK! No matter how good or bad your first draft is, you will need to do at least some editing—so just relax and let the words come to you.

In the next chapter, I discuss additional important principles of good writing—paraphrasing, avoiding excessive quoting, citing sources, and avoiding plagiarism. These writing principles are also key ethical issues, which is why they are covered in a separate chapter.

Summary

- Correct grammar and sentence structure are essential for ensuring that our writing can be understood and can impact the field as much as possible.
- Overused words should be replaced with synonyms that convey more precise meaning.
- When a term is used to refer to a specific phenomenon—such as *impaired driving*—that same term should be used each time the phenomenon is mentioned. In most other cases, it is a good idea to vary one's language (e.g., using *experiment*, *study*, and *manipulation* in a paragraph instead of using *experiment* three times in the same paragraph).
- Each paragraph should consist of a topic sentence, one to three supporting sentences, and a strong closing sentence.
- Logical leaps in one's writing should be filled in as part of the editing process. The amount of fill-in text needed depends on the size of the leap.
- Unfinished thoughts generally require one or two additional sentences at the end of the paragraph to wrap up the idea that the paragraph expresses.

- Interesting tidbits, sidebars, and sharp turns detract from the flow of one's argument and should be corrected before submitting a manuscript for publication.
- When paragraphs do not flow together, a transitional sentence or two may be needed to improve the flow.

7

Plagiarism, Citations, and Paraphrasing

Chapter Objectives

When you finish reading this chapter, you should be more comfortable with:

- How to identify and prevent plagiarism
- The concepts of paraphrase plagiarism and self-plagiarism, and how to avoid engaging in these practices
- Appropriate ways to include citations in your work
- Major citation styles (such as APA, American Sociological Association, and Chicago)

In early 2018, I was invited to visit a young scholar at another university. He had been an assistant professor there for a couple of years, and his university had invested money in bringing in established researchers to mentor and help young faculty to get started in their careers. I didn't know this young man personally, but we had colleagues in common and he was familiar with my work. He had selected me as his outside faculty member—a role that I have played with several young scholars during the course of my career. For the purposes of this book, we will refer to this young man as Dr. Y.

Less than a week before I was supposed to visit Dr. Y and his university, I received an email from another colleague, warning me never to work with Dr. Y. The colleague who sent me the email was accusing Dr. Y of having plagiarized his dissertation and publishing the plagiarized work under his own name. Worse yet, the accuser had attached a PDF copy of his dissertation—date-stamped in 2010—along with a copy of Dr. Y's article, which was dated 2018. So the accuser was clearly on solid ground and had clear evidence to substantiate his claim. He had contacted the editor of the journal that had published Dr. Y's article, and in turn the editor had contacted Dr. Y's department chair.

I emailed Dr. Y and told him I had received an email accusing him of plagiarism. I'm the kind of person who always roots for people to succeed and likes to see the best in everyone, so I was hoping that Dr. Y would somehow come back with a logical explanation for what had happened. Instead, the

The Savvy Academic. Seth J. Schwartz, Oxford University Press. © Oxford University Press 2022.
DOI: 10.1093/oso/9780190095918.003.0008

only reply I received from Dr. Y was that the whole situation was a misunderstanding, and that he had never intended to plagiarize the other person's work. (Of course, having compared Dr. Y's article with the other person's dissertation and seeing that entire paragraphs had been copied verbatim, it was difficult for me to imagine how the plagiarism could have been unintentional.) The next day, I received an email from Dr. Y's department chair, telling me that Dr. Y was being dismissed from the university and that my visit had been canceled.

In the more than 3 years since that series of events occurred, I have used Dr. Y's actions as a teaching tool in my research ethics course, and I've often wondered what could possibly have led him to plagiarize whole sections of someone else's dissertation. Plagiarism is by far the most common form of research misconduct (Juyal, Thawani, & Thaledi, 2015). Unfortunately, it is all too easy to copy someone else's words, paste those words into your paper, and submit the paper as your own work. In my classes, I have caught students plagiarizing text from the Internet, work from other students, and even the work professors in the department. A common explanation the students provide is that "I wasn't going to publish this—it was just a class project—so how can it be plagiarism?"

In short, it doesn't matter whether you are only writing an email to your friend. If you take material from someone else, you need to cite the source from which you took the material. You may have noticed that, in this book, any time I use a concept that someone else originated, I credit that person. I've credited José for all the lessons and tips I learned from him, although none of these were published and no one would have known that these ideas were not mine. The point was that, had I not credited José and others for ideas I learned from them, *I* would have known that I took someone else's ideas and passed them off as my own. I regard myself as an impeccably honest person, and I could not sleep at night knowing that I had done something that was intentionally dishonest. My father likes to say that he would cut himself shaving if he ever lied to anyone, because he couldn't look at himself in the mirror. What I am saying here is pretty much the same thing.

A small body of research has examined why people plagiarize. The most common reasons, none of which are surprising, include laziness, working at the last minute, and lack of confidence in one's own writing skills (Moss, White, & Lee, 2018). People who do not want to put forth the necessary effort to produce their own writing may instead choose to take text written by others and submit it as their own. Individuals who are extremely pressed for time may take text from others because they do not have enough time to conduct the research that is often required to generate one's own writing. People who do not view themselves as skilled writers may believe that the only way they can produce acceptable writing is to plagiarize from others.

I can offer advice for people who provide the second and third reasons for plagiarizing, but not for those who provide the first reason. Laziness is not a trait that lends itself to skilled writing. Good writing takes work, as well as sufficient patience to be willing to revise one's work over and over again. Even the most skilled writers receive critical feedback from their colleagues and from reviewers—and just when you think you have perfected your paper beyond criticism, someone will come along and offer more criticism. I've known many lazy people in my life, and very few of them ever became successful academic writers.

In terms of working at the last minute, it's probably safe to say that we have all done that at one time or another. Most high school and college students have waited until the last possible day or week to start an important project. José himself was a "Last Minute Louie" (an expression my mother taught me) for most of his career—he would come up with the concept for a grant proposal 2 or 3 weeks before the deadline, and the study team would have to work multiple overnights to finish the proposal, budget, support letters, and other materials. Eventually the university instituted policies requiring proposals to be sent to the university's research administration offices 1 week prior to the submission date (so that the administrators were not stressed out trying to proof the budget and other supporting materials)— and this policy put an end to José's days as a Last Minute Louie. I can tell you that the Last Minute Louie approach places a great deal of stress not only on the author or principal investigator, but also on everyone else on the writing or project team. Last-minute products are generally "rough around the edges" because the writing team doesn't have enough time to smooth out the writing and to ensure that the pieces all fit together—and as a result, work completed at the last minute is often not of the same quality as work completed with sufficient lead time. Moreover, having to work multiple overnights to finish the writing is not conducive to putting out the best possible product. With the exception of some night owls I know, most people don't do their best work at 3 or 4 in the morning—and most people don't work well on little or no sleep.

Because grant writing requires so many moving parts—research plan, budgets, support letters, biosketches (short curricula vitae for key study personnel), human subjects protection plan, and so forth—I have learned to work backward from the deadline so I can figure out when I need to start putting together the proposal. Some of the moving parts, such as support letters from community partners (e.g., school principals, clinic directors), are out of the writer's control and need to be planned and requested well in advance. A smooth piece of writing often requires many drafts to complete—and the iterative process of writing and editing takes time. Chris Salas-Wright and I have developed a process where we spend several hours on a teleconference and obsessively review every word in the proposal. We sometimes do this two or three times before submitting a proposal! The point here is that you cannot put out your best work when you wait until the last minute.

In terms of developing confidence in your writing, refer to the discussion in Chapter 5 about developing good writing habits. Just as I wouldn't go out and run a half marathon without completing regular training runs, I would not expect someone to be able to write an academic paper without regularly honing and sharpening their writing skills. Confidence comes from repeated practice and from showing yourself that you can do what needs to be done.

Earvin "Magic" Johnson was one of the most skilled basketball players ever. He earned his famous nickname by executing acrobatic passes that looked like magic. More than anything, however, Johnson was beloved by his teammates because he put them into the best possible position to showcase their skills. Johnson once had a teammate named Larry Kenon, who had lost his confidence in his ability to make shots. Kenon was down on himself and slumped his shoulders every time he missed a shot. So Johnson decided to build up Kenon's confidence gradually. He started passing Kenon the ball when Kenon was close to the basket—thereby allowing Kenon to attempt easy, high-percentage shots. Johnson (1993) noted in his autobiography that he watched Kenon's body language change as he began to regain his confidence—and as Kenon's confidence increased, Johnson started passing him the ball when he was a little further away from the basket. Before long, Kenon was back to making the shots that he had made earlier in his career and that he had been missing during his extended slump.

What Magic Johnson did for Larry Kenon is what good mentors do for their mentees—put them into the best possible positions to succeed.

So what does Magic Johnson's story have to do with plagiarism? My answer would be that mentors can help to prevent plagiarism among their mentees by helping them to develop confidence in their writing skills. Perhaps mentors could start by asking mentees to write sections of a paper, edit the mentor's drafts, or collaborate with more experienced mentees on manuscript writing. Then ask them to complete more and more advanced writing tasks as their writing skills progress. Helping mentees start out and build confidence in their writing skills in these ways is akin to Magic Johnson's setting Larry Kenon up for easy shots. In turn, people with more confidence in their writing skills may be less likely to plagiarize other people's work.

If you are using a team writing approach, where different people write different sections of a paper or proposal and then the lead author integrates and smooths out the sections, you need to be sure that you can trust your coauthors to write honestly and with integrity. If someone plagiarizes as part of the sections they write, you may never know about it—but if the plagiarism is caught, all authors on the paper, especially the lead author, will have their careers tainted with accusations of plagiarism. Saying "I didn't know" is not likely to work as an excuse.

I'll give you two examples to illustrate my point. First, I served on the University of Miami Institutional Review Board (IRB) for 2 years. During that time, we reviewed an annual continuing report for a study where the principal investigator's (PI's) explanations and documentation raised more questions than they answered. During one of our meetings, my IRB committee chair called the PI and requested an explanation for some of the issues that we didn't understand. The PI responded with the three words that should never be said to an IRB—"I don't know." My IRB chair's expression turned angry and his voice quickly rose. "What do you mean you don't know?" he asked, almost shouting into the phone. "You're the PI! It's your job to know!"

The PI responded that he had recently taken over the study because the previous PI had left the university and that he had not been informed about all of the study details. My IRB chair cut the PI off and replied angrily that he should have made sure he knew what he was getting himself into when he agreed to take over as PI. The PI agreed that he should have known what was happening with the study, and by the next time our IRB committee met, the PI had submitted an updated continuing report with all of the information that should have been included in the first place.

The second story occurred much more recently, shortly after I took over as editor of the *International Journal of Intercultural Relations* in early 2020. My editorial assistant runs every manuscript through a plagiarism checker, which provides a "plagiarism percentage"—the proportion of the text in the paper that is identical to text in any other source available online. Any percentage above 25% is flagged and brought to my attention. One paper that we received overlapped 35% with an article published by another group in a different part of the world. I scanned both the submitted manuscript and the article with which it overlapped, and it was clear that the authors of the manuscript had plagiarized text from the other article. I desk-rejected the manuscript (meaning that I rejected it without sending it out for peer review) and brought the plagiarism to the author's attention in my editorial letter. The author replied in less than 30 minutes, apologized for the plagiarism in his submission, and confessed that his students had written some sections of the paper. He had apparently either not reviewed what they wrote or had included it in the final submission without running it through a plagiarism checker himself. (I am not sure I would have run my students' writing through a plagiarism checker either, but I am extremely selective regarding which students I accept into my lab.) I could have reported the plagiarism to the author's department chair, but I decided not to do that. Having a paper desk-rejected because of plagiarism was embarrassing enough for this author.

These examples underscore U.S. President Harry Truman's expression, "The buck stops here." What President Truman meant by that expression was that, because he was the leader of the country, he was responsible for whatever happened—even for mistakes made by other people. The person in charge should not be "passing the buck" and blaming someone else. If you accept a position of leadership (and being first author on a paper is a position of leadership), then you also accept responsibility for whatever happens with that paper.

Effective use of citations is covered in other sections of this chapter, but an important ethical principle in writing that warrants mention here is that we must cite a source any time we use someone else's words, ideas, methods, or information. I personally tend to over-cite because I am eager to credit others for their ideas, and using too many references can sometimes annoy readers and reviewers, but I would rather advise authors to over-cite than to use someone's ideas or words without crediting that source. Integrity is extremely important in scholarly writing—we need to maintain credibility with readers, and dishonesty is a sure way to lose credibility.

When in Doubt, Cite a Source

So what exactly constitutes plagiarism? How much text can we take from a source without plagiarizing? The standard I use, and that I have often heard and read from others, is that if we copy three or more consecutive words from a source, we have plagiarized. Of course, this rule does not apply to established scientific terms and phrases. For example, using the term *unsafe sexual behavior* is perfectly acceptable even if other sources use this same term— because *unsafe sexual behavior* is an established term. However, copying more than two consecutive words of text from a source—not including prepositions and words at the beginning of a clause (e.g., who, whom, what, when, that, which)—represents plagiarism. When in doubt, paraphrase and cite the source.

Paraphrase Plagiarism

So far, the emphasis in this chapter has been on taking someone else's words and using them as one's own. A common misconception is that, if we paraphrase the original text rather than copying and pasting it, then we are not plagiarizing.

Notice that I labeled this idea a misconception. Using ideas from a source without citing that source is still plagiarism. As already noted, if someone came up with an idea and published it, that person deserves credit for the idea. A similar principle applies to methods (research procedures or analytic methods) that someone originated—other than methods that can be assumed to be common knowledge, such as analyses taught in introductory statistics classes or many research procedures taught in many introductory research methods courses. Again, when in doubt, cite the source.

Therefore, we should generally paraphrase rather than quoting directly, with very few exceptions. Sometimes the original source worded something in a way that says it better than we ever could. In that case, include the quote within quotation marks, and provide the citation and the exact page number where the quote appears in the source material. I do not recommend including more than two or three direct quotes in any manuscript.

Young writers often find themselves including a lot of direct quotes in their writing. When I was in graduate school, I taught a research methods course several times. Some students quoted sources so many times that the quotations comprised the majority of their papers. Whole paragraphs would be quoted from sources (with appropriate citations, so these students were not plagiarizing). The quoting was so extensive that I started including explicit instructions to paraphrase and to avoid using direct quotes.

As already noted, even paraphrasing a source without citing that source is plagiarism. This kind of plagiarism is *paraphrase plagiarism*; it will not be caught by plagiarism checker software, but it nonetheless involves using someone else's ideas without attribution. If I'm reading the introduction to an empirical paper, or almost any section of a theoretical or policy paper, and I don't see citations for factual statements, I assume that the writer engaged in paraphrase plagiarism. Of course, paraphrase plagiarism is not as severe an ethical issue as copy–paste plagiarism is, and reviewers and editors will often simply ask the author to include appropriate citations for the statements in question. However, you do not want to develop a reputation for taking other people's ideas and passing them off as your own.

Self-Plagiarism

Many writers don't realize that it's possible to plagiarize one's own work. If you copy text from the introductory section of one paper and paste that text into another paper, you have self-plagiarized. It is not ethical to include the exact same text (more than two to three consecutive words, unless they are part of a scientific term that you have introduced) in multiple journal articles or book chapters. Self-plagiarism is somewhat similar to duplicate or piecemeal publication, where similar work is presented in more than one article or chapter. In both cases, the literature is artificially inflated, and the same material is added to the literature multiple times.

There is one notable exception to the self-plagiarism principle. It is acceptable to copy and paste parts of method sections from one paper to another. Indeed, there are only so many ways to say who was in your study, what measures you used, or what procedures were followed. When multiple papers are written using the same data set, it is fine to use the same text in each paper—but I suggest changing some words or phrases so that the various method sections are not exactly the same. Nonetheless, self-plagiarism is far less of a concern vis-à-vis method sections than it is for other sections of a paper.

I have seen some writers "recycle" text from journal articles when they are writing a book chapter. Indeed, one reason why book chapters are less prestigious and less important than journal articles is because many contributors simply copy and paste text from their articles into the chapter. This recycling approach essentially devalues all of the chapters in the book, including those where the authors include original writing. In my estimation, this recycling is a form of self-plagiarism and should be avoided.

Why do people self-plagiarize? I suspect that common answers include laziness and not having enough time to produce original writing. It is acceptable to copy text from another paper and modify it, but in my experience, it's easier to produce original writing than it is to tinker with existing text. My advice is to generate new text for each paper you write, even if doing so requires more time and effort than self-plagiarism would require. Your scientific and ethical reputation is extremely important to maintain—and your reputation is much more important than saving a few hours of writing time.

Many years ago, I coauthored a journal article with a colleague. He was first author and did most of the writing, and I conducted the analyses and edited the text that he produced. After the article was published, I bought a book that my coauthor had written, and I was horrified to discover that entire paragraphs from the introductory section of our paper had been copied directly from the book. I wasn't sure how to handle this situation—and ultimately I never mentioned anything to my coauthor—but that experience taught me a valuable lesson. A common assumption is that plagiarism (including self-plagiarism) is committed primarily by students, postdoctoral fellows, and early-career faculty—but this assumption is false. Indeed, Martin (2013), in an editorial reviewing his experiences handling cases of misconduct in papers submitted to his journal, recounted several instances where senior scholars plagiarized (or self-plagiarized) in their submissions. So, full professors are by no means immune to the temptations of plagiarism. In fact, because they have more publications on which to draw, full professors might be more likely to self-plagiarize than younger scholars.

Citations

Chapter 5 discusses the situations where citations are needed, such as factual statements, population statistics and prevalence rates, research measures, and analytic procedures that are not commonly known. Here, we extend that discussion to cover how to include citations in your writing. Should the same source be cited repeatedly within a paragraph if we are referring to material from that source throughout the paragraph? When we are writing a sentence, do we lead with the citation, or do we lead with the concept and cite the source at the end of the sentence? How many sources should we cite for any one statement we are including in our paper?

Citing a Source Repeatedly Within a Paragraph

I believe that citing the same source over and over again within a single paragraph reads clumsily. If you find yourself citing a source repeatedly within a paragraph, I suggest citing that source at the end of the text that relies on that source—or else listing the authors' names, but not the publication year, later in the paragraph. For example, consider these two paragraphs (citations in these paragraphs are fictitious):

Clumsy: Children in two-parent homes generally evidence more favorable educational outcomes compared to other children (Sanchez, Woods, & Cho, 2017). Sanchez et al. (2017) argued that the presence of both parents provides maximal support for schoolwork and other academic activities, and that such support is often less available in homes where only one parent is present. Indeed, helping with homework, meeting with teachers, and attending school functions may be difficult for one parent to manage (Sanchez et al., 2017).

Clearer: Children in two-parent homes generally evidence more favorable educational outcomes compared to other children (Sanchez, Woods, & Cho, 2017). Sanchez et al. argued that the presence of both parents provides maximal support for schoolwork and other academic activities, and that such support is often less available in homes where only one parent is present. Indeed, helping with homework, meeting with teachers, and attending school functions may be difficult for one parent to manage.

Notice that the source is formally cited only once in the second example paragraph. The second sentence tells us what the authors of the source argued, but because the year is not included, the reference to Sanchez et al. in the second sentence is not a formal citation. *Sanchez et al.* is the subject of the second sentence. (Note: Saying "these authors" in the second sentence would have been unclear, because it is not entirely clear to whom "these authors" refers.)

Some writers tend to over-cite specific sources throughout their papers. I once read a student paper where the same source was cited more than 50 times. Such over-citing is excessive. I recommend "varying your sources" so that the same source is not cited over and over. For example, if the same author or author group published several articles, books, or chapters making similar points, I suggest citing more than one of the sources so that the same source is not over-cited. If multiple author groups have published articles, books, or chapters making similar points, I would also cite more than one of the sources.

Citing Multiple Sides of an Argument or Controversy

During a grant review session in which I participated, one reviewer scored a grant application poorly because the application cited only one side of a controversy. The reviewer had published extensively on this controversy, and the reviewer's position was opposed to the position adopted in the application. Chastising a manuscript or grant application for not citing the reviewer's own work, or insisting that the authors cite the reviewer's own work (or work done by the reviewer's colleagues), represents what Martin (2013) calls "coercive citation." Nonetheless, there was some validity in this grant reviewer's argument. Ignoring the controversy by citing only one side of the argument is somewhat disingenuous and leads readers to believe that the science is settled in the area represented by the controversy.

In most cases, we are arguing only one side of a controversy, so it is inefficient for us to "give equal air time" to both sides of the controversy. However, we should acknowledge that the controversy exists and offer a rationale for why we are addressing only one side of the controversy. Here is an example, and the citations in the example are fictitious:

> In the present study, we operationalize acculturation as the trajectory of migrants' adoption of heritage and destination cultural practices, values, and identifications (Schwartz et al., 2010). In doing so, we acknowledge that some authors (e.g., Smith & Roberts, 2013) have framed acculturation as a moment-by-moment process and have discouraged examining long-term trajectories of acculturation. However, our objective in the current study is to relate long-term acculturation trajectories to psychosocial, relational, and family outcomes.

In this paragraph, we have acknowledged the controversy, cited authors on both sides of the controversy, and have provided justification for why we are working on a specific side of the controversy. Reviewers and readers may disagree with our position, but they cannot accuse us of ignoring the controversy altogether.

In some cases, the controversy may be the topic of our paper or study—and we may include measures advocated for by both sides. In such cases, we should provide equal treatment to each side of the controversy—that is, we should be neutral—and we should allow the study results to "decide the case" (while acknowledging that a single study cannot provide a definitive verdict on a set of hypotheses). Here is an example of a paragraph setting up a study investigating a controversy (these citations are real). Note that citations are provided for both arguments:

> There is some debate in the literature regarding whether one's sense of identity is constructed or discovered (see Waterman, 1984, for a review). Berzonsky (1986) has argued that individuals construct a sense of self by making identity-related decisions and solving identity-related problems. In contrast, Waterman (1986) has postulated that individuals discover their sense of self by realizing and actualizing their best potentials. These two positions have been framed as inherently incompatible (Berzonsky, 1990). Specifically, one cannot construct a self that already exists prior to its construction, and one cannot discover a self that has not yet been constructed. In the present study, we lend empirical data to this controversy

by administering both self-construction and self-discovery measures to a sample of young adults.

Notice how we laid out both arguments and then told the reader how we plan to study the controversy. We might also give the reader a sense of how our study will help to address or resolve the controversy.

Leading With Concepts Versus Leading With Citations

One principle that I stress to my students is that, although our argument must be supported by citations, the argument should be ours. That is, citations should support—rather than drive—the argument we are building. Part of making the argument ours is leading each sentence off with a concept rather than with a citation. The sentences will flow much more smoothly when we lead with concepts instead of with citations. The following paragraphs exemplify this principle using fictitious citations:

> *Leading with Citation*: The effects of divorce on children are important to understand. Jones (2015) studied 100 children from divorced families and found that the majority of these children reported wanting more time with their fathers. Lopez and Smith (2008) interviewed 200 middle-school adolescents from divorced families and found that 70% of these youth reported experiencing distress both during and after the divorce. Roberts and Chen (2017) studied a sample of 527 college students and found that, compared to students from intact families, those from divorced families were significantly less trusting in their intimate relationships.
>
> *Leading with Concept*: The effects of divorce on children are important to understand. Children from divorced families may want more time with their fathers than they receive (Jones, 2015). Children of divorce often experience distress during and after the divorce (Lopez & Smith, 2008). Even years after the divorce, young people from divorced families may be less trusting in their intimate relationships than are their peers from intact families.

The first paragraph, which leads with citations, appears disjointed and somewhat AOTP, because it describes the methods used in each of the cited studies. It is difficult to follow this first paragraph because we focus too much on the trees (the details of the individual studies) and not enough on the forest (the overall argument that we are building). In contrast, the second paragraph is crisper, clearer, and more focused because the emphasis is on the argument, not on the details of the studies cited.

When we do describe the methods used by other studies, such description must be essential to the goal of the paper. For example, another study might have used methods that are similar to ours, or we might cite another study as justification for focusing on a specific population or age group. It is essential in these cases that the citation appear next to the mention of the study, rather than at the end of the sentence or paragraph. For example (these citations are fictitious):

> *Clumsy*: A study with adolescents demonstrated the feasibility of using wearable physical activity sensors (Sanders et al., 2017).
> *Clearer*: A study with adolescents (Sanders et al., 2017) demonstrated the feasibility of using wearable physical activity sensors.

How Many Citations Should be Included for Any Single Point?

I can remember going to a journal website many years ago to look over the journal's instructions to authors, and one guideline stood out: *Avoid long strings of citations at the end of a sentence.* That guideline matched with something my father had observed when I had given him drafts of my writing to look over—he told me that citing many sources in one place distracted him from the points I was trying to make.

Take a look at this sentence (the citations are fictitious) and see whether you agree that the citations overwhelm the text:

Research has indicated that teacher–student bonding is closely related to students' academic performance (Adams & Wong, 2015; Bustamante et al., 2018; Jones, White, & Walker, 2012; Lee et al., 2016; Rogers & Rodriguez, 2009; Thomas et al., 2017).

In this sentence, the citations account for more text than the rest of the sentence does. Clearly, some of the citations need to be removed. But how many citations are too many? Are there situations where more or fewer citations should be included?

My general rule is that we should not cite more than three or four sources for any one point that we are making—unless that point is extremely broad. If we are making a sweeping statement, we might need a couple of additional citations to be sure that we have covered our bases. However, I cannot think of a situation where more than five or six sources would need to be cited in one place—even for the most sweeping and general statement.

In scientific writing, statements should be as precise and specific as possible—so with some notable exceptions, we would not need to cite more than three or four sources at a time. Sometimes, in the opening paragraph or two in the introduction, we may wish to include a powerful statement supporting the premise and importance of our study, and such a statement might require additional citations. For example, the general statement "Intergroup processes underlie many of the political and social conflicts between and among countries" might need more citations than would a more narrow and focused statement.

Another strategy in the introduction, however, might be to include a general statement and then bolster it with a series of specific statements. In such a scenario, each of the specific statements would be supported with one or two citations, and the general statement would not need any citations (because the specific statements that clarify the broader statement are cited). With few exceptions, following a broad statement with more specific statements, and with citations for each of these specific statements, provides greater clarity than a broad statement with lots of citations. The principle I am articulating here is akin to the "make sure to finish your thoughts" principle in Chapter 6. If the broad, heavily cited statement is not followed up with more specific statements, then the thought is not finished.

Let's compare the broad, sweeping statement with lots of citations with the broad statement followed by narrower statements (as usual, all citations are fictitious):

Broad: Intergroup processes underlie many of the political and social conflicts between and among countries (Brown, 2000, 2005; Crisp, 2014; Henry & Abrams, 2017; Montealegre, Harris, & Wong, 2017; Turner et al., 1987, 2004; Williams & Jones, 2014, 2018; Young & Reed, 2014).

Narrower: Intergroup processes underlie many of the political and social conflicts between and among countries. For example, wars are often fought based on ingroup–outgroup ("us" versus "them") distinctions (Henry & Abrams, 2017; Young & Reed, 2014). Differences between "prototypical" members of national groups (e.g., Germans stereotyped as stiff and emotionless, Americans stereotyped as reckless and uncultured) may underlie conflicts between nations (Montealegre, Harris, & Wong, 2017). Nations who are regarded as mutual outgroups (i.e., each country regards the other as an adversary) are most likely to experience conflict with one another (Brown, 2000, 2005; Crisp, 2004). The contributions of social psychology and intergroup relations to dynamics between nations are therefore considerable.

Finally, as already suggested, citations should be placed directly after the statement that is being cited, not at the end of the paragraph. Citations that refer to specific parts of the sentence (e.g., citations for measurement instruments or intervention programs) should appear immediately after the names of the items to which the citations refer. Long strings of citations at the end of a sentence should be avoided.

Citation Styles

Before you begin writing, it's good to have a target journal in mind and to know which citation and reference style that journal uses. Such preparation allows you to utilize the correct citation style and helps you to avoid having to redo the citations and references in a different format later on. Of course, using Reference Manager, EndNote, or other citation software automates most of the citation and reference work for you—you can conduct a literature search and download each record directly into the citation software, and then when you want to cite a reference, you can do that directly within the software. Further, if you need to switch from one journal to another, and if the new journal uses a different style, this change can be made by clicking a button in the citation software. If you have compiled the references and citations manually, changing styles can be a tedious task.

Here I review some of the most common citation styles—American Psychological Association (APA), American Sociological Association (ASA), American Medical Association (AMA), and Chicago. Some journals have their own unique citation styles, so be sure to check the journal's Instructions for Authors (and follow those instructions carefully). More comprehensive coverage of these styles can be found in the respective style guides: American Psychological Association (2020), American Sociological Association (2019), American Medical Association (2020), and University of Chicago Press (2017).

APA Style

APA style is the most commonly used citation and reference style in psychology and behavioral science journals. In APA style, when we cite sources with fewer than six authors, the names of all authors are spelled out the first time the source is cited. For the second and subsequent times a source is cited, sources with three or more authors are cited using the first author's name followed by *et al.* For sources with two authors, both names are always listed when the source is cited. Sources with six or more authors are written as *Surname, X. X., et al.* each time the source is cited.

In APA style, the word *and* is written out before the last author's name (except for *et al.* citations) when the citation is not in parentheses, but an ampersand (&) is used in place of *and* when the citation appears in parentheses. For example:

Two authors: Jones and Rodriguez (2013) found . . .
but
It is well known (Jones & Rodriguez, 2013) that . . .
Three to five authors: initial citation: Wilson, Wong, Bryce, and Stepien (2017) found . . .
and
It is well known (Wilson, Wong, Bryce, & Stepien, 2017) . . .
subsequent citations: Wilson et al. (2017) noted that . . .
and
It has been noted (Wilson et al., 2017) . . .
Six or more authors: Davis et al. (2020) found . . .
and
It is well known (Davis et al., 2020) . . .

When shortening citations to *et al.* would lead to the same citation's being used for multiple sources, we list both the first and second authors' names before *et al.* For example, let's say we have (fictitious sources) Lopez, Wilson, Wang, and Riccio (2017) and Lopez, Jones, Drechsler, and Bryant (2017). For the second and subsequent times these sources are cited, they would be written as Lopez, Wilson, et al. (2017) and Lopez, Jones, et al. (2017).

In the reference list, entries are ordered alphabetically according to the first author's surname. When multiple entries appear for the same first author, entries are ordered according to the second author's surname. If the same authors are listed for more than one reference entry, the entries are ordered by year of publication. If two sources are cited from the same author group in the same year, letters are added to the date to distinguish them. For example, if Jones and Wilson are cited for two sources that were both published in 2019, the one that is cited first is cited and referenced as Jones and Wilson (2019a), and the second is listed and cited as Jones and Wilson (2019b). Also note that reference entries are *outdented* (i.e., they use the hanging indent), which means that the first line is flush left and subsequent lines are indented.

For journal articles, the name of the journal and the volume number are italicized. The issue number is listed in parentheses (and not italicized) only if the journal starts over at page 1 for each new issue (otherwise the issue number does not appear). No other text appears in italics. Here is an example:

Paginated by Volume:
Schwartz, S. J., & Petrova, M. (2018). Identity behind the iron curtain: Recent advances in identity research in changing contexts. *European Journal of Developmental Psychology, 15*, 1–10.
Paginated by Issue:
Schwartz, S. J., & Petrova, M. (2018). Identity behind the iron curtain: Recent advances in identity research in changing contexts. *European Journal of Developmental Psychology, 15*(1), 1–10.

For book chapters, only the name of the book is italicized, and the editors' names are listed with the editors' initials before, rather than following, their surnames:

Schwartz, S. J., Donnellan, M. B., Ravert, R. D., Luyckx, K., & Zamboanga, B. L. (2013). Identity development, personality, and well-being in adolescence and emerging adulthood: Theory, research, and recent advances. In I. B. Weiner (Series Ed.), and R. M. Lerner, A. Easterbrooks, & J. Mistry (Vol. Eds.), *Handbook of psychology, Volume 6: Developmental psychology* (pp. 339–364). New York: John Wiley and Sons.

For online sources, including online newspaper and magazine articles, we need the date of publication (if known), the article title, the newspaper/magazine title, and the website link. For example:

Cotto, I., & Chen, A. (2019, September 27). Census Bureau: Puerto Rican population in Orange, Osceola jumps 12.5% after Hurricane Maria. *Orlando Sentinel*. Retrieved from https://www.orlandosentinel.com/news/florida/os-ne-census-florida-puerto-rico-population-increase-20190927-lx3i6rxghzhehhf3md6x7hgfmu-story.html.

ASA Style

ASA style is similar to APA style in terms of general principles, but some details differ between APA and ASA styles. First, the ampersand (&) is not used in ASA style. The word *and* is used both within and outside parentheses. Commas are not used to separate the names from the publication year. For example, if we were citing Garcia, Jones, and Wong, published in 2017, in ASA style we would say (Garcia, Jones, and Wong 2017). If we were citing a direct quote from these authors on page 246, we would cite that quote as (Garcia, Jones, and Wong 2017:246).

Second, in the reference list, full first names (not initials) are listed. The first author's name is listed with the surname first, but the remaining authors are listed with the first name first. If there are more than three authors, *et al.* is used after the third author's name.

Third, unlike APA style, ASA style capitalizes all words in the article title (except prepositions, articles, and conjunctions), and quotation marks are used around the article title. In the page range, the last number is written only including the numbers that differ from the first number. That is, 115–119 is written as 115–9 and 348–371 is written as 348–71.

Here is a journal article reference entry in ASA style:

Salas-Wright, Christopher P., and Seth J. Schwartz. 2019. "The Study and Prevention of Alcohol and Other Drug Misuse among Migrants: Toward a Transnational Theory of Cultural Stress." *International Journal of Mental Health and Addiction, 17*:346–69.

Books are cited similarly. For example:

Schwartz, Seth J., and Jennifer B. Unger, eds. 2017. *Oxford Handbook of Acculturation and Health*. New York: Oxford University Press.

Book chapters are cited as follows (this entry is fictitious):

Williams, John, and Laura E. Sanchez. 2015. "How to Study Immigration." Pp. 75–96 in *Research Methods: An Advanced Textbook*, edited by A. Chen and R. K. Jackson. London: SAGE.

Importantly, in the reference list, when multiple entries appear from the same author or author group, a series of underscores replaces the author names in the second and subsequent entries:

Schwartz, Seth J., and Mariya Petrova. 2018a. "Fostering Healthy Identity Development in Adolescence." *Nature Human Behaviour, 2*:110–111.
_____. 2018b. "Identity behind the iron curtain: Recent advances in identity research in changing contexts." *European Journal of Developmental Psychology, 15*:1–10.

Finally, websites and online news articles would be referenced in ASA style as follows:

Steven Lemongello. 2019, February 8. "Venezuelans in Central Florida fret over future of their nation—and their own fates." *Orlando Sentinel*. Retrieved June 17, 2020 (https://www.orlandosentinel.com/politics/os-ne-central-florida-venezuela-20190208-story.html).

AMA Style

AMA style (also known as Vancouver or Index Medicus style) is used in most medical and public health journals. Superscripted numbers are used to denote in-text citations, and the reference list presents entries in the order in which they are cited, not in alphabetical or date order. Journal titles are generally abbreviated, and authors' initials are not followed by periods.

Here is how in-text citations would look in AMA style:

> Perceived discrimination over time, particularly in adolescence, has been linked to alteration in HPA axis activity, specifically blunted cortisol awakening response, in African Americans.[1] Far fewer studies have been conducted with Hispanics. Discrimination has also been linked with alcohol and drug use[2,3] and conduct problems.[4] In the longer term, discrimination also predicts medical conditions, including cardiovascular problems.[5]

Note that the same number should be used for a given source whenever that source is cited.

In the reference list, journal article citations appear as follows:

> 8. Aldridge-Gerry AA, Roesch SC, Villodas F, McCabe C, Leung QK, Da Costa M. Daily stress and alcohol consumption: modeling between-person and within-person ethnic variation in coping behavior. *J Stud Alcohol Drugs*. 2011 Apr 15; 72: 125–134.

Notice that the year, month, and day's date are listed—because many medical journals publish more than once per month. Journal title abbreviations can be searched at the National Library of Medicine (https://www.ncbi.nlm.nih.gov/nlmcatalog/journals/). If a journal does not have an abbreviation, the full journal name should be written out.

For book references, the AMA format is:

> 15. Ford DJ, Lerner RM. *Developmental systems theory*. Cambridge, UK: Cambridge University Press; 1992.

Book chapters are referenced using the following format (this reference is fictitious):

2. Williams AK, Mahmoody AT. Emergency health care. In: O'Callahan AL, ed. *Managing Disasters in the Emergency Room.* 4th ed. New York: Guilford; 2018: 167–186.

Websites are cited as follows:

45. Rainie L. The rise of the e-patient. Pew Research Center Internet and the American Life Project website. October 7, 2009. Accessed June 17, 2020.

Chicago Style

Chicago style is used by many political science journals. Like AMA style, Chicago style uses superscript numbers for in-text citations. However, unlike in AMA style, in Chicago style, each time a reference is cited, a new number is used—even if the same source is cited more than once. For each location where sources are cited, a single number is used, even if multiple sources are being cited.

Here is an example of a reference entry where a single source is cited:

3. Jeff Victoroff, "The Mind of the Terrorist: A Review and Critique of Psychological Approaches," *Journal of Conflict Resolution* 49 (2005), pp. 3–42.

Here is an example of a reference entry where multiple sources are cited:

6. Abdel-Khalek, "Neither Altruistic Suicide nor Terrorism, But Martyrdom," pp. 99–113; David Lester, Bijou Yang, and Mark Lindsay, "Suicide Bombers: Are Psychological Profiles Possible?" *Studies in Conflict and Terrorism* 27 (2004), pp. 283–295.

In this case, the Abdel-Khalek article had previously been cited, so only the title and page range (but not the name of the journal) are listed. The author's first name is also not listed in cases where the source had been cited previously.

To cite a whole book in Chicago style, use the following format:

40. James E. Côtê, *Arrested Adulthood: The Changing Nature of Maturity and Identity* (New York: New York University Press, 2000).

Citing book chapters in Chicago style uses this format:

75. Charry, Eric. "Music and Islam in Sub-Saharan Africa." In *The History of Islam in Africa*, edited by Nehwmia Levtzion and Randall L. Pouwels, 545–573. Athens, OH: Ohio University Press, 2000.

Finally, to cite a website in Chicago style, do it like this:

71. Herrera, Sebastian. "In Houston's Katy suburb, a Venezuelan population thrives." *Houston Chronicle*. https://www.houstonchronicle.com/news/houston-texas/houston/article/In-Houston-s-Katy-suburb-a-Venezuelan-population-11028051.php.

For book chapters and websites, if there are multiple authors, the second and subsequent authors are listed with their first names first (e.g., Wang, John, and Sarah A. Jones).

A feature of Chicago style is that if the same source (or group of sources) is cited in consecutive citations, the abbreviation *ibid.* (for the Latin word *ibidem*, which means "from the same place") is used. The use of *ibid.* obviates the need to list the same source repeatedly for consecutive citations.

Here's an example:

55. Andrea Kohn Maikovich, "A New Understanding of Terrorism Using Cognitive Dissonance Principles," *Journal for the Theory of Social Behaviour* 35 (2005), pp. 373–397.
56. Ibid.

Additionally, in Chicago style, authors are encouraged to list specific page numbers and ranges that readers should consult. For example, if I am citing findings that appear on page 121, I would write "p. 121" at the end of the reference entry. These page specifications can also be listed for *ibid.* citations. Note that these page specifications are not required, and if we are citing a source as a whole, page specifications should not be provided. Page specifications are used to direct the reader to specific material in the source that is being cited.

For example:

4. Robert A. Pape, "The Strategic Logic of Suicide Terrorism," *American Political Science Review* 97 (August 2003), pp. 343–361. See especially pp. 345–346.
5. Ibid., p. 355.

Conclusion

This chapter discusses issues surrounding plagiarism. Plagiarism is by far the most common form of scientific misconduct, and the most prominent motivations for plagiarism include laziness, working at the last minute, and lacking confidence in one's writing skills. The pressures inherent in working at the last minute can often be prevented by working backward from the deadline and allowing enough time to plan the writing project and the research needed to support the writing. Practicing one's writing skills and using the "Magic Johnson approach" (i.e., starting with small tasks and working one's way up to more complex writing tasks) can help to increase one's confidence as a writer. Laziness, unfortunately, does not lend itself to successful academic writing—and people who are predisposed toward being lazy may need to self-monitor to ensure that they are putting forth sufficient effort and not "taking the easy way out." In combination, these strategies may help to prevent plagiarism.

The chapter also discusses the need to cite sources. Citing too much is a better approach than not citing enough. People need to be credited for the ideas and contributions they have introduced into the literature, and we do that by citing their work. It is unethical to pass someone else's ideas off as our own, even if we have paraphrased their sentences. Although the most blatant form of plagiarism involves copying and pasting text from a source without crediting that source, failing to cite a source when paraphrasing that source's ideas or contributions is also a form of plagiarism.

Many younger writers don't know that authors can plagiarize themselves. Copying and pasting our own writing into another paper, without rewording the text we are pasting, is unethical because we are inflating the scientific record by publishing the same material twice. Therefore, duplicate publication is a form of self-plagiarism. Indeed, meta-analyses and other empirical methods for summarizing the literature will produce biased results if multiple papers are published using the same data. Self-plagiarism should be avoided at all costs.

Another important theme covered in this chapter is the need to be sure that we are "speaking with our own voice" in our writing. That is, we need to lead with concepts, rather than citations, so that the references support the argument (rather than driving or leading the argument). The focus should not be on what other people have said or done, but rather on the line of logic that we are tracing. Sources should be used to substantiate the points we are making. Leading with sources may cause the resulting text to be AOTP because each source cited is making different points. Our goal should be to tie the points together in our argument, rather than meandering from one source to another.

Finally, the chapter briefly reviews four common citation styles, the American Psychological Association, American Sociological Association, American Medical Association, and Chicago styles. Each of these styles prescribes different ways of citing sources and of listing entries in the reference list. It is essential to know which citation style is used by the journals to which we submit our work.

Summary

- Plagiarism is the most common form of scientific misconduct.
- It is unethical to copy someone else's words, regardless of the type of document one is writing.
- Working at the last minute decreases the likelihood that one will be able to assemble a strong written product.
- It is more advisable to paraphrase sources than to quote them directly, even when the source is cited properly.
- Self-plagiarism involves copying text from one publication and pasting it into another. This practice is unethical because it inflates the scientific record. The same information is presented in a new publication as though it were original.
- Copying text from a method section is not necessarily plagiarism (although some words should be changed after the text is pasted into the new publication).
- If one is reviewing an argument or controversy, all relevant sides of the argument or controversy should at least be acknowledged.
- Sentences should begin with concepts rather than with citations, so that the writing focuses on ideas rather than on the details of specific studies.
- When targeting a specific journal for a manuscript, it is essential to know which citation style that journal uses—and to follow that style accurately.

References

American Medical Association. (2020). *AMA manual of style, 11th edition: A guide for authors and editors*. New York: Oxford University Press.

American Psychological Association. (2020). *Publication manual of the American Psychological Association, seventh edition*. Washington, DC: Author.

American Sociological Association. (2019). *Style guide* (6th ed.). Washington, DC: Author.

Berzonsky, M. D. (1986). Discovery versus constructivist interpretations of identity formation: Consideration of additional implications. *Journal of Early Adolescence, 6*, 111–117.

Berzonsky, M. D. (1990). Self-construction over the lifespan: A process perspective on identity formation. In G. J. Neimeyer & R. A. Neimeyer (Eds.), *Advances in personal construct theory* (Vol. 1, pp. 155–186). Greenwich, CT: JAI.

Jayal, D., Thawani, V. & Thaledi, S. (2015). Plagiarism: An egregious form of misconduct. *North American Journal of Medical Sciences, 7,* 77–80.

Johnson, M. (1993). *My life*. Greenwich, CT: Fawcett Publishers.

Martin, B. R. (2013). Whither research integrity? Plagiarism, self-plagiarism and coercive citation in an age of research assessment. *Research Policy, 42,* 1005–1014.

Moss, S. A., White, B., & Lee, J. (2018). A systematic review into the psychological causes and correlates of plagiarism. *Ethics and Behavior, 28,* 261–283.

University of Chicago Press. (2017). *Chicago manual of style, 17th edition: The essential guide for writers, editors, and publishers*. Chicago: Author.

Waterman, A. S. (1984). Identity formation: Discovery or creation? *Journal of Early Adolescence, 4,* 329–341.

Waterman, A. S. (1986). Identity formation, metaphors, and values: A rejoinder to Berzonsky. *Journal of Early Adolescence, 6,* 119–121.

8
Writing a First Draft

Chapter Objectives

When you finish reading this chapter, you should be more comfortable with:

- Starting to write a first draft
- Developing intrinsic writing motivation
- Using an outline as a template for writing a first draft
- Adding citations to a first draft
- Overcoming writer's block
- Obtaining feedback and support from mentors during the writing process
- Knowing when a first draft is finished

As suggested in preceding chapters, the purpose of a first draft is to move ideas from the writer's head onto the screen. This chapter delves further into exactly how this process of transferring ideas might work and reviews some pitfalls and considerations that should be kept in mind during the process of writing a first draft. Readers should also remember that different types of papers might require somewhat different writing approaches—for example, writing an empirical article, with the four standard sections (introduction, method, results, and discussion), may proceed differently from writing a literature review or theoretical article that does not follow a standard template and does not present and interpret empirical findings. The specifics of theoretical articles, literature reviews, and position papers are covered in Chapter 16, but the present chapter touches on the process of writing first drafts of these types of papers.

As noted in other chapters, staring at a blank screen is a nerve-wracking experience for many authors. Earlier in my career, I would experience anxiety just staring at the cursor blinking—and some of my colleagues have told me about experiencing panic attacks while trying to think of how to start writing. My postdoctoral supervisor taught me to create outlines, and his technique has helped me to become a much more skilled and comfortable writer. Chapter 4 covers many of his principles for writing an effective outline that can serve as the structure for a first draft of the paper.

The Savvy Academic. Seth J. Schwartz, Oxford University Press. © Oxford University Press 2022.
DOI: 10.1093/oso/9780190095918.003.0009

Many writers often try to write the perfect first draft—as a result, they often wind up writing almost nothing. I once spoke with someone who told me that she had spent an entire day writing words and deleting them—and at the end of the day, this person's screen was blank. Nothing that she wrote was good enough (at least not to her). This person was very angry and frustrated as she recounted the story, and she ended her description by noting that "I guess I'm just not a very good writer."

My response to her was pretty much the same as what I describe in this chapter. Just write the words and don't judge them. More importantly, don't judge yourself as you write. Just get the words and ideas out of your head and onto the screen so you can edit them. As have noted elsewhere in this book, you cannot edit what is in your head.

Sometimes, when I am feeling depressed, anxious, or inspired, I will sit down at the computer and write out what I'm thinking or feeling. There is a certain power in putting thoughts and feelings into words—the amorphous thought or feeling is now encapsulated in words and can be described. We can even understand our own thoughts and emotions more clearly when they are written down.

First drafts follow much the same principle. The thought is elusive and amorphous, but the words are concrete and can be captured and more easily understood.

The first step in writing a first draft is preparing an outline (see Chapter 4 for more details on creating outlines). The outline provides a template for writing without being AOTP (all over the place). Within each section of the outline, however, we are free to write what we want; therefore, we have to allow ourselves to transfer our thoughts onto the screen. It is essential that we allow ourselves to write without censoring ourselves, judging or editing our thoughts, or worrying about how the text is flowing. Issues of flow, redundancy, logical leaps, and being AOTP can be addressed in the editing of the first draft (editing is discussed in Chapter 9).

Getting Ourselves Into Writing Shape

Although the principle of transferring thoughts onto the screen seems fairly straightforward, in many cases people need to be intrinsically motivated to write, and they need to "work themselves into writing shape." The points made in Chapter 5 apply here in terms of creating good writing hygiene, and I expand on those points here in terms of getting oneself used to the practice of transferring ideas from one's mind to the screen. Two primary domains apply here: intrinsic writing motivation and working oneself up to longer writing sessions.

Intrinsic Writing Motivation

In Chapter 5, I cite Csikszentmihalyi's (1990) concept of flow and discuss why being in a flow state is critical for being able to write effectively. Flow is characterized by being engrossed in an activity, losing track of time, and forgetting about one's worries or problems. When I am writing in a flow state, the words feel as though they are flowing through me rather than from me. My keystrokes seem automatic and do not seem to require any effort at all. Words appear on the screen almost as though they were coming from someone other than me. Effortful, critical thought generally does not occur. I am so caught up in writing that someone knocking on my door, or my dog barking, or someone calling my name will literally startle me.

It is also essential that we feel intrinsically motivated to write. Self-determination theory (Deci & Ryan, 1985, 2008) holds that autonomy—engaging in activities because we choose to—is a fundamental human need. Simply put, people are much more likely to enjoy doing something because they choose to, rather than because they are required to. Al Waterman and I, along with some of Al's student colleagues, published an article many years ago (Waterman et al., 2003) that I still use as a teaching tool around the importance of intrinsic motivation. We asked college students to list five activities that they would use to describe themselves to another person—in other words, identity-related activities. Students then rated each activity on a number of qualities, including the extent to which the activity was interesting to them, put them into a flow state, and was personally expressive (i.e., helped them to discover and realize their highest potentials). Perhaps the strongest finding from that study was that all three indicators were far higher for activities that were perceived as self-chosen than for activities that were perceived as required. Even activities that were well matched to the person and that presented an optimal balance of challenges and skills (i.e., the challenges posed by the activity were consistent with the skills that the person brought to the activity) were unlikely to be rated as interesting, to facilitate a state of flow, and to be personally expressive unless the activities were freely chosen.

What does all of this have to do with writing first drafts? The answer is *everything*.

Trying to force yourself to write—or trying to force a colleague or mentee to write—is likely to be about as much fun as pulling teeth from a horse. We have to choose to write, and we need to bring ourselves to a place where we enjoy writing enough that we look forward to sitting down at the computer and transferring thoughts from our minds onto the screen. I know, I know— some readers are probably thinking that I need to have my head examined. *How can I enjoy writing? I'm terrified of it!*

Self-determination theory also provides a continuum between autonomous (intrinsic) and controlled (extrinsic) motivation. On this continuum, autonomous motivation refers to both (a) fully self-chosen behaviors and goals and (b) behaviors and goals undertaken to be consistent with one's personal beliefs and standards (Chirkov, 2009). What this principle means is that, even if we do something because we know we have to do it, we are still likely to find it more enjoyable than we would if we were only doing it because someone else was telling us to do it. In some cases, we must offer ourselves a reward (for example, when I finish this writing session, I'm going to treat myself to some ice cream). Remember the Magic Johnson Principle—start small and build your confidence. Start by writing one page, then write two the next time, and then write three the time after that. Before long, you might find yourself writing for long stretches of time, and you will likely be far more productive than you were before.

Working Oneself Up to Long Writing Sessions

Furthermore, it is important to set goals for yourself in terms of productivity, and don't be afraid to challenge yourself. In late 2011, I had been running 5 miles three times per week, and I had struggled through a 10-k (6.2 miles) race. So what did I do? I signed up for a half marathon at the end of January 2012. I had no idea how I was going to go from running 5 miles at a time to finishing a 13-mile race, but somehow I would figure it out.

So how did I go from running 5 miles per session in early December to completing a 13-mile race at the end of January? I started adding 1 mile to my runs every 2 weeks, so that by mid-January I was running 9 miles per session. Had I tried to go from 5 miles to 9 miles all at once, I would probably have had trouble finishing my runs—and I might have gotten hurt. Instead, I finished the half marathon (and then ran another half marathon 3 weeks later).

Writing sessions can work pretty much the same way. I wouldn't expect someone who has not been writing very much to suddenly start engaging in 6-hour marathon writing sessions. That just isn't reasonable. Engaging in a single activity for long stretches of time requires not only intrinsic motivation but also a lot of practice. Distractions are inevitable, so we need to develop the ability to ignore them—or if we must attend to them, we must develop the ability to return to what we were doing once the distraction has been handled.

Another important skill for writing in long stretches is controlling over-enthusiasm. Early in my career, sometimes I would be so fired up when I sat down to write that I couldn't get my thoughts organized enough to start writing. After a few frustrating writing sessions where I couldn't focus, I started writing notes on a piece of paper so that I would remember each of the thoughts I wanted to write about. Making these notes helped me to make sure I covered all the ideas I was so excited about. (Even when we are writing within an outline, we still need to be sure that we cover all the ideas that we have in our mind.)

Using an Outline as a Template

When we sit down to start writing our first draft, a good way to start is to paste in the outline and use the outline entries as headings. This way we have a structure within which to write, and we are no longer looking at a blank screen. More or less, the outline can be used to help reduce the anxiety and "writer's block" that often prevent people from getting started with the writing process.

My PhD advisor, Bill Kurtines, used another approach that may be helpful to some writers. Bill would sketch out each paragraph within a section by writing the first few words of each paragraph. Sometimes he would write a few sentence fragments for each of the paragraphs that he had in his mind, and he would effectively map out the entire structure of each section. Then, once he had the whole section sketched out, Bill would go back and write out each paragraph.

So how much do we write within each outline heading? How do we know when we have written enough?

The answer is that we don't, and that it doesn't really matter. We are writing a first draft, not a final draft—so no matter how rough the draft is, it can be edited and refined. (Revising drafts is covered in more detail in the next chapter.)

A key principle I have learned is that no matter how bad your first draft is, it *can* be edited and refined; and no matter how good your first draft is, it will *need* to be edited and refined. Thus, trying to write the perfect first draft is not only pointless, it's impossible. When you look at your own first draft a few days after you finish writing it, you will find lots of issues to correct. If you have coauthors writing with you, they will almost always find changes to make. So don't worry about being perfect. Just write!

Even as I wrote this book, I often found myself wondering "Have I said this before in an earlier chapter?" First drafts are rarely completed in a single sitting, and in some cases, weeks or months might pass between writing sessions. If you forget what you wrote in an earlier session, don't worry about it. Redundancy is bound to occur when you write a first draft. You can clean up the redundancy later when you edit the draft—and your coauthors will suggest corrections that you missed. So, again, just allow the words to come out of your mind and onto the screen. You can edit the draft later.

In the prologue, I quote an old saying: "The perfect is the enemy of the good." Recall what I said about maladaptive perfectionism—it freezes us in place because we are worrying too much about being perfect. If you try to edit your thoughts while transferring them to the screen, you are doing yourself a major disservice! You cannot be in flow if you are thinking too much about what you're doing.

Remember that anxiety comes from judging our performance as inadequate and from worrying that the future will not work out as we hope it will. In a state of flow, we are not judging or worrying at all. We are in the present moment.

Some of you may be wondering whether it's OK to go back and look over what you've already written before you are finished writing the entire first draft. My answer is, "It depends." If you are already comfortable with your writing skills, then go ahead and look over what you have already written. But if you are still learning to be comfortable with yourself as a writer, then I advise not reading anything you've written until the first draft is done. In other words, if looking back at what you've already written is going to make you anxious or is going to lead you to judge yourself harshly, then my advice is not to look back until you finish the draft. Of course, when you sit down to write, you may need to read the last few sentences you wrote during your previous sitting so that you know where you left off. But a key principle that I suggest here is that generating new text and editing existing text are separate and distinct phases of the writing process. Finish generating new text before you start editing what you have written.

Writing is like most other skills—you can break some of the basic rules once you have mastered the skill. Someone learning to ride a bicycle should hold onto both handlebars, but an experienced rider can let go of one of the handlebars, and we have all seen expert riders take both of their hands off the handlebars. You'll know when it's OK to let go of the handlebars, because you'll know when you are confident enough in your biking skills. Similarly, you will know when you are comfortable enough as a writer to break some of the rules (such as writing without an outline). And you'll know that it's perfectly OK to try breaking a rule and then to realize that you probably still need to follow that rule. You will know when you are ready to try to break it again.

It's OK to be Anxious

If you are having feelings of anxiety, self-criticism, or worry while you are writing a first draft, please don't judge yourself for that. There is no specific way that we are "supposed" to feel while we are writing. If you're anxious, that's OK! Eventually you won't be, but judging yourself for being anxious will just increase your anxiety.

Further, it's important to be happy with small accomplishments. If you write two paragraphs the first time you sit down to write, that's just fine. You have two more paragraphs than you had when you started. Next time you can write more. It is very important not to compare your writing skills or accomplishments with those of other people. I've had students tell me "I can't write the way you do." My response is usually something along the lines of "I'm 25 years older than you and I've been writing for a living since I was in graduate school myself." My message to students and mentees is that I may be ahead of you, but I am not above you. Everything I have accomplished, you can also accomplish. But you don't need to compare yourself to me (or to anyone else, for that matter). The only valid comparison is with where you were before. If you have made progress, that's all that matters.

Adding Citations to a First Draft

A key question when you are writing a first draft is how to handle citations. Do you stop and look up sources as you are writing, or do you just keep writing and insert "(REF)" or something similar? Further, once you add a citation, do you need to enter the reference into the reference list, or should you leave that for later?

In my writing career, I have followed all three of these approaches—(1) stopping and looking up citations and entering the references into the reference list, (2) stopping and looking up citations without entering the references into the list, and (3) just writing (REF) and then looking up citations later. Each of these approaches has advantages and disadvantages that I enumerate here.

Looking Up Citations and Entering Them Into the Reference List

Looking up citations and entering the references into the reference list is clearly the most efficient method if your goal is not to leave any work for later. Whenever you find yourself making a factual-sounding statement or point, you go to your literature search engines (I use Google Scholar most of time), enter the keywords for which you need a source, and then peruse the records that come up until you find one or more that you want to cite. Google Scholar allows you to download your desired search results to EndNote or Reference Manager, or if you are creating the reference list manually, Google Scholar will give you the citation in whatever format you need so that you can copy and paste it into your reference list.

A clear disadvantage of this approach is that it is very distracting. You can lose your train of thought while you are looking up records, sorting through them to find the best citations, and entering them into your reference list. It takes practice to reach the point where you can keep your mind focused on writing while you are looking up sources. In some cases, it can take a while to find the right source to cite—and sometimes you cannot find a source for a claim you want to make. You may have to broaden or change the claim and keep looking for citations—it's possible that the claim you want to make hasn't been supported by empirical research or that no empirical research has been conducted on the specific claim you want to make. However, when you are searching the literature "in real time" (i.e., while you are writing your first draft), you can adjust your line of logic to fit the sources that are available. If you just keep writing without looking for sources, you may wind up writing in a direction for which sufficient empirical support is not available.

It can also be distracting to have to key in the full reference entry into the reference list. One trick that eliminates some of the distraction is to type in (or paste) the reference entries one after the other, and then sort them into alphabetical order after you are finished looking up sources. Most word processing programs have a sort function that will sort the entries into alphabetical order. Of course, some citation styles—such as Chicago style and American Medical Association style—don't require alphabetizing reference entries.

As already stated, a primary advantage of the search-and-enter strategy is that the in-text citations and reference list are complete as soon as the draft is finished. You don't have to go back and look for sources or type in reference entries after you finish writing the draft. Everything is done—and for those people (like me) who like closure, it is very pleasing to have a complete draft that isn't missing the reference list.

Regarding reference lists, I should note an important change that has occurred in APA style over the past few years. Many APA journals (and some journals published by other publishers as well) have begun to require digital object identifier (DOI) numbers to be listed for all journal articles and book chapters. DOIs are long strings of numbers (and sometimes letters) that uniquely identify a given journal article or book chapter. DOIs must be copied from the article itself or from a search engine record and pasted into the entry in your reference list. If you create your reference list without the DOIs and the journal to which your paper is submitted requires DOIs, you will be asked to add them. If you have a long reference list, this can be a tedious and cumbersome task, so I recommend adding the DOIs when you create the reference list.

I believe that APA style is currently the only citation style that requires DOI numbers, but this could change. I recommend consulting the style guide for whichever citation style(s) you commonly use and purchasing each new edition as it is released. As soon as a citation style is changed, journals using that style will expect authors to follow the guidelines from the newest version.

Looking Up Citations and Saving the Reference List for Later

If you have someone who can create the reference list for you, it might be a good idea to find citations and write them into your draft, but to save the full texts of the articles (or preferably PDF versions, which look exactly like the print version in the journal). I create a folder for each paper I work on, and I save the article PDFs to that folder so that I can access them whenever I need to. In fact, having article PDFs stored on my computer allows me to do a "literature search" even when I don't have access to the Internet (if I'm on a plane that doesn't have wireless access, if I'm in a doctor's office, or if I'm on a train).

So it may be possible to collect the articles and give them to the person who will be compiling the reference list. An important drawback to having someone else compile the reference list is that this person may make mistakes. I have received reference lists from students where page numbers were listed incorrectly, journal titles were misspelled, formatting was wrong, or the list was out of order. The old saying "If you want something done right, do it yourself" applies here. I have had to spend almost as much time fixing other people's mistakes on reference lists as I have spent compiling reference lists on my own.

Now, some people might ask, "It's just a reference list, so who cares if it's not entirely accurate?" I have two responses. First, anything you put your name on should be as perfect as you can make it, and second, if there are mistakes in the reference list, you will be asked to correct them when the article is copyedited (which occurs after the editor accepts your paper and sends it to the publisher for production). You will have to correct the mistakes at some point—why not do it as soon as you can?

Saving Literature Searches for Later

The third strategy involves writing the paper without looking up sources at all. You would just write "(REF)" and then look for all the citations after you finish writing the draft. The clearest advantage to this strategy is that you can just write and not worry about references at all. If you are easily distracted and lose your train of thought, this may be a good strategy for you to utilize. The disadvantages are that you may have trouble finding citations for some of the claims you make, and if you cannot find a source, you will likely have to adjust the claim to fit the sources that you are able to find.

As I stated, I have used all these strategies in the past. The strategy I use most often now is to stop and conduct a literature search each time I need to cite a source and to enter the corresponding entry into the reference list immediately. This way, once I finish writing my first draft, the citations and references are done.

Additionally, storing all of the article PDFs from prior literature searches makes it easy for me to find articles that I have already identified—that is, because many of the articles that I write are on similar topics, I often reuse sources that I cited in other papers. Of course, new literature is published regularly, so I make sure to conduct a new literature search—as well as reusing earlier sources—whenever I need to find citations. In this way, I am able to add new articles to my PDF collection while also not "reinventing the wheel." Maintaining an article PDF collection allows me to easily look up articles I have downloaded before and to cite them if appropriate.

A Note on Self-Citations

A question I have heard a lot from beginning writers—as well as from more seasoned writers—concerns self-citations. If we are writing a literature review, whether as an introduction for an empirical paper or as a stand-alone literature review article, should we cite our own prior work if it seems like a good match for the claim we are making in the current paper? How much self-citation is too much? Is it OK to cite ourselves at all, or should we avoid self-citations completely?

What I have learned from serving as a journal reviewer is that although most journals use a double-blind peer review process (i.e., the authors don't know who the reviewers are, and the reviewers don't know who the authors are), I can almost always tell who an article's authors are by looking at the reference list and seeing which names appear most often. Most authors cite themselves frequently, and if there are multiple well-published authors on a paper, chances are that each of them will be cited multiple times. Although this liberal use of self-citations might seem narcissistic, remember that we know our own work better than we know other people's work. When we make a point that relates to our own prior work, often our first instinct is to cite our own studies. After all, isn't it easier to cite our own work—which we know extremely well—than to conduct a literature search to look for other sources?

I distinctly remember an article I wrote with a group of coauthors. The paper overlapped considerably with prior work that several of us had published, so we proceeded to cite ourselves frequently. Self-citations comprised approximately one third of the total citations in the paper. (Looking back, I'm somewhat ashamed of myself for being so narcissistic.) One reviewer was quite blunt and asked us to diversify our citations. "The authors surely must know that they are not the only people who have published in this area," the reviewer wrote.

That reviewer comment felt like a bucket of ice water being dumped over my head. When I went back and read the manuscript we had submitted to the journal, I was embarrassed by the sheer volume of self-citations. The primary motivation for citing ourselves so much was not narcissism, but laziness. We simply didn't feel like conducting a thorough literature search. But after reading that reviewer comment and rereading the paper, I understood the reviewer's point. I searched the literature and quickly found many sources with which to replace some of our self-citations. The reviewer knew the literature as well as we did, and they knew that we had missed several important sources that we should have cited.

So, let's revisit the original question. Is it OK to cite ourselves, and how much self-citation is too much? First, the answer is Yes, it is OK to cite yourself, as long as the citation accurately supports the claim you are making. Second, there needs to be a clear balance between self-citations and citations of other people's work. I don't think it's appropriate to specify a percentage of citations that can be to your own work, but when you find yourself citing your work as a way of avoiding a literature search, the self-citation may be excessive. In many cases, I cite my own work in addition to other sources—so that my work is used, in conjunction with other literature, to support the line of logic I'm tracing in the paper I'm writing.

In some cases, even after searching the literature, my own work is all that I can find to support a claim I'm making. Sometimes we "have the market cornered" in a specific line of research, and few other studies have been published in this area. In such cases, self-citations are appropriate. Self-citations are also appropriate if we are directly citing a study we conducted or a theoretical model we proposed. In fact, it would be odd to see other sources cited when we are referring specifically to our own work.

When we are specifically citing our own work, there are two ways to accomplish it. We can cite ourselves in first person or in third person. For example:

First Person: We (Schwartz et al., 2010) conducted a study and found that . . .

Third Person: Schwartz et al. (2010) conducted a study and found that . . .

When we use a first-person reference, we are essentially giving away the fact that we are the authors. Journals that use double-blind peer review will generally insist that all identifying information be removed from the body of the manuscript prior to submission. In some cases, journals will require that self-citations be replaced with "Author Citation" in the body of the paper so that reviewers will not know who the authors are. (Self-citations are then restored once the paper is accepted for publication.)

Even if a journal does not have specific regulations against first-person self-citations, some reviewers might comment on first-person self-citations or request that the self-citations be converted to third person. I once had a reviewer tell me that it was "highly inappropriate" for my colleagues and me to identify ourselves as the authors of the paper. Because authors generally must satisfy all of the reviewers before their manuscript will be accepted for publication (an issue that is revisited in Chapter 12), when a reviewer asks you to remove first-person self-citations, you almost certainly must comply with this request.

In my estimation, then, it is safest to use third-person self-citations in most cases. Reviewers will be able to "read between the lines" and figure out who the authors are. If we say, "The present study builds upon work conducted by Schwartz et al. (2010), who proposed that . . .," then reviewers might start to believe that we are the authors. My colleagues and I have published more than 30 articles on our longitudinal acculturation study, in which we recruited and assessed recently immigrated Hispanic families living in Miami and Los Angeles. Because we are the only researchers who have conducted such a study, anyone reviewing papers from this study will immediately recognize my colleagues and me as authors. There is simply no way to de-identify a paper from this study—and I have made this exact argument to editors and reviewers when they have asked us to de-identify our papers.

To sum up, there is nothing wrong with citing ourselves—as long as we do not do it excessively or as an excuse not to search for other sources. Our prior published work is part of the scientific literature, and deliberately not citing ourselves when it would be appropriate to do so may be just as inaccurate as citing too much of our own work. However, I caution writers against citing unpublished work (including master's theses and doctoral dissertations). Because unpublished work has not undergone rigorous peer review, the quality of such work cannot be reliably ascertained. Theses and dissertations are reviewed by faculty committees, but this level of review is not the same as the peer review to which journal manuscripts are subjected. Similarly, it may be risky to cite manuscripts that have been submitted for publication but that have not yet been accepted. Reviewers may ask for any number of changes that can affect the results that are reported, or the editor may reject the paper after receiving the reviews. It is safest to cite work that has at least been accepted for publication.

Dealing With Writer's Block

Almost all writers have had this experience: You have been writing for a while, and you've said what you wanted to say. However, you know that the writing is not complete—there is more that needs to be said, but you are simply not sure what that is. So you sit there, staring at the screen, unsure of what else to write.

Let me assure you that I—the person writing a book about how to write for publication—have been in this situation many, many times. Even when I have an outline, sometimes I won't know how to finish writing one of the sections in the outline. Worse yet, the harder I try to come up with words and ideas, the more elusive they become.

When I am in this situation, I usually do not try to fight the writer's block directly. Trying to fight through writer's block is like banging your head against the wall. It's futile and leads to even more frustration. (My father has a great expression about this kind of frustration—when you have banged your head against the wall long enough, it feels really good when you stop.) Trying to "force" yourself to write your way through writer's block is not an approach that I recommend.

In this scenario, I use one of three strategies: I move on to another section of the paper, I take a break from working on the paper, or I send it to a coauthor and ask for help. The specific strategy I use depends on where I am in the process of writing the draft, as well as on whether I have any energy left to continue writing. One point that I cannot emphasize enough is that we are human beings, not machines—and we don't generally work well when we are tired, upset, stressed, or distracted. Sometimes, we need to stop working for the day and pick up later where we left off.

If the block seems to be centered on not knowing what to write in a specific section, the solution may be to start writing the next section. When this happens, I simply type "More Here" at the end of the section I am struggling to finish, and I move on to the next section in my outline and start writing that section. If the writer's block is specific to one section of the paper, this approach may be helpful.

If the block persists no matter what I try to write, then I may decide to take a break. Sometimes 15 minutes is all I need—just to stand up, stretch my legs, and walk around the house or the building. If it's anywhere close to lunchtime, I might go make myself a sandwich (if I'm at home) or walk downstairs and buy something to eat (if I'm in the office). If it's late in the day and I am running out of energy, I might decide to sign off for the day or go home. When my brain is exhausted and doesn't want to focus, I know it's time to stop working.

If a major writing block hits me in the middle of the day, I might find something else to do—answer emails, conduct analyses, edit other people's paper drafts, and so forth. Distracting myself with other tasks sometimes helps me to take my mind off the writer's block. Even if we are not in a good "writing place," we undoubtedly have other tasks that need to be completed. We can come back to the writing later in the day, the next day, or the next time we sit down to write.

Finally, especially early in my academic career, I sometimes didn't know what to do with a paper. I had written as much as I could, and even taking breaks didn't help. I knew that the paper was not complete, but I had no idea what to add or to change. In that situation, I would send the draft to a coauthor and ask for help. I would give the coauthor an email summary of what I was trying to accomplish with the paper, and I would outline the areas where I felt especially stuck.

I did this with José once. I was writing a theoretical paper on the confluence between prevention science and positive youth development, and even with a detailed outline, I felt stuck. I had written all I could, but the paper was bad. I read it over several times and didn't like it very much. Something important was missing, but I had no idea what the missing piece was. So I sent the paper to José, and he provided the detailed and prescriptive comments for which he was famous. After reading over his feedback, I felt much more confident about the direction in which I wanted to take the paper. When we finally submitted the paper for publication, it was accepted after two rounds of review.

Thus, receiving feedback from coauthors can help in overcoming writer's block. As I note throughout this book, writing is not a one-person activity. Writing is a team activity. I rarely write by myself because I enjoy working with other people and receiving their feedback. Regardless of how good a writer I might think I am, my coauthors help me to strengthen my writing. They point out logical leaps, incomplete arguments, internal contradictions, and other problems that I may not have noticed even when I was editing and polishing my drafts. In my opinion, writing alone is like having a conversation all by yourself—it's not very much fun, and you don't receive feedback or responses.

Even if you are writing alone (i.e., as the sole author), I would still recommend asking colleagues to read over drafts and give you feedback. Editing one's own work is very difficult—you miss many issues and errors that other people will catch—so I do not recommend submitting a paper for publication without having someone else read it first. Especially early in your writing career, it is important to solicit as much feedback as you can. We learn how to write by receiving feedback from others and from revising our papers in response to that feedback.

I cannot overstate the importance of mentors in the writing process. Writing is a skill that is developed through repeated and deliberate practice. Often, the best people from whom to solicit feedback are your mentors—your advisor if you are a student, your supervisor or principal investigator if you are a postdoc, or your faculty mentor if you are a junior faculty member. In my experience, mentoring is a lot like parenting—mentors spend a great deal of time pointing out and gently correcting mistakes, providing guidance, and offering constructive input. When I offer to mentor someone, I know that the person will be coming to me for advice, sending me drafts to review, and looking to me for guidance and input. Therefore, as you are learning the art of academic and scientific writing, make sure to consult your mentors frequently.

Several years ago, I reviewed a manuscript for a developmental psychology journal. The writing was very choppy and difficult to read. The literature review was like a roller coaster ride—here, there, and everywhere. The methods were not described in detail, and the results section was full of analyses that had little to do with the hypotheses that had been presented in the introduction. The paper didn't have a discussion section, and only a few interpretive statements were included to help the reader understand the findings and how they could be used to guide further work and applied in real-world settings.

Reviewing poorly written manuscripts is frustrating. José used to say that when he was reading a poorly written paper, he would become angry at the paper, and his comments would become increasingly critical and negative. (I experienced this negativity firsthand when I first started working with José and was learning how to write academic papers.) I thought about writing a scathing review of the manuscript and slamming the author for not knowing how to put together an academic paper. But then I caught myself. The author identified herself as "she" (indicating that this was a single-author paper) and included text suggesting that the paper was based on her doctoral dissertation. The author clearly didn't have the mentoring that she needed to learn how to write a journal article—and this was not her fault. I was a graduate student once, and I wasn't a very good writer then either. José was the person who gave me critical feedback on my drafts and really taught me how to write—and I didn't meet him until I was more than a year out of graduate school.

So I sat down and wrote a very constructive, supportive review in which I tried to offer the author some suggestions for improving her writing. I have no idea whether she followed any of my suggestions—and because the review process was double-blinded, I didn't even know who she was—but if I were she, I would have wanted to receive guidance and mentoring, not harsh criticism, from reviewers. Had this author received more involved mentoring, the paper she submitted based on her dissertation would have been far more organized, and it would have had a far better chance of being published. Unfortunately, this kind of support does not often occur in the journal review process. (The journal review process is covered in Chapters 13 and 14.)

Knowing When a First Draft is Finished

A question that I already alluded to in this chapter is, "When do I know I am done writing my first draft?" It's a very good question, especially for early-career writers who may not know what a finished draft looks like. How do we know when to stop writing, put the draft aside, and come back to it in a few days?

I'll give you two versions of the answer—the quick version and the more extensive version. The quick version is that you stop writing when you have filled in all the sections of your outline. Once you've made all the points that you set out to make, then your first draft is done. Set it aside and don't look at it for at least 3 to 5 days so that the ideas will fade from your mind. Then you can come back and start editing (see Chapter 9).

The more extensive version of the answer is that, even after you think you are finished with the first draft, you may realize that there were points you forgot to make, or you may receive a burst of inspiration suggesting additional paragraphs or sections to write. You may go back through your outline and realize that you have not emphasized some points as well as you wanted to. Maybe there were details in the method section that you meant to include, but now you realize that you didn't include them—or maybe you missed some limitations at the end of the discussion. In any case, as long as you are not trying to edit existing text (that step needs to wait at least 3 to 5 days after you declare your first draft to be finished), it's fine to go back and fill in any holes you find.

It is much easier to know when a first draft of an empirical paper is done than it is to know when the first draft of a theoretical or review article is done. As I already noted, empirical articles have a set structure (introduction, method, results, discussion) within which we create our outline and write our drafts. Theoretical and review articles do not have a set structure—the structure is whatever the authors say it is. As noted in Chapter 4, outlines are especially important for writing theoretical and review articles. Without an outline, it's extremely easy to be AOTP, to forget to cover important points, and to leave out some essential sections entirely.

Writing theoretical and review articles (as well as position papers) is covered in Chapter 16. For now, I quote Al Waterman, who told me on several occasions that "It is very, very difficult to publish theory." When we write a theoretical article, we don't have empirical data to support our arguments and conclusions. Reviewers can challenge almost anything we say. I suggest writing empirical articles as a "warm up," to help you learn how to write academic papers. Additionally, when you do start writing theory, I suggest working with coauthors. Writing a single-authored theoretical or review article is extremely challenging, and I don't recommend that beginning authors take on this kind of task by themselves.

Let me also make a note about length. Even when writing a first draft, it's important to know the specific journal and audience for which the paper is intended. If you are writing for a public health journal with a 2500-word limit, writing a 10,000-word first draft probably is not a good idea. With that said, I recommend allowing yourself to freely transfer the ideas from your mind onto the screen. If the resulting draft is way over the word or page limit for your intended journal, you might want to consider a different journal with a more generous word or page limit.

On average, each double-spaced page of text can hold approximately 250 words, so a 2500-word limit means 10 pages of text. (Make sure to check the target journal's author guidelines—sometimes the space (word or page) limit includes the title page, abstract, references, figures, and tables, but sometimes the limit includes only the body of the paper.) Importantly, your outline should fit the journal's word or page limit. Don't outline more sections than can fit within the limit.

Al Waterman, who was a journal editor or associate editor for more than 25 years, liked to say that each manuscript has an ideal length that is needed to express the ideas or to report the results. He generally didn't believe in space limits, and in cases where such limits were imposed by the journal or by the publisher, he would often grant authors considerable leeway. Most editors are not nearly as flexible as he was, and the submission portals that most journals use require authors to report the number of words and pages in their manuscripts. Editorial assistants often send papers back to the author if they exceed the space limit. Sometimes editors are willing to allow authors to exceed the space limit, but generally these exceptions are granted for revised manuscripts where the length increased as a result of responding to reviewer requests. Editors generally do not allow authors to exceed the journal's space limit for first submissions.

As is covered in Chapter 9, first drafts often contain some redundancy, where the same point appears in more than one place—and correcting the redundancy can help to reduce length. At the same time, first drafts are also often characterized by logical leaps, where a piece of the argument is missing and must be filled in. Filling in the missing pieces will increase length. Therefore, there is no guarantee that a first draft that exceeds the space limit by several pages can be cut down sufficiently without taking out some of the "meat" of the paper. You may need to cut out entire paragraphs or sections if your goal is to submit to the journal that you targeted.

Conclusion

This chapter covers techniques for writing first drafts. In general, the purpose of a first draft is to transfer ideas from your mind onto the screen. Writers need to be in a flow state to do their best writing, and writing is best undertaken when it is intrinsically motivated. It is also essential to set reasonable goals and to hold reasonable expectations—for example, someone who is just learning to write academic papers may not be able to sit and write for 6 consecutive hours. Setting realistic deadlines may mean that the draft is not completed as quickly as we might like, but we can spare ourselves a great deal of anxiety and frustration by being realistic.

This chapter also emphasizes the dangers of maladaptive perfectionism, where the need to be perfect prevents us from freely expressing our thoughts on the screen. First drafts cannot be perfect, so our goal should be creating an initial version of the paper that we can edit, sharpen, and polish later. Although length is an important consideration—writing a draft that is far longer than the page or word limit for our target journal is not a good idea—we should impose as few constraints as possible on ourselves as we write. Importantly, the writing and editing phases should be separated, so the draft needs to be completed before we start editing. It is essential to avoid anything that will increase our anxiety or self-criticism while we are still putting together our first draft. Editing needs to wait until several days after the first draft is completed.

Finally, some authors express concerns about knowing when a first draft has been completed. The most important answer is that it doesn't matter. If the draft is incomplete—which is almost always the case, because first drafts are supposed to be rough—we can fill in the missing pieces when we edit. I often tell my students that first drafts are supposed to be bad. The purpose of a first draft is to transfer thoughts from one's minds onto the screen, not to generate a perfect version of the paper.

Summary

- When assembling a first draft, we start from our outline and write within the headings we specified.
- Developing intrinsic writing motivation is an essential part of becoming a successful scholarly writer.
- It may be necessary to start with short writing sessions and build up to longer sessions.
- First drafts are supposed to be rough. The purpose of a first draft is to transfer ideas from one's mind onto the screen. It is impossible to write a perfect first draft—so it is unreasonable to expect that one's first draft will be perfect.
- There are multiple ways to add citations to a first draft. These methods are: (a) stopping to look up literature and adding citations to the reference list each time a citation is needed, (b) entering citations but leaving the reference list for later, and (c) just writing and saving literature searches for later. Each method has advantages and disadvantages.
- It is perfectly acceptable to cite one's own work when it is relevant, as long as other authors' work is also cited. Citing one's own work as a way to avoid searching for sources is generally not advisable.
- When one encounters writer's block, the best strategy may be to work on another part of the paper, or to stop trying to write and to come back to it later.
- A first draft can be considered "finished" when the outline is completely filled in. But authors may think of other points to make later. Ultimately, it does not matter whether a draft is finished—it should be sent to coauthors as soon as the lead author believes it is ready.

References

Chirkov, V. I. (2009). A cross-cultural analysis of autonomy in education: A self-determination theory perspective. *Theory and Research in Education, 7*, 253–262.

Csikszentmihalyi, M. (1990). *Flow: The psychology of optimal experience.* New York: Basic Books.

Deci, E. L., & Ryan, R. M. (1985). *Intrinsic motivation and self-determination in human behavior.* New York: Plenum.

Deci, E. L., & Ryan, R. M. (2008). Self-determination theory: A macrotheory of human motivation, development, and health. *Canadian Psychology, 49*, 182–185.

Waterman, A. S., Schwartz, S. J., Goldbacher, E., Green, H., Miller, C., & Philip, S. (2003). Self-determination, flow, and self-realization values as predictors of intrinsic motivation. *Personality and Social Psychology Bulletin, 29*, 1447–1458.

9

Editing, Filling in Gaps, and Cutting

Chapter Objectives

When you finish reading this chapter, you should feel more comfortable with:

- Editing drafts as an iterative process
- Working with mentors on revising manuscript drafts
- Identifying and correcting common problems in first drafts
- Spotting and correcting internal inconsistencies
- Avoiding overstating conclusions from a study
- Writing a strong concluding paragraph
- Cutting length from a manuscript
- Writing the abstract for a manuscript

Now we have finished our first draft, set it aside for a few days, and come back to it. What do we do now? How do we turn our first draft into a submittable paper?

The short answer is that it will take many drafts and iterations to go from first draft to submission-quality manuscript. You will make many changes in your first iteration, but the next time you look at the draft, you will find more changes to make. Editing a draft of a scholarly manuscript is similar to carving a sculpture—molding a piece of rock into a work of art takes time and effort, as well as multiple sittings. Even the best writers cannot transform a first draft into a submission-quality paper in one sitting. As you make changes and re-view the changes you have made, more changes will occur to you. Editing is an iterative process.

I once had a friend who had completed his PhD in education many years ago. He complained about his dissertation committee members' practice of "changing their own changes"—suggesting a change to the dissertation, reviewing subsequent drafts, and then suggesting additional changes. My friend didn't like that his committee members did this, but during the editing process, we change our own changes all the time, and our coauthors will change their own changes as well. Sometimes we cannot tell that additional changes are necessary until we have made the initial changes and reviewed

The Savvy Academic. Seth J. Schwartz, Oxford University Press. © Oxford University Press 2022.
DOI: 10.1093/oso/9780190095918.003.0010

them. In a way, papers "evolve" from first drafts to more polished, submittable manuscripts through multiple iterations, and there really is no way to circumvent this process.

In this chapter, I review the process I use to edit drafts of my own writing, and I sprinkle in coverage of how I edit other people's papers. Much of what I do is identical regardless of whether the draft I'm editing is my own or someone else's. The primary difference is whether I am making the changes myself or suggesting them as tracked comments, but the process I follow is the same.

I am a stream-of-consciousness editor. This means that I mark issues as I spot them, rather than reading the whole paper and then coming back to make comments. On many occasions, when I'm reading someone else's draft, I will comment that I don't understand something, only to come across the explanation a few sentences later. However, the fact that I didn't understand the concept when I first saw it may mean that the concept needs to be explained the first time it appears. We do not want readers struggling to understand our line of reasoning, even for a few minutes. José told me that well-written papers follow a straight line of logic from beginning to end, and that there are no deviations from the logic. Readers enjoy reading these papers because they are easy to understand. Simply put, the more effort readers have to expend to understand what you're saying, the less likely they are to want to read the paper.

I generally start the editing process by reading the paper from beginning to end, stopping to make changes (if I'm editing my own paper) or make suggestions and edits (if I'm editing someone else's paper). Usually, I correct problems as I spot them. When I'm editing a paper that I've written, sometimes it takes me several hours to get through the draft because I am constantly stopping to add, delete, or modify text. And each time I read through the paper, I make more changes. Commonly, I don't send the paper out to my coauthors until I am completely satisfied with it—that is, I can read through the whole paper without stopping to make changes.

Earlier in my career, it took me much longer to finish editing. I would make changes to a draft, but then I would read the draft again and would find more problems. Sometimes I would go through 20 or 25 drafts and still be making corrections, and I would still not be ready to share the draft with my coauthors. If you are having similar experiences, rest assured that this is completely normal. As your writing skills improve, it will take you fewer and fewer iterations to transform your first draft into a submittable manuscript. Currently, I can move from first draft to shareable draft (to send to my coauthors) in around 8 to 10 iterations. Regardless of how good I think my draft is, when I do share the draft with my coauthors, they usually make lots of comments. Including editing iterations undertaken in response to coauthor feedback, I can usually move from first draft to submittable manuscript in 15 to 20 iterations.

How did I learn how to become a better writer? By working with José and using his critical feedback to help me understand the writing problems that he was pointing out. As noted in Chapter 8, mentors play an essential role in helping mentees to learn how to write effectively. As a mentor, my job is to provide detailed and critical feedback to my mentees on their writing. My comments should be respectful and constructive, but I should not seek to spare my mentees' feelings. They need tough feedback to help them correct writing problems. I would not be the writer I am today—and I would not be writing this book—if not for José's critical comments on my drafts. He was never disrespectful, but he pointed out anything and everything that he spotted. As I have said throughout this book, he was the person who really taught me how to write. I see it as my job to provide this same support to my mentees.

Mentors are important not only in helping mentees to write first drafts, but also in helping them to revise their drafts. An effective mentor will sit down with the mentee and go over the mentor's comments on the draft—as a way of helping the mentee to understand the changes being suggested. The mentor should also be willing to review as many drafts as necessary before the paper goes out to coauthors, and the mentor should be willing to help the mentee respond to, and incorporate, coauthor feedback. If you are an early-career writer, I suggest that you work with your mentor (or find someone to mentor you, if you don't already have a mentor) and ask this person to provide critical feedback on your drafts.

When editing a draft, it is essential to be mindful of your outline. As you add, modify, or delete text, make sure that the structure of the paper doesn't change—unless you make a deliberate decision to change the outline. Indeed, sometimes changes to one section of the paper can lead you to realize that more sections are necessary, that an existing section needs to be divided into multiple sections, or that a section is not necessary. My point here is that such changes to the structure of the paper should be made deliberately, rather than as an unintended consequence of straying from your outline.

Common Problems to Look for When Editing a First Draft

When you are reviewing and editing your first draft, there are several problems that you will likely encounter. These include redundancy, unfinished thoughts, unjustified statements, undefined jargon and abbreviations, logical leaps, internal inconsistencies, tangents, run-on sentences, and overstated conclusions. You may also spot grammatical and spelling errors that you did not catch while writing your first draft. Each of these problems is reviewed here—both in terms of how to spot them and in terms of how to correct them.

Redundancy

Redundancy is probably the most common problem I spot in my initial drafts. Because first drafts are generally written across several sittings—and sometimes several weeks or months will pass between sittings—I don't always remember what I wrote during earlier sessions. As a result, some of the same points are introduced in multiple places throughout the paper. If not corrected, redundancy is extremely annoying to reviewers.

Sometimes redundancy can be a symptom of being AOTP (all over the place). Many beginning writers have a difficult time recognizing and correcting AOTP writing, even when they are editing their drafts. Mentors need to point out AOTP writing and help their mentees learn how to spot it on their own. Many writing problems stem from being AOTP, and although using an outline can help reduce the AOTP problem, it is still possible to be AOTP within a given section of the paper. Correcting AOTP tendencies can go a long way toward correcting a range of writing problems.

The simplest way to correct redundancy is to go back to your outline and identify the best place where the point in question should be made. Then you can copy the various pieces of text that make the same points and paste all of them into that section of the paper. After that, you will need to smooth out the text so that it flows—which will involve deleting or modifying text (and perhaps adding new text to improve flow). Here is a fictitious example where text excerpts from two sections of the paper are pasted in together and modified:

Original Excerpt 1: Because mothers and fathers often play different roles within the family system, it is essential to include both parents in research studies where possible. Failure to include both parents may provide a biased representation of parenting functions.

Original Excerpt 2: Both mothers and fathers should be included in research studies, because mothering and fathering are often quite distinct.

Pasted Together Before Integration: Because mothers and fathers often play different roles within the family system, it is essential to include both parents in research studies where possible. Failure to include both parents may provide a biased representation of parenting functions. Both mothers and fathers should be included in research studies, because mothering and fathering are often quite distinct.

Pasted Together, Some Text from Second Excerpt Integrated with First Excerpt: Because mothers and fathers often play different roles within the family system, and because mothering and fathering are often quite distinct, it is essential to include both parents in research studies where possible. ~~Failure to include both parents may provide a biased representation of parenting functions. Both mothers and fathers should be included in research studies.~~

In this example, we took some of the text from the second excerpt and integrated it into the first excerpt. We then deleted the remainder of the second excerpt. This integration allows us to extract the meaning from both instances while eliminating the redundancy. In some cases, text excerpts may duplicate each other so much that the most effective course of action may be to delete one of the excerpts. It is not always necessary to preserve text from each of the redundant excerpts—we preserve text only when it adds important meaning to the excerpt that we have decided to retain.

Whereas redundancy can be annoying to readers and reviewers if it is included without purpose, some intentional redundancy may help to drive home an essential point. For example, we might note early in the paper that findings from a study filling an important gap in the literature may have critical implications for the design and delivery of interventions. We might then review the intervention implications in the discussion. This kind of foreshadowing can be effective in terms of setting up a key point early on and then hammering it home later in the paper.

Unfinished Thoughts

Unfinished thoughts are another extremely common problem. My writing has been plagued with unfinished thoughts throughout my career. The turning point for me occurred in 1999, when my wife critically read one of my first articles and provided extensive comments. Her chief criticism was that I wasn't finishing my thoughts. When I saw her comments, I realized that I had been facing this problem for years—and her feedback taught me to watch out for unfinished thoughts as I am writing. Now I often ask myself whether I have finished my thought before I end a paragraph or section and start the next one.

Here is an example of an unfinished thought and a way in which adding an extra sentence at the end of the paragraph can help to finish off the thought:

> *Unfinished Thought*: Symptoms of anxiety and depression can undermine students' academic and social performance. It is necessary to provide counseling for students, even if they do not display any detectable signs of distress. Students may be more comfortable simply knowing that counseling services are available to them.
>
> *Concluding Sentence Added*: Symptoms of anxiety and depression can undermine students' academic and social performance. It is necessary to provide counseling for students, even if they do not display any detectable signs of distress. Students may be more comfortable simply knowing that counseling services are available to them. It is essential to offer resources to reduce the effects of anxiety and depressive symptoms on students' quality of life.

Notice how the new concluding sentence helps to tie the preceding sentences together and summarize the message of the paragraph. Without this final sentence, the paragraph is left hanging. An unfinished thought might lead readers to ask, "So what?" or "What do you mean by that?" The concluding sentence provides your answer to these questions.

Unfinished thoughts can be a problem not only for paragraphs, but also for whole sections of the paper. Ask yourself this: Does this section convey a single line of thought? Is the meaning clear? Have I completed the logic, or is the section left hanging? The final sentence in the last paragraph of the section should wrap up not only that paragraph, but also the whole section.

The paper itself should end with a concluding paragraph that summarizes the primary contributions of the study, review, or theory being presented. Without such a paragraph, the paper "drops off of a cliff." In essence, a paper without a conclusion is an unfinished thought. Here is an example of a concluding paragraph:

> In conclusion, the present results indicate that experiencing discrimination is damaging not only for one's psychological well-being, but also for one's cardiovascular and metabolic health. A key take-home message from these findings is that interventions to increase resilience against discrimination are urgently needed. Although reducing discrimination is likely not feasible at the individual level, intervention programs to help individuals cope with and manage discriminatory experiences may be able to offset the deleterious effects of discrimination on mental and physical health. We hope that these findings will inspire more research and policy efforts in this direction.

Although I do not advise doing this, a reader could conceivably read only the concluding paragraph and have a good sense of what the paper was about. The concluding paragraph is intended to hammer home the paper's primary messages—in this case, that experiencing discrimination is damaging to one's health and that developing interventions to offset the effects of discrimination represents a critical public health priority. The final paragraph is, in essence, the writer's opportunity to remind readers of the messages that they can take away from the paper. The "recency effect" in psychology—where events that occurred most recently are most likely to be remembered (Talmi & Goshen-Gottstein, 2006)—can be used to your advantage in the concluding paragraph. Tell your readers what you want them to remember.

Unjustified Statements

Unjustified statements are concepts or ideas that are included in the paper without being introduced previously. Ideas that "come out of nowhere" are very distracting to readers because they disrupt the flow of the paper. Sometimes I feel a sense of whiplash when I'm reading a draft that is AOTP, with ideas coming out of nowhere and the line of logic meandering here, there, and everywhere. Reading papers like that gives me a headache, and it is difficult to assess the quality of the ideas in the paper when the flow of ideas is poorly organized.

Although unjustified statements are often a symptom of being AOTP, sometimes we simply forget to introduce a topic during an earlier writing session and then incorporate it into the paper during a subsequent session. The most obvious solution is either (a) to introduce and define the concept where it is used, so that readers will understand it, or (b) to find an earlier location in the paper to introduce the concept. Which of the two strategies is better depends on the specific situation at hand. I provide some examples here.

If the concept is fundamental to the paper, and if much of the logic underlying the paper is dependent on the concept in question, then I advise introducing the idea as early as possible. If you read through your first draft and you notice that a key concept is not defined early on, then look for a place in the beginning of the introduction to lay out and define the concept. Remember that readers will only know what you explicitly write into your paper—they will not know what is in your head—so it is not safe to assume that readers will be aware of anything that is not clearly stated in the paper.

One question I have been asked in my publication seminars is how much to write about a key concept. It's difficult to provide a general answer to that question—it really depends on how much readers need to know and on what level of content knowledge can be assumed given the breadth versus specificity of the journal. For example, if you are writing for the *Journal of Adolescent Health*, you can probably assume that readers know about adolescent development. On the other hand, readers of the *American Journal of Public Health* cannot necessarily be assumed to know about adolescent development (because the journal's scope and readership are broader and less focused on a specific public health topic). Therefore, somewhat more basic information about adolescent development—the age range that adolescence represents, the physical, biological, emotional, and social changes that occur, and the social spheres in which adolescents live—needs to be provided in manuscripts targeting the *American Journal of Public Health* than in manuscripts targeting the *Journal of Adolescent Health*.

As is noted in Chapter 4 in the discussion of creating outlines, the purpose of the introductory section is to orient the reader toward your study, argument, or theory. Any information that the reader requires in order to be able to understand your work—such as the population you are referencing, the variables or constructs you are focusing on, and the specific research design you used—needs to be mentioned in the introduction. If you don't present a key concept in the introduction, then you will have an unjustified statement when the concept is referenced later in the paper.

Remember the principle I mention in Chapter 4—tell readers what you're going to tell them, then tell them, and then tell them what you told them. This principle applies even more to theory, literature review, and position papers than it does to empirical manuscripts—because non-empirical papers don't have set structure for you to follow. The "tell them what you're going to tell them" step allows you to set up the key points in your thesis up front, so that readers will recognize these points when you expand on them later. Even within the introductory section of an empirical manuscript, you can include a one-paragraph roadmap that "tells them what you're going to tell them." Once this roadmap is in place, you can expand on your arguments without worrying about making unjustified statements. Just remember to lay out the key ingredients of your study or argument in the first few paragraphs so that the reader is not blindsided by new concepts later.

Here is an example of a roadmap paragraph, taken from an article that my colleagues and I published, where we introduced a new model of acculturation (Schwartz, Unger, Zamboanga, & Szapocznik, 2010, p. 238):

> There are many aspects of the acculturation literature that may require rethinking, and we focus on some of those here. First, we review and contrast major

acculturation models that have been developed within cultural psychology, and we outline some of the strengths and weaknesses of these approaches. Second, we discuss the roles of ethnicity, and of similarity between heritage culture and receiving culture, in acculturation. Third, we delineate the ways in which acculturation is more or less salient, and may operate differently, for different groups or types of migrants. Fourth, we discuss the immigrant paradox, in which acculturation has been examined simplistically in relation to health outcomes, and we suggest addressing the immigrant paradox by expanding the conceptualization of acculturation. Fifth, we introduce such an expanded model of acculturation—including cultural practices, values, and identifications—that has the potential to synthesize several existing literatures and to increase the theoretical, empirical, and practical utility of the acculturation construct. Finally, we delineate context of reception as the ways in which the receiving society constrains and directs the acculturation options available to migrants, and we frame acculturative stress and discrimination under the heading of an unfavorable context of reception.

In addition to this roadmap paragraph, we needed to be sure to introduce the concept of acculturation and to define how we were using the term. On page 237 of the Schwartz et al. (2010) article, we noted the following:

> Broadly, as applied to individuals, acculturation refers to changes that take place as a result of contact with culturally dissimilar people, groups, and social influences (Gibson, 2001). Although these changes can take place as a result of almost any intercultural contact (e.g., globalization; Arnett, 2002), acculturation is most often studied in individuals living in countries or regions other than where they were born—that is, among immigrants, refugees, asylum seekers, and sojourners (e.g., international students, seasonal farm workers; Berry, 2006b).

Thus, when we referred to acculturation later in the article, readers knew what we meant. We also told readers to whom acculturation applies, thereby establishing the conceptual boundaries for our theoretical approach. Chapter 16 covers more about writing theoretical and position papers, but I will say here that it is essential to establish boundaries for one's theoretical approach so that readers know to whom the theory applies and to whom it does not apply. As we did in the 2010 article, these boundaries should be established up front so that the reader isn't left wondering about the limits of the authors' analysis or theoretical perspective later on. Indeed, sometimes authors include many unjustified statements when they limit the scope of their perspective in ways that have not been explained previously.

To repeat: *When in doubt, spell it out.* Tell your readers explicitly what you mean, rather than assuming that they know what you mean.

As you come across unjustified statements in your manuscript, you should decide on a case-by-case basis where the statements should be set up. If the unjustified statement can easily be clarified in the same location where the statement appears, then I suggest writing a sentence or two before the unjustified statement to provide the necessary background. In some cases, a whole additional paragraph may be needed to set up a complex concept—but as you contemplate adding text, be mindful of the target journal's space limit. It's okay to exceed the limit by a small amount during the editing process, knowing that you will come back later and cut length—but I do not advise exceeding the space limit by more than two pages (500 words). The more length you add, the more cutting you will need to do before you can submit. (Note: Page limits are often easier to work with than word limits, because there are creative ways to reduce lines of text. I review some of the techniques in this chapter.)

When an unjustified statement requires additional text to be added earlier in the paper, you need to identify the best location where this additional text should be inserted. My recommendation is to disrupt the existing flow of ideas as little as possible—so if there is a clear place to add the new text, add it there and then edit the surrounding text so that the ideas flow clearly. If there doesn't appear to be a clear place to insert the new text, then you will have to move the existing text around to create space for the new text. My best advice in this situation is to draft the text that you will use to set up the unjustified statement, and then insert the new text between two existing paragraphs. After that, you will probably have to start moving text around within some of the existing paragraphs and to edit some of the text in these paragraphs, so that the line of logic flows as well as possible.

Also note that, in many cases, the solution to problems with flow and unjustified statements can involve moving existing text as well as drafting new text. You may provide a wonderful explanation of a concept on page 10, but this explanation really should appear on page 4 so that readers will understand your ideas as soon as possible. Editing drafts involves moving text around at least as often as it involves drafting new text and deleting existing text. Remember, as you write your first draft, your ideas are moving from your mind onto the screen with as little editing as possible. As a result, the ideas that you have put into writing should represent what you wish to communicate to your readers. Many of the problems that authors identify in their first drafts, and that their mentors and colleagues identify when editing drafts, involve how thoughts are organized at least as much as how they are expressed. Of course, there will almost always be instances where the author, or the author's mentor or colleague, has trouble understanding the meaning that a word, phrase, or sentence is intended to convey. In my experience, however, organization is at least as much of a challenge when editing drafts. Indeed, the AOTP problem is about organization, and even if individual sentences convey their meaning quite well, poor organization can render a paper virtually unreadable.

The point is that editing first drafts is a combination of (a) rewriting and sharpening existing text and (b) moving text around to improve organization. In the case of unjustified statements, if there is no text in the paper that could be moved around to help set up the unjustified statement, then new text must be drafted. In many cases, however, existing text can be moved earlier in the paper, and then the text can be edited to improve flow and to sharpen the meaning. Therefore, when you look over your first draft and you see an unjustified statement, you might decide to look for text in that location (or elsewhere in the manuscript) that can be moved earlier in the paper and used to set up the unjustified statement.

Undefined Jargon and Abbreviations

Undefined jargon and abbreviations occur when technical terms, abbreviations, or acronyms are used without previously being introduced and defined. As with unjustified statements, determining what terms and abbreviations need to be defined depends on the specific journal and audience for which you are writing. Terms like *fMRI* (functional magnetic resonance imaging), *EEG* (electroencephalogram), and *GWAS* (genome-wide association study), for example, may be more familiar to biologically oriented audiences than to audiences in the more traditional social sciences. If you are writing for a neuroscience or genetics journal, you probably do not need to define these and other related terms. However, if you are writing for a political science or sociology journal, it's probably safest to include a definition the first time the term is used. Some acronyms are readily understood and do not need to be defined, such as ANOVA (analysis of variance) and OR (odds ratio).

If you are not sure whether an abbreviation, acronym, or term needs to be defined the first time you use it, it is safest to include a definition. At worst, reviewers will ask you to remove the definition. Remember—when in doubt, spell it out. (Note: In tables and figures, abbreviations need to be spelled out in the table notes or figure legend, even if they have been defined earlier in the paper. Tables and figures need to stand on their own, without the reader's needing to refer to the text.)

The bottom line regarding undefined jargon is that it is distracting to readers. Readers have to stop and ask themselves what the expression or abbreviation means—which takes away from the train of thought that they are following as they are reading an article. Simply put, we need to write in a way that provides as few distractions as possible for readers. José once wrote on one of my advanced drafts that he was able to "peer into the crystalline water and see my message clearly" (yes, he is a master of analogies). His comment reflects what we want from our manuscripts—to be so clear that the message is easy for readers to absorb and understand.

In essence, when we edit a first draft, we are looking for distractions and correcting them. As we correct distractions, more will become apparent—hence the need for multiple iterations of the editing process. When we can read through the paper and not be distracted by redundancy, unjustified statements, undefined jargon, internal inconsistencies, and other writing problems, then we are ready to share the draft with our coauthors. Of course, the absence of obvious distractions does not mean that we are finished editing and that we are ready to submit the manuscript for publication. There may be more advanced issues remaining, such as inadequate descriptions of the study methods, erroneous characterizations of prior literature, suboptimal analytic strategies, incorrect reporting of results, omission of key limitations, and other problems that are described in Chapter 11.

Logical Leaps

Logical leaps are instances where the paper's logic jumps from one thought to another without including a bridging statement to connect the two statements. Following the train of thought when a logical leap occurs is similar to driving over a bridge where a segment of the road is missing. On many occasions, when I come across a logical leap in someone else's writing (or in my own writing), my first reaction is, "Where did the author get that idea from?" The later statement has not been adequately set up by earlier statements.

For example, consider the following paragraph:

Well-being refers to a multifaceted construct that reflects positive affect and flourishing. Self-esteem represents a positive view of oneself and of one's personality. Subjective well-being represents being satisfied with how one's life has proceeded. Psychological well-being represents a sense of mastery and competence. Eudaimonic well-being represents seeking out challenging activities and seeking to actualize one's potentials.

In this paragraph, there is a logical leap following the first sentence. The author did not specify that well-being represents the confluence of self-esteem, subjective well-being, psychological well-being, and eudaemonic well-being. Rather, the reader is left to assume that these four indicators are components of well-being.

In this case, the logical leap is fairly small, and readers might be able to fill in the gap on their own. However, we should write in such a way that readers do not have to make assumptions about what we mean.

The following paragraph represents a larger leap:

> Interventions are often needed to redirect young people onto healthy developmental pathways. Schools often place disruptive students into separate classrooms where their oppositional behavior can be reinforced by other students' similar behavior. It is essential for all students to receive the learning opportunities that they need.

The three sentences in this paragraph convey quite different messages, and each sentence probably deserves its own paragraph. We would need to explain how interventions can redirect developmental processes and complete that thought. Then we would need to explain why placing disruptive students in separate classrooms with one another is developmentally inappropriate. Finally, we can make the statement about all students being entitled to learning opportunities—and explain what we mean.

In essence, logical leaps are a special case of being AOTP. Reading the sample paragraph above is a dizzying experience—the ideas are written down with little rhyme or reason connecting them. The sentences may go together in some way, but the connecting logic is missing. The solution is to supply the connecting logic. The extent of connecting logic needed depends on the extent of the logical leaps between and among sentences. Small leaps, like the one in the first sample paragraph, can be filled in using one or two sentences. Large leaps, however, such as those in the second sample paragraph, may require turning each sentence into its own paragraph. As a general principle, extremely disjointed paragraphs where each sentence expresses a different idea likely require using each sentence as the topic sentence for a paragraph of its own.

Let's try expanding each sentence in the second paragraph into its own paragraph. Note that citations are omitted for convenience, but if we were writing a real paragraph, citations would be needed.

Maladaptive developmental outcomes, such as disruptive behavior disorders, can be understood as outcomes of pathological developmental trajectories. Parents, for example, sometimes inadvertently promote and reinforce negative behavior, such as rewarding tantrums or engaging in shouting matches. If not redirected, these pathological developmental trajectories can lead to negative life outcomes, such as drug addiction, incarceration, and serial unemployment. Interventions are often needed to redirect these young people onto healthy developmental pathways. For older children and adolescents, such interventions are often delivered in school settings where youth can be gathered together during the day. Interventions can introduce adaptive behaviors and coping strategies and can use peers to reinforce these behaviors and strategies.

Many schools, however, sometimes address disruptive behavior in developmentally inappropriate ways. Some schools place disruptive students in separate classrooms where their oppositional behavior can be reinforced by other students' similar behavior. This "peer contagion" effect serves to worsen, rather than improve, disruptive behavior. A more developmentally appropriate strategy is needed, such as using a peer leader approach whereby youth are trained to lead group sessions where they introduce and model positive behavior. These types of interventions have been shown to be efficacious and effective in reducing disruptive behavior and in promoting prosocial behavior.

Reducing disruptive behavior is essential not only for the disruptive students themselves, but also for their classmates, whose learning may be compromised by the disruption. Providing students with optimal learning opportunities—including interacting with teachers, working collaboratively with classmates, and completing in-class projects—requires that each student be positively engaged in the learning process. Peer-based interventions may represent one way of accomplishing this goal.

Notice that the logical leaps in that single three-sentence paragraph required three full paragraphs to spell out. Thus, the amount of new writing required to fill in logical leaps depends on the magnitude of the leaps themselves. In the example above, three extremely disjointed sentences can require a large amount of text to correct.

Remember Roger Levesque's editorial guidance for papers submitted to the *Journal of Youth and Adolescence*—each paragraph needs a topic sentence, at least one supporting sentence, and a strong concluding sentence. The paragraph itself should convey a single coherent set of ideas. Any paragraph that doesn't meet these criteria is probably characterized by logical leaps—which are very distracting and aversive for readers.

Logical leaps can also occur between paragraphs. We may finish reading one paragraph and find that there is a piece of logic missing between the end of that paragraph and the beginning of the next one. In this situation, there are three options—add bridging text at the end of the previous paragraph, add bridging text to the beginning of the next paragraph, or write a new paragraph to fill in the logical leap.

The strategy that we choose in this situation will depend on where the best location is to add the bridging text. We can make this determination by identifying what ideas and content are needed to fill in the logical leap, and then deciding where this text should go. Is it best placed at the end of the previous paragraph, at the beginning of the next paragraph, or a combination of the two? If the new ideas are distinct from either the previous or next paragraphs, then a new paragraph is probably needed between the two existing paragraphs.

Let's consider an example here. There is a logical leap between the following two paragraphs:

Graduate school is a challenging yet fulfilling experience. Students often enter graduate school with only a vague idea of what they wish to do when they finish. However, by the end of their studies, most students already have identified a field to enter, and many have already secured job offers before they complete their graduate careers. Graduate school is a time when students learn to write journal articles, to present at conferences, and to come up with ideas for new studies or papers.

The academic job market can be quite challenging for students to navigate. Hiring committees often include faculty members with different interests, and the power structure within an academic department can be difficult to discern. Applicants may believe that they performed well on an interview, only to have faculty members rank the applicant poorly in committee meetings. The best approach is for students to apply to as many jobs as possible, with the hope that applying broadly will maximize their chances of receiving an offer.

Notice that the line of logic jumps from the graduate school experience to the academic job market, without filling in the gap (i.e., noting that students need to apply for jobs as they prepare to finish their graduate training). This linking text might be placed at the end of the first paragraph or at the beginning of the second.

Here we will try placing the new text at the end of the previous paragraph, and then we will try placing it at the beginning of the second paragraph. The new text is underlined.

End of First Paragraph:
Graduate school is a challenging yet fulfilling experience. Students often enter graduate school with only a vague idea of what they wish to do when they finish. However, by the end of their studies, most students already have identified a field to enter, and many have already secured job offers before they complete their graduate careers. Graduate school is a time when students learn to write journal articles, to present at conferences, and to come up with ideas for new studies or papers. <u>Of course, students must enter the job market when they finish—and the job market presents a unique set of challenges.</u>

The academic job market can be quite challenging for students to navigate. Hiring committees often include faculty members with different interests, and the power structure within an academic department can be difficult to discern. Applicants may believe that they performed well on an interview, only to have faculty members rank the applicant poorly in committee meetings. The best approach is for students to apply to as many jobs as possible, with the hope that applying broadly will maximize their chances of receiving an offer.

Beginning of Second Paragraph:
Graduate school is a challenging yet fulfilling experience. Students often enter graduate school with only a vague idea of what they wish to do when they finish. However, by the end of their studies, most students already have identified a field to enter, and many have already secured job offers before they complete their graduate careers. Graduate school is a time when students learn to write journal articles, to present at conferences, and to come up with ideas for new studies or papers.

<u>Students must also search for jobs as they are preparing to finish their degrees.</u> The academic job market can be quite challenging for students to navigate. Hiring committees often include faculty members with different interests, and the power structure within an academic department can be difficult to discern. Applicants may believe that they performed well on an interview, only to have faculty members rank the applicant poorly in committee meetings. The best approach is for students to apply to as many jobs as possible, with the hope that applying broadly will maximize their chances of receiving an offer.

As you can see, placing the linking sentence in either place—at the end of the first paragraph or at the beginning of the second paragraph—can fill in the logical leap.

Clumsy Wording
Clumsy wording can be added to the broad category of logical leaps. If your wording is unclear or otherwise difficult to understand, readers will have a

difficult time following your line of logic. Precision in language is extremely important in tracing a line of logic that readers will be able to follow without expending a great deal of effort. When you are editing your first draft, look out for clumsily or awkwardly worded sentences, and try your best to reword them. Often, while you are in the process of refining your academic writing skills, mentors and coauthors will be your best source of feedback to help you identify and correct clumsy wording.

Here are some examples of clumsily worded sentences and some possible ways to correct them:

Clumsy: According to Maslow (1943), it is strange for a human organism to change their secure if not one of the basic needs (food, shelter, safety) are missing.

Better: Maslow's (1943) hierarchy of needs holds that people will likely not pursue higher goals, such as seeking a new career or identifying new hobbies, if their basic needs (e.g., food, shelter) are not met.

Clumsy: Our findings mean that new policies have to be made to help out.

Better: Our results suggest some policy changes that may be needed to improve the lives of individuals, families, and communities.

Notice that the clumsier sentences are not only difficult to read, but also vague and unclear. The importance of language precision cannot be overstated. Remember that many readers "speed read," so it's frustrating for them to have to go back and reread a sentence several times to understand its meaning. For me as a reader or editor, having to reread a sentence multiple times not only is aversive, but also gives me headaches.

If you are not a native English speaker, you may not be familiar with the nuances of English grammar. English is one of the most irregular languages in the Western world, and even people who speak it as a first language often have trouble with sentence structure. Many of my European, South American, and Asian colleagues who speak English fluently nonetheless often make small grammatical errors that might, in some cases, change the meaning of a sentence or increase its level of clumsiness. (I have a Dutch colleague who likes to say, "You are mostly welcome" when he really means "You are most welcome.") For non-native English speakers, having a native speaker read your drafts is essential if the goal is to publish in English-language journals.

Internal Inconsistencies

Internal inconsistencies occur when we say one thing in one place, but then we say something else in another place. For example, we might say at the beginning of the introduction that no studies have examined the research questions that we propose, but later in the introduction we might cite studies that have addressed these issues. For another example, in the introduction we might describe an intervention as consisting of three sessions, but in the method section we list four sessions. Or we might cite a source for one claim early in the paper but cite this same source for a completely different claim later in the paper.

Remember that first drafts are generally written across several writing sessions that can span weeks or months, so when we sit down for a writing session, we probably won't remember everything we wrote during earlier sessions. What this means is that you will probably find some inconsistent statements in different places in the paper. If you're doing a careful read, you should be able to spot at least some of these inconsistencies and correct them.

Note that inconsistencies can also occur between the text and the tables or figures. You might report a mean in the text that is different from the mean reported in a table. You might describe a positive relationship between variables in the text, but the corresponding correlation coefficient has a negative sign in the table. A bar graph might suggest that Group A has a higher mean than Group B, but the text might say otherwise. So the text must be consistent with the tables and figures. Lack of consistency can be confusing for readers, because they will not know which set of numbers, facts, or statements is correct and which set is not.

When you are creating tables and figures, be sure to have your statistical output next to you. If possible, set up a second monitor so that you can view the output on one screen and the table or figure you are creating on the other screen. In my experience, using two monitors is far easier than trying to switch back and forth between your statistical program and your word processing program. If you don't have a second monitor, I recommend printing out the statistical output and having it in front of you when you create the table or figure.

My colleague Gordon Finley developed an editing process that he called "praying over the tables." What he meant by that is that he would carefully read through each table, compare the numbers to the statistical output, and compare the tables to numbers and patterns reported in the text. Sometimes Gordon and I would spend hours making sure that each table was absolutely correct and matched perfectly with the text. Importantly, this was not a one-time process. We would often check the tables again when working on later drafts, to ensure that we hadn't made errors when creating the tables. On several occasions, we found errors and corrected them.

An important principle is that, when information is transferred manually from one place to another—such as from statistical output to a table in a word processing file—errors are inevitable. The double data-entry method (Kawado et al., 2003) represents one way to identify and correct such errors. Two different people key the information into the table, and the numbers are compared between the tables created by the two people. Wherever a discrepancy occurs, the people must resolve it by going back to the source document (such as the statistical output file). Double entry is effective because the likelihood of both people making the same exact error is small. If you are creating multiple tables, or tables with a lot of information (e.g., means, standard deviations, correlations), the chances of making errors are fairly high. As we continue to transfer numbers, our mental precision may decrease. I do not trust myself to transfer more than a few numbers at a time, and I will go back and check my tables several times before I consider them to be finalized. As already noted, it's not a bad idea to have two people create the same table from the same numbers, and then compare the two versions of the table to ensure accuracy.

In sum, the paper must be completely internally consistent. When editing a first draft, you will probably encounter internal inconsistencies. Correcting these inconsistencies will markedly increase the readability of your paper.

Tangents

Tangents are lines of logic that you started but didn't finish, or that distract from the flow of the paper by bringing in extraneous information that is not necessary to make your case. Chapter 6 discusses interesting tidbits, sidebars, and sharp turns. These issues fall under the larger heading of tangents. A tangent can refer to a few distracting words, a distracting paragraph, or even a whole distracting section that takes away from the message of the paper. Because we don't focus on flow when we write our first draft, we will likely have sentences or paragraphs that "don't go anywhere" and that should be removed from the paper.

There are various degrees of tangents, ranging from (a) completely irrelevant text that is easy to delete to (b) text that could be relevant if the paper were framed in a slightly different way, and that could be either removed or edited, depending on how close you are to the target journal's space limit.

Completely irrelevant tangents are generally easy to spot and remove. See the sample paragraph below, where the underlined sentence is clearly a tangent.

> Now that the last white rhinoceros has died, the species is officially extinct. <u>Wild animals do not belong in the zoo.</u> White rhinoceroses were often hunted for their horns. Traders would then buy the horns from poachers and sell them to people around the world. As a result, a majestic animal has disappeared from the Earth.

The sentence "Wild animals do not belong in the zoo" has nothing to do with the remainder of the paragraph and should clearly be deleted.

In other cases, it is more difficult to decide whether to keep or discard a potential tangent. Consider the paragraph below. To what extent to do you think that the underlined sentence is a tangent and should be removed?

> Most academic journals publish only articles that are strongly endorsed by all the reviewers. Editors do have some discretion to overrule reviewers, though they seldom do so. <u>I had one paper where the editor overruled two extremely supportive reviews and rejected the manuscript.</u> Editors normally consult reviewers and then rely on their judgments. Because authors never know to whom their manuscripts will be assigned for review, the editorial process has a great deal of randomness in it.

In this case, the underlined sentence is still relevant to the paragraph, but we could delete the sentence and the paragraph would still flow well. The decision whether to keep or delete the somewhat-tangential sentence rests upon the extent to which we consider the personal anecdote to be important to the line of logic we are tracing. Perhaps the author of this paragraph wants to console readers who have had similar experiences, or perhaps the author wishes to create an argument that overruling reviewers represents an abuse of editorial power. It is difficult to render a decision without seeing the rest of the section (or the whole paper) from which this paragraph was taken. (In this case, the paragraph is fictitious, but in a real scenario, the decision to keep or discard text should be made considering how that text fits into the overall flow of the paper.)

In some cases, whole paragraphs, or even whole sections, might be considered tangents. We might decide, after writing our first draft, that we want to take the paper in a different direction than we had originally planned. Given such a change in focus or goals, text that was once central to our argument will become tangential, and new text may need to be written to move the paper in the desired direction. In my career, I have decided to change the direction of a paper on many occasions, and much of what I had written became tangential. Note that this change of direction doesn't mean that I wasted the time that I spent writing the original text. Writing is an iterative, evolving process. Had I not written the original text, I might not have realized the need to change the focus of the paper.

The iterative and evolutionary nature of writing means that the direction of a paper is constantly evolving—and even if you think that the direction of your paper is set, coauthors may suggest a change of direction. Text can become tangential at any time. However, a strategy that I use is to create a "cut text" file as I remove sentences, paragraphs, and sections from a paper. I cut the text from the paper and paste it into the cut text file, so that if I decide to switch back to the original direction (or to some version of the original direction), I can just bring the text back. I also save each draft of the paper under a different date—such as "Paper Draft July 22 2020"—so that I can easily go back to a prior draft if I decide to.

Run-On Sentences

As is covered in Chapter 6, a run-on sentence is simply a sentence that is too long. In many cases, run-on sentences contain long clauses, and some run-on sentences include conjunctions (*and, or, but*) that subsume two or more sentences within a single sentence. As we read through our first draft, we will likely find some sentences that are too long and where the message of the sentence is difficult to discern. The period at the end of a sentence signals to the reader that it's time to take a breath and summarize what the sentence means. When a sentence goes on too long, readers may have difficulty identifying its meaning. The solution is usually to break the run-on sentence into two or more separate sentences.

I find that a simple way to correct run-on sentences is to replace conjunctions with periods and break up the sentence. In the following three examples, I show a run-on sentence where *and, or,* and *but* sentences are broken up.

Run-On: Reading classic books is a wonderful way to broaden one's perspective, and reading is a great way to learn.

Broken Up: Reading classic books is a wonderful way to broaden one's perspective. Reading is a great way to learn.

Run-On: Immigration is a fascinating topic to study because immigrants are often some of the most resilient people in our society, or maybe their life experiences have forced them to become resilient.

Broken Up: Immigration is a fascinating topic to study because immigrants are often some of the most resilient people in our society. Alternatively, it is possible that their life experiences may have forced them to become resilient.

Run-On: Presidential elections are full of drama and anticipation because they represent the culmination of more than a year's worth of political theater, but many of the congressional, state, and local races are also important.

Broken Up: Presidential elections are full of drama and anticipation because they represent the culmination of more than a year's worth of political theater. However, many of the congressional, state, and local races are also important.

As these examples illustrate, *and* can be replaced with a period, *or* can be replaced with *alternatively*, and *but* can be replaced with *however* or *nonetheless*.

Additionally, you may want to look for places where you may have used a comma instead of a period, and where simply changing the punctuation can solve the problem. Here is an example:

Incorrect: High school students should start to pay close attention to their grades starting in their sophomore year, this means making sure that homework is completed and test scores are as high as possible.

Correct: High school students should start to pay close attention to their grades starting in their sophomore year. This means making sure that homework is completed and test scores are as high as possible.

José often used the word *crisp* to describe the optimal writing style. Crisp sentences are written efficiently and convey their points in as few words as possible. In crisp writing, distractions are eliminated so that even people who are speed-reading can discern the points being made without much trouble. José liked to say that crisply written papers would take him a couple of hours to read and comment on, whereas poorly written papers might take him several days. I share his sentiment—I am an obsessive-compulsive reader and I comment on every issue I see. The more mistakes I see in someone's writing (including my own), the more time it takes me to point them out, make or suggest corrections, and keep reading. It can sometimes take me a week to get through an especially poorly written draft. The point here is that authors should learn to edit their own work as much as they can—correcting the most obvious mistakes—before sending drafts to their mentors and colleagues.

Overstated Conclusions

Overstated conclusions generally refer to statements made in the discussion that clearly go beyond what the data can support. For example, an author might claim that a study's findings clearly demonstrate an effect of self-esteem on symptoms of depression—but the study was cross-sectional and was only able to suggest the presence of a correlation between self-esteem and depressive symptoms. Similarly, a discussion section might contain statements suggesting that the study's results have settled a long-standing debate. A single study cannot establish a finding as true or false—it takes a series of studies to suggest that a finding is likely true, and nothing can ever be "proven" in science. Words like *demonstrate* and *definite* are too strong for discussing scientific results. I advise using words like *suggest, possible,* and *potential,* words that leave room for revision if future work is not consistent with the findings from your current study.

Remember the discussion of the three levels of association in Chapter 2—correlation, prediction, and causation. The types of statements that can be made in a results or discussion section are very much dependent on the research design that was used in the study. If your draft contains causal-sounding terms like *effect, influence,* or *produce changes in,* but your study was not a randomized experiment (or did not use causal statistical methods, such as those outlined in Judea Pearl's Causality Blog), then your terminology is extending beyond what your data can support. Similarly, if you talk about developmental processes, or state that one variable may precede another variable, or use the word *predict,* in interpreting cross-sectional results, then your terminology is going beyond your data.

Our conclusions can also extend beyond our data if we attempt to generalize beyond the sample we studied (and the population that the sample is able to represent). A prime example of this phenomenon is the use of samples of college students to draw conclusions about the young adult population as a whole (see Schwartz, 2016, for some examples of why such generalizations can be problematic). There are important differences between college students and non-college young adults that contraindicate using student samples to support statements about young adults in general (Arnett, 2016). To make definitive statements about young adults in general, we would need to sample both college students and individuals not attending college.

In some cases, a strategy to consider is to stay very close to the data when writing discussion sections for empirical papers, and then to write a review article summarizing your program of research. Review articles are broader in scope than empirical articles are, and we can draw more general conclusions in a review article because we are not tied to a specific set of research results. For example, my colleague Jennifer Unger (2014) published a review article summarizing the longitudinal acculturation project that she had conducted and on which several empirical articles had been published. The review article allowed her to summarize conclusions across the various empirical analyses and to suggest directions for future research.

In other instances, the review article can include not only our own empirical work, but also empirical work conducted by other researchers and research groups. My colleague Chris Ferguson (2013) published a comprehensive review of research on the link between violent video games and adolescent aggression. Based on his own work and the work of other scholars in his field, Chris concluded that violent video games likely do not lead to aggressive behavior among adolescents. Review articles may be more likely than empirical studies to attract media and policy attention—simply because they are easier for non-academics to read and understand.

Indeed, as stated elsewhere in this book, one single paper doesn't create a line of research. Perhaps more importantly, a single paper doesn't *need* to create a line of research. We can write the discussion section for each paper while staying close to the data—knowing that more empirical papers will follow, and that we can write a review article to summarize across our research program (and perhaps across research conducted by our colleagues as well). My opinion is that authors go beyond their data in their discussion sections because they think they must. Earlier in my career, I tried to hit a home run every time I came up to bat—every paper had to be a major, groundbreaking contribution to the literature. Often, creating a major contribution meant drawing conclusions that my data and research design could not support.

The lesson here, as applied to reading through first drafts and correcting common errors, is that we need to stay close to the data so that the contribution of the study is clear. Because science takes baby steps, our next study can build on the present one, and the study after that can build on our next study, and so forth. Once we realize that we don't need to hit a home run with every paper, we can be more comfortable allowing each paper to make its contribution naturally.

How do we know when we have gone beyond our data? A good question to ask yourself as you read each "conclusion" statement or paragraph is, "What kind of research design would we need to be able to support a statement like this?" For example, a statement asserting that "Violent video games do not appear to predict adolescent aggression" would require a longitudinal or experimental design. (The word *predict* is inherently longitudinal.) If we were writing the discussion section for a cross-sectional study, the statement regarding prediction would be going beyond our data and research design.

Similarly, a statement claiming that "Alcohol use among young adults in the United States appears to have declined between 1970 and 2020" would require population-based samples of U.S. young adults from both years. Remember that statements about prevalence rates must be based on representative samples. Surveying a few college classrooms would not permit us to make statements about national prevalence rates. The accuracy and validity of statistical inferences—conclusions about a population that are drawn from results obtained with a sample—depend on the adequacy of the sampling approach utilized in the study (Makar, Bakker, & Ben-Zvi, 2011). Biased samples often lead to erroneous conclusions.

Importantly, if your research design and sampling frame don't support the statement you have written into your draft, then the statement needs to be revised and toned down. In some cases, using tentative language (e.g., "It is possible that," "Our data may suggest that") can help, but the safest route is probably to ensure that the statement can safely be made based on the study you conducted (or based on the methods used to collect the data set you used). For example, let's say that we conducted a cross-sectional study where we measured attitudes about seat belt safety and frequency of automobile accidents in the past year. Now let's say that we are reviewing our first draft and we find a statement in the discussion that reads as follows:

Our results indicate that more favorable attitudes about seat belt safety predict lower odds of being in an automobile accident.

This statement goes beyond our data because we measured seat belt safety attitudes and automobile accident frequency during a single measurement occasion. We cannot refer to prediction unless we measured both variables longitudinally and we can demonstrate statistically that one variable precedes the other (see Chapter 2). Instead, a more accurate statement given our design might be:

Our results indicate that more favorable attitudes about seat belt safety are associated with lower odds of being in an automobile accident.

Notice that we only changed *predict* to *are associated with*. The rest of the statement is unchanged—but now it is consistent with the study we conducted.

Further, if we describe implications of our findings for intervention or policy, the implications or recommendations should not go beyond what our study design can support. As with other claims made in the discussion section, in some cases making the language more tentative can address the issue. For example, if we are discussing the implications of a cross-sectional study for intervention design, we might say something like:

If replicated longitudinally, the current results may have important implications for the design and delivery of intervention programs.

We can then go on to describe the implications using tentative language, such as *may suggest that* and *It is possible that*. For example:

Our results may suggest that individuals who experience discrimination may be more likely to engage in problematic alcohol use. As a result, it is possible that programs designed to prevent or reduce problem drinking might focus on coping with experiences of discrimination.

Notice that the presentation of intervention implications is tentative and leaves room for revision if subsequent longitudinal results contradict the present study's findings.

Further, any study design feature that necessitates tentative language should be mentioned as a limitation in the discussion section. For example:

The present results should be interpreted in light of some important limitations. First, the cross-sectional design that we used does not permit us to draw conclusions about prediction or causation. As a result, it is essential to replicate the current findings longitudinally so as to provide greater confidence in their implications for intervention design and delivery.

Notice that, for each limitation listed, we provide a potential remedy or solution. This way, readers have a sense of what would be needed to circumvent each limitation that we list. Further, we can design subsequent studies to address the limitations of our prior work, and we can cite ourselves as justification.

A final problem to look for when reviewing a first draft involves the paper's "dropping off a cliff." Conclusions are not easy to write—I have had a lot of trouble writing them in my career, and many of the papers that I review and edit for journals need a better concluding paragraph. In most cases, the concluding paragraph appears right after the limitations section. I generally start my concluding paragraphs with "In conclusion, despite these and other limitations . . ." This structure allows me to end the paper on a positive note, rather than ending with limitations. Here is a concluding paragraph from a recent article my colleagues and I published (Schwartz et al., 2021):

> In conclusion, despite these and other potential limitations, our study has opened a line of research on micro-level acculturation processes. Our results suggest that acculturation components often shift from one day to the next, and that daily shifts in U.S. practices, collectivist values, and ethnic identity can be deleterious for well-being and internalizing symptoms. Fluctuations in U.S. identity also appear to potentiate aggression and rule breaking, suggesting that shifts in use of English at home and at work or school across days are especially unsettling. We hope that the present study will inspire additional work in this direction.

So the concluding paragraph is our chance to remind the reader what the main points of the study are, to provide some "big picture" statements about the importance of the findings, and to end the paper gently by pointing to the potential for the study to inspire additional work. Other authors have different conclusion styles, but in most cases the styles involve summing up the contribution of the study and providing a gentle ending to the manuscript.

Tips for Cutting Length

Toward the end of the editing phase, you may find yourself in a position where you are over the journal's space limit and you need to reduce length. Here I offer several tips for cutting length from a paper. The tips are somewhat different depending on whether you are dealing with a word limit or a page limit.

The most general tip I can offer is to be as economical as possible with words. I can remember a manuscript many years ago where a reviewer advised me to "be more pithy." I had to look the word up, but *pithy* essentially means economical with words. Rather than saying "The current investigation involved recruiting a sample of 200 young adults," we could say "We recruited 200 young adults." For those writers with more verbose writing styles, being pithy can require self-discipline—not necessarily on the first draft, but while you are editing and sharpening the draft. Look for longer, more flowery sentences and cut them back to the most essential message. Remove clauses that are not necessary to make your points. And active voice tends to require fewer words than passive voice does; for example, "We recruited 250 participants" is four words, whereas "Two hundred fifty participants were recruited" is six words. (Remember that we cannot start a sentence with a number written in numerical form—a number must be written as a word if it is the first word in the sentence.)

Take a look at the following sentence:

The current results illustrate the value of developing measures that assess the whole of childhood, from the earliest days of infancy through the time when adolescents finish high school.

A pithier way of writing this sentence might be:

Our findings suggest that measures need to be developed to assess children from infancy through adolescence.

Sometimes, rephrasing can allow us to cut out a couple of words. For example:

Original: Our results may have important implications for the development of interventions.
Rephrased: Our results may have important implications for intervention development.
Original: Journals are often delayed in the publication of accepted manuscripts.
Rephrased: Journals are often delayed in publishing accepted manuscripts.

I also have some "tricks" I have developed for dealing with word and page limits. For word limits, my tricks pertain largely to the reporting of statistical values in the text. Normally, we would include spaces after statistical symbols and around equals signs, such as:

The effects were statistically significant, $F(2, 216) = 5.87$, $p < .001$, $\eta^2 = .12$. (16 words)

If we removed the spaces, the sentence would look like this:

The effects were statistically significant, $F(2,216)=5.87$, $p<.001$, $\eta^2=.12$. (8 words)

So, notice that we removed eight words just by closing spaces in the reporting of statistical results. I don't generally like the look of the text without the spaces—and APA style encourages authors to include spaces next to statistical symbols and operators (e.g., equals and inequality signs)—but removing the spaces allows us to include additional words.

For page limits, a strategy I like to use is to look for "hangers"—paragraphs where the last line has only a few words on it. Try to rephrase and cut words earlier in the paragraph so that the last line is pulled up. The average double-spaced page of text, assuming you are using 12-point Times New Roman font, includes approximately 25 lines of text. If you can cut down 25 hanger paragraphs in your paper, you will cut out a page of text.

In cases where the word or page limit includes the reference list, you can cut length by taking out citations and references. Look especially for sources that are cited only once—taking these sources out will help cut text. If you have long lists of citations, see whether you can remove one or more of the citations. Again, it's easiest to remove citations to sources that are cited only once, so that the corresponding entry can then be taken out of the reference list.

A last option for cutting length when you are over a page limit is to go through your tables and figures and ensure that each of them is absolutely necessary. Can any of the tables and figures be combined or removed? Can the contents of a table or figure simply be explained in the text? Because each table and figure takes up a page (and some tables can take up more than one page), removing tables and figures can be a simple way to reduce length. In general, tables and figures that convey minimal information (such as a table with only two columns and three rows) can be removed, and the information can be presented in the text. Keep in mind that some journals impose limits on the numbers of references, tables, and figures that you are permitted to include in your manuscript.

Writing the Abstract

I have intentionally delayed discussing the abstract because the abstract is the last section to be written. Normally, I don't draft the abstract until the rest of the paper is ready to be circulated to my coauthors—and sometimes not until I am ready to submit the paper for publication. The reason for this is that the abstract needs to summarize the paper in a single paragraph, and it is difficult to summarize a paper that is still being crafted and edited.

Generally, there are two types of abstracts—the *free-form* abstract and the *structured* abstract. Each journal provides guidelines for the type of abstract it prefers and for how many words the abstract can include. I advise checking your target journal's Instructions for Authors before writing the abstract—you don't want to put an abstract together and then find that it's not in the correct format (or is too long).

Free-form Abstracts

A free-form abstract is simply a paragraph that summarizes the study or paper. Generally, free-form abstracts start with one or two sentences about the purpose of the study (or goals of the paper if it's a theoretical, literature review, or position article). These initial sentences are followed by a brief description of the methods, the primary results (without statistical text or values), and a brief conclusion. Here is an example of a free-form abstract from an article my colleagues and I published a few years ago (Lorenzo-Blanco et al., 2016):

Latino parents can experience acculturation stressors, and according to the Family Stress Model (FSM), parent stress can influence youth mental health and substance use by negatively affecting family functioning. To understand how acculturation stressors come together and unfold over time to influence youth mental health and substance use outcomes, the current study investigated the trajectory of a latent parent acculturation stress factor and its influence on youth mental health and substance use via parent- and youth-reported family functioning. Data came from a 6-wave, school-based survey with 302 recent (< 5 years) immigrant Latino parents (74% mothers, M_{age} = 41.09 years) and their adolescents (47% female, M_{age} = 14.51 years). Parents' reports of discrimination, negative context of reception, and acculturative stress loaded onto a latent factor of acculturation stress at each of the first 4 time points. Earlier levels of and increases in parent acculturation stress predicted worse youth-reported family functioning. Additionally, earlier levels of parent acculturation stress predicted worse parent-reported family functioning and increases in parent acculturation stress predicted better parent-reported family functioning. While youth-reported positive family functioning predicted higher self-esteem, lower symptoms of depression, and lower aggressive and rule-breaking behavior in youth, parent-reported family positive functioning predicted lower youth alcohol and cigarette use. Findings highlight the need for Latino youth preventive interventions to target parent acculturation stress and family functioning.

Notice that literature review material generally does not appear in the abstract. Additionally, the longest parts of the abstract involve describing the methods and outlining the most important results. One sentence at the beginning introduces the study background, and one sentence at the end provides the take-home message.

The word limit for abstracts in the *Journal of Family Psychology* (at least in 2016 when the Lorenzo-Blanco et al. article was published) was 250. Some journals impose a 150-word limit. (I have even seen a 100-word limit, which barely allows authors to say anything.) For shorter word limits, the amount of detail on the methods and results needs to be reduced. For example, Gordon Finley and I published an article (Schwartz & Finley, 2010) with a 100-word abstract. The abstract read as follows:

> This study was designed to introduce the construct of troubled ruminations about parents and to develop a brief screening instrument. An ethnically diverse sample of 1,376 university students completed the instrument and other measures of psychosocial functioning. Troubled ruminations about mothers and fathers were related to self-esteem, life satisfaction, psychological distress, and romantic relationship problems, and less strongly to purpose in life, friendship quality, and friendships satisfaction. Implications for counseling and future research are discussed.

Notice that the extent of detail on the methods and results is greatly reduced compared to the Lorenzo-Blanco et al. abstract, and the introductory and concluding sentences are extremely brief. There is only so much that you can say in 100 words!

Structured Abstracts

Some journals ask for an abstract with specific headings. Generally, these headings involve some variation on the following sequence: Purpose, Methods, Results, and Conclusions. The same ingredients that appear in a free-form abstract also appear in a structured abstract—except that there are specific headings in the abstract. Note that structured abstracts may also have word limits.

Here is an example of a structured abstract from an article that my colleagues and I published several years ago (Schwartz et al., 2015):

> **Purpose:** We sought to determine the extent to which initial levels and over-time trajectories of cultural stressors (discrimination, negative context of reception, and bicultural stress) predicted well-being, internalizing

symptoms, conduct problems, and health risk behaviors among recently immigrated Hispanic adolescents. Addressing this research objective involved creating a latent factor for cultural stressors, establishing invariance for this factor over time, estimating a growth curve for this factor over time, and examining the effects of initial levels (intercepts) and trajectories (slopes) of cultural stressors on adolescent outcomes.

Methods: A sample of 302 recently immigrated Hispanic adolescents in Miami (median of 1 year in the United States at baseline) and Los Angeles (median of 3 years in the United States at baseline) was recruited from public schools and assessed six times over a 3-year period.

Results: Perceived discrimination, context of reception, and bicultural stress loaded onto a latent factor at each of the first five time points. A growth curve conducted on this factor over the first five time points significantly predicted lower self-esteem and optimism, more depressive symptoms, greater aggressive behavior and rule breaking, and increased likelihood of drunkenness and marijuana use.

Conclusions: The present results may be important in designing interventions for Hispanic immigrant children and adolescents, including those within the present wave of unaccompanied child migrants.

Notice that, within a structured abstract, the Purpose heading allows for more detail on the study's background than is usually included in a free-form abstract.

Regardless of which format is used, the purpose of an abstract is to provide readers with enough information about your article so that they can decide whether they want to download and read it. Most readers will likely find your article through literature searches, where only the abstract is immediately available. Readers who are interested in knowing more about your study will download the full text (if it is available to them) or may contact you and ask for the full-text version. It is essential, then, that your abstract summarize the study or thesis as completely as possible.

Conclusion

This chapter explains how to edit a first draft and the most common problems to look for when editing. Because the purpose of first drafts is to move your thoughts onto the screen, the draft is likely to be characterized by several organizational and structural problems. Some of the most common organizational and structural problems found in first drafts include redundancy, unfinished thoughts, unjustified statements, undefined jargon and abbreviations, logical leaps, internal inconsistencies, tangents, run-on sentences, and overstated conclusions. Many of these issues can be symptoms of being AOTP, and as a result, editing a first draft is often largely a matter of improving the organizational structure of the paper (and of each section and subsection in the paper). In many places, thoughts may need to be finished, contradictory information may have to be resolved (e.g., stating that no literature is available but then citing literature later), logical leaps may need to be filled in, and information may need to be provided earlier in the paper so that later statements make sense. Statements in the discussion may need to be scaled back if they go beyond the research design, sample, or analyses reported in the paper. An essential take-home point from this chapter is that these issues are nearly inevitable. Writing the perfect first draft is just about impossible, because trying to be perfect conflicts with the purpose of a first draft. No matter how skilled a writer you are, you will have to correct problems in your writing as you move from first draft to shareable or submittable draft.

The chapter also discusses strategies for cutting length from a manuscript. In many cases, being pithy and economical with language can help to decrease length. Flowery, descriptive language is appropriate for novels and opinion editorials, but not for scholarly writing. Making one's points completely, and in as few words as possible, is a hallmark of scholarly writing. The process of editing drafts is likely to help improve your writing skills, and asking colleagues and mentors to provide comments to improve your writing is a strategy that I recommend for early-career writers. It is essential for early-career writers to involve their mentors in their writing. Even in cases where the mentor is not a formal coauthor, seeking guidance and feedback is strongly advised. Scholarly writing is very different from other types of writing, and the best way to learn how to write scholarly papers is to seek input from people who have already mastered this set of skills.

The chapter also covers how and when to write the abstract for a journal manuscript. Generally, the abstract should be written after the rest of the paper has been completed. Because the abstract summarizes the study or thesis presented in the manuscript, it doesn't make any sense to write the abstract until the rest of the manuscript is at least close to final form. The two general types of abstracts—free-form and structured—are discussed, and guidelines for how to write each type of abstract are provided.

It is also essential to remember that the editing process is iterative. That is, even after we finish a round of edits, we should set the draft aside for a few days and then edit it again. We will most likely find additional issues to correct and edits to make. I'll give an example here. In late 1999, I was going through my old files on my computer, and I came across my qualifying exam paper. I had submitted that paper to my dissertation committee a year and a half earlier and had essentially forgotten about it. As I read through it, I realized that the paper might be publishable with extensive revision. So I started drafting additional text to fill in some of the gaps and logical leaps in the original writing. I also needed to update some of the literature review, given that I hadn't touched the paper in 18 months. By the time I had finished writing and editing—a process that took several months—the length of the manuscript had increased substantially. However, I had provided an extensive review and integration of the personal identity literature. I had done much of the writing and editing late at night while my wife was asleep, and writing in solitude can be an isolating experience. I wasn't sure who, if anyone, would ever read what I had written. After receiving extensive feedback from my wife and two rounds of editorial review, the article was published in the first issue of the journal *Identity* (Schwartz, 2001). Over the 20 years since the article was published, people around the world have approached me (either virtually or in person) and have asked me about that article. That paper essentially helped to launch my career.

Summary

- Editing drafts is an iterative process, and you and your coauthors will discover new changes to make each time you or they review a new draft of the paper.
- There are several common problems that you will spot when reviewing your first drafts. These include redundancy, unfinished thoughts, unjustified statements, undefined jargon and abbreviations, logical leaps, tangents, run-on sentences, and overstated conclusions.
- Scholarly writing requires us to be economical with words and crisp with our sentences.
- The abstract is the last part of the paper to be written. Often, the abstract is not written until the rest of the paper is completed.
- There are two general types of abstracts, free-form and structured.

References

Arnett, J. J. (2016). College students as emerging adults: The developmental implications of the college context. *Emerging Adulthood, 4*, 219–222.

Ferguson, C. J. (2013). Violent video games and the Supreme Court: Lessons for the scientific community in the wake of *Brown v. Entertainment Merchants Association*. *American Psychologist, 68*, 57–74.

Kawado, M., Hinotsu, S., Matsuyama, Y., Yamaguchi, T., Hatsumoto, S., & Ohashi, Y. (2003). A comparison of error detection rates between the reading aloud method and the double data entry method. *Controlled Clinical Trials, 24*, 560–569.

Lorenzo-Blanco, E. I., Meca, A., Unger, J. B., Romero, A. J., Gonzales-Backen, M. A., Piña-Watson, B., . . . Schwartz, S. J. (2016). Latina/o parents' acculturation stress: Links with family functioning, youth mental health, and substance use. *Journal of Family Psychology, 30*, 966–976.

Makar, K., Bakker, A., & Ben-Zvi, D. (2011). The reasoning behind informal statistical inference. *Mathematical Thinking and Learning, 13*, 152–173.

Schwartz, S. J. (2001). The evolution of Eriksonian and neo-Eriksonian identity theory and research: A review and integration. *Identity: An International Journal of Theory and Research, 1*, 7–58.

Schwartz, S. J. (2016). Turning point for a turning point: Advancing emerging adulthood theory and research. *Emerging Adulthood, 4*, 307–317.

Schwartz, S. J., & Finley, G. E. (2010). Troubled ruminations about parents: Conceptualization and validation with emerging adults. *Journal of Counseling and Development, 88*, 80–91

Schwartz, S. J., Martinez, C. R., Jr., Meca, A., Szabó, A., Ward, C., Cobb, C. L., . . . Salas-Wright, C. P. (2021). Toward a micro-level perspective on acculturation among US Hispanic college students: A daily diary study. *Journal of Clinical Psychology, 77*, 121–144.

Schwartz, S. J., Unger, J. B., Zamboanga, B. L., & Szapocznik, J. (2010). Rethinking the concept of acculturation: Implications for theory and research. *American Psychologist, 65*, 237–251.

Schwartz, S. J., Unger, J. B., Zamboanga, B. L., Córdova, D., Mason, C. A., Huang, S., Baezconde-Garbanati, L., Lorenzo-Blanco, E. I., Des Rosiers, S. E., Soto, D. W., Villamar, J. A., Pattarroyo, M., Lizzi, K. M., & Szapocznik, J. (2015). Developmental trajectories of acculturation: Links with family functioning and mental health in recent-immigrant Hispanic adolescents. *Child Development, 86*, 726–748.

Talmi, D., & Goshen-Gottstein, Y. (2006). The long-term recency effect in recognition memory. *Memory, 14*, 424–436.

Unger, J. B. (2014). Cultural influences on substance use among Hispanic adolescents and young adults: Findings from Project RED. *Child Development Perspectives, 8*(1), 48–53.

10
Selecting a Target Journal

Chapter Objectives

By the time you finish reading this chapter, you should be comfortable with:

- Writing for a specific journal for which you are targeting your paper
- Matching manuscripts with target journals and journal prestige
- Writing for special journal issues
- Dealing with having papers rejected from journals

This chapter explores how to select the right journal for your paper. This step occurs as you are writing your first draft and editing subsequent drafts. It is most efficient to write specifically for a target journal. Journals are often idiosyncratic in terms of what they publish, and the name of the journal may not be the best indicator of the types of articles that the journal publishes. As a result, before you start your first draft, you should browse a recent issue of the journal and determine whether any of the articles are similar in scope or type to the paper you are planning to write. If they are not, you may want to consider a different journal.

There are many examples of journal titles not being completely representative of what the journal publishes. Based on their respective instructions for authors, the *Journal of Adolescent Research* almost exclusively publishes qualitative and mixed-method research, *Human Development* publishes only theoretical and review articles, and the *International Journal of Intercultural Relations* (which I edit) largely excludes research on international business. A perusal of recent issues of each of these journals would provide a good idea of what kinds of articles they generally publish.

Additionally, you should look at the journal's Instructions for Authors, which will provide the word or page limit, citation format, and other important information that will help you decide whether the journal is a good match for your paper. Papers that do not follow the author guidelines are likely to be returned to the author for revision, if not outright rejected. For the journal

The Savvy Academic. Seth J. Schwartz, Oxford University Press. © Oxford University Press 2022.
DOI: 10.1093/oso/9780190095918.003.0011

that I edit, my editorial assistant screens all submissions to ensure that they comply with the author guidelines, and papers that do not comply are sent back to the author for revision.

Journal editors often desk-reject submissions that are outside the journal's scope. (Desk-rejection occurs when an editor rejects a paper without sending it out for review.) Editors clearly explain the reasoning behind most desk-rejections in ways that the authors can understand—although some desk-rejections may appear capricious. For example, in 2019, a journal editor desk-rejected my submission because my sample consisted of various Hispanic national groups—even though that same editor had accepted articles using diverse Hispanic samples less than a year earlier. Some authors have taken issue with my desk-rejecting some manuscripts on international business, because the journal published articles on this topic under previous editors. My response is generally that editors are responsible for establishing the scope for their journals, and that an editorial transition can often prompt a change in the journal's scope. For example, when Jeff Arnett (2005) took over the editorship of the *Journal of Adolescent Research*, he shifted the journal's scope—which had previously been largely quantitative—toward almost exclusively qualitative and mixed methods research. Jeff started desk-rejecting solely quantitative papers, which came as a surprise to many of my colleagues who had been publishing in that journal for years. Subsequent editors have maintained Jeff's qualitative and mixed-methods focus, and I assume that authors have become accustomed to the journal's scope.

Thus, picking out a target journal for a manuscript involves carefully sorting through potential journal options and selecting journals that appear to be the closest matches for the paper. My best advice is to choose three or four target journals and to rank them in order from first choice to last choice. The way we rank journals for a given paper depends on our career stage, our specific goals for the paper, and how long we are willing to wait for the paper to be accepted. What is essential to know is that you must familiarize yourself with the journals that publish articles in your field—and that there is no real shortcut around the work required to learn the journals. The Web of Science (https://clarivate.com/webofsciencegroup/solutions/web-of-science/) lists journals within a given field and provides their impact factors, but it doesn't tell us about the nuances and patterns that characterize a specific journal's tendencies (in terms of the kind of work that journal is most versus least likely to publish). You have to conduct enough literature reviews so that you get a sense of what each of the journals in your field tends to publish.

Journal Prestige and Match With Article Contributions

This section considers the concept of journal prestige and how it might figure into the choice of target journals for a paper. Within any given field, it may be possible to rank-order journals in terms of how prestigious they are. The most prestigious journals are generally (but not always) those with the broadest readership, the widest scope, and the highest impact factors. Association journals (e.g., those affiliated with the American Psychological Association [APA], the American Medical Association [AMA], the American Public Health Association [APHA], etc.), and journals associated with professional societies also tend to be more prestigious and more highly ranked than other journals—but again, this is not always the case.

Take, for example, the field of developmental psychology. *Developmental Psychology*, an APA journal, has an impact factor of 2.9 for 2020–2021. The *Journal of Adolescence*, which specializes in a specific part of the life span, has an impact factor of 2.4. However, the *Journal of Youth and Adolescence*, which also specializes in a specific part of the life span, has an impact factor of 3.3. These examples illustrate the point that the journal with the broadest scope is not necessarily the most highly ranked.

Once you get to know the journals in your field, you will learn which kinds of papers are most likely to be accepted into which journals. *Developmental Psychology*, for example, tends to publish longitudinal studies from various segments of the life span. This journal employs a large number of associate editors and maintains an extremely high rejection rate (I have never been able to publish a first-authored article there). Papers are often sent out for review two or three times before the editor or associate editor handles the remaining revisions directly with the authors. Somewhat in contrast, I have had a lot of success in the *Journal of Youth and Adolescence*. Roger Levesque, the editor-in-chief, handles all submissions himself, and he consults reviewers only once. For papers that he invites authors to revise based on reviewer feedback, Roger works directly with authors to handle the remaining revisions, and he is extremely fast. If I have a paper that is appropriate for the *Journal of Youth and Adolescence*, I will almost always consider sending it there as my first choice. Roger handles the journal with amazing speed and efficiency— and I would much rather have an editorial decision in less than a month (even if it's a rejection) than have to wait several months for another journal to get back to me. Further, in my estimation, Roger is more open to a wider array of papers and methodological approaches than more traditional developmental journal editors are. On several occasions, he has accepted papers that my colleagues and I had previously had rejected by other developmental psychology journals. He knows our work, and we know his editorial style—his journal has been a natural fit for many of our papers over the years.

As the example of Roger Levesque and the *Journal of Youth and Adolescence* suggests, the impact factor is not the only index of journal desirability. As is noted in Chapter 3, impact factors tend to fluctuate across years. *Developmental Psychology* has traditionally had an impact factor above 3.0, and impact factors for the adolescent journals (including the *Journal of Youth and Adolescence*) have often fluctuated between 2.0 and 3.0. In 2020–2021, the *Journal of Youth and Adolescence* had a higher impact factor than *Developmental Psychology* had. Does that mean that the *Journal of Youth and Adolescence* is now a better journal than *Developmental Psychology* is? Maybe, and maybe not. I would assume that *Developmental Psychology* has a wider readership, both because it's affiliated with the APA and because it covers the entire life span. On the other hand, the *Journal of Youth and Adolescence* appears (at least in my estimation) to publish a greater diversity of methodological and analytic approaches—including some with which other journals may not resonate as much. Which of the two journals I choose for a given paper often depends on several factors.

Journal Readership as an Imprecise Index of Prestige

When I started publishing in the late 1990s and early 2000s, journal readership was a key consideration in deciding where to send a manuscript. Most journals still published primarily in hard copy, and journal articles were only beginning to be available online. Readers often waited eagerly for the next issue of their favorite journal to arrive in their mailboxes, and if an article title or abstract caught readers' eyes, they would likely read that article and cite it in their own work.

By the late 2010s and early 2020s, many journals had moved exclusively to online publication. Because most university libraries have access to a wide variety of journals, people generally do not need to subscribe to journals as long as they maintain a university affiliation. Many people subscribe to "contents alerts," so that they receive notification when a new issue is available (or, for some journals, when new articles are available online prior to being assigned to a journal issue). However, I suspect that the majority of article views and downloads occur through literature search engines, such as Google Scholar, PsycInfo, MedLine, Scopus, Sociological Abstracts, and the like. I personally have found useful articles from journals I had never heard of—I simply entered the keywords I wanted to search and a list of articles came up (see Chapter 1 for more details on conducting literature searches). In many cases, I have found additional articles by searching the contents of journals I had found during my literature searches. I have even subsequently submitted papers to journals I discovered through literature searches.

The point is that journal readership is less relevant now than it was in the late 1990s and early 2000s. If you publish something that is of interest to readers, they will find it and cite it—and using keywords that summarize each paper will help readers to find your work. The article I published in the first issue of *Identity*, for example (Schwartz, 2001), has now been cited almost 1,000 times despite being published in the inaugural issue of a "niche" journal. This citation count is especially remarkable in light of the fact that *Identity* has never had an impact factor. Apparently, the article was of sufficient interest to readers that they chose to download, read, and cite it.

This is not to say, however, that journal prestige isn't important. Articles published in high-impact journals may be taken more seriously, and therefore are more likely to be cited, than articles published in lower-impact journals. I am much more likely to download articles from association (APA, APHA, AMA) and professional society journals than I am to download articles from other journals. An article published in the *American Psychologist* is likely to be cited far more frequently than an article from a more specialized journal— *American Psychologist* is the APA's flagship journal, and it is known for its rigorous review process. A considerable proportion of submitted manuscripts are desk-rejected for a variety of reasons (e.g., too narrowly focused for a general psychology audience), and those submissions that are sent out for review are often sent to leaders in their respective fields as reviewers. I have reviewed for the *American Psychologist* at times when I would have turned down review requests from other journals. I suspect that other senior scholars share this sentiment. Articles published in this journal have undergone a great deal of scrutiny, and readers may be more likely to trust the articles for this reason.

Journal Prestige and Editorial Selectiveness

Generally, the more prestigious a journal is, the more selective the editorial team will be in deciding which articles to accept for publication. Among APA journals in 2019, the *Journal of Applied Psychology* maintained the highest rejection rate (92%; American Psychological Association, 2020). The journal received 1,045 submissions in 2019, and the editorial team accepted only 84 of the submissions for publication. The APA journal summary report does not indicate whether original submissions and revisions were treated as separate manuscripts, and whether revise–resubmit decisions (where the reviewers and editor like the paper but request changes) are treated as rejections. Even so, a 92% rejection rate implies that many meritorious submissions will be rejected. I advise being forewarned when submitting papers to journals with very high rejection rates—even solid papers that receive positive reviews may still be rejected.

Authors will undoubtedly perceive such rejections as unfair. In our article on the peer-review and editorial system, Byron Zamboanga and I (Schwartz & Zamboanga, 2009) cautioned against journals' rejecting papers that receive largely or unanimously positive reviews. Here are a couple of examples. In 2005, my colleagues and I submitted a paper to a well-known personality journal. The reviews were extremely supportive, and one of the reviewers expressed excitement about our submission. The associate editor, however, overruled the reviewers and rejected the manuscript. We appealed the associate editor's decision and asked him to reconsider, but he declined to do so. In 2011, my coauthors and I submitted a manuscript to a prominent developmental psychology journal. The associate editor solicited three reviews, of which two were extremely positive and the third was somewhat negative. We revised the manuscript, prepared a painstakingly detailed cover letter, and resubmitted. The associate editor sent our revision only to the negative reviewer, who simply restated the comments that they had provided on the first round of review. We were not convinced that this reviewer even read the revised manuscript. Worse yet, most of this reviewer's comments were pure speculation and were not grounded in empirical research—for example, the reviewer quoted a 20-year-old theoretical article as indicating that personal identity should not be studied in adolescents younger than 17 years old. (I have published more than 20 articles on identity among younger adolescents.) The associate editor rejected our revised manuscript based on this negative review. In both of these examples, the editor overruled the spirit of the reviews and rejected the paper – which in our view was unfair to the editorial process.

Both of these cases had happy endings: each paper was accepted for publication in the next journal to which it was submitted. The moral of these stories, however, is that the editorial review process can be unfair, especially with more prestigious journals. A colleague of mine who was an associate editor for a major APA journal told me that the editor-in-chief had mandated that 85% of all submissions must be rejected, and that the editorial team was allowed to extend revise–resubmit invitations to no more than 20% of submissions. Similarly, when I was an associate editor for a developmental psychology journal, the editor-in-chief told the editorial team that no more than 10% of submissions could be accepted. The reasons for these limitations are often based on scarcity of journal space—the publisher allocates only a certain number of printed pages for each journal per year, and prominent journals receive large numbers of manuscript submissions. Editorial decisions for highly ranked journals can be capricious and unpredictable—as one journal editor told my colleague when he appealed a rejection decision, "Some manuscripts have to be rejected." Editors are just as human as everyone else is, and they resonate more with some papers than with others. Having served as a journal reviewer, associate editor, and editor-in-chief, I can tell you that the decision whether to invite authors to revise and resubmit or to reject their manuscript is often made quickly (probably within the first few pages of reading the paper). When evaluating a manuscript for publication, reviewers and editors spend a short amount of time making up their minds, and the rest of the time trying to justify the decision they have already made.

High-, Moderate-, and Low-Prestige Journals

The difference between more versus less prestigious journals involves their tolerance for flaws in manuscripts and in the studies they report. For the sake of discussion, I will divide the universe of journals into those that are of high, moderate, and low prestige. Although this taxonomy is inexact, it is probably not difficult to identify the tier to which a given journal belongs. I'll start by defining high- and low-prestige journals, such that moderate-prestige journals are those that don't fall into either of these two categories. High-prestige journals include APA, AMA, and APHA journals; APA division journals; and the flagship journals for large international professional societies, such as *Child Development* (Society for Research on Child Development), *Psychological Science* (Association for Psychological Science), *Addiction* (Society for the Study of Addiction), and the *Journal of Adolescent Health* (Society for Adolescent Health and Medicine).

Low-prestige journals include those that don't have an impact factor or whose impact factor is below 1.5. In most cases, journals where the editor-in-chief handles all of the submissions (i.e., there are no associate editors) are low-prestige journals. (The *Journal of Youth and Adolescence* is a notable exception.) Journals that accept initial submissions without major revisions, where the editor makes decisions without soliciting reviews, or where decisions are routinely made with feedback from only one reviewer, are generally low-prestige journals. Low-prestige journals tend to receive small numbers of submissions, and in some cases there may be pressure on the editorial team to accept more papers—or even to solicit submissions from potential authors—so that there are enough articles to fill upcoming issues. Many "niche" journals—those that focus on a specific content area where the majority of work is conducted by a fairly small number of scholars—are low-prestige. Additionally, some foreign-language journals that have switched to publishing in English might be considered low-prestige. I recently published with a research group in a European country, and the article was published in a journal that had only recently begun publishing in English. The editor had reached out to my colleagues and asked them to submit an article (suggesting that the journal's manuscript flow was not sufficient to fill upcoming issues), and the article was accepted and published with no revisions. This is a classic example of a low-prestige journal.

Moderate-prestige journals are, more or less, those that fall between the high- and low-prestige categories. Some moderate-prestige journals are affiliated with smaller professional societies, whereas others are not affiliated with professional societies at all. Most moderate-prestige journals have editorial teams consisting of an editor-in-chief and a few associate editors, and rejection rates for these journals can range anywhere between 50% and 85%. Manuscript flow is generally not a concern (there are generally sufficient numbers of submissions to fill each issue without having to accept more papers than planned), but the level of editorial capriciousness is likely to be lower than authors will encounter with high-prestige journals. Moderate-prestige journals may have less pressure from the publisher and editor-in-chief to maintain a high rejection rate.

I suspect that the majority of scholarly journals fall into the moderate-prestige category. Indeed, most of my publications are in moderate-prestige journals. I prefer not to submit to low-prestige journals, and publishing in too many low-prestige journals can damage one's scholarly reputation. Hiring and promotion committees may question why someone is only able to publish in poorly ranked journals. High-prestige journals are difficult to publish in, and generally speaking, only the most rigorous and impactful studies, theories, and reviews are published in these journals. Therefore, most scholars will publish the majority of their articles in moderate-prestige journals.

Low-prestige journals can also be predatory. As defined by Jia et al. (2015), predatory journals are those that provide fast publication with little or no peer review, charge authors to publish, and distort or misrepresent the editorial team's credentials. In some cases, these journals accept publication fees from authors and never actually publish the authors' articles. Bartholomew (2014) pointed out the impossibility of the claims advanced by predatory publishers—such as being able to have an article peer-reviewed in 3 days.

Shamseer et al. (2017) analyzed sets of predatory, legitimate open-access, and traditional subscription journals. They found that predatory journals were significantly more likely than legitimate open-access or subscription journals to be affiliated with unknown or fraudulent publishers, to dishonestly report the affiliation and qualifications of the editor-in-chief, and to include spelling errors on their home pages. Open-access journals are discussed in greater detail in Chapter 17, but for now, I will only caution that if a journal looks fraudulent, it probably is. If a journal is not published by a reputable publisher, I advise staying away from it. If you receive emails soliciting manuscript submissions for journals and publishers you have never heard of, delete the email.

Let us now return to medium-prestige journals, which represent the majority of scholarly outlets and will likely serve as the final publication homes for most of a given scholar's articles. There is absolutely nothing wrong with targeting a moderate-prestige journal as the primary outlet for a manuscript you are writing. In fact, unless the paper represents a major contribution to the literature, targeting a high-prestige journal is likely to wind up wasting several months of your time. Especially for younger scholars, for whom quantity of publications is likely to be most important to hiring and tenure committees, I recommend targeting medium-prestige journals unless your mentors and senior colleagues agree that a specific manuscript has a decent chance of being accepted for publication in a high-prestige journal. More experienced scholars—especially full professors who do not need to apply for promotion or tenure—will likely be in a better position to "take a shot" at high-prestige journals, knowing that losing a few months is unlikely to hurt them in any meaningful way.

Approaches to Selecting a Target Journal

There are at least two primary ways to select target journals for a given paper. The first method is probably most appropriate for senior scholars who don't have to worry about looking for jobs or about going up for tenure or promotion. Indeed, Al Waterman used this method, which I call a "drop-down" approach. He would target high-prestige journals for most of his papers, but he would also list three or four fall-back journals to which he would submit the paper if his top-choice journal rejected it. Sometimes it would take him 2 years to get a paper accepted—in some cases he would have to try three or four journals before one would finally invite him to revise and resubmit the paper—and as a result, his publication count was not as high as I would have expected, given the number of studies he had conducted and the amount of data he had collected. However, many of Al's publications were in top personality and developmental psychology journals. (He started his first tenure-track faculty position in the early 1970s, when the pressure to publish was far less than it is now. He would likely have had to use a different journal selection strategy if he were starting his career now.)

In contrast to the drop-down approach that Al used, I utilize a more focused matching approach to selecting target journals for my manuscripts. I believe this approach is better suited for younger scholars, for whom publication count is important. I honestly evaluate the contribution that my study, review, or theory is making to the field (how I do this is reviewed in the next section). The major question I ask myself is, "Is this a major contribution, a meaningful contribution, or an incremental contribution?" (Again, I provide some examples of each level of contribution and examples from my own work in the next section.) Once I have a good idea of the contribution that my manuscript represents, I rank-order the journals in the paper's field of study and identify two or three journals that match the paper's level of contribution. At that point, I share my list of potential journals with my coauthors and ask for their input. I usually do this before I have written a complete first draft—indeed, a paper's contribution can be estimated even before it's written. The contribution is based on the findings or ideas that will be reported in the paper, and a competent editor or reviewer should be able to look at a manuscript—even if the writing needs some work—and determine whether the manuscript has the potential to represent a sufficiently important contribution to warrant publication in the journal to which it was submitted. A choppily written manuscript that conveys important ideas is more likely to be invited for revision and resubmission compared to a beautifully written manuscript that conveys unimportant ideas.

Even within a given journal tier, journals will vary based on their match with your paper. Looking at the editor-in-chief and the list of associate editors will likely give you a good idea of how well your manuscript will fit with a given journal. Is there anyone on the editorial team whose work is similar to yours? Is there anyone on the editorial team who you know to be opposed to the type of work you do? For example, Al and I had to rule out some possible journals for some of our manuscripts because the associate editor to whom the paper would most likely be assigned was on record as fundamentally disagreeing with the theoretical approach on which our work was based. Conversely, we had one article accepted in a top personality journal largely because the work reported in the article directly advanced the associate editor's research program. As I said earlier in this chapter, editors are human—they have their biases and interests just like anyone else.

In other words, there are politics in publishing. The key is to use them to your advantage. Citing an editor's or associate editor's work in your manuscript is never a bad idea. (You should be able to identify the editor or associate editor who would most likely handle your manuscript if you were to submit to a given journal.) Just make sure you cite that person's work accurately! I have reviewed and edited manuscripts that contained inaccurate citations and characterizations of my work—and I viewed these papers more negatively than I would have had they not cited me at all.

Estimating the Contribution of Your Work

It can be challenging to appraise the contribution that your own work makes to the literature. Many times, we think that our work is more important than others think it is—and on some occasions, we might judge our work as less important than others would. Let me offer some practical ways to evaluate the contribution that your work most likely offers to the literature. Just as I did with journals, I propose three general levels of contribution—major, moderate, and incremental. Matching the contribution of your work with the prestige level of your target journals may maximize your chances of receiving an invitation to revise and resubmit your paper, and hopefully an eventual acceptance for publication.

High-prestige journals generally publish major contributions. However, because of capricious and unpredictable editorial decisions, even some papers reporting major contributions may be rejected. These journals receive a large volume of submissions, and the editors can be selective about which papers they pursue for publication. Many senior scholars are willing to review for high-prestige journals, whereas they are more likely to decline review invitations from moderate- and low-prestige journals. The rigor with which submissions are reviewed is generally higher in high-prestige journals, such that major contributions are often the only papers that survive even the first round of peer review.

Moderate-prestige journals often publish both major and moderate contributions. Major-contribution manuscripts rejected from high-prestige journals are often resubmitted to moderate-prestige journals. Moderate-prestige journals also publish many moderate contributions. Further, just as moderate-prestige journals comprise the majority of academic journals, moderate contributions make up the majority of published scholarly articles.

Low-prestige journals likely publish primarily incremental contributions— although moderate contributions will sometimes appear in these journals. Papers that have been repeatedly rejected by high- and moderate-prestige journals may eventually be submitted to a low-prestige journal—a practice that I call "dumping." (That is, following a series of rejections, authors may decide to "dump" a manuscript into a low-prestige journal as a way of getting the paper published somewhere.) As already noted, peer-review practices at some low-prestige journals are often not very rigorous—I can recall that one editor accepted my manuscript with no changes at all on the first round of review, and it was not clear that this editor had consulted any reviewers at all. On another occasion, an editor sent our submission out for review, and two of the reviewers recommended rejection. However, the editor accepted our submission with no revisions! That was one of the most surprising editorial outcomes of my career.

How do we know whether our manuscript represents a major, moderate, or incremental contribution? Well, major contributions are either ground-breaking or help to change the way scholars view their field. In terms of groundbreaking work, Brody, Beach, Philibert, Chen, and Murry (2009) conducted one of the first studies examining the extent to which genetic profiles moderate the efficacy of prevention programs for adolescent be-havioral outcomes. This work was groundbreaking because it introduced a new way of looking at interventions' effects on behavior. Similarly, my col-league Theo Klimstra and his colleagues (2010) examined daily fluctuations in personal identity processes—in contrast to the much longer-term longitu-dinal studies that had been conducted previously. This research was ground-breaking because it changed the ways in which personal identity researchers and theorists thought about longitudinal research. Both of these studies were published in high-prestige journals—*Child Development* and the *Journal of Personality and Social Psychology*, respectively.

Other types of major contributions might include proposing and experi-mentally testing new theoretical perspectives. For example, Pettigrew and Tropp (2006) conducted a 515-study meta-analytic test of intergroup contact theory, which holds that individuals from conflicting social groups (e.g., po-litical liberals and political conservatives) will decrease their animosity to-ward one another, and toward the groups to which the others belong, if they spend time together and become acquaintances or friends. Arnett (2000) proposed *emerging adulthood* as a new developmental stage between ado-lescence and adulthood. My colleagues and I (Schwartz, Unger, Zamboanga, & Szapocznik, 2010) proposed an integrative theory of acculturation that brought together several disparate lines of research (e.g., ethnic identity, individualist and collectivist values, bilingualism, behavioral acculturation). All of these articles were published in high-prestige journals—specifically, the *Journal of Personality and Social Psychology* (Pettigrew & Tropp) and the *American Psychologist* (Arnett and Schwartz et al.).

In clinical psychology, the *Journal of Consulting and Clinical Psychology* is one of the highest-ranked and most highly regarded journals. Most of the studies published in this journal are randomized controlled intervention trials, although the journal does publish some therapy process studies and some etiological articles. *Developmental Psychology* and *Child Development* are two of the most highly ranked developmental journals, and these journals publish highly rigorous longitudinal research. Top social psychology journals, such as the *Journal of Personality and Social Psychology* and *Personality and Social Psychology Bulletin*, generally publish articles reporting multiple social-psychological studies. In many cases, at least one of the studies is a randomized experiment. There are high-prestige journals for almost every field of study. Often, a key criterion for acceptance in these journals is that the article must be transformative—that is, it must represent an important change or advance in the state of the field in which the study was conducted or to which the theory or review is intended to contribute.

Al Waterman used to say that the best way to find out whether one's research was transformative was to submit it to a high-prestige journal. He also believed in sending papers to high-prestige journals even if the outcome was almost certain rejection—"because you will get good reviews." His thesis was that, because high-prestige journals often recruit experienced senior scholars as reviewers, these scholars would provide the most insightful and rigorous feedback. However, Al's argument assumes that what reviewers from one journal say will be consistent with what reviewers from another journal will say, an assumption that I have found to be questionable at best. In some cases, reviewers will point out issues that other reviewers are also likely to note, but in many cases, reviewer comments are idiosyncratic. My approach has been to select journals for which my manuscript represents the best match—and in many cases, I avoid high-prestige journals when I don't think that a specific manuscript has a chance of being accepted there.

Moderate contributions are generally those that advance a field of study but are not groundbreaking or transformative. These studies may be part of a line of research, where the line of research is transformative but the individual study may not be. For example, my colleague Simon Ozer and I (Ozer & Schwartz, 2016) introduced a tridimensional model of acculturation for individuals residing in Ladakh, a remote Himalayan province of India. Most prior work on acculturation had assumed that individuals living in non-Western countries would be exposed to two primary cultural systems—the local cultural stream and the globalized Western cultural stream (spread through social media, movies, television, etc.). Simon and I, however, found that people residing in culturally distinct regions within a non-Western country—such as Ladakh in India, Hong Kong in China, and the Kurdish regions of Turkey and Iraq—would be faced with reconciling their local culture, the larger national culture, and the globalized Western culture. Our work represented an advance in the acculturation literature but was not necessarily groundbreaking—Ferguson, Iturbide, and Gordon (2014) had already introduced tridimensional acculturation models vis-à-vis immigrants from ethnic minority groups, and we were adapting their work to apply to globalization as well as to immigration. For another example, Rosario, Lance, Delgado-Romero, and Domenich-Rodríguez (2018) compared Puerto Rican and U.S. acculturation across Puerto Ricans living in Puerto Rico and in Central Florida. Although theirs was not the first study to compare acculturation profiles of Hispanic individuals living on the U.S. mainland against the acculturation profiles of Hispanic individuals in their countries or territories of origin, their study was one of the first to survey the rapidly growing Puerto Rican community in Central Florida. These two studies appear to meet the criteria for moderate contributions, and they were published in moderate-prestige journals—*International Perspectives on Psychology* and *Cultural Diversity and Ethnic Minority Psychology*, respectively.

Incremental contributions include studies that appeal to narrow audiences or that are characterized by major flaws or methodological limitations that render the paper unsuitable for publication in high- or moderate-prestige journals. The study provides a potential empirical and/or theoretical advance and appears to be worth publishing, but reviewers for high- and moderate-prestige journals are unlikely to recommend publication. For example, many personality and developmental journals have largely stopped publishing cross-sectional, self-report studies using college student samples. Manuscripts reporting these kinds of studies may be publishable primarily in low-prestige journals. The rationale for excluding these studies is that (a) college students do not represent the larger population of young adults; (b) cross-sectional studies allow for testing only of correlations, and not of prediction or causation; and (c) self-report measures are characterized by biases related to social desirability, over- or underreporting of some behaviors (e.g., substance use), and single-reporter bias (where reports of all variables are obtained from the same individual; Podsakoff, MacKenzie, & Podsakoff, 2012). As a result, scholars who do not have access to research funds may have to rely on college student samples and, depending on the type of research they conduct, may be largely relegated to publishing in low-prestige journals.

Other types of major flaws that might prevent a study from being published in high- or moderate-prestige journals include failure to measure key predictor or confounding variables, procedural mistakes that introduce error variability into the resulting dataset, collecting only post-intervention data (without collecting pre-intervention data) in an intervention study, failure to collect important demographic variables (such as gender and ethnicity), and measuring longitudinal processes retrospectively rather than prospectively (e.g., asking people to recall events from the past and using those recollections to predict current outcomes). Manuscripts reporting underpowered studies may also have difficulty being accepted in high- or moderate-prestige journals.

My advice is to design your studies carefully so that they are not characterized by major flaws. Remember the points presented in Chapter 2 regarding how to design a publishable study. What I have found as an editor, reviewer, co-author, and lead author is that most fatal flaws in empirical manuscripts come from one of two sources—(a) failure to plan the study correctly or (b) using a secondary dataset that does not have the appropriate variables, design, or other features to test the authors' hypotheses accurately. I made many of the same mistakes early in my career, and as a reviewer or editor I can recognize them almost immediately. I distinctly remember one manuscript I reviewed for a developmental journal where the authors were using a secondary dataset. They tried to put together an index of family cohesion using several items indexing obligations to family. The problem, as I pointed out in my review, is that family cohesion represents a set of close relationships among family members, not a value system that emphasizes familial obligations. I know many people who feel obligated to family members even though they do not feel close to those family members. So, in my review, I recommended rejection because the authors didn't have the data that they would have needed to test hypotheses about family cohesion. The editor agreed with my recommendation and rejected the manuscript.

I've read through low-prestige journals and have encountered studies that were severely flawed, articles that were not interesting or compelling, vastly underpowered studies, theoretical articles that were not well grounded in empirical work, and qualitative studies that appeared to "cherry pick" cases and excerpts for analyses rather than adopting a rigorous and systematic analytic approach. Is this the kind of company in which you want your articles to be embedded? Do you want your colleagues to see that your work is published in journals that don't prioritize rigorous research and theory? If you were to look at someone's curriculum vitae and see more than a handful of articles published in low-prestige journals, what would your impression of that person's scholarly skills be? Would you want to work with that person or hire them into your department?

One point I want to emphasize here—low prestige journals don't all publish sloppy science. Some are simply "niche" journals that specialize in a narrow area of scholarship. Others *do* appear to publish studies with serious limitations or major design flaws. If you have a manuscript that has been rejected multiple times and you are looking to dump it into a low-prestige journal, I suggest looking at the most current issues of that journal to see what kind of work they are publishing. If you see articles that you would not want your article to appear next to, then drop that journal from consideration.

Further, be aware that some journals charge authors to publish articles. Some of these journals are predatory, and some are not. These "open-access" journals are discussed in more detail in Chapter 17. For now, one consideration to keep in mind is that pay-to-publish journals (including some open-access journals) are not always viewed favorably by hiring and promotion committees, even if some of the journals are published by reputable publishers and do have decent impact factors. I remember an adolescent journal that ceased publication more than 10 years ago. They would publish almost any paper they received as long as it was about adolescents, but there would be a surprise along with the acceptance letter—an invoice for page charges. Dick Dunham and I published an article there once, and they charged us $400 to publish. Very early in my independent scholarly career, I submitted a paper there because I didn't have the confidence that reviewers would like it—and I had to pay the full $400 myself. When José found out about that, he told me gently that the promotion and tenure committee would not look favorably upon an article published in a journal like that. This journal had no review process, and the "editor" didn't even have a doctorate! The journal was basically a dumping ground for papers that had been rejected by other journals. It was essentially a predatory journal—and after José's warning, I never submitted there again. His point was that buying publications, or appearing to do so, is not an advisable way to build one's curriculum vitae.

Other low-prestige journals may be perfectly legitimate and may cater to limited or specialized audiences. I've seen some low-prestige journals that put submissions through a rigorous review process and where reviewer comments can be quite challenging. The primary differences between these journals and moderate-impact journals, in my estimation, appear to involve higher acceptance rates and fewer rounds of review. Papers with lukewarm reviews may be accepted in a low-prestige journal, whereas these papers would be more likely to be rejected from moderate- or high-prestige journals. Low-prestige journals may also be more likely to accept manuscripts after one round of review and revision, whereas moderate- and high-prestige journals will generally send revised manuscripts out for a second round of review.

Special Journal Issues

A key exception to the journal-matching principle I outline in this chapter involves *special issues*. A special issue is a collection of articles around a specific theme, and the special issue is often "guest edited" by people other than the journal's regular editorial team. A scholar (or group of scholars) contacts the journal editor and proposes a special issue, and the editor confers with the editorial team to decide whether to move forward with the special issue. Sometimes an editor will reach out to colleagues to invite them to guest-edit a special issue of the journal. In any case, the editor will usually provide the special-issue guest editors with a limit on the number of pages or articles that can be included in the special issue.

It is sometimes, but not always, easier to place an article in a special issue than in a regular journal issue. There are at least three types of special issues that I have seen in my career: by-invitation special issues, abstract-competition special issues, and open special issues. By-invitation special issues involve the guest editors' reaching out to specific authors or author groups and asking them to submit a manuscript for the special issue. Essentially, all the manuscripts are already accepted before they are submitted, and manuscripts will only be excluded from the special issue if they are extremely poorly written or report seriously flawed studies. For example, some of my European colleagues guest-edited a special issue of the *European Psychologist* a few years ago, and they invited my colleagues and me to write an article for the issue. The special issue was on identity in a global context, and they wanted us to write about personal and cultural identity in the United States. The manuscript was accepted after one round of review and revision—which is common for invitation-only special issues.

Sometimes special-issue guest editors decide to solicit abstracts from prospective authors and to select a handful of those to invite for submission as full manuscripts. Authors whose abstracts are selected for submission as full manuscripts are not guaranteed acceptance in the special issue, but acceptance is highly likely. I refer to this scenario as an abstract-competition special issue. The editors do not have to send full manuscripts out for review in order to select the papers they want to pursue further for inclusion in the special issue—rather, they simply must sort through abstracts (generally around 500 words each) and identify the abstracts that they would like to see submitted as full manuscripts. The journal editor generally tells the special-issue guest editors how many articles they are allowed to accept (or how many pages are allocated for the special issue), and the guest editors identify enough abstracts to fill the special issue. If the full manuscripts are placed into the journal's regular review process, the special-issue guest editors may invite a few more full manuscript submissions than they can fit into the issue, with the expectation that some submissions will be rejected.

Finally, some special issues provide an open call for papers, and submissions go through the journal's regular review process. The special issue is essentially indistinguishable from the journal's regular manuscript flow, except that articles accepted for the special issue are placed together. Larger special issues may take up a whole journal issue, whereas smaller special issues may be published as a special section within a regular issue of the journal. The special-issue guest editors may ask the editor to assign some of the regular journal articles to the special issue if they fit the special issue's theme.

If you see a special issue call for papers, should you submit a manuscript or an abstract? I recommend doing so if you have something that fits the theme and if you would want your article to appear in that journal. Some low-prestige journals will arrange special issues as a way of filling the journal's pages—and they will sometimes have to approach authors and ask them to submit papers. In that case, I would decline the offer. If a colleague or mentor invites you to submit a paper to a special issue for a high- or moderate-prestige journal, you should probably accept the offer. If someone you don't know (or don't know well) invites you to contribute to a special issue for a journal you have never heard of, I generally advise declining the opportunity.

One of a mentor's key roles is to create opportunities for mentees. Whenever I am invited to submit an abstract or a paper for a special issue, I offer first authorship to one of my students or postdocs. In this way, I can provide direct "writing mentorship" to that person. (In my opinion, the best mentorship involves more doing and less talking.) If you are an early-career person and your mentor offers you an opportunity to take lead authorship on an article for a special issue of a journal, accept the offer. Capitalizing on their mentors' expertise and datasets is a good way for young scholars to launch their careers, and mentors' relationships with special-issue guest editors may help mentees to get their papers accepted for the special issue. (As already noted, the review and editorial process can be political, especially for editorial decisions that "could go either way." When editors must make difficult decisions between rejecting a paper and inviting a revision, their personal or professional relationships with the authors may help to sway them toward offering a revision.)

I have guest-edited three special journal issues in my career. In all three cases, the editor-in-chief told me how many articles I was allowed to accept. The first time I guest-edited a special issue was for the *Journal of Early Adolescence* in 2008. I was permitted to accept five articles, and I decided to issue an open call for papers. I received 12 submissions, meaning that seven would need to be rejected. Fairness is one of my strongest guiding principles, so I allowed the strengths of the papers themselves—rather than how well I knew the authors—to decide which five papers to accept. Two of the papers I rejected were written by my colleagues, and it's not easy to write a rejection letter to someone you know! I did my best to be as collegial and kind as I could in writing the letters, but of the two colleagues whose papers I rejected, one never spoke to me again (she actually ignored me at a conference about a year later) and the other was clearly angry with me the next time I saw him—but we have since become friendly again.

My second guest-editor experience was for *New Directions in Child and Adolescent Development*, which publishes only special issues. I proposed to edit a special issue on "identity around the world," with articles covering Italy, Sweden, the Netherlands, Belgium, Germany, China, and Japan. Because the countries were already selected in advance, and because I had already worked with authors from these countries in drafting the special issue proposal, it was not possible to use an open call for papers. All the articles were "accepted" even before they were written. In this case, my role was to edit each manuscript carefully until all the articles were ready to be finalized. Because of the unique nature of this special issue—covering specific countries and written by pre-selected author groups—I handled all the reviewing myself rather than sending manuscripts out for review.

My most recent special-issue editorial experience involved a special issue of the *European Journal of Developmental Psychology* on "identity behind the Iron Curtain," focusing on the former Soviet bloc countries in Eastern Europe. I was able to accept up to seven articles, and I solicited eight, with the expectation that at least one would not survive peer review. Because the identity research community in Eastern Europe is fairly small, I solicited articles from eight author groups. One author group was not able to put together a paper, and one author group's paper received extremely negative reviews and was rejected. The remaining six papers were invited for revision and were eventually accepted for publication in the special issue. I spotted a seventh article in the journal's regular pool of accepted articles that fit with the special issue, and the editor was willing to include that article in the special issue.

My experiences with special issues suggest that connections are essential in terms of being able to publish in special issues. As the old saying goes, it's not what you know, it's who you know. More and more special-issue guest editors are soliciting abstracts or full manuscripts and sending them through the journal's regular review process—but the special-issue guest editors are still making the editorial decisions. Laband and Piette (1994) found that editors are more likely to accept papers written by authors they know personally, but that most editors do not publish subpar articles simply because of connections with the authors. Knowing the editors of the special issue helps if your paper is on par with others that have been submitted and if the editors must decide which papers to include and which to reject. It's still essential to submit your best work.

Let me address another concern I have heard from colleagues and students over the years—Are special issues less prestigious than regular issues, because special-issue articles often do not go through as many rounds of review and may not be scrutinized as carefully as regular articles are? Let me respond to the concern this way: I spent 4 years on the University of Miami's appointment, promotion, and tenure committee—and we were never told to evaluate special-issue articles differently from other articles. Further, in many cases, someone reading your curriculum vitae, or even reading a downloaded version of your article, would be unlikely to know that the article was part of a special issue. Although some special issues are paginated in a way that identifies articles as belonging to a special issue (e.g., page numbers are preceded by the letter S), not all special issues are paginated this way. So, to the extent that a special issue provides a somewhat easier opportunity to publish in a prestigious journal, I advise submitting a manuscript (provided that your paper fits with the theme of the issue). Few, if any, hiring or promotion committees will criticize you for publishing articles in special issues—especially if you also have publications in regular journal issues. (However, I might discourage you from publishing most of your articles in special issues, especially if your overall publication count is low.)

Dealing With Rejection

In Chapter 13, we discuss what to do with papers that have been rejected from a journal, but here I would like to cover how rejection affects authors and how to bounce back emotionally from having papers rejected. Let me emphasize here that the emotional process of dealing with rejection is separate from the logistical process of deciding how to revise the paper for submission to another journal. I cover the emotional components here, and the logistical components in Chapter 13.

Rejection stings many writers, but its effects may be most harmful for younger scholars. Especially if we have "hit a wall" in terms of many rejections occurring within a fairly short period of time, rejection can lead us to question our academic research and writing skills, scholarly competence, and professional identity (Horn, 2016). When a paper we're strongly invested in is rejected repeatedly, we can feel a sense of loss and pain. Hernández, Hidalgo, Salazar-Laplace, and Hess (2007) examined the concept of "place identity," where the house, state (or province), and country we live in becomes part of who we are, and Dittmar (2011) proposed that objects that we possess can also become part of our identities. Here, I extend these principles and argue that our scholarly work is also part of who we are. Our papers, grant applications, conference talks, and professional networks help to situate and define us, and we develop strong attachments to some of the work that we produce. Sometimes having a paper rejected—especially one that is central to our professional identity—can really feel like a punch to the stomach.

I have been writing academic papers since 1994, and sometimes rejections still sting me. I suspect that this is true for most scholars. In 2012, my colleagues and I wrote a paper where we reported on longitudinal trajectories of acculturation and their effects on family functioning and on adolescent behavior problems and substance use. We submitted the paper to *Developmental Psychology*, thinking that we were making a major contribution to the acculturation literature. However, the paper was rejected, with one reviewer providing an especially negative review. This reviewer pointed to all the previous longitudinal studies that had been conducted on acculturation—some of which this reviewer had conducted. The reviewer was clearly not pleased that we had characterized our study as one of the first longitudinal investigations into acculturation—and the reviewer essentially gave away his identity when he recommended that we read and cite two of his articles.

I had spent a lot of time writing that article—I had conducted the analyses myself and done almost all the writing. And then this reviewer slammed us and caused the paper to be rejected. I was angry, disillusioned, and stewing. I looked up the reviewer's name and glared angrily at his university photo. If I ever met him, I was going to give him a piece of my mind!

As I've done many times, I gave myself a couple of days to calm down. I had every right to be angry—I'd done a lot of work, and it seemed to be all for nothing. But after I had stopped feeling so angry, I downloaded the articles that the reviewer had suggested. He was right—they were quite relevant to our paper, and they should have been cited. I read the articles carefully and emailed them to my coauthors—and I admitted that I should have found and cited these articles in the original version of the manuscript. The author of the articles, who presumably was also the reviewer for our rejected manuscript, had used some very innovative statistical methods that we might be able to use with our data. So I contacted him and asked him if he might be interested in coauthoring with us and helping us to improve the paper for submission elsewhere.

To make a long story short, he agreed to collaborate with us, and eventually we published the article in *Child Development*. This negative reviewer became a colleague and pushed us to expand our literature review and to use much more rigorous methods—and the result was a far stronger article than what we had originally submitted. I did eventually meet this person at a conference, and I thanked him for helping us.

Such happy endings don't always happen, however—and even when they do, the results are almost never immediate. In the example I provided here, more than a year elapsed between the original manuscript rejection and the eventual acceptance in another journal. I've had other papers that were rejected two or three times before finally being accepted somewhere, and there were a couple papers we eventually dropped because we simply ran out of patience and interest. Scholarly publishing can be a frustrating endeavor.

I remember one paper that we eventually dropped. I ran the analyses while I was on paternity leave waiting for my older daughter to be born. I found that scores on personal identity variables were significantly different for Hispanic college students whose parents were both born in the same Hispanic country than for those whose parents were born in different Hispanic countries. Marilyn Montgomery and I wrote up the paper and submitted it to one journal after another, but it was rejected four times. Each time, the reviewers criticized us for not basing the study on strong enough theory and for not articulating why the findings were important. No matter what we added to the paper, the same criticisms kept showing up in the reviews. One key problem was that we couldn't find any literature to support why people whose parents were from the same country would differ from people whose parents were from different countries. As Al Waterman suggested when I told him about our experiences, we had results in search of a theory.

Eventually, Marilyn and I dropped the paper because we found ourselves in the impossible situation that Al described—there wasn't enough existing theory on which to base hypotheses, so there was no way to set up the research questions in a way that would highlight their importance. We probably could have dumped that paper into a low-prestige journal, but we decided that it wasn't worth our time. (Sometimes that does wind up being the best decision, as I discuss in Chapter 13.)

When these rejection experiences occurred, I was already fairly well established in my career. I knew that I could publish articles, and even though the rejections upset me, they didn't derail my career. But what about rejections occurring earlier? What about the effects of rejection on people who don't have solid mentoring or who already feel that they may not belong in academia?

I note repeatedly in this book that having José as a mentor contributed immeasurably to my career success. If I hit a stumbling block, he was always there to talk it through with me and to help me figure out how to circumvent it. Had I not had the luxury of an outstanding mentor, I probably would not had developed the resilience that I have now. Without that resilience, it would have been much more difficult for me to overcome the manuscript rejections I experienced early in my career. As I've noted several times, the importance of mentors in learning how to write cannot be overstated.

Let me say a few things about imposter syndrome—the feeling that one does not belong. I've struggled with imposter syndrome ever since I started teaching undergraduate classes in 1997. Unfortunately, some groups of people—specifically, women and people of color—are most likely to struggle with imposter syndrome (Ysseldyk et al., 2019). These same groups are also least likely to receive adequate mentoring (Buzzanell, Long, Anderson, Kokini, & Batra, 2015). As a result, women and people of color may experience more difficulties with manuscript rejection, because the rejection may reinforce feelings of being an imposter, and the person may not have a reliable mentor to help them process and overcome the rejection. Hutchins and Rainbolt (2017) found that repeated manuscript rejections may lead scholars—especially early-career scholars—to conclude that they are not "cut out" for academic writing.

I'd like to provide some reassurance for people who have found themselves in this situation. First, the majority of rejected manuscripts are eventually accepted somewhere, and more than half of all published articles were rejected at least once before they were accepted (Woolley & Barron, 2009). Second, as a colleague once told me in an email, rejection is normal, and there is no avoiding it. Given the high rejection rates that most high- and moderate-prestige journals maintain, even the most skilled researchers and writers will have papers rejected. José once joked that he was an "expert at getting rejected"—even though he has published hundreds of journal articles and has been continuously funded by the National Institutes of Health for more than 40 years. If you submit manuscripts to scholarly journals, you are going to experience rejection.

We all have "dry spells" in our careers where everything we submit seems to be rejected. One of the worst dry spells in my career occurred in 2003 and 2004—no matter what I submitted, it was rejected. Several of the editorial decisions could have gone either way—the reviews were mildly supportive, sometime even encouraging, but the editor still rejected my submission. I started to throw my hands up in despair, and I set up a meeting with José to discuss what I was doing wrong. He asked me to bring all the rejection letters and rejected manuscripts with me, and we carefully went over the reviewer and editor comments. A clear theme emerged—I was making developmental claims using cross-sectional datasets, and my interpretations were going beyond what the research design could support. Going through the various papers and the editorial feedback I was receiving was extremely instructive, and if you find yourself in a dry spell, I recommend that you follow a similar process.

José asked me to come up with an action plan for correcting these problems so that my acceptance rate would improve. I didn't have access to longitudinal data, and I could not think of any colleagues who had longitudinal datasets with the types of variables and populations I was interested in. We decided that, for the time being, I would focus on putting together more descriptive (rather than developmental) papers, and that I would target moderate-prestige journals until I was able to collect or access longitudinal data. Meanwhile, we decided that I would start looking for funding opportunities through which I could collect or access longitudinal datasets.

Almost immediately, the dry spell ended, and I started receiving more favorable editorial decisions. I took the papers that had been rejected, worked with my coauthors to revise them, and sent them to other journals—and in almost every case, we were invited to revise and resubmit. Between the summer of 2004 and the summer of 2005, I didn't receive a single rejection letter for any manuscript on which I was an author. I did submit a Mentored Scientist Award proposal to the National Institute on Drug Abuse, and the proposal was funded in April 2005. Using that grant award, I was able to access and start publishing off longitudinal datasets. I also networked at conferences and met people who had longitudinal datasets—and some of these people offered to allow me to use their data. (Conferences are a great way to meet new collaborators.)

I've also learned to handle rejection more resiliently. Academia is a difficult business, and it's important to develop a thick skin. The fact that one journal rejected your work is not the end of the world. There are always other journals you can try. As I note in Chapter 13, you should revise the paper however you can, based on the reviewer and editor feedback, before you submit elsewhere.

In some cases, there isn't much to glean from the feedback—reviewers may have simply not liked your paper, and their feedback may not be all that useful. The key takeaway regarding emotional reactions to manuscript rejections is that you have every right to be angry and disappointed. Give yourself the time you need to grieve the rejection, and then work with your coauthors to identify next steps. Once the paper is accepted for publication in a journal, no one will care about the journals that rejected previous versions of the paper.

Remember that the publication process operates much more smoothly when you have good mentorship. For example, if you're in a dry spell, you can work with your mentor to find patterns in the reviewer and editor comments you've been receiving and to devise an action plan for addressing the problems that reviewers are pointing out. If you don't have good mentorship at your current institution or in your scholarly network, you can always reach out to senior scholars in your field and ask them to mentor you. If this sounds like a strange—or even rude—thing to do, trust me that it is not. I have had many young scholars contact me and ask me to serve as their mentor, ask to use my data, or both. I am generally honored by these requests, and I don't think I have ever said no to any of them. In fact, I have assembled a group of mentees—both at my institution and at other institutions—who come to me for guidance and who analyze my data and write papers using it. As a senior scholar, I don't have as much time to analyze data and write as I would like to, so I am more than happy to share my data (and my feedback on manuscript drafts) with younger scholars who have more available time than I do. In this scenario, everyone wins—senior scholars have opportunities to mentor and to see papers written using their datasets, and the younger scholars have access to datasets that otherwise might not be available to them. If you don't have the mentorship you need, reach out to senior people in your field. You'll be surprised by how responsive and accommodating they are likely to be.

Conclusion

This chapter discusses ways to identify target journals for a manuscript. This process involves ranking the journals in the field represented by the manuscript, as well as honestly assessing the paper and the study or review that it reports. High-prestige journals generally publish groundbreaking or cutting-edge work, and these journals maintain extremely high rejection rates. Only manuscripts reporting the highest quality, most impactful work are generally given serious consideration for publication in high-prestige journals. On the other hand, low-prestige journals are generally not very selective, and some have almost no review process at all. Some low-prestige journals publish articles in narrow areas but are otherwise decent outlets, whereas other low-prestige journals will accept almost anything that is submitted, and authors sometimes will dump papers into low-prestige journals after the papers have been repeatedly rejected. Whereas some low-prestige journals publish good work in narrow areas of study, others should be avoided—especially predatory journals that charge authors to publish and whose claims are virtually impossible (such as having manuscripts peer-reviewed in 2 or 3 days). A good litmus test might be whether you would be willing to have your article appear next to the articles that have appeared in recent issues of the journal. If recently published articles in a journal are poorly written, report sloppy research, or report work that makes little or no contribution to the literature, then my best advice is not to submit your work to that journal.

Moderate-prestige journals are those that fall between the high- and low-prestige journals. The majority of scholarly journals are moderate-prestige journals; therefore, the majority of scholarly articles appear in moderate-prestige journals. These journals publish solid work and generally utilize a rigorous review and editorial process. There is no shame at all in having your work appear in a moderate-prestige journal.

The chapter also discusses special issues. Special issues can represent opportunities for young scholars to publish their work—in many cases, invitations to submit occur through senior mentors' connections, and many mentors will offer lead authorship on a special-issue paper to a mentee. Special issues vary in terms of whether articles are invited for submission from a pre-selected group of authors, abstracts are submitted and evaluated prior to full papers' being invited, or an open call for papers is issued and interested authors are asked to submit full manuscripts for consideration. Having a direct connection (or having a mentor with a direct connection) to the special-issue editors can increase one's chances of having a paper accepted for publication in a special issue—but only if the paper is of sufficient quality.

Finally, the chapter addressed dealing with having papers rejected by journals. Because most high- and moderate-prestige journals maintain high rejection rates, just about everyone will have papers rejected. Rejection can be difficult to handle emotionally—many authors will be upset or angry after receiving a rejection letter—but rejection can be especially devastating for individuals who do not have adequate mentoring and/or who experience imposter syndrome and don't feel that they belong in the scholarly publishing world. Dry spells, where one receives many rejection letters within a fairly short period of time, can lead some scholars to conclude that academic work is not the right career for them. Mentors are especially important in helping writers to identify habits and mistakes that may be contributing to dry spells.

An especially important point to underscore is that the emotional after-effects of having papers rejected must be handled separately from the logistical issues involved in deciding how to move the paper forward. Indeed, if one's confidence decreases because of a rejection or series of rejections, it is important for one's mentor to help address this loss of confidence before one attempts to return to the paper. Restoring one's confidence will help to ensure that subsequent versions of the manuscript are well written and have a greater chance of being accepted for publication in another journal. Developing a "thick skin" toward rejection is a learned skill, and younger scholars should not criticize themselves for not yet having developed that skill.

The next chapter discusses how to think like a reviewer about one's own work. Indeed, critically evaluating one's own work is one of the most difficult endeavors in the entire publishing enterprise. I provide some tips for doing it.

Summary

- Journals are often idiosyncratic in terms of what they publish. The journal title does not necessarily capture the types of work the journal publishes (i.e., the focus may be narrower than the title implies).
- Journals can be grouped into three broad tiers—high-prestige, moderate-prestige, and low-prestige journals.
- High-prestige journals generally publish only the strongest manuscripts that make the greatest contributions to the field. These journals often maintain extremely high rejection rates.
- Moderate-prestige journals publish the majority of scholarly papers. They are solid journals with rigorous editorial and peer-review processes.
- Low-prestige journals include niche journals that cater to small fields of study, as well as journals that are not very selective (some of these journals employ little or no peer review).
- Some low-prestige journals are predatory and should be avoided.
- It is advisable to create a list of three or four target journals for a given manuscript and to rank them in the order in which the authorship team will submit the paper.
- Appraising the contribution of one's work will help in selecting target journals.
- Special issues of journals can provide opportunities for authors to publish their work more easily in high- and moderate-prestige journals.

- Having papers rejected from journals can be a major blow to one's personal and professional self-esteem. Early-career writers may be especially affected by having their work rejected.

References

American Psychological Association. (2020). Summary of journal operations, 2019. *American Psychologist, 75,* 723–724.

Arnett, J. J. (2000). Emerging adulthood: A theory of development from the late teens through the twenties. *American Psychologist, 55,* 469–480.

Arnett, J. J. (2005). The vitality criterion: A new standard of publication for *Journal of Adolescent Research. Journal of Adolescent Research, 20,* 3–7.

Bartholomew, R. E. (2014). Science for sale: The rise of predatory journals. *Journal of the Royal Society of Medicine, 107,* 384–385.

Brody, G. H., Beach, S. R. H., Philibert, R. A., Chen, Y.-F., & Murry, V. M. (2009). Prevention effects moderate the association of 5-HTTLPR and youth risk behavior initiation: Gene × environment hypotheses tested via a randomized prevention design. *Child Development, 80,* 645–661.

Buzzanell, P. M., Long, Z., Anderson, L. B., Kokini, K., & Batra, J. C. (2015). Mentoring in academe: A feminist poststructural lens on stories of women engineering faculty of color. *Management Communication Quarterly, 29,* 440–457.

Dittmar, H. (2011). Material and place identities. In S. J. Schwartz, K. Luyckx, & V. L. Vignoles (Eds.), *Handbook of identity theory and research* (pp. 745–769). New York: Springer.

Ferguson, G. M., Iturbide, M. I., & Gordon, B. P. (2014). Tridimensional (3D) acculturation: Ethnic identity and psychological functioning of tricultural Jamaican immigrants. *International Perspectives in Psychology: Research, Practice, Consultation, 3,* 238–251.

Hernández, B., Hidalgo, M. C., Salazar-Laplace, M. E., & Hess, S. (2007). Place attachment and place identity in natives and non-natives. *Journal of Environmental Psychology, 27,* 310–319.

Horn, S. A. (2016). The social and psychological costs of peer review: Stress and coping with manuscript rejection. *Journal of Management Inquiry, 25,* 11–26.

Hutchins, H. M., & Rainbolt, H. (2017). What triggers imposter phenomenon among academic faculty? A critical incident study exploring antecedents, coping, and development opportunities. *Human Resource Development International, 20,* 194–214.

Jia, J., Harmon, J. L., Connolly, K. G., Donnelly, R. M., Anderson, M. R., & Howard, H. A. (2015). Who publishes in "predatory" journals? *Journal of the Association for Information Science and Technology, 66,* 1406–1417.

Klimstra, T. A., Luyckx, K., Hale, W. W., III, Frijns, T., van Lier, P. A. C., & Meeus, W. H. J. (2010). Short-term fluctuations in identity: Introducing a micro-level approach to identity formation. *Journal of Personality and Social Psychology, 99,* 191–202.

Laband, D. N., & Piette, M. J. (1994). Favoritism versus search for good papers: Empirical evidence regarding the behavior of journal editors. *Journal of Political Economy, 102,* 194–203.

Ozer, S., & Schwartz, S. J. (2016). Measuring globalization-based acculturation in Ladakh: Investigating possible advantages of a tridimensional acculturation scale. *International Journal of Intercultural Relations, 53,* 1–16.

Pettigrew, T. F., & Tropp, L. R. (2006). A meta-analytic test of intergroup contact theory. *Journal of Personality and Social Psychology, 90,* 751–783.

Podsakoff, P. M., MacKenzie, S. B., & Podsakoff, N. P. (2012). Sources of method bias in social-science research and recommendations on how to control it. *Annual Review of Psychology, 63*, 539–569.

Rosario, C. C., Lance, C. E., Delgado-Romero, E., & Domenich-Rodríguez, M. M. (2018). Acculturated and *acultura'os*: Testing bidimensional acculturation across Central Florida and island Puerto Ricans. *Cultural Diversity and Ethnic Minority Psychology, 25*, 152–169.

Schwartz, S. J. (2001). The evolution of Eriksonian and neo-Eriksonian identity theory and research: A review and integration. *Identity: An International Journal of Theory and Research, 1*, 7–58.

Schwartz, S. J., Unger, J. B., Zamboanga, B. L., & Szapocznik, J. (2010). Rethinking the concept of acculturation: Implications for theory and research. *American Psychologist, 65*, 237–251.

Schwartz, S. J., & Zamboanga, B. L. (2009). The peer-review and editorial system: Ways to fix something that might be broken. *Perspectives on Psychological Science, 4*, 54–61.

Shamseer, L., Moher, D., Madeukwe, O., Turner, L., Barbour, V., Burch, R., . . . Shea, B. J. (2017). Potential predatory and legitimate biomedical journals: Can you tell the difference? A cross-sectional comparison. *BMC Medicine, 15*, Article 28.

Woolley, K. L., & Barron, J. P. (2009). Handling manuscript rejection: Insights from evidence and experience. *Chest, 135*, 573–577.

Ysseldyk, R., Greenaway, K. H., Hassinger, E., Zutrauen, S., Lintz, J., Bhatia, M. P., Tai, V. (2019). A leak in the academic pipeline: Identity and health among postdoctoral women. *Frontiers in Psychology, 10*, Article 1297.

11

Thinking Like a Reviewer

Chapter Objectives

When you finish reading this chapter, you should be more comfortable with:

- What reviewers consider when they are evaluating a manuscript for publication
- "Thinking like a reviewer" about your own work
- Evaluating the fit of your paper with your target journal
- Recognizing major flaws in your work, and how to frame them in your writing
- Primary criticisms that reviewers often include regarding each section of a manuscript
- Ways to "head off" specific reviewer concerns and comments

In my career, I have served as a journal reviewer or editor for hundreds of manuscripts. As I read through a manuscript, I look for specific strengths and weaknesses that I can note in my review. I look primarily for the contribution of the study, review, or theory being presented and for potential problems that could interfere with the presentation of the study's contribution. For an empirical manuscript, I ask: Does the introduction set up the study? Are the methods described in a way that would allow readers to replicate the study if they chose to? Are the hypotheses tested fully, such that every hypothesis is tested and every result corresponds to a hypothesis? Does the discussion cover all the findings, including those that don't support the authors' hypotheses? For literature reviews, I consider: Is the relevant literature reviewed fully and objectively? Are the authors ignoring literature that might contradict their closely held assumptions? For theoretical and position papers, my concerns include: Is the theory or argument set up well enough in the introductory section? Do the authors make the case for why their new perspective or direction is needed?

However, there is also a deeper level of review with which reviewers are charged. I call this the "30,000 feet approach"—imagine yourself looking out

The Savvy Academic. Seth J. Schwartz, Oxford University Press. © Oxford University Press 2022.
DOI: 10.1093/oso/9780190095918.003.0012

an airplane window and seeing the ground below. From this viewpoint, you have a much more comprehensive and "big picture" view of the landscape than you would if you were standing on the ground. This analogy applies well to evaluating manuscripts for publication—more or less, in the big picture, what is this paper contributing to the literature? Is it able to make the impact that the authors argue for, and is this impact sufficient to warrant publication?

For empirical manuscripts, are there design or methodological flaws that cannot be fixed through revision? What is the magnitude of the study's contribution? What have we learned from this study or set of studies, and how much of an advance does this contribution represent for the field? For literature review papers, is this review really needed? At this point in its evolution, what does the field gain from a review of this type? Have other reviews been published recently, and do these reviews undermine or lessen the contribution of the current manuscript? For theoretical and position manuscripts, how novel is the theory or viewpoint being advanced? How much does it contribute beyond what we already know? Is this perspective going to change how the field views itself? Will it change how future research is designed, conducted, and interpreted?

As an editor, I use the 30,000 feet approach to decide whether a manuscript is a serious candidate for publication in my journal. What do we, as a journal, gain by publishing this paper instead of another paper that was submitted for consideration? How will the paper benefit the field in which the paper was written? Is the article likely to be read and cited? (Remember how the impact factor works—the numerator is the number of citations to the journal in a given year.) How will publishing this paper contribute—or not—to maintaining the journal's prestige?

It's much easier to ask these questions about someone else's work than it is to ask them about our own work. The inherent difficulty involved in critically and objectively evaluating one's own work is why I decided to include a chapter on "thinking like a reviewer." Overall, when you think like a reviewer about your own work, you are pretending that you are evaluating someone else's manuscript. Remember that a reviewer's job is to identify flaws and problems in manuscripts and in the work that they report. Van Lange (1999) referred to this reviewer job description as stressing the limiting aspects of manuscripts (SLAM). He found that, not surprisingly, scholars are more critical of other people's papers than of their own papers, and that reviewers are more likely to agree with editors' rejection decisions than authors are.

This chapter aims to turn van Lange's characterization into an advantage. That is, we can use the SLAM approach to help us assess our own work honestly. What are the limits of our own manuscript and of the study, theory, position, or review it reports? What would a critical reviewer say if that person read our paper? If an editor were looking for a reason to reject our manuscript, what reasons would that editor use? Using this "devil's advocate" viewpoint, are there specific statements that we can insert into our manuscript to help insulate ourselves against the concerns and criticisms that we are anticipating? Drawing on the information provided in Chapter 10, are there certain journals that we should avoid, given our frank and objective assessment of our manuscript and of the work it is reporting?

It is easy—and quite often unproductive—to assume that our work is excellent and has essentially no flaws. Such a perception might lead us to overvalue the contribution of our paper and to send it to a journal that is almost certain to reject it. I remember talking with a colleague of mine who was an associate editor for a prominent developmental psychology journal. He told me about a submission he was handling—the authors had conducted a cross-sectional study using a college student sample and had used their results to draw developmental inferences. I offered to review the paper for my colleague, and when I read the manuscript, it was clear that the authors had not engaged in much critical reflection about their work. The paper had essentially no chance of being accepted in the journal to which the authors had submitted it, and in trying to make their study fit with a developmental audience, they had stretched their discussion far beyond what their research design could support. In my review, I noted all of these issues and recommended rejection.

Had these authors evaluated their work critically, they probably would have surmised that a premier developmental journal was not going to consider seriously their cross-sectional college student sample. They likely would have reported and interpreted their findings in terms of associations among variables—and might have included some very tentative statements about the findings' being potentially suggestive of developmental trends. They might have inserted statements cautioning readers to interpret their results in light of the cross-sectional design and of the inclusion only of college students in the sample. Given these important limitations, they would likely have targeted a moderate-prestige (or even low-prestige) journal. In short, they would have asked themselves how a reviewer might assess their work—and they would have proceeded accordingly.

A Reviewer's Job Description

Before we discuss how to think like a reviewer, it's important to go over what reviewers are asked to do when they agree to review a manuscript. What exactly are we looking for from reviewers? What kind of feedback are they supposed to provide? What do reviewers contribute to the process of evaluating a manuscript for publication, and how does their input help authors and editors?

The most basic function of peer review is to prevent flawed, sloppy, or otherwise inadequate work from entering the scientific literature (Alberts, Hanson, & Kelner, 2008). Reviewers are expected to read the manuscript critically and to comment on anything that they find troubling, confusing, or otherwise problematic. In theory, reviewers should also praise aspects of the paper that they believe are well done—but as van Lange (1999) noted, reviewers generally devote most of their comments to shortcomings and problems. Reviewers therefore serve as "gatekeepers" for science and help to ensure that substandard work is not published—or at least is not published in reputable journals.

When I review manuscripts, I generally attend to three levels of review—(1) whether the paper warrants further publication consideration in the journal to which it was submitted, and why or why not; (2) major addressable concerns and limitations; and (3) more minor writing issues. Clearly, the first level will largely determine the fate of the paper; editors are far more likely to reject a manuscript when even one reviewer recommends rejection (Schultz, 2010). Level (2) encompasses "major revisions" (i.e., those changes that are likely to improve the quality of the paper substantially). Level (3) encompasses "minor revisions"—word changes, grammatical corrections, and small points that the authors may have overlooked or missed. Some reviewers don't provide comments at this lowest level unless the writing is noticeably poor—and if the writing is poor, it may be difficult for reviewers to understand the study or arguments reported in the manuscript.

Reviewers also submit a confidential publication recommendation to the editor. Authors generally do not see these recommendations unless the editor or reviewer includes them in their feedback to the author. These confidential recommendations may help to explain why some editors will reject a paper where reviewers' comments to the author are fairly benign or even moderately supportive. I remember one journal editor telling me that he would never offer authors an invitation to revise and resubmit their manuscripts if any reviewer had recommended rejection. When I am serving as editor, I place far more weight on the manuscript's review narratives than on the reviewers' official recommendations (see Schwartz & Zamboanga, 2009, for a more in-depth discussion of this editorial approach). I've seen reviewers recommend rejection and then provide largely supportive comments. As an editor, I see the decision regarding publication as mine. As another editor told me once,

"The reviewers don't get to decide; they provide their best judgment and I get to take the responsibility."

Notwithstanding that editor's—and my—philosophy on editing, it remains a truism that manuscripts that receive largely negative reviewer feedback are highly unlikely to be accepted for publication in the journal to which they were submitted. Editors usually make "judgment calls" only when the reviewers disagree with one another on the merits of the paper. When I am acting as editor, if all of a manuscript's reviewers have recommended rejection, I generally only scan the paper and identify the most major issues to comment on in my editorial letter. Reviewers generally do most of the "heavy lifting" involved in the editorial review process. This is why I advise writers to "think like a reviewer" more than to "think like an editor."

I was recently invited to review a manuscript for the *Journal of Child and Family Studies*, and the instructions I received were among the most informative and prescriptive that I have seen in a review invitation letter. I include them here, because they provide an excellent summary of the reviewer's job description:

Please provide an evaluation of its scientific merit: conceptualization and rationale, methods, reliability and validity, clarity of presentation, implications, and contribution to the field. The rigor of the work is critical; however, the paper must also make an important conceptual or empirical contribution to the literature in order to merit publication in JCFS. We are particularly interested in translational works that inform not only research but also policy and practice and ask you to encourage authors to make their work accessible in this manner.

Effective editorial reviews are informed by a careful review of the paper, are unbiased, and are absent comments likely to be experienced as demeaning by the author(s). We invite you to make constructive and critical comments about any aspect of the paper and ask that you frame your feedback in the form of observations ("the ms lacks a clear articulation of . . .") and requests ("in a revision, please provide . . ."). Kindly provide the authors with constructive feedback so that they can improve on their efforts in future research and/or incorporate your suggestions in a revision.

If you assess a paper to have "fatal flaws"—such as design/methods that cannot be improved through revision or reanalysis—please recommend rejection of the manuscript at the first round of review. In so doing, you are welcome to share your appraisal in the "confidential comments to editor" and to the author(s) as well (for example, by stating that the paper in its current form does not meet the standards for the journal, and why). Comments directly to the author(s) are expected when undertaking a review; when possible, suggest improvements that might benefit subsequent research or improve the likelihood of acceptance of the paper to another journal.

If you believe that a paper is likely publishable contingent on revision, please provide specific instructions or guidelines as to where and what must be done to make the paper acceptable. Our aim is not only to publish papers of high quality but also to encourage our colleagues to enhance the quality of their research.

So, in essence, reviewers who recommend that a paper be revised and resubmitted should be as clear as possible about the potential they see in the paper, what issues they would like to see addressed, and what successful resolution of those concerns might look like. Serving as a reviewer is not an easy task, and it should not be taken lightly. I have had reviewers provide one- or two-line reviews of my manuscripts, and in those instances I have been surprised that the editor even allowed the reviewer comments to be passed along to the author. Indeed, as an editor, I have removed reviews from a manuscript—meaning that they were not shared with the authors and were not factored into my editorial decision—if they were inadequate, contained personal attacks on the authors, or otherwise went against the collegial spirit that the *Journal of Child and Family Studies* recommended in their instructions to reviewers.

How to Think Like a Reviewer About Your Own Work

Let's extrapolate the reviewer job description back to our own work. At the 30,000-feet level, what would you say is the primary contribution of your paper and of the research it reports? What are the two or three take-home points that you would want readers to remember from your paper? What is the message you are aiming to send? Now consider the journals that you have targeted as outlets for your paper. How do your take-home points match up with the prestige level, focus, and scope of the journal you have targeted? At the broadest level—not considering any potential design flaws in your study or logical flaws in your theory or position—are the take-home points from your paper in line with the journal you are targeting?

Even if the contribution represented by your paper matches up with the prestige level of the journal you are targeting, you need to think about how reviewers for that journal might evaluate the topic of your paper and the ways in which you have framed your arguments. I provide two examples here. First, many personality journals focus heavily on certain personality typologies, such as the Big Five (Costa & McCrae, 1995) and Dark Triad (Furnham, Richards, & Paulhus, 2013) models of personality. Studies not using such typologies may be difficult to publish in some personality journals. Second, using a longitudinal design may not be sufficient to warrant publication in a developmental journal—the study needs to be framed developmentally. That is, you need to ground the work in a developmental theoretical perspective. Remember that readers of personality journals will be looking for research and theory that draws upon the predominant models used in personality psychology, and readers of developmental journals will be looking for research and theory that draw upon developmental models. And remember that the reviewers whom the editor or associate editor recruits for your paper will likely be drawn from the people who have published in the target journal, who read the target journal, or both.

At the next level—level (2) in the review criteria—list your research questions and hypotheses, one at a time, and think critically about the specific research designs that you would need to test each hypothesis. If your paper presents a literature review, theoretical perspective, or position, think critically about the type and extent of empirical evidence and logical steps that would be required to support and substantiate your argument. As is discussed in Chapter 1, think carefully about how novel your work is. To what extent does it duplicate, or build only incrementally on, prior work? Even if the work you have conducted matches well with what would be expected or required given the hypotheses or goals you have enumerated, if reviewers conclude that "this has been done before," then your paper is likely to be rejected. Overall, your paper has to report solid work and advance the literature if it is to be seriously considered for publication in a high- or moderate-prestige journal.

Next, think carefully about anything in your study design, argument, or theory that reviewers might consider a fatal flaw. If you are evaluating the efficacy or effectiveness of an intervention, have you used an "intent to treat" design (see Dawson & Lavori, 2015) where all cases are assessed through the end of the study even if they drop out of the intervention? Have you used random assignment or a statistical technique (e.g., propensity score matching; Guo & Fraser, 2014) that allows you to compare the active and control conditions and draw causal conclusions? If you are comparing means, correlations, or other statistical values across naturally occurring groups (e.g., gender, ethnicity, nationality), have you conducted invariance analyses (Putnick & Bornstein, 2016) to verify that the factor structure of the variable you are comparing is equivalent across groups? If you are conducting survival analyses, have you examined whether your data satisfy the proportional hazards assumption, where the effect of each predictor on the hazard function (likelihood of observing the event of interest) is consistent across time (Xue et al., 2013)?

On a conceptual level, have you cited key theories, studies, and research traditions in your field of study? Would a reviewer take issue with how you have framed your study? Are there important people in your field whom you have not cited (or have not cited sufficiently)? As already noted, the review process is at least somewhat political. Your paper is likely to be reviewed by people who are leaders in your field—or by their colleagues or students. Not citing the "big names" in the area represented by your paper can upset some reviewers. Are there important lines of research in your area that you might have left out?

I remember one paper that my colleague and I submitted to a journal almost 20 years ago. We were reporting the results of a personal-identity-based intervention on college students' sense of identity and well-being. We cited what we thought were the most important names in the personal identity literature and grounded the intervention in their work. However, one reviewer criticized us extensively for not citing, and grounding our program in, a theory of college student identity that I had never heard of. However, when I conducted a literature search on identity theory and research published in that journal, many of the articles I found used the theoretical perspective that this reviewer had criticized us for not adopting. Clearly, we had not done our homework on this journal.

Thus, it is essential not only to think like a reviewer in general, but to think like a reviewer for the specific journal that you are targeting for your manuscript. What theoretical perspectives tend to be used most often in that journal (at least for articles published in your field of interest)? Are there specific research methodologies that are most often used? For example, some social-psychology journals strongly prefer experimental designs. If you write a paper that reports results of a cross-sectional study, and you are considering submitting the paper to a social-psychology journal, I recommend that you consult recent issues of the journal—and talk to colleagues who have published in that journal recently—to determine whether your paper is likely to resonate with the reviewers for that journal.

Almost all journals list the editor-in-chief, the editorial team (including associate and assistant editors), and the editorial board on the journal's home page. In many cases, the editorial board consists of individuals who have committed to review a certain number of manuscripts per year for the journal in question. Editors and associate editors often rely heavily on editorial board members to provide reviews—so I suggest scanning the editorial board and looking for people who publish in your field of study. At the very least, make sure that your paper doesn't contradict or undermine their work. If you can find ways to cite their work, that would be even more favorable if editorial board members wind up reviewing your manuscript.

Editors also often invite their close colleagues to serve as reviewers. Most reviewers I invite to review papers for me wind up declining the invitation. I've had papers where I had to invite 11 or 12 reviewers just to get two completed reviews. So, often I have "aces in the hole"—mentees and close colleagues whom I know will accept a review invitation when I really need a reviewer. If you can figure out who is likely to be the action editor for your manuscript after you submit to your target journal, look up that action editor's publications and see whether they have frequent coauthors whose work is in your area of expertise. Those coauthors may well wind up reviewing your manuscript.

Reviewers often criticize authors for not measuring or controlling for key covariates. If you are studying immigrants, for example, it's important to assess and control for the age at which they arrived in the destination country. If you are studying a group whose members migrate back and forth between the heritage and destination countries or regions—such as Puerto Ricans moving back and forth between the mainland United States and Puerto Rico (Acosta-Belén & Santiago, 2018)—you might also control for the total number of years spent in the destination country or region. Failing to control for some index of exposure to the destination culture might represent a fatal flaw for some reviewers. Similarly, in studies of posttraumatic stress symptoms after natural or human disasters, it is critical to measure and control for extent of exposure to the traumatic event (Weems et al., 2010). Without knowing whether a given respondent was in the middle of the event, watched it on television or social media, or heard about it from someone else, we cannot properly ascertain the associations of other variables with extent of posttraumatic stress symptoms. Thinking like a reviewer involves ensuring that you account for key covariates in your analyses. If the study is already completed and you didn't measure a key covariate, thinking like a reviewer involves (a) explaining why you could not, or did not, assess the key variables or control for their effects or (b) listing the covariates as important limitations that should be overcome in future work.

Chapter 2 discusses how to plan a publishable study. Part of the planning includes identifying and assessing important covariates. If you were not able to assess the covariates, or if you are using a secondary data set where they were not measured, then listing them as limitations is probably the best course of action. However, be prepared for reviewers to recommend rejection—especially with high-prestige journals—when important predictors, outcomes, or covariates are not included in analysis. Similarly, when authors' statistical analyses are confounded by variables whose effects cannot be effectively controlled, reviewers might also recommend rejection. I remember reviewing a paper many years ago where the authors were comparing two preventive interventions. Rather than randomly assigning participants to one of the two conditions, these authors compared one intervention delivered in one city to a second intervention delivered in a different city. Because the effects of intervention condition could not be uncoupled from the effects of geographical location, I recommended rejection—and the editor ultimately rejected the manuscript. In this case, the use of two different interventions in two different cities was a fatal flaw.

I don't know this for sure, but it's possible that the authors had access to two different intervention data sets and decided to compare them. Sometimes, authors spot opportunities like that and decide to capitalize on them, despite the possible presence of fatal flaws. My best guidance in this situation is drop down to a lower journal tier. You may need to target a low-prestige journal, especially if your paper has already been rejected from two or more journals. (What to do with rejected manuscripts is discussed in Chapter 13, but if you have received similar reviewer comments from multiple journals, you may need to consider "dumping" the paper into a low-prestige journal.) It is often an uphill battle to publish manuscripts from fatally flawed studies in high- or moderate-prestige journals.

But what if there are no obvious flaws? Are there certain kinds of statements that may help to increase the likelihood that reviewers will respond favorably to your paper? In my estimation, the answer is a clear Yes, and I provide some tips in this chapter, but remember that my examples are just that—examples. You may have to adapt them for your specific papers and fields of study.

The third level of review has to do with the writing itself. The points made in Chapter 6 about principles of good writing apply here. Just as molecules are comprised of atoms and cells are comprised of molecules, sections are comprised of paragraphs and paragraphs are comprised of sentences. Sentences must be structured properly and flow well in order for paragraphs to flow well. In turn, paragraphs must flow well for sections to flow well and have maximum impact. Beyond sentence, paragraph, and section flow, it is essential to ensure that each section sets up, explains, and interprets the study, theory, review, or position being reported. Next, I proceed section by section of a paper and note some issues that I (and other reviewers and editors) have often found in manuscripts that we have evaluated. This discussion pertains primarily to empirical manuscripts (both quantitative and qualitative), but some of the points I list here also apply to theoretical, position, and literature review manuscripts. (You will notice that these points reiterate what Chapters 7 and 9 outline about the ingredients of each section in the manuscript.)

Introduction

The primary criticisms I have seen (and provided) on introductory sections include the following:

- The introduction section is poorly organized. It is not clear what the paper is about or what arguments the authors are trying to set up.
- The introduction does not adequately set up the study. There is not enough introductory material covering some of the key study constructs.
- Covariates are used in analyses, but the importance of these covariates is not set up in the introductory section. The reader does not know to expect these covariates to be measured and accounted for.
- The study is not grounded in a clear theoretical framework. The study hypotheses do not logically come out of an established theoretical perspective.
- No testable hypotheses are listed in the introduction. I had a lot of trouble understanding what exactly was being tested in this study.
- The authors state that they are grounding their work in a specific theoretical perspective, but many of their statements in the introduction are not consistent with that perspective.
- The authors contradict themselves in the introductory section.
- Some of the claims and citations that the authors include in their introductory section are not accurate.

Method

Criticisms I have seen, and provided, on method sections include:

- Did the study receive approval from an ethics committee or Institutional Review Board?
- The sampling strategy is not clear. How were participants recruited? Were they compensated in some way? If so, how much?
- Why were some of the exclusion criteria used? It is not clear why participants would be excluded for these reasons.
- What was the participation rate? How many individuals were approached, and how many of these individuals agreed to participate?
- What was the attrition rate? Do the authors know why participants dropped out of the study?
- Did the authors ask for additional demographic information beyond what is reported in the manuscript? If not, why not?

- How were participants recruited? Did the authors use printed flyers, social media announcements, or something else?
- Please describe all the study activities in which participants were asked to engage. Did any participants decline to engage in any of these activities? If so, how many? Do we know why participants declined to engage in some of the study activities?
- Were the study procedures pilot-tested prior to being used in the study? If not, why not?
- Some key variables (predictors, outcomes, or covariates) appear to be missing from the assessment battery.
- *For experimental studies*: Did the authors make sure that participants were blinded to their condition assignment? If so, how was this accomplished?
- *For experimental studies*: Were data collectors blinded to participants' condition assignment?
- Who administered the surveys, conducted the interviews, or collected the biological samples? What were these individuals' qualifications to conduct these activities? What training did they receive?
- *For behavioral intervention studies*: What were interventionists' qualifications? How were they trained? Was supervision provided? Did the study team assess interventionists' adherence or fidelity to the intervention manual or protocol? If so, how was this done? If not, how do we know that the intervention was delivered properly?
- *For online studies*: How was the study website set up? Was it pilot-tested prior to use? How were participants' data and responses kept secure?
- *For studies involving interviews or focus groups*: Were interviews or focus groups recorded? How were they transcribed? Did multiple transcribers listen to the recordings and compare notes to ensure that the transcription was accurate?
- *For studies involving material translated across languages*: What translation procedure was used? Did multiple translators work together to ensure translation accuracy?
- *For studies where the same procedures were utilized across multiple sites*: How did the study team ensure that the same procedures were followed across sites? What kinds of checks were used?
- *For longitudinal studies*: What procedures were used to retain participants across time? What was the retention rate? If the study was conducted across multiple sites, did the retention rate differ significantly across sites? Did any demographic or study variables significantly predict retention versus attrition?

Results

Criticisms I have seen, and provided, on results sections include:

- Not all the analyses correspond to hypotheses that were presented in the introduction. There appear to be some "stray" analyses reported in the results section.
- Did the data satisfy all the assumptions for the analyses that were conducted?
- Why did you use the specific types of analyses that you used?
- The results are difficult to follow without tables and figures.
- Why did the analyses not control for additional covariates? (Reviewers often list the covariates they would have wanted to see you control for.)
- Confidence intervals should be reported along with test statistics, p-values, and effect sizes.
- The authors need to indicate the extent to which each of their results provides support for the study hypotheses.
- Did the analyses control for effects of multilevel nesting (e.g., patients in hospitals, children in schools, time points in individuals)?
- *For cross-sectional and longitudinal studies*: A table of correlations among study variables should be included.
- Statistical values are presented, but it is difficult to understand what the results mean. The text of the results section needs to augment the statistical values much more clearly.
- *For qualitative and mixed-method studies* How did the authors select cases and excerpts to analyze? I am concerned that the authors may have "cherry picked" their quotes to support their existing theory.
- *For qualitative and mixed-method studies*: What approach and coding system was used to analyze the data? Did multiple coders provide ratings? What was the level of interrater agreement?

Discussion

Criticisms I have seen, and provided, on discussion sections include:

- The discussion just restates the results and does not interpret them.
- The discussion needs to offer a verdict on each of the study hypotheses. Which hypotheses were supported, which were not supported, and which were partially supported?

- The discussion refers to variables and constructs that were not included in the analyses.
- The discussion includes conclusions that the data and research design cannot support.
- The discussion is vague and does not clearly interpret the findings.
- The discussion section does not include limitations of the study.
- The discussion doesn't interpret all the results. It appears to interpret only the results that the authors had hypothesized. This selective interpretation makes the study look like a fishing expedition.
- *For journals that are oriented toward clinical, counseling, or community practice*: The discussion needs to include implications for practice. How do the present results help to inform intervention design and delivery?
- The discussion section presents new results. Results do not belong in the discussion section.
- The conclusions in the discussion section appear to come out of nowhere and are not connected to the findings presented in the results section.
- The discussion section is too brief. The authors don't help the reader to understand what the results mean for further research and for intervention.
- The discussion section does not place the present findings back within the context of the literature that was reviewed in the introduction.
- Even after reading the discussion, I did not get a sense of why these findings are important. What do the authors see as the primary contribution of this study?
- The discussion section provides too many broad and sweeping generalizations. These are unhelpful. More specific and targeted statements are needed to help the reader understand and apply the findings.

There are also several criticisms that may be levied against the paper as a whole. As I did with the section-by-section criticisms, I focus primarily on empirical articles—but I also note some criticisms that might be directed at theoretical, position, and literature-review articles.

- The paper is poorly organized. The writing is choppy, and I found the paper to be very difficult to follow.
- The study does not make a clear contribution to the literature.
- This study largely duplicates past work and is not really needed.
- It is not clear what the authors are trying to say in many parts of the paper.
- The field has moved beyond the methods used in this study.
- The grammar and sentence structure throughout the paper were very hard to read.

- Throughout the paper, the authors present their ideas as original, when in fact many of the ideas came from prior literature. Citations are needed; otherwise, what the authors are doing borders on plagiarism.
- I am sympathetic to the authors' attempts to present their study as a major contribution. However, the study represents a far more incremental contribution. That is to say, the authors appear to have overstated the importance of their work.
- The authors need a native English speaker to go through their manuscript and help them improve the writing.
- Why is the authors' new theory necessary? The theory reads like a rehashing of existing work.
- Why is it important to review this body of literature? The authors don't really make the case for why their analysis is needed.
- This manuscript reads like a poorly written dissertation literature review. The authors are all over the place, and there is no clear thesis or message.
- I cannot tell exactly what the authors are arguing for. The authors contradict themselves repeatedly.
- Although this manuscript is supposed to be an integrative review of the literature, the authors ignore whole lines of literature. They appear to be biased in terms of the work that they have decided to include.
- There is little rhyme or reason in what literature the authors include in their review. Literature reviews are supposed to be systematic, but this one is clearly not.
- The authors' theory is not sufficiently grounded in empirical literature.
- Why are the authors arguing for the position they are advocating for? They never provide a reason why their arguments are important or what they contribute to the literature.

Of course, the reviewer comments I provide here are only a sampling of those that I have received from reviewers on my own papers, that I have provided as part of reviews of submitted manuscripts, or that I have received about manuscripts that I was handling as action editor. My goal here is to help you to look at your own work more critically in light of what reviewers have commented about other authors' manuscripts. I advise looking at your own papers and asking yourself whether any of the reviewer comments I have listed here might apply.

Note that each of your coauthors should also be given the opportunity to "think like a reviewer" about the manuscript. One of José's greatest contributions to my writing abilities—and to my skills in setting up and planning studies—was serving as a de facto reviewer on just about every manuscript draft I ever sent him. He would ask the kinds of questions, and make the kinds of comments, that I have listed here in this chapter. By the time I submitted a manuscript for publication with José as a coauthor, the paper (and the study it reported) had been through several rounds of highly rigorous review. Largely as a result, more than 50% of the editorial decisions on our papers were positive—an extremely respectable rate given the high rejection rates for many of the journals to which we submitted our work.

Chapter 14 says more about working with coauthors, but for now, the point is that coauthors can help you think like a reviewer about your own work. Coauthors who challenge you and "keep you honest" are the most valuable coauthors to have. If there are flaws in your study, and the flaws cannot be corrected (i.e., because the data have already been collected), you want to make sure that you know about the flaws so you can mention them as limitations. The last thing you want to have happen is for a reviewer to blindside you with a weakness that you were not aware of.

In some cases, you might spot a weakness in your study design, but you might decide that this weakness is not important enough to mention and draw attention to in your manuscript. That is, your belief might be that, if you don't call attention to the issue, reviewers may not notice it or regard it as important enough to mention in their comments. Al Waterman referred to this kind of intentional omission as "benign neglect." Of course, there is an inherent risk in this approach—namely that reviewers will treat the issue as more important than you thought they would, and that the issue might factor into the reviewers' recommendations and the editor's decision whether to invite a revision or reject the manuscript. In my experience, however, calling attention to fairly small issues is more likely to lead to more reviewer criticisms than would have occurred had the issue not been mentioned in the manuscript.

Heading Off Major Criticisms

One final set of observations and recommendations is important to thinking like a reviewer. The most important reviewer criticisms to "head off" are those that are directed toward the manuscript or study as a whole. That is, reviewers are more likely to recommend rejection based on "big-picture" issues that pertain to the entire manuscript than they are to recommend rejection based on specific sections. Such big-picture issues might pertain to the absence of a clear justification for the study, theory, position, or review; a belief that the manuscript does not make an important enough contribution to the literature; difficulty understanding the key arguments presented in the manuscript; questioning the grounding of the study, theory, or position within extant literature; concerns that the authors have omitted important lines of research from their review, theory, or position; and omission of key variables or procedures from a study. There may be strategic ways to place statements in the paper to help avoid some of these criticisms, as I outline in this section.

Concerns pertaining to the importance of the study, review, theory, or position can be avoided by placing statements in the beginning of the manuscript. These concerns usually relate to the gap in the literature that we are seeking to fill. One strategy that I often use is to place an "importance paragraph" in the first few pages of the introduction section. Here is an example from a recent empirical article that my colleagues and I published (Schwartz et al., 2021, p. 123):

> There may be important disparities among Hispanic college students. Hispanic students who report experiencing microaggressions or other forms of discrimination tend to report lower well-being, and higher levels of externalizing symptoms, compared with Hispanic students who do not report such culturally stressful experiences (Schwartz et al., 2021; Nadal, Wong, Griffin, Davidoff, & Sriken, 2014). However, it should be noted that the vast majority of these studies have been cross-sectional. It is therefore imperative to identify cultural processes that predict well-being, internalizing symptoms, and externalizing problems over time among Hispanic college students.

In this case, notice that we map the specific phenomena that are important to study, state the limitations of prior work (i.e., that prior studies examining the phenomena in question have been cross-sectional), and argue for the importance of the design and type of study that we report in the article. In this way, we were able to insulate ourselves against reviewer comments questioning the importance of our study.

The contribution of the manuscript to the literature should be noted in the discussion section (for empirical manuscripts) or toward the end of the paper (for theoretical, position, and review manuscripts). The reader should finish the paper with a good idea of what the study, theory, review, or position has added to the literature. The contribution statement should build on earlier statements about the importance of the question on which the paper is based. For example, in that same article (Schwartz et al., 2021), we end the paper with the following paragraph (p. 139):

> In conclusion, despite these and other potential limitations, our study has opened a line of research on micro-level acculturation processes. Our results suggest that acculturation components often shift from one day to the next, and that daily shifts in U.S. practices, collectivist values, and ethnic identity can be deleterious for well-being and internalizing symptoms. Fluctuations in U.S. identity also appear to

potentiate aggression and rule breaking, suggesting that shifts in use of English at home and at work or school across days are especially unsettling. We hope that the present study will inspire additional work in this direction.

So, here we tell the reader what we are adding to the literature—in this case that we have opened a new line of research on daily acculturation processes. We also summarize the biggest-picture findings so that the reader leaves the article with a clear sense of what we found. In my estimation, these bottom-line summaries represent an important way of communicating the study's contribution.

Grounding the work in theoretical and empirical literature is accomplished through citations of current literature—including both theory and empirical work. As is argued in Chapters 2 and 3, theory is essential—the hypotheses must come from somewhere, and "dust bowl empiricism" (the words used by a reviewer to describe one of my papers) is not an acceptable way to establish a set of research questions and hypotheses. Although prior research can give us hints about what we might expect to find in our study, we need a systematic analysis of the relationships and effects that might be expected to exist (and this systematic analysis is what theory provides). Papers that include factual statements without citations are concerning to reviewers because, without citations, it is not clear how we know what we are stating in our manuscript.

Remember also that, with the exception of major breakthroughs (such as the introduction of functional magnetic resonance imaging in the 1990s; Casey et al., 1997), science proceeds in small steps. We review where the field is currently, and we detail how our current work will move the field forward. Citations to recent scholarship help us to ground our current efforts in the literature and to tell the reader how our work adds to, and extends, the literature. Without this grounding, it is difficult—if not impossible—for readers to tell where the literature was prior to our current work and where our work is taking the literature.

Particularly in theoretical, position, and literature-review manuscripts, it is essential to establish boundaries for the analysis. Tell readers what literature you will cover and what literature you will not cover and provide compelling reasons. Your manuscript may be reviewed by people who are heavily invested in the literatures you are omitting from your analysis—so a compelling rationale for which literatures you include, and which ones you exclude, is critical.

Here is a description, from a review article that my colleagues and I published several years ago (Schwartz, Zamboanga, Luyckx, Meca, & Ritchie, 2013, p. 98), detailing the specific literature we planned to review:

In this article, we review three primary models that have their roots in Erikson's work. The majority of the present article is devoted to the identity status perspective (Marcia, 1966), recent extensions of identity status theory, and related research conducted within specific identity domains (e.g., politics, religion/spirituality, and gender/sexuality). We also review work conducted within (a) the identity style perspective (Berzonsky, 1989), which began as an extension of identity status but has now established its own literature, and within (b) narrative approaches to identity (e.g., Bauer & McAdams, 2010; McAdams, 2013).

And here is an excerpt from an article (Schwartz, Montgomery, & Briones, 2006, p. 2) where my colleagues and I discuss literatures that will not be included in our analysis:

> The concept of acculturation has been used to refer both to immigrant people and to nonimmigrant ethnic groups (Pope-Davis, Liu, Ledesma-Jones, & Nevitt, 2000; Saxton, 2001; Suleiman, 2002). Nonimmigrant ethnic groups are faced with acculturation challenges not because they have chosen to enter a new society, but rather because they have been involuntarily subjected to the dominance of a majority group (often on their own land). Examples of such nonimmigrant ethnic groups include African Americans and Native Americans in the United States, Palestinians in Israel, and Catholic Irish in Northern Ireland. Acculturation among groups such as these is quite different from acculturation among voluntary immigrant people or refugees because their status as "minorities" or "ethnic groups" within the receiving culture is involuntary. As such, acculturation among members of nonimmigrant ethnic groups involves issues that are beyond the scope of the present analysis (Markus, Steele, & Steele, 2000).

Notice that we provided a rationale for not including nonimmigrant minority groups—namely that we were focusing on processes related to immigration. Reviewers did not take issue with our decision to exclude nonimmigrant minority groups from our analysis—but had we not included this paragraph, a reviewer might well have questioned why we did not include these groups.

Generally, the best way to address omitted variables (variables that probably should have been included, but on which data were not collected) in empirical manuscripts is to acknowledge the omission as a limitation in the discussion section. Of course, acknowledging omitted variables is a double-edged sword; authors must decide whether it is more likely that (a) not mentioning the limitation will invite criticisms from reviewers or (b) mentioning the limitation will draw attention to an issue that reviewers otherwise would have ignored.

Because it is impossible to know who will review a given manuscript when it is submitted for publication, authors must venture their best guess. My advice is to ask yourself what you would say if you were reviewing your manuscript for a journal. Would you criticize the authors for not measuring a given variable and for not mentioning the omission as a limitation? Or would you be more likely not to notice the omission if it was not mentioned?

Here is an example of a limitation statement pertaining to an omitted variable (Schwartz et al., 2018, p. 32):

> Third, we did not ask where in Venezuela participants had migrated from. Although some research has examined the effects of immigrating to large cities versus rural areas, far less work has considered the urbanicity of the areas in which immigrants resided prior to migrating.

In this example, the omitted variable was where in Venezuela participants had resided prior to migrating to the United States or to Colombia. Assumedly, individuals from urban areas in Venezuela would have experienced their new countries of residence quite differently compared to individuals from rural areas. The fact that we did not ask participants where in Venezuela they were from is a clear limitation of our study.

Other issues involving confusion about what your paper is saying or arguing for can be addressed through careful editing, as is noted in Chapter 10. It is essential that your coauthors have the opportunity to read through the paper and offer comments. If coauthors give the paper "the summer vacation treatment" (an expression I borrowed from Jeff Arnett), then I would ask them to please provide a more careful read. If you are an early-career scholar, I advise asking your mentor to read through the paper. If your eyes are the only eyes that have seen your paper, then it is not ready to be submitted for publication. Editing one's own work is extremely difficult—often we overlook our own writing mistakes or see what we intended to say rather than what the paper actually says—so it is critical to have as many coauthors or colleagues as possible read your paper and provide feedback. You can think like a reviewer about your own work only to a certain extent, and beyond that, you need your coauthors, mentors, or colleagues to help you.

Conclusion

This chapter introduces the idea of thinking like a reviewer about one's own work. If you were a reviewer for your paper, what would you say in your review? (Reviewers almost never say "This paper is perfect—publish it now," so be mindful that, regardless of how carefully you edit and polish your manuscript, reviewers will have something to say about it.) Would you comment on the research design, the organization of the manuscript, the analytic plan, or the structure of the discussion? Would you point out variables that you probably should have included in your data collection and/or analysis? If your manuscript is a literature review, theoretical treatise, or position paper, would you as a reviewer criticize the scope of the analysis? Would you recommend that the authors specify the boundaries of their analysis more clearly? Would you ask the authors to emphasize the importance of the topic and the nature of the contribution their paper is making to the literature? Might you say that the key points need to be specified more clearly? Whatever you think you might say about your paper should be addressed before you submit it for publication.

It is also essential to assess your paper honestly and to match it with a journal tier (and with specific journals within that tier). There are multiple approaches to selecting journals, but in my experience, reviewer comments are idiosyncratic enough that "sending a paper to a top journal just to get good reviews" may not be an especially efficient strategy. If you know that your paper's contribution is not strong enough to warrant publication in a high-prestige journal, then I advise selecting a moderate-prestige journal as your starting point. As is noted in Chapter 10, there is no shame in publishing in moderate-prestige journals. Most manuscripts will eventually find a suitable journal home even if they are rejected initially—and being realistic about the contribution your manuscript offers, as well as matching the manuscript with a set of target journals, is an advisable way to decrease the amount of time (and rounds of review) necessary to publish your paper.

Keep in mind that I am not saying not to take chances. I'm saying to take smart chances. Sports teams often design higher risk plays or sets to target opposing teams' specific weaknesses. Similarly, if you know that a high-prestige journal has recently published articles similar to yours, then your paper might be a potential fit for that journal even if the contribution is not as substantial as you might want it to be. Several years ago, my colleagues and I submitted a manuscript to a top personality journal because the paper was an excellent match with the associate editor who would likely be handling it. The associate editor and reviewers resonated well with the paper, and the paper was eventually published in that journal—even though the contribution was likely smaller than what that journal typically publishes. This was a targeted, high-risk, high-reward submission where we saw an opportunity and seized it.

The chapter also enumerates common criticisms that reviewers offer about various sections of a manuscript, and about manuscripts in general. Many of these criticisms can be prevented through carefully placed statements, through careful editing and organization, and by reading your paper through the eyes of a reviewer. Engaging coauthors and mentors (as well as other colleagues) is also essential—the more sets of edits and comments you receive, the better. A principle I have adopted is that I would rather receive criticism from a coauthor than from a reviewer.

A final point is that one of the best ways to learn how to think like a reviewer is to be a reviewer. Journal editors and associate editors are always looking for reliable reviewers, so I expect that volunteering to review will lead to manuscripts' being assigned to you for review. I learned to be a better writer—and to anticipate reviewer comments—by serving as a reviewer myself.

Now that we have discussed how to think like a reviewer, the next two chapters cover the journal review process. Chapter 12 advises on how to interact with reviewers and editors, and Chapter 13 discusses what to do with rejected manuscripts.

Summary

- When reviewers evaluate manuscripts, perhaps the most important assessment they are asked to provide is the paper's overall contribution to the literature.
- Secondarily, reviewers also note major concerns and limitations, as well as smaller writing concerns.
- It is essential to identify the take-home points from your work and to emphasize them in your manuscript. Authors need to assess honestly what their work contributes to the literature and to highlight that contribution in the discussion section.
- The take-home points from a paper should be matched with the journal to which it will be submitted.
- Design flaws in the study being reported should be identified and considered when writing the manuscript and choosing a journal.
- Key literature (including major contributors to the field of study) should be cited, and covariates relevant to the population under study should be included in analysis.
- Statements can be included in various sections of a paper to head off potential reviewer criticisms.
- Mentioning design flaws as limitations may lead reviewers to be more forgiving than they might have been had you not mentioned the flaws, but sometimes authors may choose to ignore small issues rather than drawing attention to them.

References

Acosta-Belén, E., & Santiago, C. E. (2018). *Puerto Ricans in the United States: A contemporary portrait* (2nd ed.). Boulder, CO: Lynne Rienner.

Alberts, B., Hanson, B., & Kelner, K. (2008). Reviewing peer review. *Science, 321*, 15.

Casey, B. J., Trainor, R. J., Orendi, J. L., Schubert, A. B., Nystrom, L. E., Giedd, J. N., . . . Rapoport, J. L. (1997). A developmental functional MRI study of prefrontal activation during performance of a go-no-go task. *Journal of Cognitive Neuroscience, 9*, 835–847.

Costa, P. T., Jr., & McCrae, R. R. (1995). Primary traits of Eysenck's P-E-N system: Three- and five-factor solutions. *Journal of Personality and Social Psychology, 69*, 308–317.

Dawson, R., & Lavori, P. W. (2015). Design and inference for the intent-to-treat principle using adaptive treatment. *Statistics in Medicine, 34*, 1441–1453.

Furnham, A., Richards, S. C., & Paulhus, D. L. (2013). The Dark Triad of personality: A 10-year review. *Personality and Social Psychology Compass, 7*, 199–216.

Guo, S., & Fraser, M. W. (2014). *Propensity score analysis: statistical methods and applications* (2nd ed.). Newbury Park, CA: SAGE.

Putnick, D. L., & Bornstein, M. H. (2016). Measurement invariance conventions and reporting: The state of the art and future directions for psychological research. *Developmental Review, 41*, 71–90.

Schultz, D. M. (2010). Are three heads better than two? How the number of reviewers and editor behavior affect the rejection rate. *Scientometrics, 84*, 277–292.

Schwartz, S. J., Martinez, C. R., Jr., Meca, A., Szabó, A., Ward, C., Cobb, C. L., Cano, M. A., Unger, J. B., & Salas-Wright, C. P. (2021). Toward a micro-level perspective on acculturation among US Hispanic college students: A daily diary study. *Journal of Clinical Psychology, 77*, 121–144.

Schwartz, S. J., Montgomery, M. J., & Briones, E. (2006). The role of identity in acculturation among immigrant people: Theoretical propositions, empirical questions, and applied recommendations. *Human Development, 49*, 1–30.

Schwartz, S. J., Salas-Wright, C. P., Pérez-Gómez, A., Mejía-Trujillo, J., Brown, E. C., Montero-Zamora, P., . . . Dickson-Gomez, J. (2018). Cultural stress and psychological symptoms in recent Venezuelan immigrants to the United States and Colombia. *International Journal of Intercultural Relations, 67*, 25–34.

Schwartz, S. J., & Zamboanga, B. L. (2009). The peer-review and editorial system: Ways to fix something that might be broken. *Perspectives on Psychological Science, 4*, 54–61.

Schwartz, S. J., Zamboanga, B. L., Luyckx, K., Meca, A., & Ritchie, R. A. (2013). Identity in emerging adulthood: Reviewing the field and looking forward. *Emerging Adulthood, 1*, 96–113.

Van Lange, P. A. M. (1999). Why authors believe that reviewers stress limiting aspects of manuscripts: The SLAM effect in peer review. *Journal of Applied Social Psychology, 29*, 2550–2566.

Weems, C. F., Taylor, L. K., Cannon, M. F., Marino, R. C., Romano, D. M., Scott, B. G., . . . Triplett, V. (2010). Post-traumatic stress, context, and the lingering effects of the Hurricane Katrina disaster among ethnic minority youth. *Journal of Abnormal Child Psychology, 38*, 49–56.

Xue, X., Xie, X., Gunter, M., Rohan, T. E., Wassertheil-Smoller, S., Ho, G. Y. F., . . . Strickler, H. D. (2013). Testing the proportional hazards assumption in case-cohort analysis. *BMC Medical Research Methodology, 13*, Article 88.

12

The Journal Review Process

Decision Letters, Reviewer Comments, and Author Responses

Chapter Objectives

When you finish reading this chapter, you should feel more comfortable with:

- The steps in the journal review process
- Submitting manuscripts through submission sites
- How editors conduct initial screening and decide whether to send papers out for review
- How action editors and reviewers are assigned to manuscripts
- What initial editorial decisions often look like
- Revising a manuscript in accordance with reviewer feedback
- Constructing a response letter for a revised manuscript
- Responding to a reviewer request without complying with the request
- Handling reviewer comments that conflict with other reviewer comments
- Integrating text added or modified in response to reviewers with text from the original version of the paper
- What happens during the second round of review (after you revise and resubmit)
- Provisional acceptance decisions on manuscripts
- Reviewing page proofs and answering publisher queries for accepted manuscripts

So now we have submitted our manuscript to a journal for publication. What happens then? How long do we have to wait for the journal editor to decide whether to reject our paper or invite us to revise and resubmit for further consideration? When we receive feedback from the journal, what will that feedback look like—and what do we do with it?

To many beginning authors, the journal review process is shrouded in mystery. The review process seems like a "black box" between the time we press "Submit" on the journal's manuscript submission site and when we receive

The Savvy Academic. Seth J. Schwartz, Oxford University Press. © Oxford University Press 2022.
DOI: 10.1093/oso/9780190095918.003.0013

an email from the journal with editorial feedback. Therefore, this chapter unpacks the process and lays it out, step by step. Figure 12.1 provides a "cheat sheet" that you can use throughout the chapter—the figure lays out the entire process so that you can understand where your manuscript is in the process.

This chapter follows the journal review process in great detail, using Figure 12.1 as a roadmap. The process starts with submitting your manuscripts to a journal, which has become somewhat complex with the advent of manuscript submission sites. We then discuss the steps in the editorial process: (a) how editors screen manuscripts and assign them to associate editors, (b) how peer reviewers are selected, (c) how editors reach decisions to reject manuscripts or to invite authors to revise and resubmit, (d) tips for revising manuscripts, and (e) how editors handle revised manuscripts and reach final decisions.

Let me start with a word of advice: if you have questions about the suitability of your manuscript for a specific journal, I suggest emailing the editor. Some journal websites provide links for authors to send inquiries to the journal editor. There is no harm in emailing an editor, describing your paper, and asking the editor for feedback on how well your submission fits with the journal. I've had editors respond enthusiastically and encourage me to submit, and I have had editors tell me that their journal is not the right outlet for the paper I described. Some editors give vague answers that are not especially helpful (in which case the author must make a judgment call about whether to submit the manuscript to that journal). The bottom line is that editors are accustomed to receiving and responding to inquiries from authors.

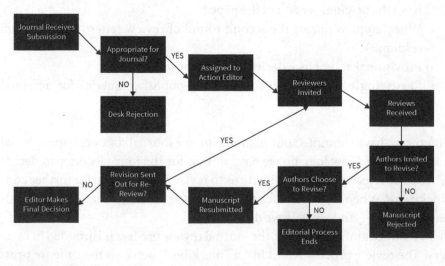

Figure 12.1 The journal review process.

Manuscript Submission Sites

The journal review process begins when you submit your manuscript to the journal. Almost all journals use submission sites, such as Editorial Manager, EVISE, and ScholarOne. Authors must initiate the manuscript submission on whichever site the journal uses. In most cases, you will be asked to choose the format you want to submit (I explain more about the formats in a moment). You will also be asked to enter the title, to copy and paste the abstract from the manuscript, to select a set of keywords, to enter the names of your coauthors, and to upload the manuscript files. You will also be asked to approve the PDF version of the manuscript—with all the files merged—before you can submit. This PDF is what reviewers will see, so be sure that it's accurate. I have spotted many mistakes in PDFs, in which case I have had to go back, modify the word processing documents, and re-upload them to the journal submission site. Always remember that it's better to catch and correct errors than to have reviewers read a version of your manuscript that includes mistakes.

Formats

The most common article formats that journals publish are full-length articles and brief reports. In general, full-length articles report new findings or introduce new theoretical perspectives. If your manuscript represents an advance that is commensurate with the prestige level of the journal, then I advise submitting it as a full-length article. On the other hand, if your manuscript reports a replication study or an interesting set of findings that probably don't warrant a full-length article, then I suggest submitting it as a brief report. Keep in mind that word limits will differ between these two formats, with brief reports being considerably shorter than full-length articles. Certain academic departments may also assign less credit toward tenure and promotion for publishing brief reports versus full-length articles—but brief reports in high-prestige journals may still be highly valued.

In general, theoretical and literature-review manuscripts should be submitted as full-length articles unless the journal allows authors to select literature review or theory as a format. Meta-analyses are also generally submitted as full-length articles, and some journals provide a more generous word count for meta-analyses. Some journals also allow extra words for manuscripts that report multiple studies. Figure 12.2 provides a sample journal submission site where authors are asked to choose the type of manuscript they are submitting.

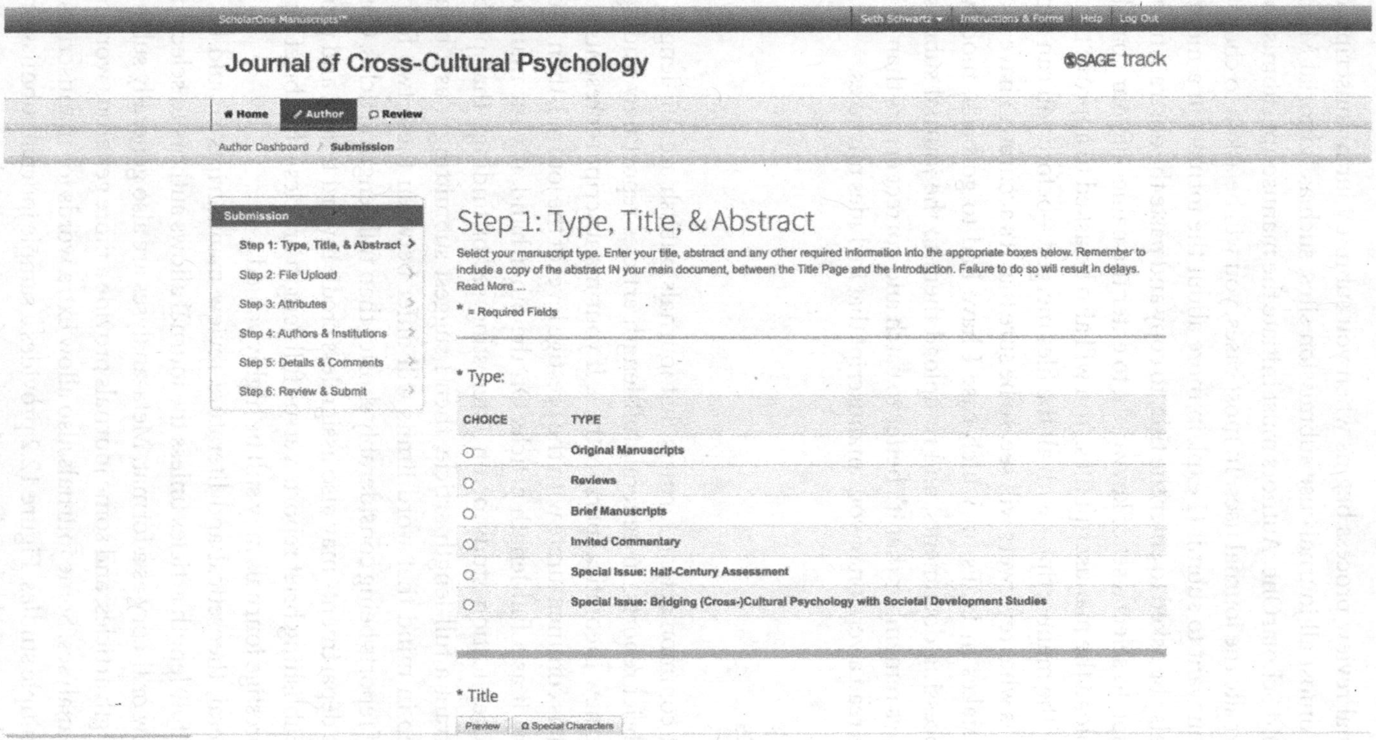

Figure 12.2 Journal submission site format-selection page.

I cannot overemphasize the importance of reading the journal's instructions to authors. In addition to length limitations, the instructions will tell you whether you need to do one or more of the following (note that this list is not exhaustive):

- Blind all self-citations (i.e., replace self-citations with "Author Citation" and remove the corresponding references from the reference section);
- Include a Highlights page with a bulleted list of the major contributions that the manuscript adds to the literature;
- Include a public significance statement indicating how the findings advance the public interest;
- Provide the word count on the title page; and/or
- Include specific statements regarding your study's, theory's, or review's implications for practice or policy.

If you do not follow the journal's instructions to authors, the journal's editorial assistant will return your manuscript to you so that you can make the necessary corrections. Given that editorial assistants can sometimes take several days to perform their checks on new submissions, not following the journal's instructions to authors can cost you up to a week. I have seen cases where a manuscript was returned to the authors three or four times before it was finally forwarded to the editor for processing.

Cover Letter

Almost all journals require authors to upload a cover letter as part of the submission process. Cover letters for initial submissions are generally brief, providing a short description of the manuscript's major contributions and thanking the editorial team in advance for considering the submission. Here is a sample cover letter that I wrote for a first submission:

You may also want to use the cover letter to ask the editor not to select specific people as reviewers. If someone in your field has disagreements with you that would prevent that person from reviewing your work objectively, you should let the editor know about this potential conflict. I had to do that with someone in my field earlier in my career after this person created major disruptions in two or three of my articles. I would write the following sentence into my cover letters: "I would like to request that you not invite Dr. A to review my manuscript. He and I have serious philosophical disagreements, and I do not believe that he is capable of reviewing my work

Box 12.1 Sample Cover Letter

December 10, 2013

Jeffrey J. Lockman, Ph.D.
Editor, *Child Development*
Department of Psychology
Tulane University
2007 Percival Stern Hall
New Orleans, LA 70118

Dear Dr. Lockman:

My colleagues and I are pleased to submit our manuscript, "Developmental Trajectories of Acculturation: Links with Family Functioning and Mental Health in Recent-Immigrant Hispanic Adolescents," for publication in *Child Development*. Our paper reports a five-wave longitudinal study of acculturation, using a multidimensional model, in a sample of recently immigrated Hispanic adolescents from Miami and Los Angeles. We find that adolescents whose cultural practices and values change following immigration report the most favorable mental health and family relationships, whereas those whose practices, values, and identifications do not change following immigration report the poorest mental health and family relationships. These findings appear to have important implications for promoting biculturalism among immigrants.

We thank you and your editorial team in advance for considering our submission.

Sincerely yours,

Seth J. Schwartz, Ph.D.
Associate Professor

objectively." Importantly, no editor ever denied this request after I asked, but it is important to make this kind of request only when it is necessary. The fact that someone is a "tough" reviewer doesn't mean that you should ask for that person not to review your work.

As an editor, I generally read authors' cover letters, and occasionally the study description causes me to take special notice. However, in most cases I simply glance at the letter and then proceed to the manuscript itself. I advise making sure the cover letter provides a general summary of the paper, but don't spend more than a few minutes composing the cover letter. It is essential, however, to ensure that you list the editor's name and degree correctly and to use the correct salutation. In my experience, *Dr.* is the correct salutation for most professors (regardless of rank) in the United States and Canada, but in most other parts of the world, full professors should be addressed as *Professor* rather than as *Dr.* In some European countries, full professors are addressed as *Prof. Dr.* Do not use *Ms.* or *Mr.* unless you are positive that the editor does not have a doctoral degree. I advise taking the time to find out how to address the editor properly so that you don't inadvertently insult this person during the process of submitting your paper. (If you don't know how to address the editor, use *Dr.* [for editors in the United States or Canada] or *Professor* just to be safe.)

Some submission sites require authors to copy and paste the cover letter into a text field and to upload the cover letter as a separate file. Be sure that you provide all the necessary files and material so that the editorial assistant does not send the manuscript back to you for corrections.

Keywords

Your choice of keywords is extremely important, as many editors will use the keywords to select reviewers. In general, most journals ask for four to six keywords. Keywords should refer to the population you are studying (e.g., African Americans, adolescents, nurses, college students), the methods you used (e.g., randomized experiment, longitudinal study, implicit cognition), and the key constructs you focused on (e.g., self-esteem, social rejection, therapeutic alliance). If the statistical methods that you utilized are a major part of the story that the paper tells, then these methods should be included as keywords (e.g., if you are focusing on predictors of initiation of a given event or behavior, then you might list survival analysis as a keyword). I usually provide the maximum number of keywords that the journal allows so that reviewers can be most closely matched to the manuscript I'm submitting. It is important to ensure that reviewers have the necessary expertise to evaluate your paper—including the content area, the population, the methods, and the statistical analyses. Figure 12.3 shows a keyword selection page.

Some journals allow authors to type in their own keywords, whereas other journals ask authors to select keywords from a list. If a keyword you are looking for doesn't appear on the journal's list, then you should look for the closest approximation. For example, if you studied self-concept, but *self-concept* is not one of the keywords listed for you to choose from, you may have to select *identity* or *self-esteem*. Again, consult the journal's instructions to authors to see how you are expected to select keywords.

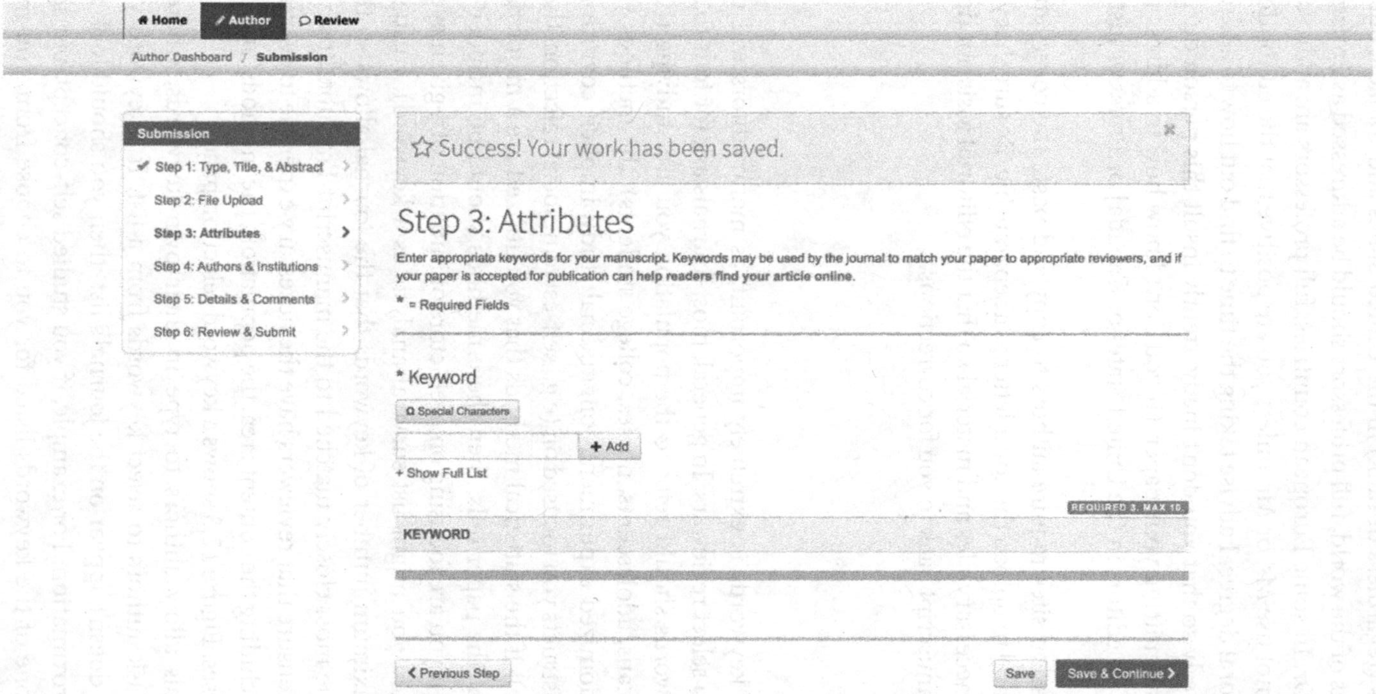

Home / Author / Review

Author Dashboard / Submission

Submission

Step 1: Type, Title, & Abstract
Step 2: File Upload
Step 3: Attributes
Step 4: Authors & Institutions
Step 5: Details & Comments
Step 6: Review & Submit

☆ Success! Your work has been saved.

Step 3: Attributes

Enter appropriate keywords for your manuscript. Keywords may be used by the journal to match your paper to appropriate reviewers, and if your paper is accepted for publication can help readers find your article online.

* = Required Fields

* Keyword

Q Special Characters   + Add

+ Show Full List

KEYWORD

REQUIRED 3, MAX 10

< Previous Step

Save   Save & Continue >

Figure 12.3 Journal submission site keyword-entry page.

Uploading Files

Figure 12.4 shows a sample file upload page. When you upload the manuscript files, pay attention to the instructions to authors. Note that the title page must be removed from the manuscript and saved as a separate word processing file. For some journals, tables and figures must be removed from the manuscript and uploaded as separate files. In general, I upload the manuscript (without the title page) as a single file unless the instructions to authors indicate that tables and figures need to be uploaded separately. Once the files have been uploaded, make sure they are listed in the order in which you want them to appear—title page first, manuscript body second, tables third, and figures last.

Online Supplemental Material

Some journals allow authors to upload additional tables and figures as "online supplemental material." When the article is published, a link will be provided so that readers can view the additional tables and figures. The online supplemental material feature essentially allows authors to exceed the journal's page limit or to include more tables and figures than the journal normally permits. However, note that the online supplemental material does not appear with the rest of the article—readers have to click on a link to view the additional tables and figures. I personally do not include online supplemental material unless a reviewer or editor asks me to—and I almost never provide online supplemental material with an initial manuscript submission.

Online supplemental material often must be uploaded in a different place from where other manuscript files are uploaded. The cover letter is also uploaded on a separate page. Make sure to upload the various files in the correct place.

Initial Editorial Review and Desk Rejection

Once the manuscript has been submitted and the editorial assistant has passed it along to the editor, the editor will conduct an initial screening to ensure that the paper is appropriate for the journal. If the editor concludes that a manuscript does not fit within the journal's scope or that the paper is too weak to have a reasonable chance of surviving the peer-review process, the editor will likely "desk-reject" the manuscript. Desk rejection occurs when the editor-in-chief rejects a manuscript without assigning it to an associate

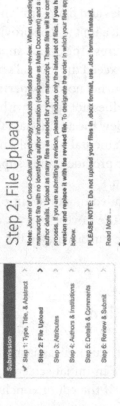

Step 2: File Upload

Note: *Journal of Cross-Cultural Psychology* conducts blinded peer-review. When uploading your manuscript you will need to upload a manuscript file with no identifying author information (designate as Main Document) and a separate title page (designate as Title Page) with author details. Upload as many files as needed for your manuscript. These files will be combined into a single document for the peer review process. If you are submitting a revision, please include only the latest set of files. If you have updated a file, please delete the original version and replace it with the revised file. To designate the order in which your files appear, use the dropdowns in the "order" column below.

PLEASE NOTE: Do not upload your files in .docx format, use .doc format instead.

Read More ...

* = Required Fields

Files

ORDER   ACTIONS   FILE   * FILE DESIGNATION   UPLOAD DATE   UPLOADED BY

0.00 OUT OF 97.66 MB

No files uploaded

| ↻ Update Order | Remove All Files |

File Upload

SELECTION	FILE DESIGNATION
⬈ Select File 1 ...	Choose File Designation ... ⌄
⬈ Select File 2 ...	Choose File Designation ... ⌄
⬈ Select File 3 ...	Choose File Designation ... ⌄

Submission

✔ Step 1: Type, Title, & Abstract	˅
Step 2: File Upload	˄
Step 3: Attributes	˅
Step 4: Authors & Institutions	˅
Step 5: Details & Comments	˅
Step 6: Review & Submit	˅

Figure 12.4 Journal submission site file-upload page.

editor or sending it out for peer review (Craig, 2010). Desk rejection is a form of triaging where associate editors' and reviewers' time and effort are saved for the strongest and most meritorious submissions. Desk rejection often occurs quickly—I have had papers desk-rejected in under 3 hours—and allows authors to submit their work elsewhere with minimal delay.

Generally, the editor-in-chief is responsible for desk-rejecting manuscripts. I perform this function for the journal that I edit (the *International Journal of Intercultural Relations*). Most of the articles that I desk-reject are outside the journal's scope—for example, manuscripts focusing on single cultural groups, papers outside of psychology and closely related fields, and articles that do not adopt a clear intercultural focus. I have desk-rejected papers that include immigrant samples (and therefore have the potential to be intercultural) but where the theoretical focus of the manuscript is grounded in social psychology, in international business, or in anthropology. Just as using a longitudinal design does not make a paper developmental, using an immigrant or expatriate sample does not make a paper intercultural.

I also desk-reject manuscripts that are poorly written or organized, where the methodology is weak or unclear, or where the contribution to the literature appears to be negligible. I recently desk-rejected a manuscript that reported a set of quantitative analyses with a sample of 25 participants. The authors also focused heavily on immigrants in their literature review, but nearly 75% of participants were born in the United States. Although I was initially excited by the title of the manuscript, the study itself was underwhelming, and I did not believe that it had any realistic chance of surviving peer review. I also desk-rejected a paper whose introduction section was only one page, where the method section was four paragraphs, and where the discussion section was only seven lines long. This was simply not a journal-quality manuscript.

When editors desk-reject a paper, they will usually provide a rationale for doing so. I have had papers desk-rejected because the journal to which I had submitted did not publish studies using convenience samples. Another journal desk-rejected my paper because we had used a cross-sectional design. In some cases, editors will vaguely say that they receive a large volume of submissions and are only able to forward a small number of manuscripts for peer review. Sometimes desk rejections can appear capricious, and it may be worthwhile to write a respectful email to the editor asking for the desk rejection to be reconsidered. (I discuss appealing rejection decisions later in this chapter.)

The likelihood of desk rejection depends on the journal's prestige level and manuscript flow. An editorial team can be reasonably expected to handle only a certain number of submissions per year. Simply put, the more manuscripts a journal receives per year, the greater the likelihood that a given submission will be desk-rejected. My experience with one developmental journal, where the editor-in-chief handles all submissions himself as action editor, is that he desk-rejects a lot of submissions. However, submissions that he sends out for review have a good chance of eventually being accepted for publication. In contrast, other journals utilize a much more lenient policy regarding desk rejections, and therefore having a submission sent out for review is not a good indicator of the likelihood of eventual acceptance.

Action Editor and Reviewer Assignment

Once the initial editorial screening has been completed, the next step of the journal review process involves assigning an action editor to manage the review process. Some journals use a system where every manuscript that is not desk-rejected is assigned to an associate editor, and where the editor-in-chief does not generally handle manuscripts. In other cases, such as the journal I edit, the editor-in-chief handles some submissions and assigns other submissions to associate editors. In either of these cases, the editor-in-chief determines who will handle the review process for a given manuscript.

The ways in which editors-in-chief make these determinations also vary across journals. Some journals use a random system where submissions are randomly assigned to associate editors, whereas other journals assign papers to action editors based on the match between the paper's focus and the editorial team's expertise. When Al Waterman was the North American associate editor for the *Journal of Adolescence*, he handled all submissions from authors based in the United States or Canada, and the editor-in-chief (who was based in London) handled submissions from authors based in other parts of the world. Once a manuscript was assigned to Al, he had the option of desk-rejecting it, assigning it to an assistant editor (he had a set of assistant editors working under him), or handling it himself. Al generally chose to handle papers falling within his own areas of expertise, and he assigned the others to assistant editors.

In many cases, when a new editor takes over a journal, that editor will change the journal's scope, editorial procedures, and editorial team. When I took over the *International Journal of Intercultural Relations* in 2020, I sought to broaden the types of papers that the journal considered, as well as to move the journal's scope away from international business. A new editor may impose or relax space limitations, may designate new types of articles that the journal will publish, and may change the journal's extent of emphasis on practice and policy. Most journals announce editorial transitions on their websites a few months prior to the transition—so authors submitting articles will know that the transition is taking place.

Journals also differ in terms of who handles in-process manuscripts following an editorial transition. In some cases, the outgoing editorial team will continue to handle papers that were submitted prior to the transition, so that, even after the new editorial team takes over, papers assigned to an outgoing associate editor will continue to be handled by that editor until they are accepted or rejected. In other cases, the new editorial team will assume control of all manuscripts, regardless of where they are in the editorial process. Al Waterman and I received a revise–resubmit decision from an outgoing associate editor in 2002, and when we resubmitted, the incoming editor-in-chief handled the manuscript himself and accepted our revised version. Similarly, when I took over the *International Journal of Intercultural Relations* in January 2020, I had to make editorial decisions on papers that the previous editor had sent out for review. I also evaluated revised versions of manuscripts that she had handled on the first round of review. In the interest of fairness, I generally held these authors to the same standards that the previous editor had established. I didn't think it would be fair to force these authors to "shoot at a moving target" by changing the rules in the middle of the editorial process. Manuscripts submitted to the journal under my editorship have been handled using my editorial standards. I've retained the same editorial team that the previous editor established, which has helped to maintain continuity for the journal. Not all editors do this, however—some incoming editors choose to bring in their own editorial team.

Once an action editor has been assigned to manage the review process for a manuscript, the next step is for that action editor to select reviewers. Action editors will sometimes read papers carefully as soon as they receive them, and action editors are often permitted to desk-reject papers if they so choose. However, in most cases, action editors simply select reviewers based on the abstract and keywords, and they read the manuscript more carefully after the reviews have come in. As Byron Zamboanga and I (Schwartz & Zamboanga, 2009) argued in our position article on the peer-review process, action editors who do not read papers carefully before sending them out for review may wind up wasting authors' time if they decide that they don't like the paper after the reviews come back—even when the reviews are positive. This scenario happened to Byron and me multiple times—leading us to include this issue in our position article.

Action editors generally select reviewers in one of two general ways—(1) inviting reviewers whom the authors suggested when they submitted and

(2) choosing reviewers on their own (see Wager, Parkin, & Tamber, 2006, for a review of these two reviewer selection methods). Some journals require authors to suggest reviewers as part of the submission process—Wager et al. found that these author-suggested reviewers are more likely to recommend positive editorial decisions than are reviewers whom the action editor chooses independently of author recommendations. Authors may recommend their colleagues or may suggest reviewers who are sympathetic to the authors' theoretical or methodological approach.

When action editors select reviewers on their own, they generally do so in one of four ways. Sometimes they invite their colleagues to serve as reviewers—as is noted in Chapter 11, I keep a list of people on whom I know I can rely when I need a review. Editors can also use manuscript management systems to search for reviewers using the keywords that the authors entered when they submitted. I am regularly invited to review for journals I have never heard of, and I suspect that the editors found my name through a keyword search. A third way to identify reviewers is to search the authors' reference list and look for names that are cited repeatedly. (Al Waterman used this method often when he needed to find reviewers for a manuscript.) The fourth way to identify reviewers is to follow the suggestions that prospective reviewers offer when they decline the review invitation.

My editorial team's experience with finding reviewers suggests that, in some cases, more than 10 reviewers must be invited in order to secure two completed reviews. Sometimes the search for reviewers feels like a "wild goose chase"—person A declines the review invitation and suggests person B, who in turn declines and suggests person C, and so on. By the time we arrive at person I or person J, we no longer have the keyword or expertise match that we were seeking. The person who finally accepts the review invitation may have only tangential expertise in the topics on which the manuscript focuses. Indeed, in their survey of researchers at a U.S. government funding agency, Resnik, Gutierrez-Ford, and Peddada (2008) found that reviewer incompetence was the primary complaint that participants reported. In my publishing career, I have occasionally received reviews that contained factually incorrect statements, although in most cases, reviewers commenting on my papers have provided excellent reviews. My contention is that action editors need to be prescriptive in communicating to authors which reviewer comments are most important to address, and that the action editor, not the reviewers, should be the person making the decision on the paper.

My experiences as an editor, along with my communications with editors who have handled my manuscripts, suggest that most of the delays that occur in peer review are due to difficulties finding reviewers and to reviewers' not returning their reviews within the agreed-upon amount of time. I've had weeks where I received as many as 10 reviewer invitations from journals—such that, if I accepted all these invitations, I would spend all my working time reviewing manuscripts. Many of my colleagues have reported similar experiences—which suggests to me that scholars are overloaded with review requests. Quite simply, there are not enough potential reviewers to handle all the manuscripts being submitted to scholarly journals. The number of submissions to many journals is increasing—Table 12.1 reports numbers of submissions to 11 of the most prominent APA journals in 2019 versus 2010 (American Psychological Association, 2011, 2020). On average, across these selected journals, submissions increased by 25% over the 9-year period. Of the 11 journals, the numbers of submissions increased for nine and decreased for the other two. For the nine journals for which the number of submissions increased, the magnitude of the increase ranged from 5% to 60%. The take-home message from these numbers appears to be that the demand for reviewers is increasing—but it is not clear that the reviewer workforce is necessarily increasing in kind. Editors are having to invite more potential reviewers to obtain the required number of completed reviews (generally two or three), and as a result, authors are having to wait longer to receive editorial feedback. When reviewers are not expert in the content area represented by the paper, authors may also receive reviewer comments that are inaccurate or misinformed.

Table 12.1 Differences in Numbers of Submissions for Selected American Psychological Association Journals, 2019 versus 2010

Journal	Submissions in 2019	Submissions in 2010	Percent Increase
Psychological Assessment	663	414	60%
American Psychologist	234	152	54%
Psychological Bulletin	326	230	42%
Psychological Methods	291	205	42%
Psychology of Addictive Behaviors	411	312	32%
Journal of Family Psychology	522	399	31%
Journal of Applied Psychology	1,045	930	12%
Developmental Psychology	711	651	9%
Journal of Personality and Social Psychology	897	857	5%
Journal of Consulting and Clinical Psychology	425	442	−4%
Journal of Abnormal Psychology	468	497	−6%

Initial Editorial Decisions

Once the reviewers have completed and submitted their reviews, the next step is for the action editor to read the reviews and to render a decision on the manuscript. One would hope that the action editor will also read the paper before rendering a decision, but it is not always clear that this is the case. Especially for journals with large numbers of submissions, it seems infeasible that action editors would be able to read every manuscript assigned to them. Indeed, once the reviews have been completed for a manuscript, my usual practice is to scan the paper (especially the methods and results) and then read the reviews carefully. In cases where the reviewers' impressions differ from my own, I will go back and carefully read the sections on which the reviewers' opinions diverge from mine. I will then render a decision that takes into account both my impressions and those of the reviewers.

Editorial Styles

In my experience with scholarly publishing, I have identified four primary editorial styles—the passive editor, the interpreter, the extra reviewer, and the meddler. It is important to figure out which style the action editor for a given manuscript is using—the revision process will take a somewhat different form for each of these different editorial styles. The editorial styles differ in terms of how much influence the reviewers and the action editor exert on whether the manuscript is ultimately accepted or rejected for publication.

The Passive Editor

The passive editor is by far the most common style I have encountered in my publishing experience. In some cases, the editor appears to take a vote count among the reviewers, and papers are only invited for revision and resubmission when all reviewers recommend this course of action. In other cases, the editor acts on the content of the reviews, rather than on the reviewers' official recommendations, but the decision is still essentially made by the reviewers rather than by the action editor.

The hallmark of the passive editor is found in the editorial letter, where the editor simply tells the authors what the decision is and then proceeds directly to the reviews (see Figure 12.5). Passive editors generally don't provide any feedback of their own in their editorial letters. In many cases, the decision letter itself is a form letter, and the editor doesn't modify the boilerplate language. Perhaps of greatest concern, it is not clear that the editor has even

Please revise and resubmit

Schwartz, Seth J
Wednesday, November 19, 2014 at 7:19 PM
Show Details

Ref.: Ms. No.
Trajectories of Cultural Stressors and Effects on Mental Health and Substance Use Among Recently Arrived Hispanic Immigrant Adolescents

Dear Dr. Schwartz:

Thank you for submitting your manuscript, "Trajectories of Cultural Stressors and Effects on Mental Health and Substance Use Among Recently Arrived Hispanic Immigrant Adolescents," to the Journal of ▮. I would like to ask you to revise your manuscript and resubmit it for our review.

For your guidance, reviewers' comments are appended below.

If you decide to revise the work, please address each comment, query and critique contained in the reviews. Also, please submit a list of changes or a rebuttal against each point that is being raised when you submit the revised manuscript.

To submit a revision, go to ▮ and log in as an Author. You will see a menu item call Submission Needing Revision. You will find your submission record there.

Please note that we expect revised manuscripts to comply with our author guidelines. Finally, in order to keep our publication process moving forward, please submit your revised manuscript within one month (December 19, 2014).

Yours sincerely

Figure 12.5 Passive-editor decision letter.

looked at the paper—the editor could just as easily have read the reviews and rendered a decision without consulting the manuscript at all. Figure 12.5 presents a passive editor's decision letter.

Passive editors are by far the easiest editorial style to respond to when revising a manuscript. The authors can essentially ignore the editor and simply respond to the reviewer comments. Assumedly, acceptance for publication is conditioned on satisfying the reviewers, and the editor is almost certain to send the revised manuscript back to the reviewers for a second round of review. The editor will accept the manuscript for publication only once all the reviewers have indicated that they are satisfied and that the revisions have been responsive to their concerns.

The Interpreter

The interpreter is also a somewhat passive style, except that the editor singles out the reviewer comments that are most important for the authors to address. In some cases, the editor will explicitly tell the authors that the comments listed in the editorial letter represent only a selection of the reviewer comments and that the authors are expected to respond to all the reviewer concerns in their revision. However, the fact that the editor singled out these specific reviewer comments suggests that the authors might want to place special emphasis on responding to these specific comments (while addressing all the concerns expressed by the reviewers). Figure 12.6 displays a sample interpreter decision letter.

Like passive editors, editors using the interpreter style may be likely to insist that all reviewers endorse publication before they will accept a manuscript. They will also likely continue to send revisions back to reviewers until the reviewers are satisfied—so it is essential to be sure to respond fully and completely to every reviewer concern. I have seen editors send papers back out for review three or four times before finally accepting them for publication. In my opinion, such a strategy is a poor use of reviewer time and effort—reviewer input is most valuable on new submissions, and reviewers' value decreases with each successive round of review. As Ed Diener (2006, p. 3), founding editor of *Perspectives on Psychological Science*, noted in his opening editorial,

> Many journals now make it necessary to go through many rounds of revisions before they publish an article. Both the editor and reviewers make numerous and detailed suggestions for revisions, and over successive revisions new reviewers are often brought in and provide even more suggestions for revisions. Essentially, publication is often based on trial-by-revision and is a test of whether the author can persevere. Further, the editor and reviewers in a sense become coauthors of the article.

Dear Dr. Schwartz:

Thank you for submitting your manuscript to the Journal of ████. I have read over two evaluations. Based upon my own reading and the recommendations of the reviewers, I'm recommending to the editor that the manuscript undergo revisions.

Reviewer comments are attached. A revised manuscript will be sent to original and/or new reviewers. If you choose to revise the manuscript, please attend to and address the detailed feedback.

In your re-submission, please create and upload a separate, blind document noting how the comments were addressed. It would also be helpful to note the changes within the manuscript itself (e.g., highlighted text).

I'm interested in the concept of this study in that it examines acculturation from a micro-level. However, as noted by Reviewer 1, as currently written, it appears that the premise is that acculturation fluctuates daily. Is it components of acculturation that is fluctuating or is it the person who is choosing a specific values, beliefs, or behaviors that is fluctuating? My thought is that the ability to fluctuate is based on an established level of acculturation. For instance, an individual who is low acculturated and doesn't know or speak English couldn't chose to fluctuate between Hispanic and US practices as measured by the daily items listed in the study.

The reviewers ask similar questions that I had in mind when I read over the manuscript. I'm interested in seeing how these are addressed.

I wish you the best in your future research and hope you will continue to consider the Journal of ████ as an outlet for your work.

Sincerely,

Figure 12.6 Interpreter decision letter.

Nonetheless, as is explained in the section on revising manuscripts and responding to reviewer comments, we need to deal as effectively as possible with whatever editorial style we encounter with a given manuscript and journal.

The Extra Reviewer

Some editors like to add their own comments to those of the reviewers, and in some cases, it seems as though the editor is serving as an additional reviewer (hence the name I have assigned to this editorial style). The editor's decision is a function of both the reviewers' impressions and recommendations and the editor's own reactions to the manuscript. Overall, authors must respond to all the reviewer comments, and to the editor's own feedback as well. Figure 12.7 presents an extra reviewer's decision letter.

Editors using the extra-reviewer editorial style may be less likely than those using the passive or interpreter styles to consult reviewers repeatedly, although I have seen extra-reviewer editors send manuscripts back to reviewers several times before accepting a final version. As an author, you will need to satisfy the editor's own revision requests as well as those provided by the reviewers.

The Meddler

The least common editorial style is the meddler, where the editor essentially disregards the reviewer feedback and provides an independent review of the manuscript. Editors who overrule positive reviews and reject a submission are essentially meddlers. I've also seen editors explicitly tell authors to disregard specific reviewer comments, or else indicate that the editor's own concerns are more important to address than the reviewers' concerns are. See Figure 12.8 for a sample meddler editorial letter.

In many cases, an editor using a meddler style will not send the revised manuscript back to the reviewers for a second round of evaluation, because the editor has overruled the reviewers' recommendations. This is not always true, however, and a meddling editor may decide to reverse course on subsequent rounds of review if reviewers provide negative comments on the revised paper. In my experience, editors using the meddler style are most likely to be capricious and unpredictable in their decision-making—such as rejecting a revised manuscript even though the authors have addressed all the concerns expressed in the initial decision letter and reviews. When you are dealing with a meddler, be especially careful to attend to all the editor's requests and provide responses that are extremely deferential. (Preparing editorial response letters is discussed later in this chapter.)

Dear Dr. Schwartz,

Thank you for considering the *Journal of* ███████████████ as an outlet for your manuscript, *Biculturalism dynamics: A daily diary study of bicultural identity and psychosocial functioning.*

I received reviews from two individuals with expertise related to your study; their comments are appended below. After my own independent and thorough reading of your manuscript, I concur with both reviewers regarding the potential contribution of your work to the literature on biculturalism, both in regards to the theory on cultural identity and the methodological approach. However, I also agree with them that there are a number of issues that need to be addressed before the contribution of this study to the existing literature can be fully assessed. Thus, although I cannot accept your manuscript for publication, I encourage you to consider reviewers' detailed comments and submit a revised manuscript, if you believe you can address all comments successfully.

Rather than reiterating the reviewers' comments here, I would like to emphasize the most critical issues noted by reviewers; but ask that you consider all of their feedback carefully.

The first critical issue is the lack of grounding of the study and discussion of findings in relation to the realities of U.S. Latino college students and/or within a developmental framework. Given the interest of our readership, please consider framing your study within the development of identity in the early adulthood, as well as within the unique socio-cultural context of the study (i.e., the cultural groups you are including and the general socio-cultural context of their lives). Reviewer 2, in particular, provides helpful suggestions for you to consider.

The second critical issue is the lack of clarity of the construct under investigation. So, while the study intends to examine bicultural identity, key measures assessing cultural identification (i.e., BIIS-2 and MISS) contrasts nationality (i.e., feeling American) with ethnicity (i.e., feeling Hispanic). This is problematic as individuals, when contrasted with being/feeling American, might identify more strongly with their country of origin (e.g., Cuban or Colombian) rather than with the label Hispanic depending on both individual and national group immigration histories). Therefore, please provide further clarification on the concepts of nationality, ethnicity, and cultural group as these are used in the study.

The third critical issue, noted by both reviewers, is the lack of clarity and alignment between research questions, hypotheses, and findings, thereby obscuring the main contributions of the study. I describe below recommendations for each section that address this main problem:

In the introduction/literature review, you need to provide a clearer and more concise,yet more thorough review, of past work in this area. In addition, please highlight theoretical tensions to help situate the study and thus appreciate its unique contribution. I also urge to read through the introduction carefully to make sure that assertions about cultural processes are clear and supported by evidence. For instance, as a rationale for the study you suggest that for Latino youth integrating societal and home culture might pose a challenge given the difference in cultural orientations (i.e., individualistic vs.collectivist). This is a big claim that requires some evidence and further elaboration.

With respect to the methods, both reviewers found essential information missing regarding your sample (see Reviewer 2 comments) and the use of diaries (see Reviewer 1comments). In particular, I echo the remark of Reviewer 2 about the unevenness in the generational status of your sample. Please justify the inclusion of 2.5and 3rd generation participants, especially given your operationalization of immigrants, as well as provide more information about the completion of the diaries.

Figure 12.7 Extra-reviewer decision letter (first page).

30-May-2015

Hi ████

Re: ██

After 25 years of editorial experience, first with the Journal of ████████ and then with ████, manuscripts inevitably have a strong organic/aesthetic structure for me. When the aesthetics are "off", this serves as a cue for me that something is problematic about a ms.

There is a rather well known quote that I have seen attributed to several different playwrights that goes: "Never put a gun on the wall in the first act unless you intend to use it in the third act." The analogy with respect to a ms. is when it starts off in one direction, then abandons that vector to go someplace else. This was the problem I encountered with your original submission and it was what prompted my detailed initial letter of editorial feedback. This problem continues to exist in the current version and, thanks to your cover letter, I now have a better understanding of it.

As I now see it, you wish to take this ms. in three, more likely four, separate directions and those directions are not easily compatible. (See the Addendum to this e-mail.) It may be possible to achieve this outcome, but it will be necessary to show how these destinations are somehow linearly connected. You did not accomplish this in either the original or the current versions.

The Title of the ms. and the opening paragraph suggest that the first direction/goal is a demonstration that being Jewish is an ethnicity that make Jewish American emerging adults somehow different from White American emerging adults who are not Jewish. You seek to do this by comparing Jewish American college students with White American college students (who are not Jewish) with respect to American identity and religiosity. This is alright as far as it goes but in my view does not go far enough. Aesthetically, my problem is that having gone that far, the ms. then starts off in a whole different direction.

One the face of it, the second direction the ms. takes involves comparisons of Jewish American emerging adults with emerging adults of four other ethnicities (inclusive of White Americans who are not Jewish) with respect to religiosity. As interesting as the finding you have to report is, I do not see how it bears on the matter as to whether Jewish Americans are "not quite white". At least with respect to religious behaviors they are apparently not quite Asian, Black, or Hispanic either . . . but I not think anyone was serious entertaining the possibility that they were these ethnicities. As suggested in the Addendum, I am currently of the view that this is not material that is germane to this presentation.

One reason for this conclusion can be found in a very important point made in your cover letter:

. . . if the focus of the study was completely on comparisons among the ethnic groups, I would agree. However, the focus is on the Jewish American subsample being treated as an ethnic group and investigating if they have similar patterns as the established relationships in the literature.

Figure 12.8 Meddler decision letter (first page).

Editorial Decisions

When the editorial letter arrives in the author's email inbox, it is likely to convey one of the following outcomes: unconditional acceptance, acceptance with revisions, revise-and-resubmit, rejection with the possibility of resubmission, and outright rejection.

Unconditional acceptance is extremely rare on the first round of review and occasionally occurs on the second round of review. In my career, I have had only one manuscript that was accepted without any requests for revisions on the first round of review. Most journals that accept papers without revisions are low-prestige journals. In my career as a reviewer, I cannot remember ever recommending unconditional acceptance on the first round of review, and on only one occasion have I seen a reviewer recommend acceptance with no revisions. As an author, you should plan to revise your manuscripts at least once (and likely more than once) before they are accepted for publication.

Acceptance with revisions is also rare on the first round of review, but it is more common on the second round of review. Excluding papers that I submitted to low-prestige journals early in my career, I have had only two manuscripts that have been accepted with revisions on the first round of review. One of the papers had been previously rejected by another journal on the second round of review—so the paper was reasonably polished by the time we submitted it to the journal where it was ultimately published. The other paper received extremely favorable reviews, and the editor accepted it with only a couple of requested revisions.

Revised manuscripts are discussed in greater detail later in this chapter, but in most cases, a revision that is responsive to reviewer concerns may be accepted with revisions on the second round of review. Reviewers are often grateful and appreciative when their concerns are taken seriously and are incorporated into authors' manuscripts, and in many cases, reviewers have thanked me and my coauthors for our attentiveness to their comments. Reviewing manuscripts is a thankless service—almost all journals blind reviewers' identities (so that reviewers can be candid in their evaluations of manuscripts), and reviewers are almost never paid for their service. Reviewing for journals is a service to the profession, and reviewers are often gratified to know that their work has helped to improve the quality of scholarly publications.

Revise–resubmit is usually the most favorable decision that authors can expect on the first round of review. Essentially, a revise–resubmit decision indicates that the reviewers and editor see promise in the manuscript, but that major revisions are necessary before the paper can be published. These major revisions can include citing additional literature, reorganizing and spelling out ideas and subsections, providing additional methodological details, conducting and reporting additional analyses, expanding the interpretation of results in the discussion, and acknowledging additional limitations, among many other revisions that can be requested. In many cases, the revisions requested can seem overwhelming, particularly to early-career authors. Reviewers can seem harsh even when they see promise in a paper and are requesting revisions.

Here are the reviewer comments on a manuscript that has since been published. You will notice that the reviewers commented on almost every aspect of the paper.

Reviewer 1

1. It may be worth clarifying the authors' use of "micro" and "macro" level in this context (e.g., where it comes from; what it means in this area of study), as most persons may not be familiar with the use of the terms in this area of study. I would guess that these terms are more widely understood (as in sociology or social work) to refer to levels of societal analysis (e.g., micro-, meso-, macro-).

2. While no one would take issue with the statement that acculturation occurs in part through day-to-day interactions, the authors appear to infer that this alone is justification to treat acculturation as a daily fluctuating, or otherwise relatively dynamic, variable (similar to mood or emotions). However, both research and theory describe acculturation to be a relatively stable, slow-to-change variable—as indicated by some of the stable constructs purported to comprise it (e.g., identity, values). Thus, the theoretical argument for examining daily fluctuations in acculturation is weak.

3. The literature review on extant research examining acculturation over time may serve to confuse the issue further. The author presents studies wherein acculturation or ethnic identity is measured as a static variable, or wherein processes related to identity formation are measured. These are appropriate uses of the variables in question but do not support an argument for examining daily fluctuations in acculturation.

4. If in fact it is important to examine the extent to which acculturation exhibits daily fluctuation, then it would seem highly relevant to report and interpret the indices of variability computed by the authors. This would also give more context to the analyses involving the acculturation variables.

5. Table 2 lists the items used to measure daily fluctuations in "accultura-tion." It is unclear from what published scale these items were extracted, but an informal read of them suggests that at least the first four items appear to be tapping into acculturative stress rather than acculturation.

6. The analytic approach is not well-articulated, but the manuscript does NOT appear to indicate that either a hierarchical linear modeling or growth modeling approach was taken. The analytic approach should be better articulated, and it should be one appropriate for nested data.

7. The last two figures likely can be omitted.

Reviewer 2

This study uses daily diaries to examine fluctuations in acculturation measures with mental health variables. The study provides an interesting look at how daily appraisals can impact well-being. The study seems to expand existing work and could be improved in several ways.

1. The term *Hispanic* is problematic. While there is a small justifica-tion embedded in the methods, within the literature there has been a move to use the term *Latinx*. NLPA (National Latino Psychological Association) has an entire article discussing the move to this termi-nology (Cardemil et al, 2019). I urge the authors to review the more recent work in this area and to explore what might be the most appro-priate term.

2. A larger issue is that the introduction does not adequately justify the premise of the study. The first parts of the introduction focus on immigrants in general rather than focusing on the population of focus. Further, the justification for examining mental health variables and the link with acculturation is lacking. The discussion on page 5 (line 8) needs to be further fleshed out. This is the only section that discusses the DVs [dependent variables] and should be much more prominent in the study justification.

3. Greater detail for the justification of the daily assessment is needed. Why does Doucerian suggest daily experiences shape acculturation? This would seem appropriate to include in your micro-level section but is not present there.

4. You mention just-in-time interventions and that should be fleshed out further. Additionally, this seems like something that would be appro-priate to incorporate in your discussion or future directions. There isn't any context provided for including this and then it is never addressed again in the paper.

5. One question that remains unclear in the introduction is why the fluctuations have such a negative impact. There is some discussion of Erikson as a justification, but this needs to be fleshed out more. Specifically, is someone who has these fluctuations in identity process worse off than someone who has consistently low ethnic identity and why? The Kilmstra and Schwartz studies cited reference poorer outcomes, and I am assuming this is compared to those who do not fluctuate, but this isn't completely clear. The theoretical justification needs to be bolstered.

6. Overall, the introduction seems to provide justification for why the study should be done, but it doesn't dive into the specific hypotheses proposed in the present study section. There is minimal coverage on U.S. and Hispanic practices and how they impact well-being in the introduction. There isn't a hypothesis for how fluctuations in values will impact well-being, yet that appears to be something being examined. The introduction minimally addresses gender and generational status and specifically generational status for Latinx populations.

7. It is mentioned that there were multiple cohorts: How many? What was the time frame of data collection (i.e., over the course of how long)?

8. In terms of missing data, were there any students who did not complete a baseline or final assessment. It was mentioned that all cases were kept, so am I to assume everyone had that final assessment?

9. Several variables included in the demographic questionnaire were not included in the demographic tables (skin color, ethnic neighborhood composition). Further, why was ethnic neighborhood composition not controlled for in the mode as the other variables were? Also, the issue of gender is not addressed. Did all participants identify as male and female? Did anyone not answer this question? Were there non-binary options provided for participants? Discuss this in your limitations as well. There is a brief discussion of gender in the introduction, but this should be covered further in the introduction, methods, and discussion.

10. It would be helpful to have a visual of the SEM model with all variables.

11. The discussion of results ends without a sense of the clinical implications of this work. What is the clinical value of this work? Interventions are mentioned in the introduction. How might those interventions be utilized given the findings? What can a clinician do with these findings? What can we do about the language switching? A section on implications would help identify the application of these findings in the real world.

This chapter discusses how to revise a manuscript in accordance with reviewer comments, but here it is important to note that one of the first steps is to glance at the reviews and put them away for a few days. They will seem far less daunting later than they do when you first see them. The bottom line is that editors don't generally invite authors to revise and resubmit manuscripts where the likelihood of eventual publication is extremely low. In fact, over the course of my career, approximately 75% to 80% of revise–resubmit editorial decisions resulted in a revised version eventually being accepted for publication. The key, of course, is to figure out how to revise the paper in a way that is responsive to the reviewer comments and requests.

Some revise–resubmit decisions involve a great deal of work and can be exhausting. I remember one paper where the editor forwarded four reviews along with his decision letter. Because each reviewer will likely offer comments that mostly don't overlap with the comments provided by the other reviewers, responding to four reviewers resulted in a response letter that was nearly 50% longer than the manuscript itself. The first round of revision for that paper took me well over a month—and I pride myself on working quickly and efficiently. The editor sent our revised manuscript back to the reviewers for a second round of review, and, as is often the case, the volume of second-round comments was dramatically lower than the volume of comments from the first round. The editor offered us a conditional acceptance (acceptance with revisions) after the second round of review, and he accepted the paper unconditionally after we addressed the remaining reviewer concerns.

Rejection With Recommendations to Resubmit

A revise–resubmit editorial decision indicates that the manuscript has a good chance to be accepted, provided that the authors successfully address the reviewers' concerns. When reviewers see some promise in a paper but believe that drastic revision is needed—often involving additional data collection and a complete rewrite of the paper—they may recommend that the current manuscript be rejected and that the authors be encouraged to "try again." That is, the editorial process for the current paper is closed, but the "door is left open" for the authors to rework the project and/or the paper and to submit a new manuscript. Such an editorial outcome falls somewhere between a revise–resubmit decision and an outright rejection (where the journal is not willing to consider a new or revised version of the manuscript).

Generally, revise–resubmit decisions involve requests for additional analyses and for rewriting, but not for additional data collection. If the reviewers and editor believe that the authors need to collect additional data, the paper will usually be rejected with the possibility of submitting a new manuscript.

(Occasionally I have seen reviewers and editors ask authors to collect new data as part of a revise–resubmit decision, but such requests are fairly uncommon in revise–resubmit editorial outcomes.) Papers that are poorly written but where there is some promise of a noteworthy contribution might also be rejected with the possibility of resubmitting a new manuscript.

Unlike a revise–resubmit editorial decision, rejection with the possibility of submitting a new manuscript does not guarantee that any of the same reviewers will be invited to evaluate the new paper once it has been submitted. In fact, in my experience and in the cases I know about, in most cases where the authors submitted a new manuscript after a previous version had been rejected, the new version was rejected as well. At best, when an editor rejects a paper but offers to consider a new manuscript based on the same general set of ideas, eventual acceptance in that journal should be viewed as a long shot.

Outright Rejection

Outright rejection is by far the most common editorial outcome for most journals. The reviewers either recommend rejection or raise major and potentially unaddressable concerns, and the editor decides that the manuscript is not an appropriate fit for the journal. Manuscripts can be rejected for any number of reasons: The methods may be flawed, the reviewers may not like or resonate with the theoretical approach underlying the study or argument, the questions guiding the study or argument may not be considered novel or important, or the reviewers and editor simply may not have liked the study or argument that the paper was reporting. I remember one paper that Al Waterman and I submitted to a prominent personality journal. The study was based on Al's theory of intrinsic motivation, which postulated a set of predictors and indicators of when activities would be experienced as enjoyable and fulfilling (see Waterman, 2008, for a review of this theoretical perspective). One of the reviewers made a comment that bordered on a personal attack, claiming that "the Waterman theory" was not important enough to be tested. The associate editor rejected our submission but did not provide any feedback of her own, so we were not able to ascertain the extent to which that specific reviewer comment might have figured into her decision. Nonetheless, we concluded that the reviewers and editor were simply not interested in the work we were reporting—especially given that few or no methodological weaknesses were mentioned.

When editors reject a manuscript, they may or may not provide a rationale for doing so. The "service to the profession" approach to journal editing suggests that editors should tell authors why their papers are being rejected— rather than simply using a form rejection letter and referring the author to the reviews for details. However, busy editors and associate editors often don't invest very much time in papers that they know they are rejecting. I have encountered many editors and associate editors who don't really engage with a paper until the second round of review—they let the reviewers do the heavy lifting on the first round and offer their own feedback only when a manuscript is close to acceptance. When a paper is being rejected, many editors adopt the approach that the paper isn't their problem anymore. (With that said, however, some action editors really do go "above and beyond" in laying out the problems that led them to reject a manuscript.)

Easy Rejections and Close Calls

Rejection decisions can be divided into two general categories—the easy rejections and the close calls. An *easy rejection* refers to a scenario where the reviews are uniformly negative and recommend against publication, and where the editor doesn't need to spend much time deliberating. A *close call*, however, refers to a situation where (a) reviews are lukewarm, (b) the reviewers are split between recommending rejection and inviting a revision, or (c) the reviews are positive, but it isn't clear whether the paper's contribution meets the standards of the journal. In these cases, the editor has to make a judgment call. If the editor decides to reject the paper, the rejection letter should clearly explain why the paper is being rejected. Indeed, the authors are likely to read the reviews and wonder why they were not invited to revise and resubmit. Sometimes editors will explain that their own judgment is closest to that of a reviewer who recommended rejection, or that the paper doesn't represent an extensive enough contribution to warrant publication in the journal to which it was submitted. In other cases, editors may spot flaws that the reviewers overlooked, and they may note these flaws as their reason for overruling the reviewers' recommendations.

As is discussed in Chapter 13, close calls are the type of rejections that authors are most likely to appeal, and in my experience, the appeals can be successful in some cases. In essence, a close call could have gone either way, and sometimes the editor can be convinced to consider reversing the decision. Al Waterman used to say that close calls indicated that there was a "constituency" for the manuscript, and that the authors should therefore be given a chance to revise their paper. However, if the editor's contention is that the paper does not represent a strong enough contribution to warrant publication in the journal, then pointing out how reviewer comments can be successfully addressed may not be sufficient to convince an editor to reverse a rejection decision.

In most cases, the best course of action following a rejection decision is to incorporate whatever reviewer and editor feedback seems relevant, and then to send the manuscript to a different journal. Most manuscripts will eventually find a home, even if doing so requires trying several journals. (Again, what to do with rejected manuscripts is covered in greater detail in Chapter 13.)

Revising Manuscripts: Turning a Revise–Resubmit Into an Acceptance

Revising a manuscript in accordance with reviewer feedback is one of the most challenging aspects of scholarly publishing. A revise–resubmit decision is essentially a "foot in the door" with the journal—the reviewers and editor see promise in your manuscript and are interested in pursuing it for publication, but now the onus is on the authors to make the requested changes. I have developed a system for revising manuscripts—a system that has generated a success rate greater than 80% over the course of my career—and I lay out this system for you here in this section.

Key Principles for Revising Manuscripts

Before we discuss the mechanics of revising manuscripts, I'd like to go over some basic principles. The most basic principle of revising manuscripts is that the response letter is essential. Although readers won't see the response letter when the article is published, the action editor and reviewers will see it—and a carefully crafted response letter can greatly increase the likelihood that the editor and reviewers will respond positively to the revised manuscript. The functions of a response letter are to show the editor and reviewers how you have responded to their concerns, to decrease the amount of work they must do to find the changes you have made, and to demonstrate clearly to them that you have taken their concerns seriously and have complied with their requests.

A carefully crafted response letter is often as long as—and sometimes longer than—the manuscript itself. As is detailed in this section, I list each reviewer comment in italics, followed by a narrative description of how my colleagues and I have modified the paper in response to the comment. Where applicable, I also include the exact text added to or modified in the manuscript in response to the comment, and I provide the page number(s) on which this text appears in the paper. Overall, I want to make it as easy as possible for the reviewers and the editor to see that I've done what they asked me to do.

A second principle to keep in mind is that, as an author, you are in a "one-down" position. Hardré (2013) provides an excellent framing of the relationship between authors and reviewers, a relationship that is essentially centered on gatekeeping. In most cases, reviewers must recommend publication before the action editor will accept your manuscript for publication. Although authors don't necessarily have to comply with every reviewer request, they must respond to every request. (I detail the distinction between compliance and response later in this section.)

The one-down position means that authors should not respond angrily or defensively to reviewer comments, should not "blow off" reviewer concerns, and should do their best to adopt the reviewer's perspective (i.e., "I may not agree with this comment, but I want to understand why the reviewer thought this about my paper, study, or argument"). Remember that readers may interpret your statements, arguments, and interpretations in the same way that reviewers interpret them—so if something in your manuscript is unclear to a reviewer, it may well be unclear to readers as well. I advise adopting the position that there is at least a kernel of truth in every reviewer comment, even if the comment is worded strongly or awkwardly. My strategy is to give reviewers at least some of what they are asking for—even if I ultimately choose not to make all the changes they are requesting. My strategy is to respond deferentially and collegially, even in cases where I disagree with the concern that the reviewer is expressing.

A third principle is that responding to reviewer comments almost always improves the manuscript. I have found this to be the case with every article I have ever published. Reviewers point out logical inconsistencies, suggest new analyses that strengthen the message of the paper, and help authors to identify and address flaws in their work. Even when a revision takes me a long time, and a lot of effort, to complete, I am thankful and grateful to the reviewers for helping to improve the manuscript and to communicate its messages more clearly. I express this gratitude in my response letters— and I know that reviewers appreciate seeing their work acknowledged. As already noted, reviewing is a service to the scholarly profession, and reviewers often derive great satisfaction from helping authors to improve their work.

Starting the Response Letter

As Hardré (2013) noted, starting a revision can be intimidating for many early-career authors. Starting a revision can be just as difficult as staring at a blank screen when one is sitting down to write a first draft. Just as José taught me to write the method section first so that I would no longer be looking at a blank screen, Dick Dunham taught me to begin assembling the response letter as the first step in the revision process.

I start a response letter by copying and pasting the reviewer comments from the journal's email into a blank document. I separate the comments according to who provided them—for example, I list all of Reviewer 1's comments together, all of Reviewer 2's comments together, and so on. Then I number each reviewer's comments consecutively. Numbering reviewer comments is essential because it allows you to refer to them by number (e.g., "See our response to Reviewer 1, comment 6"). I then read the comments carefully to see whether a reviewer might have combined several comments into one—in which case I will separate the comments and renumber accordingly. For example, consider the following comment:

4. The authors need to consider country of origin in their analyses. A better case needs to be made in the introduction for examining these specific groups. And the findings for these various country-of-origin groups need to be interpreted more clearly in the discussion.

I might separate this comment into three separate comments as follows:

4. The authors need to consider country of origin in their analyses.
5. A better case needs to be made in the introduction for examining these specific groups.
6. The findings for these various country-of-origin groups need to be interpreted more clearly in the discussion.

After the comments are assembled, I italicize them and put in a placeholder for the response. For example:

4. The authors need to consider country of origin in their analyses. RESPONSE HERE
5. A better case needs to be made in the introduction for examining these specific groups. RESPONSE HERE
6. The findings for these various country-of-origin groups need to be interpreted more clearly in the discussion. RESPONSE HERE

I then sort through the comments and label them according to (a) the extent of revision required and (b) the primary section(s) in which changes are requested. In terms of the extent of revision required, I usually delineate among major, moderate, and minor revisions. Major revisions include changing or reframing the overall message of the paper, incorporating new theoretical perspectives, restructuring or reorganizing sections of the paper, and conducting new analyses. Moderate revisions include creating new tables and figures, adding new sentences or paragraphs to existing sections of the paper, clarifying methodological or analytic details, and reviewing and incorporating additional literature. Minor revisions include word changes, adding missing references, correcting typographical errors, and ensuring that numbers reported in tables and figures match up with numbers reported in the text. Overall, major revisions will likely change the bottom-line messages that the paper is conveying, moderate revisions involve clarifying and sharpening the paper, and minor revisions involve small corrections.

Of all the major revisions that reviewers request, new analyses have by far the greatest potential to "make or break" the paper. If the new analyses that reviewers are requesting don't produce significant results, then the paper may be "dead" unless the authors can come up with a way to salvage it. It may be possible to push back against reviewer requests for new analyses, but such pushing back should be based on the logic underlying the authors' original analyses and how that logic is not compatible with the new analyses that reviewers are asking for. Authors should not push back against requested analyses simply because the new analyses don't produce significant results (or because the new analyses produce results that alter the original set of findings). In my estimation, the bottom line is that, if the analyses that the reviewers are requesting are scientifically sound, they should be conducted and reported. If the new analyses cause the results to become nonsignificant, then the authors need to think carefully about whether—and how—the paper can be salvaged while still giving the reviewers at least some of what they are requesting.

Because conducting new analyses has the potential to change the overall message of the paper, I suggest conducting the new analyses before making any of the other requested changes. If you conduct the analyses and find that the new results have altered the paper's message, then many of the other changes you made or need to make may become obsolete. Further, if the new analyses cause the results to become nonsignificant, and if you and your coauthors cannot find a way to salvage the manuscript, then you might have to drop the paper (or abandon the revision for the current journal and submit elsewhere). Only after the new analyses are completed, and after you and your coauthors have discussed the impact that the new findings might have on the message of the paper, should you start making the textual changes that reviewers have requested.

Once the new analyses have been completed, I suggest adjusting the analytic strategy and the results section to include the new analyses and results. I would take these steps before making any other requested changes. It's essential to ensure that the new results are incorporated into the paper first—so that other changes (especially changes to the discussion section) can take the new results into account. Even some parts of the introduction may have to be rewritten to set up the new analyses. For example, if a reviewer asks you to use survival analysis instead of structural equation modeling, then the introduction would have to be rewritten to focus on initiation and time to event occurrence rather than predictive associations among study variables.

Reviewer requests for new analyses raise some key ethical issues. Chapter 3 discusses the scientific method and cautions against HARKing (hypothesizing after the results are known). That is, we specify our hypotheses before conducting analyses, and we do not conduct analyses and then come up with a set of hypotheses to match the results we obtained (Kerr, 1998). However, when reviewers ask us to conduct new analyses, or to control for new covariates within our existing analyses, they are effectively asking us to HARK. We did not plan to conduct the analyses or include the covariates that the reviewer is asking for, but we do need to include a justification in the introduction to set up the new analyses. So we likely need to incorporate additional theoretical statements—and perhaps introduce additional hypotheses—that the new analyses would test.

As is outlined in greater detail in the next section, it is possible to conduct a set of requested analyses and include the results in the response letter but not include those analyses in the manuscript itself. In my style of responding to reviewers, conducting the requested analyses and reporting them in the response letter represent a "show of good faith"—especially if the authors offer to include the analyses in the manuscript if the reviewer and editor would like them to do so. (In my experience, reporting the results in the letter is usually sufficient—reviewers and editors generally do not ask for these results to be incorporated into the paper unless the new analyses are central to the reviewer's critique of your paper.) Conducting the requested analyses and reporting the results in the response letter are a way of pushing back against the requested analyses while still showing the editor and reviewers that you put forth a good-faith effort to respond to their concerns. So, when I genuinely do not want to include a set of requested analyses in a manuscript—either because the new analyses are too far astray from my research questions and hypotheses or because I am not comfortable with the HARKing that including the new analyses would require—I report the results in the response letter. Again, however, if the new analyses are central to the reviewer's critique, you may have to integrate them into your revised manuscript.

Revising the Manuscript and Constructing the Response Letter

Generally, when revising a manuscript, I address the major revision requests first. A reviewer request to rewrite the introduction section, for example, takes precedence over another reviewer request to add a sentence to the introduction or to correct a typographical error. Once you have rewritten the introduction section in accordance with the reviewers' requests, the request to add a sentence to the original introduction section may no longer be applicable.

So, go through the major revisions that are requested and identify the request that you believe should be addressed first. (Remember that new analyses should be conducted, and their results reported in the manuscript if you decide to include them, before you attend to any other revision requests.) Unless some revisions are dependent on other revisions—for example, a request to include new ideas in the introduction should be addressed after you have addressed a request to reorganize the whole introduction section—the order in which you address the revision requests likely does not matter. Most reviewers organize their comments according to the sections to which they apply, so comments on the introduction will often appear first. As a result, I usually start by revising the introduction.

How to Address Each Reviewer Comment

First, read the text of the comment carefully. I suggest reading the comment multiple times so that you don't miss any nuances or subtleties in what the reviewer is saying or requesting. Once you believe that you understand the spirit of the comment, ask yourself the following questions:

- What specific subsections or paragraphs does the comment apply to? Is there specific text that the reviewer is referencing in the comment?
- What issues is the reviewer identifying with those subsections or paragraphs? Just as a doctor would diagnose a medical problem by examining the affected area, I suggest that you examine the text that the reviewer is referencing and identify the problem(s) that the reviewer is asking you to correct.
- What is the best strategy for making the corrections or changes that the reviewer is asking for? Does the solution involve drafting new text, modifying existing text, deleting existing text, or some combination thereof?

- If the solution involves drafting new text, what should that text say? What is the message that the new text needs to communicate? (Don't worry as much about the specific words—those can be drafted in rough form and then smoothed over in later iterations—but be sure to have in mind the intended message that you want the new text to bring across.)
- Similar considerations apply to modifying existing text. What does the text need to say? How is that different from what the text says now? What is the best way to change the existing text so that it says what it needs to say? Should you insert new sentences or paragraphs? Should you change existing wording? Should you do some of both?

Once you have identified the problem to which the reviewer comment refers and have come up with a strategy for addressing that problem, you should start drafting the new text. Just as you would do when writing a first draft, allow the ideas to flow from your mind onto the screen. Moreover, when you are beginning the revision process, don't worry about length. You can always cut text later—or, if necessary, you can email the action editor and ask for more space. Requests for additional space are far more likely to be granted for revised manuscripts than for new submissions, especially in cases where reviewers are asking for a lot of new information.

Keep in mind that reviewer comments, especially requests for major revisions, often require drafting, removing, and/or revising text in multiple locations in the paper. For example, a request to clarify results may require not only modifying text in the results section, but also clarifications to the discussion section. Similarly, because the introduction section traces a line of logic from the broad opening statements through the statement of the study purpose and hypotheses, adding or revising text in the introduction is likely to disrupt that line of logic. Once you finish responding to all the comments, you should smooth out the sentences and paragraphs so that the line of logic is clear. In general, the more extensive the revisions are to the introduction, the more work that will be required to restore the line of logic that this section requires.

When you have finished responding to a comment, go back to the response letter and write a description of how you have addressed the comment. Then paste in the text you drafted in response to the comment. You should use a wildcard character (I use a bolded x) to specify the page number of the manuscript on which the new text appears. After the revised manuscript has been finalized and approved by all your coauthors, you will replace the wildcard characters with page numbers. And if you cite references in your narrative response, include those references in your response to the comment.

Because some manuscript submission sites provide only a text box for the response letter and don't allow formatting in this text box, I usually put the word *RESPONSE* in front of my narrative response, and I place quotation marks around the copied and pasted text excerpts. It might also be a good idea to manually indent each paragraph (using two or three spaces) rather than using the indent function in your word-processing software—just in case you are not able to submit the response letter with formatting. (The reviewer comments will not be italicized if you cannot use formatting—that's why I include the word *RESPONSE* to separate each comment from my response to that comment.)

Here is an example of a reviewer comment, a response narrative, and copied and pasted text from the manuscript:

6. I think it would be necessary to, early in the manuscript, define/operationalize the terms and potential differentiation between culture, race, and ethnicity.

RESPONSE: We have now added a section titled "Rethinking the 'One Size Fits All' Approach: The Role of Migrant Type, Ethnicity, and Cultural Similarity in Acculturation." In this section, we question the "one size fits all" approach that is prominent in the acculturation literature, where the same model and assumptions are thought to apply to all migrants.

The first three paragraphs of this section are devoted to outlining the importance of—and defining—culture and ethnicity (pp. 9–10):

"A further criticism of the acculturation literature is that it adopts a "one size fits all" approach (Rudmin, 2003). That is, according to Berry's (1980) model, and other similar approaches, the same two acculturation processes, and the same four acculturation categories, characterize all migrants equally—regardless of the type of migrant, the countries of origin and settlement, and the ethnic group in question (Berry, Phinney, Sam, & Vedder, 2006). Many psychological approaches to acculturation (e.g., Berry, 1980; Phinney, 2003) have examined migrants in isolation and have used terms such as "acculturation strategies," which implies that individual differences in acculturation outcomes are the result of specific choices made by migrants. Although migrants likely *are* at choice regarding some aspects of their acculturation, other aspects are constrained by demographic or contextual factors. A more nuanced approach—based on Berry's model but adjusting for the many variations among migrants and among their circumstances—may have more explanatory power and broader applicability compared to a "one size fits all" perspective (Chirkov, 2009).

Indeed, to understand acculturation, one must understand the interactional context in which it occurs (e.g., Rohmann, Piontkowski, & van Randenborgh, 2008; cf., Crockett & Zamboanga, 2009). This includes the characteristics of the migrants themselves, the groups or countries from which they originate, their socioeconomic status and resources, the country and local community in which they settle, and their fluency in the language of the country of settlement. Two acculturation-relevant terms that may require some definition and clarification are *ethnicity* and *culture*. Because so many contemporary migrants to the United States and to other Western countries are from non-European backgrounds (Steiner, 2009; Suárez-Orozco, Suárez-Orozco, & Todorova, 2008), ethnicity has become an integral aspect of the process of acculturation and migrant reception—where ethnicity refers to membership in a group that holds a specific heritage and set of values, beliefs, and customs (Phinney, 1996).[1]

Because acculturation refers to cultural change, it is essential to specify how culture is defined. Culture refers to shared meanings, understandings, or referents held by a group of people (Shore, 2002; Triandis, 1995). Rudmin (2003) contends that the similarity between the receiving culture and the migrant's heritage culture can help to determine how much acculturation is needed to adapt to the receiving culture. Culture is sometimes, but not always, synonymous with nations and national boundaries."

Footnote 1 reads "Pan-ethnic groups, such as Black, Asian, or Middle Eastern, can serve either as racial or ethnic categories, depending on the criteria used to assign group memberships to individuals (i.e., physical or cultural; Phinney, 1996). We do not use the term *race* in our manuscript, given arguments against the use of race as a psychological or behavioral construct (Helms, Jernigan, & Mascher, 2005; Hirschman, 2004). We use *ethnicity* instead (cf. Hitlin, Brown, & Elder, 2007). Whereas *ethnicity* refers to a group that holds a specific heritage and set of values, beliefs, and customs, *race* refers to a group characterized by a specific skin color or phenotype (Helms & Tallyrand, 1997)."

Where possible, you should include citations in your responses—especially in cases where you are electing not to comply with a specific reviewer request. An empirically based reason for not making a requested change generally places you on the most solid ground. If no empirical evidence is available, then you can state and defend your preference not to comply with a reviewer request.

One word of caution—as already noted, even when you choose not to comply with a request, be sure that you fully respond to the request. That is, provide a clear and thoughtful justification for not making the change that the reviewer is requesting. Be sure that your response is not defensive or disrespectful, and that you are not "blowing off" the reviewer. Notice how extensive my response was to the reviewer comment in the example above. If a comment touches on multiple issues, be sure that you address all the issues. (Separating complex comments into multiple simpler comments helps to ensure that all the issues are addressed.)

Another word of advice: I strongly suggest that you comply—at least partially—with all requests for major revisions. When reviewers request major revisions, these requests are often make-or-break issues that will lead to your revised manuscript's being rejected if you do not comply. Remember the one-down principle—reviewers often must recommend publication before the editor will accept your paper. (If the action editor uses a meddler strategy, then you need to satisfy the editor's comments first—but where reviewer comments don't conflict with specific editor comments, be sure to address the reviewer comments fully and completely.)

Using Limitations to Address Reviewer Comments

If a reviewer asks for a change that you are unable to make—generally involving covariates or predictor variables that are not available in your data set—then the strategy I recommend is to incorporate the variable as a limitation. A good approach might be to describe the importance of the omitted variable and to suggest that future studies incorporate this variable into their assessment batteries.

Here is an example of a reviewer comment and an author response—including the text inserted into the paper in response to the comment.

4. *When studying immigration, it is essential to control for the age at which individuals migrated to the destination country. Did the authors assess and control for this?*

RESPONSE: Unfortunately, we did not ask participants how old they were when they arrived in the United States. We now list age at arrival as a limitation of our study and recommend that future studies assess and control for this variable (page x):

"Fifth, although all participants in our sample were born outside the United States, we did not ask participants how old they were when they arrived. Research has found that acculturation and other immigration-related variables operate differently for individuals who migrate as young children, as adolescents, and as adults (Cheung, Chudek, & Heine, 2011). As a result, it is essential for future research to assess age at migration."

Because we did not assess the requested covariate, the best we can do is to list this omission as a limitation. On most occasions, reviewers appear to be satisfied with this approach, but occasionally in the second round of review, after learning that the authors didn't measure an important predictor or covariate, a reviewer will recommend rejection. In my experience, reviewers are most likely to balk at the exclusion of variables that they deem essential to testing the specific theory and/or hypotheses guiding the study. For this reason, when you are designing a study, it is critical to survey the literature to identify essential predictors and covariates. Similarly, if you are using a secondary data set for a purpose other than that for which it was designed, you need to think carefully about whether the data set includes all the variables you need to test your theory and hypotheses.

Responding to Reviewer Comments in the Cover Letter Rather Than in the Manuscript

As already noted, one way to push back against a reviewer request (especially a request for new analyses) is to conduct the requested analyses and report the results in the response letter. Here is an example:

8. On page 14 you note the "low levels of convergence between parent and adolescent reports of family functioning." Please provide the correlations that led you to conclude that the levels of convergence were low.

RESPONSE: The following table displays correlations between adolescent and parent reports of family functioning, separately by gender, at each time point. We have not included this table in the manuscript but would be happy to do so if the reviewer and editor would like us to.

Timepoint	Baseline	6 Months	12 Months	24 Months	36 Months
Boys	.13	.22*	.25**	.31**	.35***
Girls	.36***	.25**	.21*	.29**	.31**

So, we are providing the information that the reviewer is requesting, but we have reported it in the response letter rather than in the manuscript. We are letting the reviewer and editor decide whether they would like us to add this information to the paper. (This reviewer did not ask us to add the table to the paper—indeed, the reviewer recommend acceptance on the second round of review. The editor used an interpreter approach and never provided any comments of his own, beyond what the reviewers had noted and requested.)

Responding to Positive Reviewer Comments

Although it may be tempting to list only the reviewers' negative comments and concerns, it's also essential to list and respond to positive comments. There are two primary reasons for doing this. First, listing positive comments reminds reviewers of the praise they gave your paper in the previous round of review. Second, listing positive comments tells the editor and other reviewers that reviewers saw merit in your manuscript, study, theory, review, or position. In the second round of review, your response letter will allow each reviewer to see what the other reviewers said and how you responded. Seeing that other reviewers praised your manuscript may predispose a given reviewer to view your revised manuscript more positively as well.

My response to positive comments is simple—usually I say something like, "We thank the reviewer for these positive comments" or "Thank you so much for your positive assessment of our manuscript." Remember that reviewing is a thankless job, so receiving a "Thank you" often means a lot to reviewers. I also say, "Thank you for catching this" when reviewers point out typographical or grammatical errors. If you think back to Dale Carnegie's (1936) classic book *How to Win Friends and Influence People*, showing appreciation for others is a great way to convince them to help you. In this case, showing appreciation for reviewers' time and effort can predispose them toward endorsing publication of the manuscript. I've thanked reviewers in almost every response letter I've written, and I can confidently say that this strategy works.

Responding to Reviewer Comments That Require Changes in Multiple Locations in the Paper

In some cases, reviewer comments require text to be inserted or modified in multiple places in the paper. In my experience, this occurs in at least two scenarios. The first occurs when a reviewer asks you to correct a pattern of errors in the paper. For example:

22. When summarizing the findings and connecting them to past studies, please make sure it is clear to what extent these findings are novel and how they extend current research.

RESPONSE: We have now added text in a number of places.

Page 23: "These methods advance the biculturalism literature because they allow us to examine directionality and daily fluctuations among biculturalism components, as well as how these fluctuations (as an index of instability) predict later levels of well-being. Such advances are important because most prior research on biculturalism has been cross-sectional or experimental, with few longitudinal studies available. Information about this natural progression and interrelationships is essential to informing the design of interventions to promote biculturalism in Hispanic college students, as well as other groups of young people."

Page 25: "The cross-lagged panel analyses permitted us to *move beyond prior cross-sectional work* and examine the sequencing among the biculturalism dimensions." (Italics denote new text.)

Page 25: "Again, these results go beyond prior work in specifying directionality among biculturalism components."

Pages 27–28: "Although prior studies (e.g., Nguyen & Benet-Martínez, 2013) have examined links between biculturalism and well-being, the present study is the first to do so longitudinally, with controls for earlier levels of well-being so as to permit us to assume directionality."

Here is another example with a similarly broad comment:

16. I suggest integrating the results and discussion into theory and previous studies in a more focused manner.

RESPONSE: We have now done this. We have incorporated more prior theory and research into our interpretation and discussion of the findings.

Page 25: "The finding that both Hispanic and U.S. cultural indices appeared to change in similar directions across all three acculturation domains (practices, values, and identifications) was somewhat consistent with Knight et al. (2009), who found that U.S. and Hispanic cultural practices tended to change similarly over time. Knight et al.'s (in press) study of changes in cultural values, however, found highly divergent patterns of change in U.S. versus Hispanic values over time. Our study was among the first to examine longitudinal trajectories of both ethnic and U.S. identity."

Page 27: "In cross-cultural psychology, such a phenomenon is referred to as the 'frame of reference effect' (Smith, Fischer, Vignoles, & Bond, 2013). Cultural practices are often taken for granted when one is operating within a context where those behaviors are normative, but those behaviors are viewed as "cultural" when one is operating within a new context where one's typical behaviors are different from the norm. Berry (1997) hypothesized that acculturation results from contact with others who are culturally dissimilar from oneself, and he suggested that such contact would cause the person to examine her/his own cultural attitudes as well as those held by others. At least in adolescence, and within bicultural contexts that encourage endorsement of both one's cultural heritage and of the receiving culture, acculturation may be likely to manifest as similar patterns of change in endorsement of both cultural streams."

Page 28: "Kiang and Fuligni (2009) have found that associating with coethnic friends, and with family members who have lived in the United States for longer periods of time, may help to maintain or increase one's endorsement of ethnic identity over time. It is also possible that ethnic identity increases following immigration as adolescents begin to emphasize themselves as Cuban, Mexican, Colombian, et cetera, within the United States. For example, individuals living in Colombia likely do not spend a great deal of time thinking of themselves as Colombian, but the frame of reference effect suggests that identification as Colombian might increase following immigration to the United States. Experiences of discrimination or social marginalization may also cause ethnic identification to increase (Armenta & Hunt, 2009) . . . It is important to note that none of the classes we found involved decreases in U.S. or Hispanic practices, values, or identifications. Acculturation components either increased or remained stable throughout the study period. Such a pattern of findings may suggest that exposure to a new cultural context tends to be an additive, rather than subtractive, experience. That is, adolescents can incorporate a second cultural stream into their cultural repertoire. Such a finding is consistent with Cheung et al. (2010), who found that childhood and adolescence represent a "sensitive period" for cultural adaptation. Our findings also support Nguyen and Benet-Martínez (2013), who identified biculturalism as the most advantageous approach to acculturation across a variety of life outcomes."

Page 29: "If acculturation among recent-immigrant adolescents is represented as *increases* over time in one or more cultural domains, then lack of change in any of these domains (i.e., the SSS class) may be analogous to Berry's (1997) marginalization category (where the person rejects both the heritage and receiving cultures). Marginalization is often associated with the poorest psychosocial outcomes (Berry, Phinney, Sam, & Vedder, 2006)."

Page 31: "Theories of ethnic identity may also help to explain the somewhat modest role of identifications in the present results. Ethnic identity (and by extension, U.S. identity) consists of both an affective component and a behavioral component (Phinney & Ong, 2007; Umaña-Taylor et al., 2014). That is, identifying with one's heritage cultural group, the United States, or both involves thinking about the meaning of the group membership, as well as participating in activities reflective of the group. The behavioral component of ethnic identity may overlap with cultural practices, such that only the affective component contributes uniquely to predicting outcomes."

In other cases, a reviewer comment might require changes to multiple sections of the paper. For example, in this next case, a reviewer comment required us to make changes to both the introduction and the discussion:

3. The authors appear to equate identity, as commitment and reconsideration processes, with self-concept clarity which appears to be, by definition, a trait.

RESPONSE: The reviewer makes an excellent point. Self-concept clarity refers to the extent to which one possesses a positive and coherent sense of who one is. Thus far, no published longitudinal studies have been conducted on self-concept clarity—in fact, a search of the PsycInfo literature database from 1990 (when the term was first used) through September 2011 yielded 71 records, all of which were cross-sectional or experimental studies. As a result, the reviewer has inspired us to clarify that longitudinal research on self-concept clarity is needed. We now note in the introduction (pp. 8–9) that

"A notable limitation of extant research on self-concept clarity is that no published longitudinal studies have been conducted on this construct. A search of the PsycInfo literature database from 1990 (when the term was first used) through September 2011, seeking records with the term "self-concept clarity" in the title, abstract, or keywords yielded 71 records, all of which were cross-sectional or experimental studies. The functions of self-concept clarity *over time* are therefore in need of study. The definition of self-concept clarity—a coherent, positive, and firm sense of who one is—suggests that it might be more of a trait than a developmental process, but longitudinal research is needed to examine this issue. Erikson's (1968) notions of identity coherence and confusion are conceptually similar to self-concept clarity, and Eriksonian measures of coherence and confusion (e.g., the Erikson Psychosocial Stage Inventory; Schwartz, Zamboanga, Wang, & Olthuis, 2009) contain items that are quite similar to those on Campbell et al.'s (1996) Self-Concept Clarity Scale. According to Erikson (1950), identity synthesis is characterized by consistency and integration among one's various roles and commitments —suggesting that making commitments is associated with, but does not guarantee, a synthesized sense of identity and a clear sense of self. Further, Schwartz, Mason, Pantin, and Szapocznik (2009) found developmental change in identity confusion over time—suggesting that self-concept clarity might also represent a developmental construct."

Additionally, in the Discussion (page 26), we note that

"Indeed, longitudinal findings have suggested that patterns of identity development—especially patterns of commitment making and maintenance— may be quite consistent over time (Meeus et al., 2010)— suggesting that they may be more "trait-like" than "state-like." In the present study, the stability of commitments and self-concept clarity over time suggests some degree of within-person consistency in these processes. Further, our rank-order stability findings suggest that commitment and self-concept clarity become more stable and "trait-like" over time. Indeed, some adolescents may maintain higher levels of commitment and self-concept clarity over time compared to other adolescents, even notwithstanding temporal fluctuations in the strength of a given adolescent's commitments and in the clarity and coherence of her or his self-concept."

The point is that, for each reviewer comment, it is essential to consider all the ways in which you can respond appropriately to the comment. Changing one section of the paper in response to the comment may create inconsistencies between that section and other parts of the manuscript. These inconsistencies, in turn, need to be corrected by adjusting the other sections. Similarly, a reviewer comment may pertain to various places in the manuscript. In these cases, consider the comment as an opportunity to correct multiple potential problems within a single response.

Responding to Multiple Iterations of the Same Reviewer Comment, and Dealing With Conflicting Reviewer Comments

Sometimes reviewers repeat themselves, or multiple reviewers bring up the same points. Rather than copying your response from the first iteration of the comment and pasting it into the response to the second iteration, I advise simply stating "Please see our response to Reviewer 1, comment 5." This approach saves you time, and it also makes the editor's job easier—all the editor has to do is go back to your response to Reviewer 1, comment 5, to see how you're responding to Reviewer 2, comment 10.

An associate editor who handled one of my papers many years ago noted in his action letter that "reliability among reviewers is a rare thing." Empirical evidence supports his contention—Kravitz et al. (2010), for example, found that reviewers' agreement on whether to recommend rejection or revise–resubmit ranged from 11% to 23%. Reliability of individual comments is likely even lower than that. In my experience both as an author and as an editor, reviewers often bring up largely idiosyncratic issues, and the overlap between reviewers in terms of issues raised is negligible. There may be a few issues that are raised by multiple reviewers, but I wouldn't count on very many of them for any paper you are revising.

What do we do in the opposite situation—when reviewers are asking for opposing changes? For example, I can remember a manuscript in the early 2000s where the first reviewer asked for more detail on the methods, but the second reviewer wanted the overall length of the paper reduced by 40%. Other than deleting whole subsections from the introduction and discussion, I could not think of a way to satisfy both reviewers. If we complied with one reviewer's request, we would be going against what the other reviewer was asking us to do.

In this scenario, my advice is to give both reviewers at least some of what they are asking for. For example, in this case Reviewer 2 was asking for the large cut, so we replied to this reviewer as follows:

1. Although the paper is well written, it is not concise. At 25 pages it is rather long and should be cut quite considerably. I would recommend trying to be around 15 pages. The Introduction can be cut considerably and so can the Methods section, particularly the description of the intervention's implementation. The Discussion is also too long.

RESPONSE: We have attempted to shorten the paper according to this reviewer's recommendation. In the Introduction, we have summarized our own work much more concisely. In the Method, we have moved the intervention implementation section into a table and have deleted that material from the text. In the Discussion, we have also worked to eliminate the redundancy and extraneous material. Given the amount of additional information requested by Reviewer 1, we were unable to perform the full 40% cut that Reviewer 2 recommended. However, we have reduced the body of the paper by 25% (from 36 pages to 27).

Then we replied to Reviewer 1's individual requests for additional information. For example:

2. *In addition to participatory learning, what was the theoretical frame for the intervention?*

RESPONSE: We now note (pages 5–6) that the intervention is based on ecodevelopmental theory (Szapocznik & Coatsworth, 1999):

"This integrative program is multilevel, addressing processes operating at varying systemic levels: increasing parental investment within the family, fostering proactive connections between the family and other important systems such as the peer network and school system, and garnering external support for parents. The multilevel nature of our intervention draws upon ecodevelopmental theory (Szapocznik & Coatsworth, 1999), which proposes that risk and protective processes operating at varying systemic levels compound one another to create an overall profile of risk and protection. By promoting protective factors within the family and between the family and other important systems, our integrative prevention program represents an attempt to address risks at multiple systemic levels and to prevent those risks from compounding one another."

So, as this example demonstrates, it is usually possible to give both reviewers some of what they are asking for—which will increase the chances of both reviewers' endorsing publication when you resubmit. Remember that you do not want any of the reviewers to feel left out, ignored, or disregarded by your responses. Always assume that the action editor is going to send your revised manuscript back to the reviewers when you resubmit. If the editor chooses to render a final decision without consulting the reviewers again, consider yourself lucky. That doesn't happen very often. Some journals mandate sending revised manuscripts back out for a second round of review—and some passive editors will keep sending revised papers back to reviewers repeatedly until all reviewers are completely satisfied.

Revising Based on Editorial Style

Remember the four editorial styles—the passive editor, the interpreter, the extra reviewer, and the meddler. If you are dealing with a passive editor or an interpreter, you should plan that your revised manuscript will be sent out for review again and again until all of the reviewers have recommended acceptance. I remember a paper that Byron Zamboanga and I wrote with one of our colleagues several years ago. The action editor provisionally accepted our manuscript for publication on the second round of review, and we then proceeded to make all the changes that the reviewers requested. When we resubmitted, the editor sent our paper out for review again, although she had already granted us a provisional acceptance! In the article we published a couple of years later (Schwartz & Zamboanga, 2009), Byron and I called on editors to take control of the editorial process and to render a decision, rather than ceding control of the process to reviewers. Nonetheless, when you are dealing with a passive editor, you must respond adequately to every reviewer comment.

Editors adopting the extra-reviewer or meddler styles may be more likely to take control of the process after the first or second round of review. I remember one editor whose responses to my coauthor's and my manuscript became more and more negative as the reviewers expressed increasing satisfaction with our revisions. This editor was clearly a meddler. When we revised and resubmitted following the second round of review, the editor sent our revision to a "trusted advisor" who looked over the previous reviewer comments and our responses and recommended publication. The trusted advisor's review stated that "This manuscript has gone through a process of review, revision, review, and revision. The authors have pretty much complied with all the requests made. As a result, I am recommending publication."

This editor was ideologically opposed to the argument that we were advancing in our manuscript—even though our argument was supported by our data. I have never seen another editor send a paper to a trusted advisor to verify that the authors had complied with all the editor and reviewer requests. I can only speculate that the editor's philosophical disagreement with our position led her not to want to accept our paper on her own, so she brought someone else in to make the decision for her. This approach clearly reflects a meddling style—this editor essentially overruled the reviewers, who became more enthusiastic about our work after we resubmitted—and she was willing to accept our manuscript for publication only after her trusted advisor recommended acceptance.

Understanding the type of editor who is handling your paper is a critical part of crafting your response letter. As our experience with the meddling editor and her trusted advisor suggests, when you are dealing with a meddler editorial style, the editor's comments are paramount to address, and if there are any points of conflict between the editor's and reviewers' requests, the editor's requests should be prioritized. The extra-reviewer style is generally more balanced than the meddler style is, suggesting that the editor and reviewer comments should be weighted equally. There is no style where the reviewer feedback is disregarded entirely, but reviewer feedback is weighted most strongly for passive editors and interpreters, somewhat less strongly for extra reviewers, and least strongly for meddlers.

Making Revisions Fit With Existing Text

Inserting or modifying text in response to reviewer requests will likely disrupt the flow of text in the manuscript. Revisions may also create redundancies in the paper, especially when the text you draft in response to reviewer comments repeats some of the points from the original version of the manuscript. You may also find that revisions made later in the paper may become unjustified statements if the ideas introduced in the new text weren't set up earlier in the manuscript. So, the editing principles outlined in Chapter 9 will likely need to be revisited as part of the revision process. Some "smoothing over" will be necessary to make the paper flow and read well again.

Importantly, when you draft new text in response to reviewer requests, the paper must continue to speak with your voice. The reader should not be able to tell which parts of the paper were part of your original submission and which parts were inserted or modified in response to reviewers. Furthermore, the paper should not read defensively—as Al Waterman told me once, readers will have no idea what you are defending yourself against. Remember that readers will not see the response letter—all they will see is the paper itself— so all statements in the paper should be assertive rather than defensive. Even when you mention limitations, I suggest you do so assertively—for example, "One key limitation is that we did not ask participants what kind of work they performed for a living." Such a statement is preferable to "We do not believe that asking parents about their work is important." As Al noted, the reader would have no idea why such a defensive statement was included in the article.

A final point involves the journal's space limit. Reviewers often ask for additional details that will cause the manuscript to exceed the journal's space limit. As already noted, my practice is to draft responses that are complete but pithy—that is, covering all the points I think need to be covered, but as briefly as possible. I generally draft the text without worrying about the journal's space limit, and once I'm done revising, I check to see how far we are over the space limit. If I can cut length to bring the manuscript back below the space limit, I do that—and if the paper is still over the limit, I will then reach out to the action editor and ask for more space. Generally, the most I've been able to request successfully has been 500 extra words or two to three additional pages. (Some editors genuinely don't care about space limits for revised manuscripts, but you need to ask permission before you submit a revised manuscript that exceeds the space limit. The editorial assistant may not pass the submission to the editor unless you can document that you have permission to exceed the limit.)

Choosing Not to Revise

Occasionally, authors will run into situations where they are simply not able to address the reviewer comments, and rather than trying to revise and resubmit for the current journal, they either decide to submit elsewhere or to discard the paper entirely. Sometimes, the reviewers want to take the paper in a direction that the authors don't agree with, or sometimes the authors conclude that they cannot fulfill the reviewers' requests. If you believe that you cannot satisfy the reviewer requests, it might be best to submit elsewhere. The time required to revise the manuscript may not be well spent if the likely outcome is rejection after you resubmit.

A colleague and I ran into this situation in 2019. We had submitted a manuscript to an educational psychology journal, and the editor invited us to revise and resubmit the paper. However, the reviewers were asking us to reanalyze the data in ways we were not comfortable with. The new analyses would have completely changed the message of our paper, and the message that the reviewers wanted us to convey was not the message that we wanted to send. So we decided to submit the paper to a different journal, and the paper was ultimately accepted for publication in that journal.

Making Sure You Speak With Your Own Voice

When I was revising a manuscript in late 2009 and early 2010, I was having trouble with some of the reviewer comments. The reviewers were asking me to take the paper in a different direction than I had planned, and I wasn't sure what to do. I emailed my coauthors, including José. His response was exactly what I needed to hear—he told me that I was allowing the reviewers to lead the revision process rather than using their comments to guide me in revising the paper using my own voice. José's response reminded me of Ed Diener's (2006) opening editorial for *Perspectives on Psychological Science*, where Diener outlined an editorial policy that reviewers would not be consulted repeatedly and that, after the first round of review, the author and editor would work directly together to develop the final version of the paper.

Even if other editors don't follow Diener's approach, authors still have room to inject their own style and voice into their responses to reviewer comments. Reviewer comments are generally broad—for example, reviewers will say that the arguments in the introduction need to be clarified, but the content of that clarification is determined by the author. A good reviewer makes suggestions but doesn't give orders—reviewers are essentially consultants who help editors decide which papers to pursue for publication, and when revise-resubmit decisions are issued, reviewers help authors to strengthen, streamline, and clarify their manuscripts. Remember that it's acceptable for authors to push back against reviewer requests as long as their reasoning for doing so is thoughtful and empirically (or theoretically) based. Providing a well-thought-out, comprehensive reason for not making a requested change will, in most cases, be palatable to reviewers. (Of course, there are exceptions—some reviewers will insist that their requested changes be incorporated into the paper.) Giving reviewers at least some of what they are asking for will usually satisfy them unless they have strong feelings and preferences about their requests.

What reviewers often find troubling is when authors don't respond to their requests. I recall a manuscript that I reviewed many years ago. The author responded defensively (or didn't really respond at all) to many of my and the other reviewer's requests. The revised manuscript wasn't all that different from the original version, despite our requests for major revisions. The other reviewer and I both recommended rejection, and the editor rejected the revised manuscript. Had the author of that revised manuscript taken our suggestions into account and considered them seriously, his paper would probably have been published in that journal—even if he had pushed back against some of what we were asking him to do. Pushing back thoughtfully and meeting reviewers "in the middle" is quite different from simply blowing off reviewer requests.

The Second Round of Review

When you are finished revising the paper, and once your coauthors have signed off on the revision and agreed that it's ready to resubmit, then you need to go back to the journal's manuscript submission site and submit the revised manuscript. (Of course, your revised paper and response letter should be shared with your coauthors for their review and approval before you resubmit.) The resubmission process is almost exactly like the original submission process, except that you also have to upload your response letter. The response letter should be formally addressed to the action editor, much like the cover letter for the original submission. The cover page—which should appear on your professional letterhead—is usually "short and sweet," and is followed by the response letter that you crafted while you were revising the manuscript. Here is a sample cover letter I have used with a revised manuscript:

January 28, 2020

Linda G. Castillo, Ph.D.
Associate Editor, *Journal of Clinical Psychology*
Department of Educational
Psychology Texas A&M University
801 Harrington Tower
College Station, TX 77843

Dear Dr. Castillo:

Thank you so much for inviting us to revise and resubmit our manuscript JCLP-19-028, "Toward a Micro-Level Perspective on Acculturation among Hispanic College Students: A Daily Diary Study," for publication in the *Journal of Clinical Psychology*.

The reviewers' comments have truly helped us to improve and strengthen our paper, and we are grateful to them and to you.

In the pages that follow, we list each reviewer comment in italics, followed by a narrative description of the revisions that we have made to the manuscript in response to the comment. Where applicable, we also include the exact text added or modified in response to the comment.

We hope you will find our revised manuscript acceptable for publication in the *Journal of Clinical Psychology*.

Sincerely yours,

Seth J. Schwartz, Ph.D.
Professor

Another important step is to be sure that all the page number references in the response letter match where the text appears in the manuscript. When I'm ready to resubmit, I go to the response letter, search for the bold x's I put in place of the page numbers and replace them with the correct page numbers from the final version of the revised manuscript. It is essential that you do this before you resubmit.

Many of the manuscript submission sites I have encountered over the last few years—Editorial Manager, ScholarOne, and EVISE—require authors both to upload the cover letter as a word processing document and to copy and paste the cover letter into a text box. The formatting will be lost when the text is pasted into the text box, so be sure to indent paragraphs manually in the text box. If you have tables in the response letter, you will have to reformat them manually using spaces so that the numbers or words line up correctly in each table.

If you have added coauthors during the revision process, make sure that their names are listed on the authorship, both on the title page and on the manuscript submission site. You may have added a statistical colleague to help you respond to requests for new analyses, or you may have added someone with expertise in specific theories that reviewers asked you to cite or acknowledge. The point is that anyone who was added to the authorship needs to be listed when you resubmit.

On the File Upload page on the manuscript submission site, you should remove the files from your original submission and replace them with the files from your revised manuscript. If the title page hasn't changed (i.e., the title is still the same and you have not added or removed anyone from the authorship), then you can leave the title page from your original submission. However, I suggest deleting the tables and figures from your original submission and replacing them with the tables and figures from your revised paper.

Even if you haven't changed some of the tables or figures, you may have added or deleted tables or figures—which would cause at least some of the existing tables or figures to be renumbered. You don't want to confuse reviewers by having two tables labeled Table 3, or by referring to Table 2 in the text when you really mean Table 4. These small details are important to attend to and to resolve before you resubmit. Removing existing tables and uploading new ones is akin to the old saying, "Better safe than sorry."

If you are uploading the entire manuscript (without the title page) as a single file, then make sure that the tables and figures are numbered consecutively both where they are referred to in the text and where they appear at the end of the manuscript. In addition, you should double-check that the callout for each table and figure in the text matches the correct table or figure in the manuscript. Again, if you refer to Table 3 in the text, make sure that you are referring to the Table 3 supplied at the end of the manuscript.

Also remember to review the PDF proof carefully before you click the Submit button. Make sure that your cover letter appears exactly as you want it to appear, and that all the manuscript files are correct. The PDF proof is what the editor and reviewers will see. The last thing you want is for the editor or reviewers to be confused by something that is missing from, or out of place in, the PDF. As already noted, I have caught many errors in PDFs when I was submitting or resubmitting. If you spot an error, you need to go back to the word-processing files, correct the error, and re-upload the manuscript file(s) where you made changes.

Once you have resubmitted, an email will be sent to you and each of your coauthors confirming the resubmission. After that, you just have to wait to receive a decision letter on your revised manuscript. As noted, most action editors will send revised manuscripts back out for review. In some cases, editors will want the original reviewers to "sign off" on the changes you have made in response to their comments. In other cases, editors will also invite new reviewers to comment on your revised manuscript. In my estimation, bringing in new reviewers on the second round of review is fundamentally unfair and forces authors to "shoot at a moving target." New reviewers may bring up issues that were not raised in the first round of review, and they may try to take the paper in a different direction than what you intended. Especially if the action editor adopts a passive approach, the editorial process can start to feel like a roller coaster ride.

Several years ago, a former PhD student and I coauthored a paper on adolescent sexual behavior. The editor invited us to revise and resubmit, and we addressed all the reviewer comments. On the second round of review, however, the editor sent our revised manuscript to two new reviewers, who asked for completely different changes than had been requested on the first round (neither of the original reviewers reviewed our revised paper). Again, we made all the requested changes and resubmitted—and again the editor brought in two new reviewers. The editor did this twice more before we finally wrote him a polite but firm email asking why he continued to invite new reviewers rather than asking the reviewers from the previous round to re-evaluate our paper. He never answered our email, but the next time we resubmitted, he accepted our revised manuscript for publication.

If you are an active scholar and are submitting manuscripts to journals often, you will experience many different types of editors and editorial processes. You will be able to collect and recount stories similar to those that I present in this book. Two of the lessons I have learned from my publishing experience are that (a) no paper can be counted as "accepted" until the editor uses the word *accept* in an editorial letter and (b) it's always safest to assume that a revised manuscript is being sent back to reviewers unless the action editor tells you otherwise (e.g., "I will handle your revised manuscript myself and will not send it back out for review"). You may be pleasantly surprised with a provisional or final acceptance letter when you were not expecting one, but wait until you receive at least a provisional acceptance before you add a paper to your curriculum vitae.

Sometimes a thorough and comprehensive response letter can convince an editor to accept your paper without sending it back out for review. When Jennifer Unger, Byron Zamboanga, José, and I resubmitted our manuscript to the *American Psychologist* in January 2010, we expected the action editor to send our paper back out for review. She had indicated in her original editorial letter that she was going to send our revision back to the reviewers. However, less than a week after we resubmitted, she sent us an acceptance letter. She explicitly acknowledged that our thorough response letter (22 pages long) had convinced her that we had responded appropriately to the reviews. I was very surprised that our manuscript was accepted for publication in the APA's flagship journal after only one full round of review. (I do not expect that to happen again, but it was a wonderful surprise.)

Asking for Extensions to Resubmission Deadlines

In many cases, when an action editor invites you to revise and resubmit a manuscript, the decision letter will specify a date by which your revised manuscript is due. In most cases, you should try your best to resubmit your manuscript before that deadline. If you know that you will be delayed beyond that date, contact the journal's editorial assistant (and copy the action editor on this communication), letting them know when you anticipate being able to deliver your revised manuscript. Provide a reason for the delay if you can—unless doing so would divulge someone's private information (e.g., if one of your coauthors is going through a divorce, you might just tell the editorial assistant and action editor that members of your research team are facing personal challenges).

In my experience, action editors are generally willing to grant the first request to extend the resubmission deadline, as long as you don't request more than an extra month or two. Requests for a second extension may be less likely to be granted—I remember one editor who told me that he needed to keep manuscripts moving along within the editorial process, and if I could not resubmit within a month of the originally proposed deadline, I would have to resubmit my paper as a new manuscript. In most cases, however, editors will give you between 1 and 3 months to complete your revision.

Outcomes of the Second Round of Review

The outcomes I have received and observed on the second round of review include final acceptance, provisional acceptance, a second revise–resubmit decision, and outright rejection. In some cases, reviewers will read over your revised manuscript and response letter, conclude that you have addressed all their concerns, and recommend acceptance. This has happened several times in my publishing career. More likely, however, reviewers will be largely satisfied with your responses but will provide a few remaining concerns. Depending on the volume and magnitude of the concerns, the action editor will likely offer either a provisional acceptance or a second revise–resubmit. The key difference is that a provisional acceptance is granted when the requested revisions are minor and the editor plans to handle the revised manuscript rather than send it back out for review again. (However, remember my experience when a passive editor granted us a provisional acceptance but still sent our revised manuscript back out for review.) A second revise–resubmit generally involves more extensive changes and the likelihood that the revised manuscript will receive a third round of review. In either case, my usual practice is to follow the same revision procedures that are outlined earlier in this chapter.

The final possibility is that your revised manuscript is rejected. Even with my highly responsive style, I have still had revised manuscripts rejected. In general, this has happened when a reviewer didn't like our original manuscript, but the editor invited us to revise and resubmit, and the reviewer didn't "budge" despite our attempts to be as responsive as possible to that person's concerns. I can remember two occasions on which that happened. On the first occasion, the action editor invited three reviewers to comment on our original manuscript. Two of the reviewers recommended that we be invited to revise and resubmit, whereas the third reviewer was extremely critical. We did our best to respond to all three reviewers, but the action editor sent our revised manuscript to only the most critical reviewer—who was unmoved by our responses and recommended rejection. The review stated, "My concerns from the previous round of review still stand, and despite the authors' attempts to revise the manuscript, the major issues I raised in my initial review have not been addressed."

Many of the comments that this critical reviewer raised were speculative—such as citing a 20-year-old review article claiming that personal identity should not be examined in youth under age 17. (Many other sources, some of which we cited, have contradicted the claim that the reviewer cited.) However, in situations like this, the best—and often only—course of action is to start over again with another journal.

The other scenario involved a journal that allows only two rounds of review—meaning that, if reviewers provide more than superficial comments on the second round of review, the revised manuscript is rejected. This was the scenario that happened to us. Two of the three reviewers were satisfied with our revisions, but the third reviewer provided some substantive (but addressable) comments on the second round. The editor proceeded to reject our revised submission—and he was not willing to reconsider that decision when I appealed it. Again, our only option was to submit the paper to another journal.

In my experience, revised manuscripts are most likely to be rejected when the initial revise–resubmit decision was *pessimistic* (some journals use this term in decision letters). A pessimistic revise–resubmit is an editorial decision that could easily have been a rejection, but the editor decided to give the authors a chance. In these cases, there is often one reviewer who was strongly critical of the manuscript and at least one reviewer whose evaluation was more positive—and, especially when the action editor adopts a passive approach, eventual acceptance appears to be conditioned on satisfying the more critical reviewer. I have seen cases where the critical reviewer was persuaded by the authors' responses and revisions, as well as cases where the critical reviewer was unmoved by the revisions. Some reviewers are fairly rigid in their evaluation of manuscripts, where there is only a small range of approaches that they are willing to endorse for publication. Unfortunately, you probably will not know whether such a reviewer is evaluating your paper until after your revised manuscript is rejected. Such reviewers may not be persuaded by even the most accommodating revisions. So, in essence, a pessimistic revise–resubmit may, in some cases, be a trap. It's up to individual authors to decide whether a pessimistic revise–resubmit looks like a trap. Just as my colleague and I decided not to revise and resubmit to the journal where the reviewer requests were not consistent with our objectives, you can make a similar decision with your manuscript. The key questions to ask when you receive a pessimistic revise–resubmit are: Can we address these concerns successfully? Will doing so take our paper in a direction in which we don't really want to go? Is the critical reviewer making reasonable points, or do the disagreements seem ideological and idiosyncratic? The answers to these questions should be decided by the authorship team.

Of course, having revised manuscripts rejected is extremely frustrating and disheartening because of the amount of time and effort that the authors have invested in the journal that rejected the paper. You essentially have to start over with a new submission to a new journal—which will involve a new set of reviewer comments. Given how idiosyncratic reviewers can be, it is certainly not guaranteed that being invited to revise and resubmit for one journal will predict receiving a similar invitation from another journal.

Once you are past the initial anger and disappointment about the rejection, you should reassess the paper and examine the reviewer and editor comments carefully. Do the reviewers and the editor raise valid points? To what extent are the comments idiosyncratic, representing reviewers' own preferences—and to what extent will reviewers for another journal raise similar issues? You may not know the answer after only one set of reviews, but you and your coauthors should venture a guess. If you can use the reviews to improve the manuscript, you should do so.

As is discussed in Chapter 13, there is also the possibility of appealing the rejection decision. Appeals are a low-yield strategy, because most editors are not willing to reconsider their decisions, but if they are, there may be specific ways to frame the argument so that the editor will be most likely to give the appeal serious consideration. Keep in mind that appeals are most likely to be successful when the decision was a close call and could have gone either way. If your revised manuscript was soundly rejected—that is, the reviewers and editor were primarily negative in their assessments—you may not have much of a case for an appeal.

Provisional Acceptance

If your revision elicits only minor reviewer comments—or if the editor decides that the next version of your manuscript doesn't need to go out for review—the editor will likely provisionally accept your manuscript for publication. Broadly, a provisional acceptance indicates that, as long as you address the remaining editor and reviewer comments, the editor will accept your paper and send it to production.

A provisional acceptance is obviously good news—and it's time to add the paper to your curriculum vitae as soon as you're finished revising. The primary caution at this stage is that this is likely your last chance to make major changes to the paper. Once the manuscript is accepted and sent to production, further changes are usually limited to minor corrections (e.g., correcting typographical errors, inserting words into a sentence, updating in-press citations that have been published). You and your coauthors should read carefully through the paper and make any changes that you think need to be made. Once you resubmit the paper, it will likely be accepted and sent to production.

Note, however, that assistant and associate editors' ability to accept manuscripts differs across journals. For most APA journals, as well as many other journals, action editors can provide an acceptance letter and send manuscripts directly to production. For other journals, however, assistant and associate editors offer recommendations to the editor-in-chief, who then renders a final decision. So, action editors can recommend acceptance, but the editor-in-chief is the only one who can formally accept a paper for publication.

In most cases, the editor-in-chief "rubber-stamps" the action editor's recommendation and accepts the manuscript. However, I submitted two papers to a journal where the editor-in-chief was well known for making additional requests even after the associate editor had recommended acceptance. In an email, the associate editor told me that the editor-in chief often "gets in a few good zingers before accepting a final version." I saw that firsthand—the editor-in-chief caught some statistical mistakes we had made, and he then sent our revised manuscript out for another round of review before he finally accepted it for publication. At one point, the editor-in-chief told us that he would be "forced to reject" our manuscript if the errors were not corrected. So having an assistant or associate editor recommend a manuscript for publication doesn't necessarily mean that the editorial process is completed.

After Acceptance

Once your manuscript has been accepted for publication, the editor will send it to the publisher for typesetting and production. Within a couple of months of acceptance, you will receive proofs from the publisher. You will be asked to check the proofs for errors (you will not be able to make any changes to the article after you have returned the proofs to the publisher) and to answer queries from the copy editor. Copy editors' queries often include entries missing from the reference list, references that are listed but not cited in the text, author affiliations, unclear sentences, and numbers that don't match between tables and text. Be sure to answer all the queries—if you don't, then your article will be published with errors.

Errata and Corrigenda

Once the article appears online, no further corrections can be made. If you catch an error after your article is already online, you should contact the editor. If the editor decides that the mistake is important enough to correct officially, then the most likely step will be to publish an erratum or corrigendum. Errata and corrigenda are short (usually only a couple of lines) and simply list the corrections being made to a previously published article. A link is usually then added to the webpage for the additional article letting readers know that an erratum or corrigendum has been published.

Retractions

If you discover a major error in a published article, then you should contact the editor and request a retraction. Retraction essentially involves "de-publishing" an article. Although the original article still appears online, the word *RETRACTED* will appear on the article website—alerting readers not to read or trust the article. Retracted articles are embarrassing for authors, and once an article has been retracted, editors may not trust that author's work (Kuroki & Ukawa, 2018). Kuroki and Ukawa document that retraction is often utilized in response to scientific misconduct.

Sometimes, informal retractions are used when honest mistakes are discovered after an article has been published. Miller, Fan, Christiansen, Grotevant, and van Dulmen (2000) used a national data set to examine differences in behavioral outcomes between adopted and non-adopted adolescents. They later discovered that a group of adolescents appeared to have labeled themselves falsely as adoptees and to have provided extreme scores on behavior problem variables. This author group published a second article (Fan, Miller, Christiansen, Park, Grotevant, & van Dulmen, 2002), in a different journal, excluding these adolescents from analysis. Unlike the original article, the second article reported few significant differences between adopted and non-adopted adolescents. In this case, the second article was not a formal retraction, and no notice appears on the webpage for the original article informing readers about the irregularities in the data set. Although the error was not the authors' fault, it would be much more helpful to readers if a link to the second article were to appear on the webpage for the first article.

Copyright Issues

Academic social media sites like ResearchGate and Academia.edu enable scholars to share their work with other scholars around the world. These platforms allow authors to post abstracts of their articles and to upload full-text versions of the articles that other scholars can download. Many other scholars maintain personal websites where they post full-text copies of their published articles. Although posting articles allows for widespread sharing of scholarly information, such posting may violate copyright laws. In 2018, Elsevier, one of the largest academic publishers in the world, sued ResearchGate for copyright infringement (Else, 2018). Most copyright agreements allow authors to post the final accepted manuscript version of their article, but not the final typeset version, online. Authors are, however, allowed to email copies of published articles to others upon request. So, overall, if someone asks you for a copy of your article, you are allowed to send it to them—but you cannot post the final published copy online.

Conclusion

This chapter reviews the journal publication process from start to finish—from uploading the manuscript onto a journal submission site to final acceptance, checking proofs, and correcting errors that are identified after the article is published. It covers how editors assign action editors and reviewers, how action editors make decisions on manuscripts, and how to respond most effectively to reviewer comments. It discusses ways to push back against reviewer requests without blowing off the reviewer, as well as the importance of the response letter in helping the editor and reviewers to identify and appreciate the revisions the authors have made to the manuscript. It mentions why editors might choose to reject revised manuscripts and about some ways to avoid such an outcome.

Summary

- The review process starts with manuscript submission sites.
- It is essential for authors to read the target journal's instructions to authors.
- Editors often use manuscript keywords to select reviewers.
- Editors often desk-reject manuscripts that are outside the journal's scope or that they do not believe are competitive for publication.
- In most cases, initial editorial decisions (following peer review) include revise–resubmit, rejection with recommendation to resubmit, and outright rejection. Outright or conditional acceptance is rare on the first round of review.
- Editors can be classified into four general styles, and each style requires somewhat different types of author responses when revising manuscripts.
- The response letter is a critical component of convincing editors and reviewers that a manuscript is ready to be accepted for publication.
- Responses to reviewer comments should be respectful and comprehensive. Even if the authors choose not to comply with the reviewer request, they must fully respond to the request. Reviewer comments should never be ignored.
- The response letter can be started by copying the editor and reviewer comments and pasting them into a word-processing document. Responses to each comment will then be added.
- Comments should be prioritized by the magnitude of the revisions requested (major, moderate, minor). Requests for major revisions (especially new analyses) should be addressed first.
- The response letter can be used to report information that authors do not wish to put into their manuscript (especially results of analyses that the authors see as tangential).

References

American Psychological Association. (2011). Summary report of journal operations, 2010. *American Psychologist, 66*, 405–406.

American Psychological Association. (2020). Summary report of journal operations, 2019. *American Psychologist, 75*, 723–724.

Carnegie, D. (1936). *How to win friends and influence people.* New York: Pocket Books.

Craig, J. B. (2010). Desk rejection: How to avoid being hit by a returning boomerang. *Family Business Review, 23*, 306–309.

Diener, E. (2006). Editorial. *Perspectives on Psychological Science, 1*, 1–4.

Else, H. (2018. October 5). Major publishers sue ResearchGate over copyright infringement. Retrieved from https://www.nature.com/articles/d41586-018-06945-6#:~:text=Two%20journal%20publishers%20have%20launched,in%20their%20journals%20freely%20available

Fan, X., Miller, B. C., Christiansen, M., Park, K. E., Grotevant, H. D., & van Dulmen, M. (2002). Questionnaire and interview inconsistencies exaggerated differences between adopted and non-adopted adolescents in a national sample. *Adoption Quarterly, 7*(2), 7–27.

Hardré, P. L. (2013). The power and strategic art of revise-and-resubmit: Maintaining balance in academic publishing. *Journal of Faculty Development, 27*, 13–19.

Kerr, N. L. (1998). HARKing: Hypothesizing after the results are known. *Personality and Social Psychology Review, 2*, 196–217.

Kravitz, R. L., Franks, P., Feldman, M. D., Gerrity, M., Byrne, C., & Tierney, W. M. (2010). Editorial peer reviewers' recommendations at a general medical journal: Are they reliable and do editors care? *PLOS One, 5*, Article e10072.

Kuroki, T., & Ukawa, A. (2018). Repeating probability of authors with retracted scientific publications. *Accountability in Research, 25*, 212–219.

Miller, B. C., Fan, X., Christiansen, M., Grotevant, H. D., & van Dulmen, M. (2000). Comparisons of adopted and nonadopted adolescents in a large, nationally representative sample. *Child Development, 71*, 1458–1473.

Resnik, D. B., Gutierrez-Ford, C., & Peddada, S. (2008). Perceptions of ethical problems with scientific journal peer review: An exploratory study. *Science and Engineering Ethics, 14*, 305–310.

Schwartz, S. J., & Zamboanga, B. L. (2009). The peer-review and editorial system: Ways to fix something that might be broken. *Perspectives on Psychological Science, 4*, 54–61.

Wager, E., Parkin, E. C., & Tamber, P. S. (2006). Are reviewers suggested by authors as good as those chosen by editors? Results of a rater-blinded, retrospective study. *BMC Medicine, 4*, Article 13.

Waterman, A. S. (2008). Reconsidering happiness: A eudaimonist's perspective. *Journal of Positive Psychology, 3*, 234–252.

13
What to Do With Rejected Manuscripts

By the time you finish reading this chapter, you should feel more comfortable with:

- Incorporating reviewer comments into rejected manuscripts and submitting elsewhere
- Appealing rejection decisions
- Options to consider when a manuscript is rejected repeatedly
- Deciding when to dump a paper into a low-prestige journal or drop it entirely

All authors—from undergraduate students to full professors—will find themselves in the unenviable position of having manuscripts rejected by journals. The question is therefore not whether you will have papers rejected, but rather what you will do with those papers after they are rejected. As mentioned in Chapter 11, more than half of all published articles were rejected at least once before they were accepted by the journal in which they appear. Some of the articles I'm proudest of were rejected by other journals, and some were previously rejected by the journal that eventually accepted them. In my career, I've had only a handful of papers—no more than 10—that my coauthors and I eventually dropped because we were not able to get them accepted in scholarly journals. In other words, persistence pays off in scholarly publishing.

As stated in Chapter 12, there are two broad types of manuscript rejections—easy rejections and close calls. Easy rejections are those where the reviews are unanimously negative. The most logical next step for authors following an easy rejection is to read the reviews carefully, to make whatever changes are possible based on the editor and reviewer comments, and to submit the manuscript to another journal.

Close-call rejections present a somewhat different scenario. At least one reviewer was positively inclined toward the paper. In these cases, appealing the decision may be an option, and it may also be worth asking the editor whether submitting a new manuscript that addresses the reviewer and editor comments is an option.

The Savvy Academic. Seth J. Schwartz, Oxford University Press. © Oxford University Press 2022.
DOI: 10.1093/oso/9780190095918.003.0014

There are also manuscripts that seem to be "cursed"—that is, they have been rejected by several journals, and no matter what you do, the paper keeps getting rejected. Al Waterman and I had a paper like this—it was rejected three times before finally being accepted in a fourth journal. After the third rejection, I remember Al telling me in an email that "all we need is the right editor in the right mood—eventually." So, there is the question of how long to keep trying with a cursed manuscript—especially if reviewers keep pointing out the same flaws repeatedly. At what point do you simply dump the paper into a low-prestige journal, or drop the paper altogether?

So, this chapter covers three primary issues: revising papers that were soundly rejected and submitting them to a new journal, appealing close-call rejection decisions, and what to do with cursed manuscripts that have been repeatedly rejected.

Revising Rejected Manuscripts for a New Journal

In most cases, even the most negative reviewer comments offer some suggestions for how to revise, recast, or even repackage the manuscript for submission to another journal. Reviewers may have "slammed" you for not controlling for an important covariate, or they may have taken issue with the theoretical approach you adopted, or they may not have liked your experimental design. Reviewers can recommend rejection for any number of reasons, including fatal flaws, fundamental disagreements, and idiosyncratic preferences. Fatal flaws are problems with the research methodology that cannot be addressed through reanalysis or through textual revisions—and these flaws generally lead reviewers to recommend rejection (Lovejoy, Revenson, & France, 2011). Fundamental disagreements are philosophical differences between authors and reviewers, such as inclinations toward or against specific theoretical perspectives or methodological approaches. Idiosyncratic preferences are a specific reviewer's beliefs that may or may not be based on empirical evidence. Some reviewers' idiosyncratic preferences can be so resistant to change that even the most accommodating revisions will not satisfy them.

Generally, the best you can do with fatal flaws is to acknowledge them as limitations and drop down to a lower status journal than the one that rejected your paper previously. Failing to measure an important covariate, or not randomizing participants to conditions, or not measuring outcome variables at all time points, is a clear design flaw and will not permit a full and rigorous test of the study hypotheses. Low-prestige journals, and some moderate-prestige journals, may have more tolerance for these flaws if they are listed as limitations.

Some fatal flaws have to do with the combination of design and analytic considerations. For example, tests of mediation—where variable A is hypothesized to predict or cause variable C through variable B—require longitudinal or experimental designs (O'Laughlin, Martin, & Ferrer, 2018). Cross-sectional tests of mediation are likely to yield biased estimates of mediated effects because earlier levels of mediating and outcome variables cannot be statistically controlled (Maxwell & Cole, 2007). For this reason, cross-sectional studies testing mediational hypotheses must be framed as exploratory or speculative, and some reviewers and editors are not willing to endorse or accept manuscripts reporting cross-sectional tests of mediation. Spector (2019) provides recommendations for writing manuscripts based on cross-sectional data.

So how do you plan the recasting and revision of a rejected manuscript for another journal? Several years ago, José gave me a terrific idea—to draft a response letter as though I were revising the paper, and then to use the responses as a roadmap for recasting the paper. Here is an example of a reviewer comment (in italics) and a draft response:

You need to justify your comparison of African American and Latino (Hispanic) youth. I would expect more specific hypotheses about ethnically related patterns of association among your study variables, and an explanation of the cultural basis for these hypotheses. Below I suggest some references on which to base hypotheses. In short, the study remains seriously underconceptualized, relying upon a general framework that does not address the specific dynamics that you intend to examine.

Response: We now include only Hispanics in our study. We agree that including two ethnic groups introduces a degree of complexity that is not warranted.

In the family microsystem, Hispanics would be expected to report elevated levels of conflict because of differences in acculturation. In the peer domain, we now specify that Hispanics would likely have more problems because their parents may not understand the need to monitor effectively (cf. Coatsworth, Pantin, & Szapocznik, 2002; Pantin, Schwartz, Sullivan, Coatsworth, & Szapocznik, 2003). In the school domain, Hispanics have the highest dropout rates of any American ethnic group (American Council on Education, 2002). Therefore, we now specify that school disinterest would be elevated for Hispanics.

These differences would translate into clear hypotheses for the study: negative ecodevelopmental processes would be positively associated with internalizing and externalizing problems, whereas positive ecodevelopmental processes would be less strongly associated.

Regarding self-concept, we would expect that it would contribute significantly to both internalizing and externalizing problems over and above the contributions of ecodevelopmental variables.

Although we were not revising and resubmitting for that same journal, we wanted to glean whatever insights we could from the reviews and to use those insights to improve the paper before submitting it to another journal. As Stivers and Cramer (2017) note, ignoring the reviews you just received from reviewers is not wise, because reviewers for another journal may well bring up some of the same points that the previous reviewers raised. It's possible that a prior reviewer may even be invited to review the paper again when you submit to a new journal. In most cases that I have seen, reviewers will decline the invitation to review a paper that they have already reviewed for another journal—but we do not know whether all reviewers would decline. Simply put, taking reviewer feedback seriously is generally a smart decision.

There may be some idiosyncratic comments, however, that you and your coauthors decide not to address. Because you are not going back to the same journal when you submit next, you can choose which comments to address and which comments to ignore. Generally, you need to decide which suggested revisions would help improve the manuscript and to incorporate them. Fatal flaws that prior reviewers pointed out should be listed as limitations in the new version that you submit to the next journal.

It's possible that you may not find any of the reviewer comments to be particularly useful as you prepare to submit to the next journal. Al Waterman and I had this experience once—the reviewers simply didn't like our theoretical approach and were not interested in the work we were reporting. There were no criticisms of our methods or analyses—the reviewers just did not resonate with the study and the manuscript. When Al and I spoke over the phone to debrief and to plan our next move, we decided that none of the reviewer comments would be helpful in improving the paper. We reread the manuscript carefully, made some cosmetic changes, and submitted to the next journal.

In terms of choosing journals, as is recommended in Chapter 10, you may have created a list of target journals for your manuscript and rank-ordered them from first choice to last choice. In most cases, the highest-prestige journals on your list will be listed first, and the prestige level will decrease as you go down the list. A simple method for choosing the next journal is simply to move to the next journal on your list—as long as the reviewer feedback that you received does not contraindicate submitting to that next journal. For example, if reviewers criticized you for examining mediation using cross-sectional data, you might not want to submit to another journal where you will be similarly criticized for this design and analytic approach. If you were criticized for your method of randomizing cases to conditions or for your method of delivering your intervention, then you should probably avoid journals where reviewers are likely to provide similar criticisms. You can look in recent issues of your target journals to get a sense of the kinds of design and analytic choices that the journal is likely to publish.

When you do decide on your next journal, be sure to consult the instructions to authors. The new journal may have a shorter (or more generous) space limit, may use a different citation style, and may have other preferences that you should know about. Journals may prefer specific types of papers—such as qualitative research, experimental studies, or randomized trials. Some journals expressly encourage or prohibit specific types of statistical analyses—such as *Basic and Applied Social Psychology*'s ban on all use of *p*-values and confidence intervals (Fricker, Burke, Han, & Woodall, 2019). Some journals, such as *Psychological Review*, accept only theoretical manuscripts (American Psychological Association, n.d.-a), and some, such as *Psychological Bulletin*, prefer literature reviews and meta-analyses (American Psychological Association, n.d.-b). Don't blindly submit to a new journal without examining what that journal is looking for. Importantly, do not include any information suggesting that your paper has been submitted to (and rejected by) another journal prior to being submitted to the current journal.

I want to reiterate that having manuscripts rejected is part of being an active scholar, and that often the most effective strategy is to make whatever revisions are possible based on the reviews you received and to submit elsewhere. Deciding where to submit next, however, should be a thoughtful and reasoned decision. Remember that a round of review normally takes 3 to 4 months on average. Impulsively submitting without making changes and reviewing the new journal's preferences will likely lead to another rejection. If you have a strong sense that the flaws that the previous reviewers pointed out may be raised again if you submit to a journal with a similar level of prestige, then the most advisable course of action may be to drop down to a lower journal tier. Especially if you are in a position where your publication count is important—for example, if you are preparing to go on the job market or to submit for promotion or tenure—time is probably an important consideration. Ask yourself what the highest ranked journal is that would give your paper fair and serious consideration for publication, and then be sure to look at that journal's preferences and requirements before you submit there.

Appealing Rejection Decisions

If the rejection decision was a close call, you can appeal the decision if you choose to. As already noted, such appeals are a low-yield strategy. (In my career, I've succeeded in about 20% to 25% of appeals that I have attempted.) Some journals have a formal appeals process, but most do not. In most cases, the only option is to email the editor and ask for an appeal. Regardless of how appeals are considered, the letter of appeal needs to be thorough, empirically based, and designed to convince the editor or appeals committee that the reviewer and editor comments you received can be addressed successfully.

If you are appealing directly to the action editor who rejected your paper, keep in mind that there are considerable individual differences between and among editors in terms of their willingness to consider appeals. Some editors flatly refuse to reconsider their decisions at all—they will reply to your email and tell you that their decision is final. Other editors will take your appeal under consideration. In any case, you should know that the likelihood of your appeal being granted is low, and that you will probably have to submit your paper to another journal (see the previous section for details on preparing your manuscript for submission to a new journal).

The letter of appeal should be structured the same as a response to reviewers. Provide a clear plan for how you will respond to each reviewer comment— and how your paper will benefit from these responses. As with a response to reviewers, the appeal letter should convey gratitude, appreciation, and optimism. Take each reviewer comment seriously and view it as a chance to improve your manuscript.

The response letter that I provide below pertains to a manuscript that my colleagues and I submitted to the *American Psychologist* in 2014. The action editor rejected the paper based on the comments of one reviewer who believed that our manuscript did not go far enough beyond a previous article that had been published. Based on the comments, it was clear to us that this reviewer was probably the person who had published the article to which the reviewer had referred. The appeal was successful, and the article was eventually accepted for publication (Schwartz, Lilienfeld, Meca, & Sauvigné, 2016). Here is the text of the appeal letter:

July 4, 2014
John F. Disterhoft, Ph.D.
Associate Editor, *American Psychologist*
Department of Physiology
Northwestern University
Ward Building Room Ward 7-158
303 East Chicago Avenue
Chicago, IL 60611

Dear Dr. Disterhoft:

Thank you for the decision letter that you provided to us in response to *American Psychologist* ms. 2014-3365. We greatly appreciate the feedback that the reviewers offered us, and it is clear that we need to more clearly and forcefully highlight the unique contribution of our paper. It is also clear that we may have tried to cover too much ground in the second half of the paper, and we will address this organizational issue in our future work on the manuscript.

The basis of your decision to reject our paper appeared to rest largely on Reviewer 2's conclusion that our paper did contribute uniquely beyond the valuable Miller (2010) article in *Perspectives on Psychological Science*. For several reasons, we are respectfully asking you to reconsider your decision. Reviewer 2 appears to be either Dr. Gregory Miller himself or one of his close colleagues (the reviewer even corrected Miller's middle initial in our reference section), and this reviewer's criticisms seem to center largely on the claim (which we dispute; see below) that our article does not make a sufficiently significant contribution above and beyond an article that he wrote. This reviewer also asked us to be sure to go beyond what Scott Lilienfeld has written in his prior papers. Given that Dr. Lilienfeld is my coauthor, I am quite confident that we can do that. We should note that we have great respect for Dr. Miller's contributions to neuroscientific approaches to psychology, but we sharply disagree with Reviewer 2 that our article does not go sufficiently beyond what Dr. Miller and others have written. We should also note that several of Reviewer 2's opinions, such as his/her perceptions of RDoC (which many scholars beside ourselves do not share; e.g., see Berenbaum, 2014, *Journal of Abnormal Psychology*), strike us as better suited to a commentary on our article than as reasons to reject it, as these views are grounds for legitimate debate.

As we note below in this letter, we believe that there are many new points that our paper makes beyond Miller (2010) and other prior work. Our paper also serves to bring together information that is published in various other sources and synthesize it in a distinctive manner for the AP readership. It would seem to us that the flagship journal of the American Psychological Association would want to publish a paper on such an important topic with so many implications for the future of psychology, including research, hiring, and teaching priorities for the next generation of scholars. Not only do we believe that our paper makes important points that have not been made before and that it synthesizes existing information in one of the most important journals in our field, but we are excited about strengthening the paper so that it makes an even more distinctive and important contribution.

Below, we provide a bulleted list of contributions that our paper makes beyond what other works have contributed. If you will permit us to revise our paper for consideration at AP, we believe that we can elaborate further on these contributions and delineate their significance beyond past work:

- Elucidating the ties between funding agency priorities (which are both scientifically and politically motivated) and hiring practices in psychology departments. Reviewer 2 seems to regard the hiring issue as a byproduct of the other issues that we raise (and that Miller raised in his 2010 article), but the hiring trends hold deeply important implications for the future of psychology that have not been previously discussed to our knowledge. At the same time, these trends need to be documented quantitatively and empirically. We would be happy to do this in a revised version of our article.
- Definitions of "science" and "health," both of which have become increasingly biological in the psychological literature. The point needs to be made that science is not a content area, but rather an approach to evaluating evidence; and that "health" includes psychological as well as biological outcomes. These points have not been made in prior work to our knowledge
- Making the point that, although neuroscience generally and brain imaging specifically are extremely useful and important approaches to psychology, there are limits to what conclusions it can support. As the reviewers note, we are able to identify the brain regions that are activated when people are displaying prejudice. However, it is not at all clear how this information can help us to prevent or reduce prejudice—or to help people who have experienced it. Similar conclusions can be reached regarding stress experienced when one is laid off from a job, the process of developing a sense of identity in adolescence and emerging adulthood, and adjusting to life in a new country following migration. We can identify neural correlates of these processes, but there may also be essential information about the psychological *experiences* involved that cannot be gathered through brain imaging. Again, we would be happy to elaborate on this issue in a revised version of the manuscript.
- Proposing an event horizon between the cellular/neural and experiential levels of analysis. Such an event horizon would explain how agency and purposive action can operate at the experiential level but not at the neural level. The event horizon concept has been used in physics, but not in psychology.
- The hardware/software analogy has not been widely used to explain the relationship between brain functioning and human experience. Miller (2010)

did not address this analogy in his article, and Lilienfeld has not used it in his published work.

- The reviewers are correct that mental health is not necessarily the backbone of psychology, but it is central to many fields of psychological inquiry. Health psychologists often examine the links between mental and physical health; clinical and counseling psychologists examine threats to mental health and ways to improve mental health; and so forth. The increasingly biological definitions of mental health, which we would be happy to document (partially through the reorganization of the National Institute of Mental Health under Dr. Thomas Insel), have pushed psychological research, hiring practices, and training of students toward more of a "hardware" orientation and away from a "software" orientation.

- Training of students: This is an issue that has not been discussed in previous work on the trend toward hiring brain imaging specialists and away from hiring individuals with other types of expertise. Psychology has always been a broad field, and training of students has reflected this breadth. If our hiring practices are not reflecting this diversity of substantive and methodological viewpoints, what will be the implications for the forthcoming generation of psychological researchers? For example, many of the methodological approaches associated with "software" research—such as psychometrics—will be passed down to students only if we have the appropriate expertise in our departments to teach these approaches. None of this is to deny the scientific value of brain imaging approaches, which is substantial; rather, we aim to raise important but largely neglected questions concerning the implications of current trends for future psychological research. In a revised version of the article, we would be happy to elaborate on issues of training and teaching of students in greater detail.

Again, the reviewers have offered extremely valuable feedback, and we will follow their guidance in strengthening the paper and in bringing out its unique contribution to the field of psychology. Specifically, we are convinced that we can use many of the reviewers' suggestions to sharpen our arguments and more clearly highlight their relevance to the profession of psychology. In light of these considerations, we very much hope that you will reconsider your decision and allow us the opportunity to do so. We believe that a revised version of our article will raise a number of novel issues that are extremely relevant to the broad readership of *American Psychologist*, and that it will advance ongoing debates concerning the future of our profession.

Thank you in advance for considering our request; we will look forward to hearing from you.

Sincerely yours,

Seth J. Schwartz, Ph.D.
Professor

Although we didn't list each individual comment in this letter of appeal, we summarized the themes from the reviews and indicated how we planned to modify the manuscript in response. We clearly laid out why we believed we could respond to the reviewers and how these responses would help strengthen the paper. The editor read our appeal letter and granted the appeal.

On several other occasions, however, editors have chosen to remain with their original rejection decisions. Some of these editors have provided thoughtful, reasoned explanations for denying our appeal, whereas others have simply told us that the appeal was denied. As already, most editors are not willing to reconsider their decisions, and some may even seem annoyed by the request. One editor never even responded to my detailed, point-by-point appeal letter after he had rejected my manuscript.

It is vital that your appeal letter be respectful and deferential. I have usually started out by thanking the editor for carefully evaluating my paper and by respectfully requesting that the editor reconsider the decision to reject the manuscript. My practice is not to write the letter of appeal just after receiving the decision, when I'm still angry—I wait to write the letter until I have calmed down. One editor who denied our appeal nonetheless thanked us for approaching him in a respectful manner. He alluded to other authors who had responded to rejection letters in aggressive or accusatory ways. Remember that editing a journal, or serving as an assistant or associate editor, is a difficult job. Jeff Arnett (2005, p. 3), in his opening editorial, noted that editors are likely to "make more enemies than friends" because of low acceptance rates. As an editor, I know that most of my decisions on manuscripts are going to be disappointing to authors. An angry letter from an author is highly unlikely to convince me to change my mind.

Another tactic to avoid involves going over an action editor's head and approaching the editor-in-chief. This can happen when an author doesn't like the action editor's decision or is upset that the action editor denied the author's appeal, so the author contacts the editor-in-chief in hopes that the editor-in-chief will reverse the action editor's decision. This strategy is likely to upset both the action editor and the editor-in-chief—the action editor will not appreciate the authors' action, and the editor-in-chief is extremely unlikely to overturn the action editor's decision. The only reason even to contemplate going over an action editor's head is if that action editor appears to have committed serious editorial misconduct. I know of only two cases where this approach has been successful. In both cases, the action editor had rejected a manuscript despite unanimously positive and enthusiastic reviews, and the action editor had essentially written their own review of the manuscript and rejected the paper on the basis of that review. After unsuccessfully appealing the decision directly to the action editor, the authors approached the editor-in-chief with a thoughtful, well-reasoned request for the manuscript to be assigned to a different action editor. In one of these cases, the editor-in-chief overruled the action editor and took control of the manuscript herself—and in the other case, a different action editor was asked to evaluate the reviews and render a decision. The manuscripts were eventually accepted in both cases.

In most cases, however, the editor-in-chief will support the action editor's decision. In my incoming editorial (Schwartz, 2020), I explicitly noted that I would not overrule an associate editor's decision, and authors who approach me to appeal an associate editor's decision will be asked to submit their appeal directly to that associate editor. Al Waterman once told me, "If an editor overrules an action editor, they might as well fire the action editor." I don't completely agree with that statement, but I understand the point that Al was making. Appealing an action editor's decision by going over that person's head and approaching the editor-in-chief is a risky move. Remember that academia, and scholarly work in general, is a small field. Many people know each other, and the last thing anyone (especially young scholars) wants is a reputation for being disrespectful.

Repeatedly Rejected Manuscripts

Having a paper rejected once is disappointing. Having a paper rejected three or four times is aggravating and demoralizing. Authors may feel tempted to drop a paper that has been rejected repeatedly, believing that there is no point in continuing to revise the manuscript and target more journals. Authors may also feel inclined to find a low-prestige journal where they can dump the manuscript—to ensure that it is published somewhere. Coauthors may disagree on what to do with manuscripts that have been repeatedly rejected—some coauthors may want to drop or dump the paper, whereas others may want to keep trying with moderate-prestige journals. In short, repeatedly rejected manuscripts often represent dilemmas, and a source of great consternation, for authors.

A particular source of frustration may occur when reviewers for one journal provide a set of recommendations, the authors incorporate the recommendations into their paper and submit to another journal, and reviewers for the second journal offer an opposing set of recommendations. I had this experience a couple of years ago. I was writing a paper with a group of colleagues from several different countries. Our paper was based on an international conference on immigration. All of us were psychologists, and we observed that much of the published literature on international migration was authored by sociologists, anthropologists, political scientists, and other nonpsychological fields. So I offered to lead a manuscript on the role of psychologists in international migration research. After spending several months drafting and editing the paper, we submitted it to a prominent psychology journal. Reviewers recommended rejection based on the premise that the article would not be of much interest to psychologists, and that the most appropriate audience for the paper would be a migration studies or sociological journal. The reviewers offered no substantive comments on the structure or content of the manuscript, so we reformatted the paper into American Sociological Association style and submitted to a migration studies journal. Reviewers for that journal, in turn, told us that the paper was not appropriate for the journal and that it would be better placed in a psychology journal. Collectively, my coauthors and I threw our hands up in frustration. (We did eventually publish the article in another migration studies journal.)

In this kind of situation, one suggestion (Fatheirahman, 2015) is to send the paper to an open-access journal (open-access journals are covered in detail in Chapter 16). Essentially, open-access journals charge authors to publish articles—and their review processes may be different from the review processes for traditional subscription journals. Although reviewers for open-access journals are asked to comment on manuscripts, their recommendations are not binding—editors are permitted to continue inviting reviewers until they can find two reviewers who will endorse publication. In some cases, reviewers may be asked to comment only on technical issues (e.g., design, analyses) and not to comment on the potential impact of the manuscript on the field. Legitimate, nonpredatory open-access journals may therefore represent a "fallback option" for authors when their manuscripts have been repeatedly rejected by subscription journals. Open-access journals published by Frontiers, BMC, and PLOS, among others, are generally regarded as respectable.

In cases where authors do not want to (or are unable to) pay several thousand dollars to publish their paper, the question becomes what to do next. Is it best to try another moderate-prestige journal, or is it time to dump the paper into a low-prestige journal? The answer to this question depends on several factors, including (a) how many times the paper has been rejected, (b) whether the same issues have been brought up by reviewers for more than one journal, (c) where the first and second authors are in their careers, and (d) how much patience the authorship group (collectively) has for continuing to send the paper to moderate-prestige journals. Sometimes the author group will plan to submit to three or four high- or moderate-prestige journals before giving up and dumping the paper into a low-prestige journal. If that is the case, then this agreement should be honored before any alternative decisions are considered.

I've had several manuscripts that have been rejected by three or more journals, and only a handful of them were dropped and no longer pursued for publication. I do not advise you to drop or dump a paper that has not been rejected at least three times. Yes, I know rejection is upsetting, but scholars need to develop a thick skin. Mentors are extremely helpful in encouraging young scholars to persevere in the face of repeated rejection. In my estimation, after the third rejection, the authorship team should meet and discuss the best course of action for the paper. If a paper is written in a field where there are lots of journals—substance use, personality, and aggression are some examples—it may be worth trying several of these journals before giving up and deciding to drop or dump the paper. On the other hand, if the paper is written in a field where journal options are scant, then it may be more prudent to re-evaluate the authorship team's plans after the third rejection.

If the same flaws continue to be mentioned by reviewers for multiple journals, then it may be time to consider dumping or dropping the paper. I can remember one manuscript that was rejected four times before my coauthors and I finally dumped it into a low-prestige journal. Reviewers for the first four journals all brought up the same problems, and no matter what caveats and limitations we put into the paper, reviewers kept criticizing us for the same issues. Finally, we decided to dump the paper and move on. Our experiences with the first four journals told us that the paper was not publishable in a high- or moderate-prestige journal.

Remember, different strategies apply to early-career and senior scholars. Al Waterman was able to utilize a top-down approach to journal selection, and to continue submitting papers to moderate-prestige journals despite repeated rejections, because he was a tenured full professor and wasn't concerned about looking for a job or applying for tenure. He could afford to take as long as he wanted to publish articles—and Al prided himself on not allowing external forces to dictate the direction he took with his research program. I, on the other hand, was a young scholar for much of our collaboration, and I needed to build up my curriculum vitae. Al and I came to an agreement that, for the papers where he was lead author, he would use his approach to selecting journals—and for the papers where I was lead author, I would use my approach. (This agreement served us well throughout our collaboration, during which we published 13 articles together.)

So early-career scholars—whom I define as undergraduate and graduate students, postdoctoral fellows, and assistant professors (or equivalent ranks for non-academic institutions)—should focus on publication count as a way of building a curriculum vitae. There is an important caveat here—José always said that one article in *Science* or *Nature* was worth 20 articles in most other journals. I'll expand his point to suggest that a smaller number of articles in high-prestige journals may be equivalent to a larger number of articles in moderate- and low-prestige journals. As an adolescence and young adulthood researcher, I would say that the three first-authored articles I've published in *Child Development* are more prestigious than all the articles I have published in other developmental journals. At the same time, and in some degree of contrast to José's point, if my only publications were those three articles in *Child Development*, I would have a difficult time finding an academic job. I also need my other publications in other developmental journals to complete my curriculum vitae. In scholarly publishing, the most effective way to build a curriculum vitae is through a combination of quantity and quality.

Persistence Can Pay Off

Although the usual strategy is to drop down in journal prestige each time a manuscript is rejected, sometimes you can move up in prestige and publish the paper. One of the manuscripts from my dissertation represents a good example of this strategy. My colleagues and I had tried two low/moderate-prestige journals because the findings weren't overly striking, and both journals soundly rejected the paper. The four reviews we received from these two journals were unilaterally negative. In reading the reviews, we concluded that the reviewers weren't really understanding our points. They were criticizing us for not grounding our work in theories that had nothing to do with the study we had designed. We realized that we had been submitting the paper to journals that didn't have the expertise to review the work. We needed to find a journal that matched the theoretical perspective we were adopting.

We then selected a journal where several scholars from our field were on the editorial board. The reviews were strongly supportive, and the associate editor provisionally accepted the manuscript after one round of revision. Ironically, the journal where the paper was eventually published had a better impact factor than either of the journals we had tried previously. So, in this case, the issue was not fatal flaws in the manuscript, but rather a poor match between the theoretical orientation guiding our work and the journals to which we were submitting.

There is an important lesson to be learned from this example. If you are receiving reviewer comments "from out of left field," the issue may be that reviewers just aren't resonating with your work. If a journal doesn't have anyone on its editorial board who is a good match for your paper, chances are that it's not the right journal for your manuscript. There are some notable exceptions to this principle, such as measurement and psychometric papers, where reviewers will likely focus primarily on the methods and statistical analyses rather than on theoretical and conceptual issues. High-prestige journals may also be exceptions because their readership and reviewer base are broad. However, for moderate-prestige journals—especially those that specialize in particular theoretical approaches, age periods, or subfields of study—the best matches for your paper are generally those where you can identify editorial board members who match well with the work that the paper reports.

Furthermore, if reviewers are giving you different criticisms each time the paper is rejected, there may be hope for the paper. Al Waterman's quote that "all we need is the right editor in the right mood" applies to this type of situation. The fact that you keep receiving different types of comments speaks to the idiosyncrasies of the journal review process, and it suggests that you will eventually find an editor and a set of reviewers who resonate with your work. There is a far greater need for concern when you continue to receive the same comments over and over. Given the idiosyncratic nature of peer review and the low agreement rates between and among reviewers, receiving the same comments repeatedly is an especially strong sign that the work reported in your manuscript is fatally flawed. This conclusion is especially applicable when your paper reports empirical findings and reviewers continue to recommend rejection because of problems with your methods. In this type of situation, you need to listen to what the reviewers are telling you—this work is not publishable in a high- or moderate-prestige journal.

If your manuscript is a theoretical, position, or literature-review paper, receiving the same negative comments repeatedly may indicate that the perspective you are adopting does not resonate with the field—at least not now. In some cases, your ideas might be countercultural—that is, they "go against the grain" and challenge beliefs that your field regards as sacred. I have published many countercultural articles, and I can tell you that it's an uphill battle. Many reviewers are not willing to support ideas that go against the field's prevailing wisdom. In these cases, I advise adopting José's "standing on the shoulders of prior work" approach, rather than criticizing prior or existing theory or research. (I say more about publishing theory, position, and literature-review papers in Chapter 16.)

Sometimes repeated rejections occur because the authors adopt an overly combative approach. Remember that reviewers for your manuscript are likely to be scholars whose work is similar to yours, and adopting a combative approach will likely lead reviewers to become defensive. I know one author whose career was based largely on criticizing and poking holes in the predominant theories in his field. His papers were often rejected by journals because he had used extremely strong language (words like *wrong*, *illogical*, and *errors*) to describe existing theory and research. I emailed with this person once and found him to be quite resistant to constructive criticism—a trait that doesn't work well in scholarly publishing. Scientific humility would have helped this person greatly. If you do need to criticize existing work, my advice is to do so gently and in such a way that the authors of that work are able to save face.

Dump or Drop?

A key question regarding repeatedly rejected manuscripts involves what course of action to follow when you have decided that it is not worth continuing to pursue publication of a given manuscript in high- or moderate-prestige journals. For whatever reason, you and your coauthors have not been successful in publishing your manuscript in any of the journals you had targeted. You have reached the end of the line with the paper, and the only remaining decision is whether to dump it into a low-prestige journal or to drop it entirely.

In my career, my colleagues and I have followed both courses of action. We have dumped some papers into low-prestige journals, and we have dropped other papers entirely. In many cases, the decision whether to dump the paper into a low-prestige journal or to drop it entirely is predicated on the importance of that paper to your career trajectory and to your line of research (see Figure 13.1). If a paper is essential in establishing your career trajectory, it may be important to publish somewhere—even if the journal where it appears

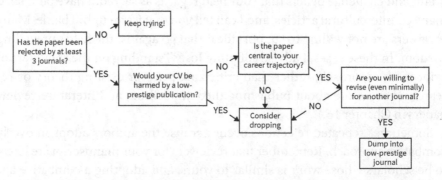

Figure 13.1 Flowchart for dumping or dropping a repeatedly rejected paper.

is not as prestigious as you would have hoped. For example, my colleagues and I (Schwartz et al., 2012) wrote an article describing the development and validation of a new measure of national identity. We tried a couple of journals, but none of the reviewers seemed interested in the work—so we sent the paper to an identity-focused journal. The journal doesn't have an impact factor, but it's a respectable outlet that publishes work on various aspects of identity. We needed an article that we could cite when we used the measure—and this journal provided us with an opportunity to do so.

On the other hand, we had another paper that we tried to publish but were unsuccessful in doing so. We tried one journal where we were invited to revise and resubmit, but one reviewer wasn't satisfied with our revision and recommended rejection. We then tried two other journals, but the paper was soundly rejected. I became so frustrated with the paper that I essentially dropped it. One of my colleagues has done some work on it, but she hasn't had the time to devote to it—so the paper has not been touched in over 4 years. As I write this in November 2020, I have very little motivation to return to that paper. As this example illustrates, sometimes the decision to drop a paper is not necessarily reached intentionally. Sometimes you can become so frustrated and disillusioned with a paper that even thinking about it becomes aversive.

If your total publication count is low, you may be better off publishing in a niche journal (niche journals tend to be low-prestige journals but respectable) than dropping the paper. People who have more publications can afford to drop papers that are rejected repeatedly, whereas people who need to build up their curriculum vitae might be better advised to dump repeatedly rejected papers into low-prestige journals. As noted in Chapter 10, you can judge journals based on the types of articles that they publish. If you look at recent issues of a journal and the articles seem solid, then that journal might be a potential home for your manuscript. Niche journals often have low impact factors—or no impact factor at all—because their readership and audience are small. Publishing in these journals will likely not hurt your career or reputation as long as you do so only occasionally. Be mindful also that different academic departments have different standards regarding how journal articles are evaluated in terms of promotion, tenure, and other types of career advancement. If your department—or the type of department that you would like to be hired into—places a lot of weight on impact factors as an index of prestigious publications, then it might be better to drop papers that are rejected repeatedly and that you and your coauthors have concluded are not publishable in high- or moderate-prestige journals.

Here is a hypothetical scenario: Let's say that faculty member A published 10 articles in a given year. One of the articles was dumped into a low-prestige journal, two were accepted for publication in high-prestige journals, and the other seven were published in moderate-prestige journals. On the other hand, faculty member B published only three articles in that same year, and one of them was in a low-prestige journal. Publishing one article in a low-prestige journal will hurt faculty member B considerably more than it will hurt faculty member A—largely because faculty member A has enough other publications to offset the low-prestige journal article. When I served on the University of Miami's appointment, promotion, and tenure committee, I reviewed many faculty members whose curricula vitae primarily listed articles in low-prestige journals. My recommendations regarding these faculty members' hire, promotion, or award of tenure were rarely supportive. If only low-prestige journals are willing to publish someone's work, what conclusions might a hiring committee or tenure reviewer draw about that person? Would that person likely be able to compete successfully for grant funding? Therefore, when you are deciding whether to dump or drop a paper, you might wish to consider how this additional entry on your curriculum vitae might affect the balance of high/moderate-prestige versus low-prestige journals on your scholarly record.

Of course, keep in mind that, as long as you are working in a scholarly network, many of your publications will be collaborative—so the pressure to publish in high- and moderate-prestige journals may, at least to some extent, be offset by coauthored publications. Earlier in my career, before I had the confidence to submit first-authored articles to high-prestige journals, I relied on my coauthors to submit papers to top journals. Working with José and his various research teams provided me with lots of opportunities to coauthor articles in high-prestige journals—and working with these colleagues helped me to learn how to navigate the review process for these journals. When I started to gain access to high-quality longitudinal data—both my own data sets and data sets collected by my colleagues—the learning curve was somewhat less steep than it would have been had I not received exposure to high-prestige journals earlier in my career.

Sometimes, rather than choosing to drop a paper, we can decide to set it aside for some period of time. Have you ever noticed that taking a break from a frustrating activity can help you to approach that activity with a clearer head later? Scholarly manuscripts are no different—sometimes you may need a break from a paper that has been rejected several times so you can return to it with a fresh perspective later. One warning, though—you need to provide a reminder to yourself so you don't wind up inadvertently dropping the paper.

Repeated Rejections and Self-Confidence

I want to return to the emotional impact of repeated rejections on authors' self-confidence (see also Chapter 10). Albert Bandura (1977) wrote that *self-efficacy* is one's belief that one is able to perform an activity successfully. If I have high self-efficacy for speaking in public, I will likely be a much more effective speaker than I would be if I had low self-efficacy for public speaking. Self-efficacy applies equally well to scholarly writing—Huerta, Goodson, Beigi, and Chlup (2017) found that writing self-efficacy was significantly and negatively related to writing-related anxiety, suggesting that people who believe that they can write successfully are likely to be more successful and prolific writers than people who do not view themselves as successful writers.

For some writers—especially those with less experience and documented success in writing—rejection, and especially repeated rejection, can damage their self-efficacy (Horn, 2016). When people are repeatedly told that they cannot do something correctly—which I suspect is how many young writers interpret rejection—they may conclude that they are not capable of performing that task or behavior properly. I cannot emphasize enough the importance of mentors in learning how to write successfully for publication. Without adequate mentorship, the process is less likely to turn out positively. I know many people who tried to write journal articles, had their articles rejected repeatedly, and simply gave up.

I've also known many young writers who decided to team up with other young writers and to publish together. In so doing, they established a writing support group and helped to encourage and support each other through the process of publishing their work. I am currently collaborating with three young scholars who worked together during graduate school and into their postdoctoral fellowships and junior faculty careers. The three of them taught each other how to write—and as any one of them was receiving mentorship in writing, they would share that wisdom with the others. All three of them have now become prolific scholars.

Another important point is that everyone will have manuscripts that seem cursed. No matter what you do, the paper keeps getting rejected. Sometimes there is a consistent theme to the rejections, and sometimes there isn't. Having people whom you can approach for support and guidance is essential, especially early in your career. Writing is not a solitary activity—indeed, the single-authored article is quickly becoming obsolete as team science becomes increasingly common. Rejection stings, and I doubt that anyone enjoys having manuscripts rejected from journals. The point is to develop resilience so that you are able to persist in your efforts to publish your work despite the rejections. Maintaining a writing support network—which will often double as your network of collaborators—is essential.

Conclusion

This chapter covers options to pursue when manuscripts are rejected by journals. When papers are soundly rejected—the "easy rejections" from an editorial point of view—the most effective course of action is generally to incorporate into the paper whatever wisdom you can extract from the reviewer comments and to submit the paper to a different journal. When a rejection decision is a close call, appealing the decision may be an option if a well-reasoned, theoretically based (or empirically based) rationale can be developed to support the appeal. It is critical to word the appeal neutrally and deferentially rather than aggressively, and appeal letters should not be written while you are angry or upset about the rejection. It is important to know that appeals are a low-yield strategy because the action editor who rejected your paper is most likely also the person who will be deciding the fate of your appeal. If the appeal is denied, then the paper should be revised and submitted to a new journal. Unless there is reason to suspect that serious editorial misconduct has occurred, going over an action editor's head and asking the editor-in-chief to reverse the action editor's decision is generally not advisable.

The chapter also discusses what to do when manuscripts are repeatedly rejected. Repeated rejections where reviewers provide different sets of comments during each round of review are qualitatively different from repeated rejections where you receive similar comments from each set of reviewers. In cases where the idiosyncrasies of peer review appear to be responsible for the repeated rejections, authors should be encouraged that they will eventually find a sympathetic editor and set of reviewers. However, when different sets of reviewers keep pointing out the same methodological flaws repeatedly, it may be time to dump the paper into a low-prestige journal or to drop it altogether. The decision to dump or drop a paper should be reached considering how important the paper is to your career trajectory—papers that are instrumental to your work should probably be published somewhere, whereas it might be a better idea to drop papers that are not essential. Especially for authors with relatively few publications, publishing in low-prestige journals can signal to others that the author's work is not worthy of publication in high-prestige and moderate-prestige journals.

Papers can also be rejected because they were submitted to the wrong journal. Being criticized for not citing theories that are not relevant to your work is a clear sign that the reviewers are "speaking a different language" than you are. If you cannot find editorial board members who appear to be well-matched with your work, and if you cannot find articles in recent issues of the journal that are conceptually similar to your paper, then the journal you are considering may not be a good fit for your work.

Finally, it is helpful to assemble a writing support group. Such support groups can supplement mentors, because they provide opportunities to publish with other scholars who are also getting started in scholarly writing. Given the increasing emphasis on team science in the scientific research community, learning how to collaborate is an essential component of a successful research and scholarly writing career, and the next chapter gives more detail about working with coauthors.

Summary

- When manuscripts are soundly rejected, the best option is to incorporate whatever reviewer suggestions seem relevant and then to prepare the paper for submission to another journal.
- Rejections that were close calls can sometimes be appealed—but the likelihood of a successful appeal is low.
- When an article is revised for a new journal, design flaws should be listed as limitations. Authors may choose not to submit to journals where these flaws would likely be considered fatal.
- Some manuscripts are cursed—that is, they are rejected repeatedly.
- When papers are repeatedly rejected but the reviewer comments are different each time, authors may wish to keep submitting to more high- or moderate-prestige journals.
- When papers are repeatedly rejected and the same reviewer concerns appear over and over, authors may wish to consider the possibility that the paper is not publishable in a high- or moderate-prestige journal.
- Repeatedly rejected papers might be dumped into a low-prestige journal, or they might be dropped entirely.

References

American Psychological Association. (n.d.-a). *Psychological Review*. Retrieved from https://www.apa.org/pubs/journals/rev.
American Psychological Association. (n.d.-b). *Psychological Bulletin*. Retrieved from https://www.apa.org/pubs/journals/bul.

Arnett, J. J. (2005). The vitality criterion: a new standard of publication for *Journal of Adolescent Research*. *Journal of Adolescent Research, 20*, 3–7.

Bandura, A. (1977). Self-efficacy: Toward a unifying theory of behavioral change. *Psychological Review, 84*, 191–215.

Fatheirahman, A. I. (2015). Rejection of good manuscripts: Possible reasons, consequences, and solutions. *Journal of Clinical Research and Bioethics, 6*, Article 1.

Fricker, R. D., Jr., Burke, K., Han, X., & Woodall, W. H. (2019). Assessing the statistical analyses used in *Basic and Applied Social Psychology* after their p-value ban. *The American Statistician, 73*, 374–384.

Horn, S. A. (2016). The social and psychological costs of peer review: Stress and coping with manuscript rejection. *Journal of Management Inquiry, 25*, 11–26.

Huerta, M., Goodson, P., Beigi, M., & Chlup, D. (2017). Graduate students as academic writers: writing anxiety, self-efficacy and emotional intelligence. *Higher Education Research and Development, 4*, 716–729.

Lovejoy, T. I., Revenson, T. A., & France, C. R. (2011). Reviewing manuscripts for peer-review journals: A primer for novice and seasoned reviewers. *Annals of Behavioral Medicine, 42*, 1–13.

Maxwell, S. E., & Cole, D. A. (2007). Bias in cross-sectional analyses of longitudinal mediation. *Psychological Methods, 12*, 23–44.

O'Laughlin, K. D., Martin, M. J., & Ferrer, E. (2018). Cross-sectional analysis of longitudinal mediation processes. *Multivariate Behavioral Research, 53*, 375–402.

Schwartz, S. J. (2020). Incoming editorial: Advancing intercultural research and standing on the shoulders of giants. *International Journal of Intercultural Relations, 74*, 1–6.

Schwartz, S. J., Lilienfeld, S. O., Meca, A., & Sauvigné, K. C. (2016). The role of neuroscience within psychology: A call for inclusiveness over exclusiveness. *American Psychologist, 71*, 52–70.

Schwartz, S. J., Park, I. J. K., Huynh, Q.-L., Zamboanga, B. L., Umaña-Taylor, A. J., Lee, R. M., . . . Agocha, V. B. (2012). The American Identity Measure: Development and validation across ethnic subgroup and immigrant generation. *Identity: An International Journal of Theory and Research, 12*, 93–128.

Spector, P. E. (2019). Do not cross me: Optimizing the use of cross-sectional designs. *Journal of Business and Psychology, 34*, 125–137.

Stivers, J., & Cramer, S. F. (2017). From rejected to accepted: Part 2—Preparing a rejected manuscript for a new journal. *Journal of Faculty Development, 31*, 63–65.

14
Working With Coauthors

Chapter Objectives

When you finish reading this chapter, you should be more comfortable with:

- The concept of team science and the trend toward working in large research teams
- What coauthors are expected to do when they collaborate on manuscripts
- Handling politics and infighting in an authorship team
- Incorporating coauthor feedback into drafts
- Differences between active versus passive coauthoring
- Collaborations between senior and junior scholars
- Working in large authorship teams
- Handling difficult or resistant coauthors
- Leaving a toxic collaboration
- Mentor–mentee collaborations
- Student-led collaborations with faculty members

As noted in various places in this book, team science has expanded greatly since the dawn of the 21st century. Team science is exactly what the term implies: Groups of experts from various disciplines, sometimes also in partnership with community members and leaders, come together to pursue knowledge, equity, and social change (Tebes, 2018). Team science provides several advantages over traditional discipline-bounded work, such as providing multiple perspectives on scientific and social problems (e.g., psychologists and social workers working together to prevent substance use). Viewing a problem from multiple disciplinary angles adds voices to the conversation and may help to overcome disciplinary blind spots that can impede progress toward finding solutions to important challenges (Hall, Feng, Moser, Stokols, & Taylor, 2008).

Team science also brings challenges. Among the challenges is working with coauthors. Coauthors can add a lot to your work by providing critical feedback and ideas that you might not have thought of on your own. They can read your writing and catch errors that you overlooked. They can offer

The Savvy Academic. Seth J. Schwartz, Oxford University Press. © Oxford University Press 2022.
DOI: 10.1093/oso/9780190095918.003.0015

new ideas and perspectives when you feel stuck in your writing progress. At the same time, however, coauthors can be slow, unresponsive, and inflexible. I've had coauthors hold up papers for months (and even years) because they were not willing to compromise with other coauthors. Coauthors can sometimes be aggressive and confrontational when you don't follow their suggestions. Coauthors can also disagree strongly with one another—and these disagreements can spill over into the collaborative work. I provide examples of all these scenarios in this chapter.

Working with large numbers of coauthors can be challenging even if everyone is cooperative. Receiving large numbers of comments and having to reconcile them can be difficult. Coauthors may offer suggestions and edits that conflict with suggestions provided by other coauthors, and sometimes coauthors' input is not consistent with the direction you envision for the manuscript. This chapter presents ways in which I have handled these issues.

This chapter covers all these themes regarding working with coauthors. First, I provide a "coauthor job description" that outlines what coauthors are expected to do. I offer my own experiences as a coauthor—and as a first author—and I suggest some Dos and Don'ts for coauthors. Second, I provide guidance on incorporating coauthor feedback and for working on large authorship teams. Third, I offer suggestions for dealing with difficult, inflexible, or resistant coauthors. In this third section, I also discuss handling power imbalances between and among coauthors (e.g., the imbalances that occur when students are collaborating with professors). Further, what should you do if a coauthor is holding up or blocking the progress of a paper? What if coauthors are insisting that the direction of the paper must follow their directions or visions? What if you are lead author and some of your coauthors are arguing or vehemently disagreeing with other coauthors? What is your role, and what are your responsibilities, in managing this type of conflict in a collaboration that you are leading?

A Coauthor Job Description

If someone asks you to coauthor a manuscript with them, what does that mean? What are you being asked to do? If you ask someone else to coauthor a paper with you, what are you asking them to do? There are clearly multiple answers to this question, but many professional societies maintain a list of criteria for who is entitled to coauthorship. The National Academy of Sciences (2009) specifies that a coauthor is someone who conceptualizes the paper or project, writes drafts of the manuscript, conducts in-depth literature reviews, provides substantive edits (e.g., going through drafts and suggesting changes or decisions that need to be made), and/or conducts the statistical analyses to test the study hypotheses. So, coauthors must make essential contributions to the paper. Someone who performs language editing (e.g., grammar checks, suggesting punctuation) would not be a coauthor—that person would be acknowledged and thanked in an author note. Similarly, someone who compiles references or creates tables and figures would be acknowledged but would not be listed as an author.

As I tell my students in the research ethics class that I teach, my primary point of disagreement with these authorship guidelines involves project directors. For complex projects, such as longitudinal studies and randomized trials, a project director is needed to oversee the daily conduct of the study. This person coordinates activities like recruitment, assessment, intervention delivery, and participant follow-up and retention. Project direction requires a specialized set of skills that are not easy to find. Although data collectors— people who administer surveys, conduct experiments, or collect biological samples—can be hired, trained, and replaced fairly easily, the project director is an essential and indispensable member of the study team. I have had to switch project directors in the middle of a study, and in many cases the study must essentially stop until the new project director is ready to take over. I have offered authorship to project directors on all my studies—without these people, we would not have our data.

When you think of a coauthor, however, you're probably thinking about someone who offers comments and edits on manuscript drafts. My primary focus in this chapter is on this kind of coauthor. In my experience, although statisticians and project directors are also coauthors, they seldom offer substantive comments on manuscript drafts. So, I restrict my discussion in the remainder of this chapter to coauthors who provide comments and edits. When I discuss the job description for coauthors, this is the kind of coauthor to whom I refer.

When I'm invited to coauthor a paper with someone, I assume that my responsibilities will include the following:

- Reading drafts closely and providing substantive feedback (I explain what I mean by "substantive feedback" later in this section);
- Pointing out flaws (both fatal and nonfatal) and suggesting ways to explain or address them;
- Suggesting alternative directions in which the paper could be taken— including new theoretical approaches, analyses, and discussion points;

- Pointing out wording that is unclear or vague;
- Indicating statements with which I disagree or to which I object; and
- Providing "food for thought" for the lead author to consider.

One of the most important lessons José taught me was how to work with coauthors. His rule, which I have adopted for use with my coauthors as well, is that the first author makes the call. That is, a coauthor's job is to advise the first author regarding suggested edits, ideas to consider, potential directions for the paper, and flaws that must be explained. The first author's job is to digest and integrate the coauthors' recommendations and to revise the manuscript in a way in which the first author feels most comfortable, but that hopefully also incorporates the majority of feedback from coauthors. As first author, you have to make many judgment calls regarding whether to include specific suggestions that your coauthors have offered. Remember that the authorship team is just that—a team—and that everyone's feedback should be viewed as attempts to strengthen the manuscript and to head off potential reviewer criticisms.

So, the coauthor's job is to comment on any and all issues that they notice. One of my favorite sayings regarding coauthors is that I would rather have a coauthor raise an issue than have a reviewer raise it. José was one of my favorite coauthors because he would comment on everything. Once he was satisfied with a paper, I knew it had a good chance of being invited for revision and resubmission. I have adopted his style—I read every word of manuscripts I'm coauthoring, and I suggest any and all changes (and raise any and all potential issues) that I can find. From there, it's up to the first author to decide which changes and comments to incorporate and which ones to ignore. I see my role as pointing out whatever I notice in the paper and in the work it reports—and then ideally the first author will seriously consider my suggestions (along with everyone else's) and generate an improved version of the paper.

In any collaborative endeavor, the goal is to ensure that the paper is published, that the grant is funded, or that the project is otherwise successful. An important aspect of a coauthor's job is therefore to subjugate their own ego to the good of the team and to the goal of the collaboration. If the first author doesn't incorporate one of my suggestions in the paper, but the paper is ultimately published, then I need to be satisfied with that. Yes, I have seen coauthors grumble about their feedback not being included in the final version of an article after the article has been accepted for publication. This scenario reminds me of basketball players complaining about their individual statistics even though their team won the game. For me, this kind of attitude is not conducive to collaboration.

Of course, I'm not saying that all coauthor grievances are illegitimate. I've seen situations where some coauthors' suggestions were largely, if not completely, ignored. This kind of first-author behavior is also not conducive to collaboration. If you are a first author and you disagree with the majority of someone's suggestions, I advise you to reach out to that person and ask them to explain their feedback. Maybe there is a miscommunication somewhere—remember that most face-to-face communication is nonverbal, and therefore the written word doesn't provide the nuances and clues that we often need to understand what someone is telling us. So, we may not completely understand someone's comments, and a conversation with a coauthor is preferable to simply ignoring that person's feedback. If you as a coauthor feel that your feedback is being ignored by the lead author, then reach out to that person and request a conversation.

Remember also that your coauthors are generally people with whom you have chosen to collaborate—and in many cases they are (or have the potential to become) long-term colleagues. As a result, I suggest "treading lightly" when communicating to coauthors that you don't like or understand their feedback (and likewise when coauthors are telling the first author that they feel their feedback has been ignored). The saying "You catch more flies with honey than you do with vinegar" applies here. Voice your complaint or question gently and respectfully and be sure to listen carefully to the person's response. In most cases, coauthor feedback is intended to help improve the paper, and I genuinely believe that most first authors want their papers to be as strong as possible when they are submitted for publication. Of course, there are exceptions to these assumptions, and we cover some of them in the final section of this chapter.

Of course, any time you bring a group of people together, politics emerge. Some people may gravitate toward one another, whereas other people may be less positively inclined toward others. The emergence of politics among a group of people is normal and is difficult, if not impossible, to avoid. With that said, however, politics must be managed if a collaborative team is to accomplish their goals. If there are both junior and senior people on a writing team, then I would expect the senior people to take their junior colleagues gently aside and nudge them back toward the collaboration if they are behaving in ways that are not collaborative. However, senior scholars are not immune to politics, and I have seen senior people behaving in ways that are not conducive to collaboration. This kind of situation can become difficult for younger colleagues—it may not be advisable for students or mentees to take their senior colleagues aside and tell them that they are not behaving collaboratively. Junior scholars may also not have the option of leaving the collaboration without severely damaging their careers. (We return to this last scenario in the final section of the chapter.)

Agreeing on Authorship Arrangements in Advance

One of the most predictable mistakes I have seen scholars make—indeed, I have committed this error myself—is not discussing authorship arrangements in advance. In my opinion, the more parameters that can be agreed upon in the beginning of the collaboration, the happier everyone is likely to be later. Some of these parameters include:

- Who will be first author, and why;
- What the remaining authorship positions will be (note that first, second, and last are the most prestigious positions on the authorship—last author is generally reserved for the lab director or other senior scholar);
- What decision-making system will be used (e.g., "first author makes the call" versus "all decisions must be made collaboratively");
- Who will carry out which tasks (e.g., writing the introduction, conducting the analyses, creating the tables, compiling the reference list); and
- How many rounds of coauthor review will be needed before the manuscript is submitted for publication (or how the first author will be able to decide whether further coauthor review is needed).

In my experience, when these parameters are not decided upon in advance, members of the authorship team will often make assumptions regarding how the process will unfold. If these assumptions prove to be false—for example, someone is listed as sixth author when they believe they deserve to be second or third—conflict may emerge between or among coauthors. If this conflict is then not resolved amicably and proactively, resentments can build up and damage the relationships among the coauthors. I have seen collaborative relationships become strained and even severed based on "surprises" that occurred during the authorship process for a paper.

A student I know had a situation like this happen to her. Her master's degree mentor asked her to lead the writing and analyses for a paper the mentor was working on. The student went well above and beyond what she was asked to do, and her mentor complimented and praised her on multiple occasions. Her mentor promised her second authorship—but when the article was published, the student was listed as fifth author. The mentor had inserted three of her own colleagues, none of whom had done very much on the paper, in front of the student who had done so much of the work. Because of the power imbalance between students and their faculty mentors, this student decided not to address the situation with her former mentor. She did, however, decide not to engage in any further collaborations with her former mentor. (I am involved in many projects with former students and mentees—so having hard-working and productive mentees decide to stop working with their former mentors is a major loss for both parties.)

Thus, it is essential to discuss and agree on as many of the authorship parameters as possible before starting the work. A strategy I advise is to put the agreements into writing—through email or by having the authors sign a contract with one another. Most scholars are busy people, and they may not remember what they agreed to—so having the agreement in writing can help to avoid conflicts among authors later. My belief is that the long-term future of a collaboration is at least as important as—if not more important than—any individual paper that the group writes together.

Reasonability and Flexibility Are Essential

Within any given collaboration, disagreements are likely to occur. A coauthor may not agree with a statement that the first author has included in a manuscript draft, or the first author may not agree with comments or edits that coauthors have provided. In both scenarios, it is essential for all parties to be reasonable and flexible with each other. Reasonability and flexibility refer to several types of attitudes and practices. First, I suggest being open and understanding rather than defensive. Assume that the lead author or coauthor has the best interests of the manuscript and project in mind, and that their statements, edits, and comments are provided with these best interests in mind. (Of course, there are exceptions where someone is trying to further their own interests to the detriment of the collaboration. I address these situations in the last section of this chapter.)

The reasonability and flexibility criterion suggests that you should approach coauthors respectfully when their suggestions or edits are confusing or troubling to you. Ask them what they meant and allow them to clarify. Perhaps they spotted something in the paper that concerned or confused them. Always offer your coauthors the benefit of the doubt unless they give you a convincing reason not to. Try to keep in mind that everyone on the authorship team most likely wants to see the manuscript published and to ensure that it is as impactful as possible.

When you are a first author, reasonability and flexibility also mean that you should be open to your coauthors' suggestions—even if you initially disagree with them. Often, coauthors can anticipate what reviewers might say about a manuscript, and you can use coauthor feedback and suggestions to "head off" potential reviewer comments. I can remember a paper I was writing early in my career, where one of my coauthors provided some extremely critical feedback. His primary statement was that, if he were a reviewer for the journal we were targeting, he would not like the paper very much. I was taken aback by his strong statements and probably didn't incorporate as much of his feedback as I should have. When we submitted the manuscript, reviewers indeed provided some of the same comments that my coauthor had offered.

One experience I have had many times is simply not wanting to put in the effort to make the changes that coauthors are recommending. The feeling doesn't necessarily imply laziness—rather, it represents feeling content with the paper as it is and not wanting to make extensive revisions, conduct new analyses, or bring in new theories or streams of literature that coauthors are suggesting. Although the first author generally has veto power in terms of whether to incorporate coauthors' suggestions, a litmus test to consider is whether a given suggestion will strengthen the manuscript and increase the likelihood that reviewers will respond positively to it. If the answer is Yes, then I advise you to make the change, even if you don't really "feel like" doing it. Again, remember that your coauthors have spent their time and energy helping you to sharpen the manuscript.

I generally treat coauthor comments the same way I treat reviewer comments. That is, I try to be as responsive as I can, and I almost always incorporate the requests for major revisions. I might ignore word changes I disagree with, but if I have an issue with a larger change or recommendation that a coauthor is suggesting, I will generally reach out to that person and request a meeting. Blowing off coauthor suggestions is not a great way to encourage people to want to keep working with you.

Of course, there may be times when coauthors will provide contrasting recommendations. One coauthor may recommend spelling out the methods more extensively, whereas another coauthor may suggest that you reduce the description of the methods. In that case, you as first author need to make the call, and if you have decided not to incorporate major revisions that someone suggested, I encourage you to reach out to that person and explain why. Perhaps you can say that various coauthors provided contrasting suggestions, and that you decided to follow a specific course of action for reasons that you are explaining.

As is discussed in the next section, large collaborations—which I define as those with six or more authors—require the first author to exercise a great deal of patience and thoughtful consideration. As first author, you will have to sort through and reconcile several sets of comments, and you will have to decide which input to incorporate and which input to ignore. Even with smaller collaborations—those with three, four, or five authors—you will still need to sort through multiple sets of comments and suggestions. When you have finished, you should send a group email to your coauthors thanking them for their input—and be sure to note that you considered everyone's comments and had to make some difficult decisions. Diplomacy is very important when working with coauthors—you can deliver the same message in an empathetic and caring way or in a dismissive and hostile way.

Margin Comments or In-Text Edits?

The coauthor job description involves providing comments, edits, and "food for thought" for the first author to consider, and I have encountered two primary ways in which coauthors can provide this input. The first way is to provide margin comments and suggestions—essentially leaving it to the first author to make the changes that coauthors are suggesting. For example, a coauthor might read a sentence, find it to be awkwardly written, and provide a margin comment saying "This sentence is awkwardly written. Please rephrase." The first author is then tasked with finding a way to reword the awkward sentence. Similarly, a coauthor might think that a specific theoretical perspective should be incorporated into the introduction, and this person might insert a margin comment saying, "You should consider incorporating Theory X into how you frame the study." Again, in this scenario, the coauthor is assigning this new thinking and writing to the first author. I refer to this kind of coauthoring as passive coauthoring.

A second approach is for coauthors to edit the manuscript directly. For example, instead of inserting a margin comment suggesting that a sentence needs to be reworded, the coauthor would rewrite the sentence directly (using the tracked comments function in the word processing software). A coauthor might draft text introducing a specific theory that might be relevant to the manuscript and tying that theory into the study, perspective, or review that the paper is reporting. I refer to this kind of coauthoring as active coauthoring.

As a coauthor, I utilize both active and passive coauthoring strategies. In situations where I can think of the text I would want to see added to, or modified in, the paper, I draft it myself and either insert it directly or suggest it in a margin comment. In situations where something seems "off" about a sentence, paragraph, or section, but where I cannot point out exactly what that is, I will note this observation in a margin comment. I also use margin comments when I'm not sure what a phrase or sentence is trying to communicate. I do try to use an active coauthoring style wherever I can—I find that some coauthors use a passive style when they really could fix the sentence themselves or suggest text to make the point that they are recommending. As a first author, I find this type of passive coauthoring to be somewhat frustrating.

As a first author, if you want your coauthors to draft and revise text actively rather than passively inserting margin comments, you should state this expectation explicitly when you share the manuscript draft with your coauthors. I was part of a working group several years ago, and one of the group's policies was that anyone who had a suggestion should make the changes they were recommending rather than leaving margin comments for someone else to address. On many occasions, we had to remind people who had left margin comments that they were supposed to insert or modify the text themselves. Over the course of my career, I have found passive coauthoring to be more common than active coauthoring, so you may need to remind your coauthors to use an active style.

Expecting active coauthoring also involves giving your coauthors permission to change the messages you have put into the manuscript. Some coauthors may not feel comfortable altering your message, and they may be more comfortable with making suggestions and letting you incorporate them as you see fit. As suggest regarding other coauthorship issues, it is critical to clarify everyone's expectations and parameters prior to initiating the collaborative project. If you haven't clarified your preferences, then your coauthors may not do what you are expecting them to do.

Indeed, perhaps the authorship group should draft a "list of coauthor expectations" at the beginning of the writing process. Creating a written document that everyone contributes to and agrees to would help to minimize conflict and resentments later on. If the group decision is that coauthors should actively revise text, this agreement should be specified in writing. If the decision is that, in an ongoing collaboration where several papers will be written, first authorship should rotate among members of the author group, then this should be specified in writing as well. Remember that unwelcome "surprises" are not conducive to continuing the collaboration.

Collaborations Between Senior and Junior Scholars

A specific type of collaboration that is important to mention involves collaborations between and among scholars who are at different stages in their careers. In many cases, such collaborations occur within mentoring relationships (e.g., professors mentoring students and postdoctoral fellows). In these types of collaborations, the balance of power is unequal—and mentees may not feel comfortable speaking freely with their mentors (Sanfey, Hollands, & Gantt, 2013). In these cases, it is imperative that the mentor explicitly communicate to the mentee that it is safe to speak freely without fear of reprisal or other unwelcome consequences.

When I begin a mentoring relationship with someone, I like to set the ground rules as soon as possible. I tell my mentees that they can express their concerns—in terms of comments on coauthored papers or interpersonal issues within the collaboration—and that I will listen and will support the mentee as much as I can. As a mentor, it is essential to communicate to mentees that you will treat them as equals and allow them to push back against your suggestions (respectfully, of course) without fear of reprisal.

Publications arising from student theses and dissertations are a special case of mentor–mentee collaborations. Most professional societies specify that students are entitled to first authorship on manuscripts based on their theses and dissertations (Oberlander & Spencer, 2006). That is, even if the thesis or dissertation was based on the mentor's research program, and even if the thesis or dissertation was a collaborative project between the mentor and the student, the student should be listed as first author. However, more than a fourth of the students whom Sandler and Russell (2005) surveyed reported that their mentors had not permitted them to be first author on articles stemming from their thesis or dissertation. I once knew an academic couple who were famous for committing ethical violations against their students. On several occasions, they took a student's thesis or dissertation, converted it into a journal manuscript, and submitted it for publication without the student's name on it. I often wondered why this couple's publications had only their names listed as authors—I don't know very many full professors at major universities who collect their own data, review the literature themselves, conduct their own analyses, and do all the writing on their own. I spoke with several of their students, and the stories they told me were consistent—the two professors had been leaving their students' names off papers that were based on the students' dissertations.

Because there is often no formal grievance process through which students can advocate for their rights without fear of retribution, it is essential for mentors to understand what they are "getting themselves into" before they take on mentees. Taking on mentees is the scholarly equivalent of bringing children into the world—you are responsible for them until they can take care of themselves. They need you to advocate for them—which includes helping them to build their curriculum vitae. My practice is to offer first authorships to students and other mentees whenever possible—as a tenured full professor, I don't need first-authored publications because I don't have to worry about being evaluated for tenure or promotion. My mentees, on the other hand, need as many first-authored articles as possible. They are preparing to search for jobs, to submit for tenure and/or promotion, or to apply for career development grants (for which first-authored publications are extremely important). I will take first authorship on papers where I have done most of the work and where none of my mentees is interested in being lead author—but if I have a mentee who is willing to be first author (and is willing to assume the responsibilities that first authorship entails), then I will give first authorship to that person.

Mentors might also adopt a different balance of active versus passive coauthoring when working with mentees than when working with other colleagues. I generally use more active coauthoring techniques when working with new writers, so that they can see how I write. Passive coauthoring, which requires the first author to generate or modify text on their own, may be less helpful with new writers who need more guidance.

Students who are first-authoring manuscripts with their mentors (and with other senior colleagues) should endeavor to be as responsive as possible to the mentor's comments and edits. Senior colleagues generally know how to publish, and they are usually familiar with the types of statements that are more versus less effective in each section of a manuscript. You may become frustrated when you think that your paper is ready to be submitted but your mentor keeps making more and more comments and asking for more and more changes. Try to remember that, in most cases, your mentor's goal is the same as yours—to submit the best possible version of the manuscript for publication. You might find yourself wondering when your mentor will finally sign off on the paper and indicate that it's ready to be submitted. Just remember that editing—whether you are editing your own work or someone else's—is an iterative process. I may not spot a problem in a manuscript until other problems have already been corrected. Revisions may raise new issues in your mentor's mind. (This may occur with other coauthors as well.) So, I advise you to be patient with the publication process. It's better to take a few more weeks to perfect the paper than to submit a less polished version earlier. Assuming that the action editor invites you to revise and resubmit, the time from initial submission to acceptance is likely to be between 6 and 12 months—and quite likely more than that. So, losing a few weeks because your mentor keeps asking for changes is quite inconsequential.

I cover unresponsive coauthors more in the last section of this chapter, but I'd like to say a few things about unresponsive mentors and the delays they can cause for students. I have known many students who have waited for months to receive feedback from their mentors on drafts of their manuscripts, theses, or dissertations. One student I know waited over a year for her mentor to provide comments on a draft she had sent him. She reminded him many, many times to provide feedback, but he continued to ignore her. This student had to stay in her PhD program beyond the end of her funding because her mentor took so much time to comment on her drafts.

Unfortunately, there isn't much that students can do in these situations. As a student, you are dependent on your mentor to help you progress through and finish your program. However, I have served as an informal mentor for many students, postdoctoral fellows, and assistant professors who weren't receiving the mentoring they needed. Many people have reached out to me and asked me to coauthor with them, asked to use my data, or asked me to serve as their mentor for a career award application. I have almost never said no to any of these requests—and if anything, I have helped to provide relief for overwhelmed mentors who didn't have time to respond to their mentees' requests for comments on drafts. Some mentors are territorial and don't want anyone else working with their mentees, but at least in my experience, most mentors are more than happy to let someone else publish with their mentees. The mentee's formal mentor may also appear as a coauthor on these publications—so in this scenario, everyone wins. I can list at least 10 "informal" mentees where the arrangement (the mentee is publishing with me, but their formal mentor is also a coauthor) has benefited everyone. So, I advise mentees to seek out informal mentorship if their formal mentors are not giving them what they need. I advise such mentees to be sure that their mentor approves of this kind of arrangement before they reach out to a prospective informal mentor.

The Point of Diminishing Returns

A key principle I learned early in my career is that there are always more changes that can be made to a manuscript. More words can be changed, more points can be spelled out, and more redundancy can be eliminated. However, at a certain point you reach what my colleague Gordon Finley called the "point of diminishing returns." The manuscript is unlikely to be appreciably improved through further editing—and each round of coauthor review beyond the point of diminishing returns is likely to yield few or no benefits. Once all your coauthors have agreed that the paper has reached this point, then it's time to submit for publication.

If you believe that your paper has reached the point of diminishing returns, but one or more of your coauthors still believe that more changes are necessary, I suggest scheduling a meeting with those coauthors to discuss their remaining concerns and to develop an action plan to incorporate their feedback and to prepare the paper for submission. I should note that, in my experience, compared to more experienced writers, younger writers are much more likely to believe far earlier that their paper has reached the point of diminishing returns. A younger writer may be satisfied with the paper, but a more senior colleague might suggest lots of corrections and edits. Again, the most effective way to learn to write is to collaborate with experienced writers. As you gain experience, it will take longer to reach the point of diminishing returns. I've reached the point in my career where my coauthors often reach the point of diminishing returns before I do.

Working in Large Authorship Teams

Large authorship teams can be especially challenging because of the sheer volume of comments that the first author must resolve and incorporate into the manuscript. (I've been involved with papers that had more than 15 or 20 authors.) Even if some of the authors don't provide much feedback— such as project directors and statisticians—the majority of authors will send comments, and the task is then to decide how to reconcile the many different comments, edits, and suggestions. The first time I was first author on a manuscript like this, I was overwhelmed—but after a while I became more comfortable leading papers with lots of authors.

In this section, I discuss the challenges involved in large writing collaborations, both from a first-author perspective and from a coauthor perspective. Clearly, the first author faces the most daunting challenge, but being a coauthor in a large collaboration is similar to trying to ensure that one's voice is heard in a crowd of people. Some coauthors' voices will be louder than others, and other coauthors' input might be less likely to be incorporated into the final version of the manuscript.

The First-Author Perspective

As first author, I've used two general strategies when working with large authorship teams. The first is to incorporate each set of comments as it comes in. This approach requires me to compare each new commented draft with the current version of the paper, so that I can see what the person commented on (or what text they added or modified). As I incorporate comments from each coauthor, the current draft of the paper changes and improves—and I effectively have to deal with only one set of comments at a time. The disadvantage of this approach is that I must keep comparing the next commented version of the paper against the current version with previous sets of comments already incorporated—and some of the text on which the next set of comments is focused may already have been deleted, modified, or moved. So, I sometimes have to hunt for the text in the current version that the current set of comments is targeting. This approach is best implemented with a split screen or with multiple monitors, where you can display the current draft on one monitor (or on one side of the screen) and the next set of comments on the other monitor or side of the screen.

The other approach I've used is to wait until all the commented drafts come in and merge them. I then have everyone's comments in one place, and I can address everything at once. The major downside of this strategy is that dealing with so many comments at one time can be overwhelming. I recently worked on a manuscript with 15 sets of comments, and it took me several working days to get through everything. Sometimes one coauthor would recommend one course of action but someone else would suggest something else—and I had to make many judgment calls. The whole paper was a mass of tracked edits and comments, and looking at all the colored highlighting gave me a headache!

A variant of this second approach involves coauthors' "taking turns." Coauthor A goes through the paper and then sends it to Coauthor B, who then goes through it and sends it to Coauthor C—and so on. This strategy is useful because coauthors are able to see what other coauthors have said, and they can agree or disagree with prior comments. You, as first author, can then have more information—in this case, how coauthors have reacted to other coauthors' feedback—to help you decide what course of action to follow. Of course, for this strategy to work effectively, each coauthor needs to work off the most recent version that the previous coauthor sent. Some coauthors work off your original draft, which then creates more work for you. (It may also be possible to use Google Docs or another collaborative platform so that multiple people can edit the paper at the same time.)

Regardless of which strategy you use, you will have to make lots of judgment calls. Different coauthors may suggest different courses of action, and in the end it's up to you to decide how to proceed. Chances are that you will not be able to incorporate every comment from every coauthor—so there is a chance that some coauthors may be unhappy with some of your decisions (I provide some examples in this chapter). I have received unpleasant feedback from coauthors on many occasions during my writing career.

As noted in the previous section, I advise interpreting each coauthor comment and deciding what requested changes to make based on your goals for the paper. Optimally, you will have communicated these goals to your coauthors—in this case, coauthors should be able to anticipate why you would have made the decisions you made regarding their input. In cases where coauthor recommendations conflict, you can use your goals for the paper to help you decide which course of action to follow. In most cases, the best course of action may be to incorporate some of what each of the conflicting comments are suggesting. For example, let's say you are reporting a study on alcohol use among combat veterans. One coauthor suggests that you should say more in the introduction about alcohol use among active-duty military personnel, but another coauthor suggests that you should focus more on trauma and post-traumatic stress and their links with alcohol use. Clearly, you can do both, and you probably should cover both topics in a paper about alcohol use among veterans—but you need to decide how much coverage to devote to each of these topics. In this situation, I would return to my outline and decide on the most important points to address vis-à-vis each of these topics. Ultimately, the decision is yours as first author.

When you are working on a large authorship team, many authors will be concerned about—or at least interested in—where their names will appear on the authorship list. As already noted, for papers with many authors, the most important authorship positions are first, second, and last. Over the course of my career, I have written many papers with six or more authors, and in many of these cases, at least one coauthor has asked me where their name will appear on the list of authors. In some cases, these concerns are related to preparing to submit for tenure or promotion, to going on the job market, or to applying for grants, all cases where appearing toward the front of the author list is important. In other cases, full professors have complained about their authorship position even though they were already tenured and didn't have to worry about tenure or promotion. Further, although authorship positions other than first, second, and last essentially don't matter very much (Cals & Kotz, 2013), some people may be bothered by their position on the authorship. As mentioned, disputes regarding authorship (including authorship position) have the potential to disrupt or even end collaborative relationships.

In most cases, these disputes can be avoided by discussing and agreeing upon the authorship order at the beginning of the collaboration and renegotiating this order if necessary (e.g., if someone contributed more or less than expected). However, some situations are difficult to anticipate. For example, I was involved in a manuscript several years ago where we brought in two additional, statistically oriented coauthors because reviewers were asking for new analyses that none of the original authors knew how to conduct. The new analyses played a critical role in getting the paper accepted for publication, and as a result, my colleague who was lead author decided to give the two new coauthors the fifth and sixth positions on the authorship (there were a total of 15 authors on the paper). Insertion of the new coauthors caused some of the other coauthors to be "bumped down." One coauthor was bothered by this change in the authorship order, and he sent the first author a scathing email accusing him of unprofessionalism. We had not thought that moving from eighth to tenth author was important enough to seek this coauthor's approval, but he was clearly angered by the change. The result of this accusatory exchange was that this coauthor was not invited to collaborate with us on any subsequent papers.

So, there are several touchy situations that can arise in large authorship teams. On a smaller team, most of the authors likely know each other—but on a team with 15 authors, the likelihood is high that at least some of the authors will not know one another. As a result, negotiations among authors are likely to be funneled through the first or last author—and the first or last author may then be tasked with resolving disputes between and among authors. In essence, then, serving as first author on a large team may represent a combination of culling through multiple sets of comments, following up with unresponsive coauthors, and resolving disputes among coauthors.

The Coauthor Perspective

As a coauthor on a large writing team, your task is to comment on drafts that the first author has sent out for coauthor review. My approach to coauthoring is to read every word and comment on anything and everything that looks out of place. In other words, I want to provide the first author with as much input as I can so that the first author can decide which feedback to incorporate. When I agree to coauthor a paper, I take this role very seriously, and I see myself as committing to doing whatever I can to help move the paper from early draft to submittable draft. As already described, I use a combination of active and passive coauthoring strategies—I generate new text when I think I know what the first author is trying to say and I can think of a more effective way of saying it, but I use margin comments when I am not sure what the first author is saying or when I want to share an idea with the first author but I don't want to impose it on the paper without the first author's consent. In effect, I am thinking like a reviewer as I go through the paper, pointing out anything that might attract a reviewer's critical attention.

When I receive a draft on which other coauthors have already commented—or when the authorship team is using a shared editing platform like Google Docs—I also take the opportunity to add to, or comment on, edits or comments that other coauthors have inserted. I might say "I agree" in response to a coauthor comment (to signal to the first author that multiple coauthors share the sentiment expressed in the comment), or I might offer a different perspective than the other coauthor has expressed. If I do offer a different perspective, I will do so gently and respectfully and will not directly contradict the other coauthor. For example, if another coauthor suggested that a paragraph could be deleted, I might state "I actually like this paragraph. I think it expresses some important ideas. I do agree with Coauthor X, however, that it could be shortened."

Another important coauthor responsibility is to support the first author by being a team player. If some of your comments are not incorporated into the version that is submitted for publication, do not say anything to the first author unless you believe that the omissions were explicitly and personally targeted at you. Chances are that the first author had to sort through many sets of comments and couldn't satisfy everyone. Further, I avoid complaining to the first author about other coauthors unless necessary. No one likes to play referee—it's a difficult position to be in, and you are asking the first author to choose sides. Remember that the first author likely chose all the coauthors on the paper and probably doesn't want to have to choose between you and another colleague.

I remember one paper a couple of years ago where one coauthor started taking "pot shots" at a theoretical perspective that another coauthor had developed. The purpose of the study we were reporting was to integrate the models that the two coauthors had developed. The coauthor taking pot shots was criticizing the other coauthor's model as a way of favoring and promoting her own model—and because all the coauthors were copied on the emails, I had to try to resolve the dispute. The coauthor whose model was being criticized was clearly upset by the other coauthor's comments and mentioned dropping out of the paper. The situation really had me in a bind. I didn't want to lose either of them from the paper, and the situation was causing me a great deal of stress and anxiety.

It took several diplomatic and carefully worded emails from me—including one where I told both coauthors that I was lead author and I was going to determine the direction of the paper—to end the dispute. I am normally very democratic in my style and don't like to take charge, but in this situation, one of my coauthors wasn't leaving me much choice. When I emailed the group telling them that I had decided on a course of action, both coauthors replied, "Sounds good." The lesson here is that a democratic approach is normally quite effective, but occasionally the first author has to take control of a situation where coauthors are arguing and triangulating the first author into their disagreement. From a coauthor's perspective, it is not a good idea to create a situation where the first author must play referee.

Remember that the goal is to get the paper published. If you, as a coauthor, disagree with the direction of the paper, then I suggest asking for a meeting or conference call where you can discuss the disagreement respectfully. Taking pot shots at other coauthors through email doesn't solve anything—it only creates tension that the first author has to resolve. Email is not an effective means of communicating about important disputes or disagreements. These issues should be discussed in person or through video chat, and all of the parties in the disagreement should attend and be afforded opportunities to express their views.

So, in essence, coauthors should support the first author and provide whatever feedback they can to help improve the paper. In large collaborative writing projects, coauthors should also support other coauthors by building on their comments, respecting their viewpoints, and refraining from disparaging other coauthors. The first author has more than enough work to do without having to arbitrate disputes between and among coauthors.

Difficult Coauthoring Situations

Several topics are covered in this section: dealing with difficult and resistant coauthors, excusing oneself from a collaboration, and students leading collaborations with mentors and other faculty members.

Dealing With Difficult and Resistant Coauthors

Let me start by specifying what I mean by difficult and resistant coauthors. Briefly, I am referring to coauthors who don't return comments within a reasonable time frame, coauthors who try to block submission or publication of papers, and coauthors who attempt to harass or intimidate other authors. I have witnessed, and heard about, all of these types of coauthor problems—and I will provide ideas to avoid and resolve them.

Slow Coauthors

Coauthors who are painstakingly slow can be frustrating, but I would not place them in the same category as coauthors who try to sabotage a manuscript or intimidate other authors. Nevertheless, slow coauthors can be a major source of delays in getting a paper finalized and submitted, and there may be ways to encourage them to pick up their pace. Of course, part of the solution involves understanding why these coauthors are slow. Do these people have impending grant submission deadlines? Are they buried under a heavy teaching or administrative load? Do they have young children at home (especially in the case of single parents and people who don't have access to childcare)? Are they facing difficult family situations, such as serious illnesses, separations or divorces, or economic disruption? Are they not good at time management? Do they often agree to collaborate and then not follow through? If someone has a temporary situation that prevents them from commenting on your draft, such as a grant submission deadline, then you may just need to wait for the deadline to pass. If the person is buried under a heavy teaching or administrative load, then you may need to decide whether it's realistic to wait for comments from that person. I have colleagues who work at small teaching colleges, and they are often able to dedicate large blocks of time to manuscript writing only during the summer. I know that, if I invite these colleagues to collaborate on papers during the academic year, I will likely have to wait several weeks—or longer—to receive comments on a draft. I've declined opportunities to coauthor because I was too busy, and I hope that other people would extend the same courtesy to their colleagues. It's difficult, and frustrating, to have to turn down collaborations because you don't have time, but declining is the most respectful course of action when you would likely wind up delaying the progress of the paper.

When people are faced with serious family illnesses, potential or actual family dissolution (e.g., severe marital problems, separation, divorce), or economic disruption, they may not respond to your emails or comment on your drafts. Urgent life situations and crises take precedence over work commitments, and if you have emailed someone repeatedly and have not received a response, I suggest that you leave that person alone. They will likely reach out to you once their life situation has stabilized.

With that said, however, some people tend to offer excuses rather than producing results. I've had colleagues come up with all sorts of excuses for why their work was not completed as promised. There is a major difference between people who have legitimate life situations and people who make excuses—if you notice someone has a pattern of unreliability and broken promises, then I advise that you not continue collaborating with the person.

I can remember a paper I was writing that was really important to me. I had a strong feeling that the paper would be an important contribution to the literature. One of my coauthors, however, was extremely slow. At one point this person took 6 months to return comments on a draft I had sent. I emailed repeatedly to remind the person to please look at the draft. At one point the response was, "I will get to this as soon as I possibly can; I know you are eager." But the person's comments were slow in coming—and even when the coauthor did send comments, they didn't comment on the whole draft. About 70% of the way through, the coauthor left a comment saying, "I think I need to quit on this now." As you can probably imagine, I was not pleased, and after that manuscript was accepted for publication, I did not write with this person again. Unreliability and unreasonable delays are not desirable characteristics in coauthors.

However, once you have started writing a paper with someone, you should do your best to finish that paper. You may decide not to work with that coauthor again, but pulling out in the middle of a collaboration is generally not a good idea (although there are times when you may need to withdraw, as I cover later in this section). Remember that academia—and scholarly research more broadly—is a small community, and it is essential to maintain a positive reputation with your colleagues and in the field.

Coauthors Who Try to Block Publication or Sabotage the Manuscript

Although most coauthors' goal is to contribute to getting the paper published, some coauthors appear to be more interested in advancing their own self-interests. These coauthors may insist that the paper say only what they want it to say, and nothing else, and they may refuse to sign off on submission until their demands are met. Sometimes this attitude reflects rigidity and dichotomous thinking, where the person is only willing to accept a narrow range of ideas that fit the person's view of the world, and sometimes this type of attitude can be rooted in Machiavellianism, the tendency to use others to achieve one's own objectives without regard to the other person's well-being or goals (Jones & Paulhus, 2009). In either case, the first course of action I recommend is to engage in dialogue with the coauthor and try to map out a path forward for the paper. If that strategy fails and the person is not willing to negotiate or compromise, then the other coauthors (as a group) may need to develop a united strategy and present it to the resistant coauthor. If the coauthor continues to resist, then the other authors might simply tell that person that they have been outvoted (and then proceed with the course of action that the group has decided). At that point, the resistant coauthor has two options—accommodate to the wishes of the group or drop out of the authorship altogether.

I had an experience with a coauthor like this when I was in graduate school. My master's thesis integrated streams of work conducted by two senior professors, so Ron Mullis, Dick Dunham, and I reached out to these two people to invite them to coauthor. The experience was extremely difficult, and it took 3 years to get the paper accepted—because one of these senior professors was extremely rigid and was not willing to compromise with the other professor. The rigid coauthor—let's call this person Dr. A—pushed back on any and all attempts to proceed with the manuscript. We then initiated a conversation with Dr. A where we offered to compromise but made clear that we were not willing to give in completely to Dr. A's demands. Dr. A continued to insist that his approach was the only reasonable course of action and insisted that he would not sign off on submitting the paper unless all his requests were incorporated. Eventually, we told Dr. A that the four other authors were overruling and outvoting him. Almost immediately, Dr. A decided to withdraw from the authorship.

Dr. A behaved the same way toward several other student coauthors—and on one occasion, Dr. A was serving on a student's dissertation committee and refused to approve that student's dissertation unless she changed all her analyses. The analyses that Dr. A was requesting were completely self-serving—Dr. A wanted the analyses to completely support his theory—and the result was that the student became exasperated and left academia altogether.

People like Dr. A are fortunately uncommon, but they do exist. Dr. A didn't seem Machiavellian, but he did have a very limited range of ideas that he was willing to accept. His insistence on always being right led him to block submission and publication of several manuscripts that I know about, and his obstructionist behavior effectively chased a graduate student out of academia. Thankfully, I had three senior professors to support me in dealing with Dr. A—had I not had their support, that paper probably would never have been published.

Coauthors Who Harass and Intimidate Other Authors

On some—thankfully rare—occasions, coauthors may harass, intimidate, or threaten other authors. On most occasions, this behavior is intended to coerce the other authors into incorporating the person's ideas or viewpoints into the paper. The coauthor who is doing the harassing may be in a position of authority over the first author (and perhaps over other coauthors as well), and the person may use this authority as a way of pushing their ideas onto the other authors.

Whereas resistant coauthors are often rigid and inflexible, coauthors who harass and intimidate others are more likely to be Machiavellian. They use and manipulate others as a way of achieving their own goals. These people are likely to abuse their authority over others for their own personal gain—and in my experience, they often believe that they cannot be held accountable for their actions. Working under someone like this is not especially pleasant, and coauthoring with someone like this can be quite aversive.

A senior professor, whom we will call Dr. B, sabotaged the work of graduate students and assistant professors unless they incorporated her ideas into their papers and listed her as first author. Dr. B was in a leadership position in her academic department and used this position to coerce younger scholars to write papers for her. Dr. B often insisted on being first author on papers where she had not earned that authorship position. In fact, Dr. B would not sign off on papers unless she was listed in the most advantageous authorship position that she could justify for herself. Thus, she managed to get herself tenured and promoted to full professor by intimidating her colleagues into writing papers for her and listing her as first author.

Dr. B was an example of a Machiavellian coauthor who used her position of power in her department to intimidate her younger colleagues into doing work for her. Unfortunately, it is difficult to push back against someone who has authority over you—and students, postdocs, and early-career faculty members may essentially have to comply with the Machiavellian person's wishes. The best course of action—if it's possible—is to remove yourself from collaborations with these people. Such a strategy is often not feasible with mentors, so you may need to finish the mentored experience and then end the collaboration.

There is an old saying that it's often better to lose the battle and win the war than vice versa. This saying applies well to difficult mentors, supervisors, and other "non-optional" colleagues whom you cannot remove from the authorship of your paper (or from whom you cannot remove yourself). In my career, I have worked successfully with many difficult people, and one of the strategies that has worked best for me is to challenge the person very gently—and never directly. I might ask something like, "Have you thought about maybe doing it this way?" I also praise the person effusively, using only compliments that I know to be true. I may tell the person that I really need their guidance because of their vast experience in the field and expertise in the area of study represented by the paper. (Note that I don't say anything that isn't true—but I do "stroke" the person as a way of helping them drop their guard.) I will stop and ask the person how they feel about each major decision I've made for the paper. And if something goes wrong, I generally take the blame. I'm careful never to confront the person directly or to accuse them of anything. You don't want a difficult person to get defensive—that's a sure way to create problems with that person.

As Dick Dunham told me once, the purpose of a master's thesis or doctoral dissertation is to get it done so you can move on with your life and career. If you have to appease your mentor, department chair, graduate program director, or anyone else in order to secure their approval and consent for your work to move forward, then I suggest doing that. The sooner you finish your thesis or dissertation, the sooner you can advance to a place where your difficult mentor, chair, dean, or graduate program director no longer has control over you.

But while you are working with difficult coauthors who are trying to block submission of your paper—including Machiavellian people who may be aiming to use others for their own personal gain—I suggest trying to explore what their concerns are. In some cases, such as Dr. A, the coauthor may be willing to endorse only a limited and narrow range of ideas. If the ideas that your paper presents fall outside that range, the coauthor may become resistant and attempt to block you from submitting the paper. In other cases, such as Dr. B in the second example, the coauthor may be trying to block submission for reasons that have nothing to do with the content of the paper. The person may not be comfortable with their position on the authorship, or they may have more nefarious motives. I remember a student whose advisor discouraged her from pursuing a project for her dissertation. The advisor came up with all sorts of reasons why the project was likely to fail, but the real reason he was discouraging the student was because of his own greed and ambition. When the student became frustrated and gave up on the dissertation project, the advisor stole the idea, completed the project on his own, and published the findings himself.

In some cases, you may be able to appease these people sufficiently to get your work submitted and published. However, please know that there are some situations where a first author who is not senior enough (especially students, postdoctoral fellows, and beginning assistant professors) simply cannot win a fight against a senior coauthor who is engaging in Machiavellian tactics. If you can withdraw from the collaboration without damaging your career, then I advise doing that. Another strategy might be to state that you don't see a way forward for the paper given the concerns that have been raised. Coauthors may decide to rethink their opposition if they know that it may cause the paper to be dropped. Of course, as with the greedy advisor described in the previous paragraph, some coauthors might actually want a junior colleague to abandon a paper so that they can take it over. Unfortunately, students, postdoctoral fellows, and other mentees and supervisees may not have any recourse against a mentor, supervisor, or other authority figure who is blocking a paper from being advanced.

In some cases, the mentor may not be blocking the paper per se but may be blocking the mentee from advancing in general. I was once friends with a PhD student at another university. She was from another country and had come to the United States to pursue her graduate degree. She was working with the academic couple I mentioned earlier in this chapter—the couple who regularly denied their students the opportunity to publish papers based on their master's theses and doctoral dissertations. My friend called me crying on many occasions because the academic couple were blocking her attempts to advance in the PhD program and to use their data for analyses and writing. After almost a year of being manipulated and lied to, she finally left the program and returned to her native country. (Unfortunately, my friend's story is not unique—I have heard other stories just like hers.)

If you are working with a toxic mentor or supervisor, my advice is to stick it out if you can. Finish your degree, your postdoc, or whatever other mentored experience you are in, and move on with your life and career. When Dick Dunham started to become difficult at the end of my time at Florida State, I vowed to finish my master's degree and leave. I wasn't going to let the way Dick was behaving keep me from achieving my goals. There are, however, some situations that are unbearable or where the person chooses to walk away. Mentees who are being sexually harassed, threatened, stalked, or otherwise having their rights violated by their mentors may have little choice but to end the mentoring relationship. Unfortunately, in many cases taking this step is likely to endanger the mentee's academic future. Machiavellian mentors and supervisors are well known for retaliating (or trying to retaliate) against people who defy or leave them.

Leaving Toxic Collaborations

Sometimes, when a collaborative project has become toxic, the best course of action is to leave the collaboration altogether. A first author might decide to abandon a paper or to hand it off to someone else, or a coauthor might decide to drop out of the collaboration. (For the record, I have done both things.) Such decisions might be reached because other authors are behaving in counterproductive or unethical ways, because of infighting among the authors, or because of serious disagreements that appear insurmountable. Although withdrawing from a collaboration seems like a form of quitting, in some cases it is probably the best decision for the author who is leaving the paper, and perhaps also for the paper and for the collaboration as a whole.

I'll give you a couple of examples of times when I (or other people I know) have withdrawn from manuscripts. The first example occurred at the end of my postdoctoral fellowship, when the mutual dislike between me and the research group I'd been working with had reached its peak. My chemistry with this group had never been good, and after I announced that I had taken a faculty position and was leaving, the tension became almost impossible for me to bear. I had been leading a manuscript using the group's data, and once I announced my impending departure, the feedback I was receiving on drafts became increasingly harsh. It became clear to me that this paper was never going to be submitted with me as lead author—the group wasn't going to allow that—so I told my supervisor that I was withdrawing from the collaboration. (To her credit, even after she had assigned another postdoctoral fellow to take over the paper, she asked him to reach out to me and invite me back onto the authorship before the paper was submitted for publication.)

The second example occurred several years ago when José and I were collaborating with two junior colleagues on an empirical manuscript. The two junior colleagues, who were first and second author (I was third author and José was fourth and last), spent several weeks bickering with one another over email, and before long, the bickering became personal. The first and second authors started berating one another so viciously that José threatened to drop out of the authorship if these attacks didn't stop. I echoed José's position and told the first and second authors that, although they clearly didn't like each other, the goal of the collaboration was to publish the paper. "The two of you never have to speak to each other after this paper is finished," I wrote in an email. "But our priority is to get the paper accepted. Please stop attacking each other and get the writing done." After I sent that email, the bickering stopped, and we got the paper accepted in a top journal.

Important questions that some readers may have in their minds concern when, how, and why to withdraw from a collaboration. My answer is fairly simple and straightforward—when you begin to feel uncomfortable with the direction the paper is taking, with how the first author is incorporating (or not incorporating) your feedback, with the interpersonal dynamics among the authors, or with potentially unethical decisions or behavior taking place around the paper or the project it is reporting, you should voice your discomfort. Speak directly with the first author or request a meeting among the authors and let them know what your concerns are. Don't leave the paper at the first sign of discomfort; rather, do so only after it's clear that your concerns are not being taken seriously or that they are not going to be addressed. If you do decide to withdraw, it's essential to do so respectfully and in a way that allows the remaining authors to save face. If you are first author, make sure to arrange for one of the other authors to take over the paper. I definitely do not advise dropping out of a paper angrily or leaving the other authors "hanging." Remember that academia, and scholarly publishing more generally, is an extremely small world. Damaging professional relationships is never a good idea.

Coauthoring Issues for Students and Other Mentees

Mentor–Mentee Collaborations

I know I have been providing some very extreme and ominous examples of toxic mentors in this chapter. I'd like to emphasize that the vast majority of mentors are highly supportive, encouraging, and collaborative with their mentees. Even so, mentor–mentee collaborations can be tricky because of the power differential between mentors and mentees. Indeed, as already noted in this book, mentoring is like parenting in many ways. This analogy also suggests that mentors often wield the same authority that parents do. As a mentee, how would you go about asking to use your mentor's data, asking to serve as first author on a manuscript that you are coauthoring with your mentor, or pushing back against feedback that your mentor has offered on a manuscript? How would you take these steps while remaining mindful of your mentor's position of authority?

I suggest approaching these situations using a strategy similar to the one I use with difficult people. (I am not suggesting that your mentor is difficult—I am simply suggesting that this approach works with most people.) Make suggestions rather than pronouncements and ask for guidance rather than pushing back directly. Asking "Have you thought about . . ." and then offering your ideas is likely to keep your mentor from becoming defensive. If your mentor offers a suggestion or comment on a manuscript and you don't agree, you may want to offer a suggested course of action and ask for your mentor's thoughts. You know your mentor and the communication styles that work best with that person—so please take my ideas as suggestions and add your own "spin" to them.

Let's now turn to the "nuts and bolts" of working with mentors. The first suggestion I offer is to set up weekly (or biweekly) meetings with your mentor. These meetings can take place in person, through video chat, or however else you both are comfortable meeting. Especially if you are actively writing, managing projects, or otherwise interfacing with your mentor's work, you should be meeting regularly. If you don't meet regularly, weeks and months can pass without sufficient progress on your projects. Especially if your mentor is a really busy person, it is essential to keep yourself and your work on your mentor's radar.

Second, I suggest initiating a "ground rules" conversation with your mentor. Ask whether your mentor prefers having you physically present in the office or whether it's acceptable for you to work from home some of the time. (I suspect that, given that almost everyone in academia and other scholarly fields has been working from home during the coronavirus pandemic of 2020 and 2021, working from home will remain common and accepted even after the pandemic ends.) Ask how accountable your mentor wants you to be with your time—some mentors want to know what their mentees are doing during the day, whereas other mentors are primarily concerned with deliverables and are less concerned with when and where the work is completed. Find out whether there are other arrangements that your mentor would like you to maintain.

Third, in the PhD program I used to direct, each mentor–mentee pair was required to sign a contract where deliverables, timelines, and meeting arrangements were specified. I countersigned all the. contracts, so that I was able to arbitrate disputes by referring to the terms of the contract. Using the contracts, both the mentor and the mentee were expected to specify their expectations for one another and for themselves. For example, when the mentee sends the mentor a draft, how much time does the mentor need to return comments? When the mentor asks the mentee to complete a task, how much time does the mentee need to complete that task? How often will the mentor and mentee meet, and is there a specific format that those meetings will take? Will a formal agenda be required for the meetings? What deliverables (e.g., manuscript drafts) is the mentee expected to produce in each semester?

Notice that I have not mentioned writing very much in this subsection on mentor–mentee collaborations. I have done this by design—focusing more on structural issues within the collaboration and less on the writing. Once the necessary structural arrangements are in place, mentors and mentees can work together just as any other pair of coauthors would. (Of course, Machiavellianism and rigidity can also serve as impediments to mentor–mentee collaborations.) Here I am assuming that the mentor has the best interests of the mentee—and of the collaboration as a whole—in mind, and that the mentor is flexible enough to accommodate differences of scientific opinion. As long as the mentor treats the mentee with respect and as a colleague, and as long as the mentee takes the work seriously and puts sufficient time and effort into it, the odds of a successful collaboration should be fairly high. Most mentor–mentee problems occur when one or both of these two assumptions are not satisfied.

As a mentee, you are best served when you stay in touch with your mentor and seek your mentor's support and input whenever you feel stuck. If you are writing a draft and you're not sure what to write next, let your mentor take a look and provide feedback. Be sure not to "disappear" for long periods of time, and if you agree or promise to deliver a work product by a specific date or time, it is essential that you keep your word. If you miss a deadline that you and your mentor agreed on, try to avoid making excuses for why the work wasn't done on time. Simply take responsibility for the error and dedicate yourself to delivering on time in the future. If the work you submitted to your mentor was not your best effort, take responsibility for that and dedicate yourself to putting forth your best effort in the future. Although mentoring is like parenting in many ways, unlike parents, mentors are not required to continue working with you if you habitually disappear, make excuses, or deliver subpar work. Mentoring you needs to be a source of fulfillment and generativity, rather than a source of frustration, for your mentor.

As a mentor, remember that your mentees are learning from you and that they do not yet know how to write scholarly papers on their own. Especially early in their training, mentees may submit writing that is choppy, disorganized, and difficult to read. (One of my students likes to describe her early writing as "word vomit.") Your role as mentor is to gently correct and edit your mentees' writing and to help them to improve their scholarly writing skills. Try your best not to lose patience with your mentees when their writing needs more editing from you than you hoped it would need. Point out the writing mistakes (e.g., AOTP, unfinished thoughts, logical leaps) that mentees seem to make most often and suggest ways for them to correct these problems. Keep in mind that mentees may need more feedback, and more rounds of edits, from you than your colleagues would. (You should treat your mentees like colleagues in terms of the respect and regard that you offer them, but your expectations of them should be developmentally appropriate for where they are in their graduate training and in their evolution as scholars and writers.)

Just like parenting, mentoring involves gently and supportively correcting mistakes. Mentees may submit work that is not as polished or as complete as you would like. It's essential to use such occasions as teachable moments where you point out exactly what you are not happy with and how the mentee's performance can improve in the future. Try to avoid belittling, criticizing, or reprimanding mentees the first time they make a mistake or submit subpar work. Of course, if the same mistakes continue to occur repeatedly, you should gently—but firmly—point out the pattern of mistakes and remind the mentee exactly what your expectations are. If the problems continue even after repeated conversations with the mentee, you may want to explore the possibility that this mentee is not well matched with you and that another mentor might represent a better fit. Of course, if the mentee is experiencing serious life or family difficulties, these issues should be factored into your evaluation of the mentee.

Patterns of disappearing, excuse making, and subpar work should be pointed out and discussed with the mentee. If a mentee continues to come up with "reasons for reasons" without really explaining the behavior, it may be helpful to try and point that out. However, the mentee may become defensive regarding the pattern of behavior you are describing; if that occurs, further discussion may yield only frustration for both of you. If the pattern of unreliable and disappointing behavior continues, the best course of action may be to end the mentoring relationship in as supportive a way as possible. Try to help the mentee find another mentor if possible. You might want to suggest that the mentee seek help (such as mental health services) if you believe that such services might be beneficial.

So let me sum up my observations and recommendations regarding mentor–mentee writing collaborations. The most effective collaborations appear to be those where the mentor is invested in the mentee, respects the mentee as a colleague, and is available to meet the mentee's needs, and where the mentee is accountable, reliable, and invested in their own development. In such an arrangement, having the mentor and mentee specify the parameters of their working relationship, including their expectations of one another and of themselves, may help to facilitate productivity. The more parameters that can be worked out in advance—including meeting frequency and modality, working arrangements (e.g., working from home versus having "face time" in the office), and deliverables—the smoother the working relationship is likely to be.

Students Leading Collaborations With Faculty Members

A special case of student–mentee collaborations involves students, postdoctoral fellows, or other mentees who are leading collaborative projects with multiple faculty members. I did this multiple times during my career as a mentee (including the paper that Dr. A was trying to block from being published), and I have also served as a faculty-level collaborator on papers led by students and postdoctoral fellows. Optimally, these collaborations are

hugely advantageous for mentees, because they provide the mentee with access to input and collective wisdom from multiple people who know how to
publish.

I have a colleague who has been very successful in this kind of collaboration. Although at the time of this writing (October 2020) he is only a postdoctoral fellow, this person has led several collaborations with multiple full
professors. He reached out to each of us individually; and he put together the
ideas, data sets, or arguments. Most of all, his humility, openness to feedback
and constructive criticism, and outstanding writing and conceptual skills
have impressed all the full professors who have been fortunate enough to publish with him.

I've had other student and postdoctoral colleagues who have led similar
collaborations with multiple faculty members. In almost all the cases, the
person's mentor or advisor also participated in the collaboration and advocated for the junior person when necessary. Having the mentor play the role of
advocate helps to eliminate the power differential between the student, postdoctoral fellow, or other mentee and the faculty-level collaborators. In turn,
eliminating the power differential allows the mentee to lead the collaboration
most effectively.

In my experience, most faculty members enjoy collaborating with young
scholars. I know I do. Our role is to support the young scholar in writing the
paper and in pushing forward fresh and innovative ideas. In many cases,
writing with faculty-level collaborators helps young scholars to connect with
postdoctoral fellowships and job opportunities later on—for example, while
I was writing articles with the colleague I just mentioned, I connected him
with another colleague of mine who became his postdoctoral supervisor. I've
done the same for another young scholar who impressed me (and others) immediately with her strong conceptual and writing skills.

Faculty collaborators can also serve as informal mentors for young
scholars. I have done this for several young scholars who have reached out to
me and asked to collaborate. When I was a student, I connected with several
faculty-level colleagues at conferences, and I invited them to write with me.
Most of them agreed, and I used these opportunities to "build my Rolodex"
(to borrow my father's expression). In this regard, it's important to be fear-
less when reaching out to faculty members—both at your own institution and
elsewhere—who might represent potential collaborators for you. A principle
I use is that, if you don't ask for what you want, the answer is already No. By
asking, you can change that answer to Yes. The worst-case scenario is that
the person declines your request. My only caveat in this regard is that you
should keep your mentor, advisor, or supervisor in the loop in terms of other

collaborators to whom you have reached out. As already noted, your mentor can advocate for you in these collaborations.

If conflicts emerge as part of a collaboration between a young scholar and a group of faculty-level collaborators, the young scholar's mentor should help to resolve the conflict. If you are a faculty-level scholar and you collaborate with students, postdoctoral fellows, and other mentees, please keep in mind that these young scholars may not be aware of some of the "unwritten rules" of academia and scholarly publishing. If a young scholar (who is not a mentee of yours) does something that you believe is inappropriate, I suggest reaching out to that person's mentor and addressing the issue with the mentor. It is generally not appropriate to contact the young scholar directly unless you have established a close working relationship with that person. If you are the young scholar in this situation and a faculty collaborator contacts you directly with critical feedback regarding something you said or did, I suggest reaching out to your mentor and asking for help in addressing the situation.

Conclusion

This chapter covers issues involving coauthors. It provides the coauthor's job description, reviews issues involved in working in large authorship teams, and introduces difficult coauthoring situations. The coauthor job description includes providing comments and edits on the materials that the first author has provided. Coauthors often use both active and passive coauthoring methods, where active methods involve writing and revising text directly in the paper, whereas passive methods involve inserting margin comments for the first author to address. It's essential for the authorship group to agree on their desired combination of active and passive coauthoring styles, so that coauthors don't become upset with each other for not contributing sufficiently to the collaboration.

With each passing year, working in large teams is becoming more the norm and less the exception. Team science has helped to break down disciplinary barriers that once prevented scholars from working together across fields, but increasing numbers of coauthors pose challenges for first authors, including having to sort through many sets of comments that may contradict one another. Coauthors may also not work together well, and in some cases the first author may have to play referee between and among coauthors. Large numbers of coauthors may provide an advantage, however, in that errors, internal inconsistencies, and other issues are more likely to be caught and corrected when there are more people reviewing drafts. It is therefore essential for young scholars to gain experience working on large authorship teams.

In terms of difficult authorship situations, slow coauthors are probably the most common problem. Professors and other scholars face more demands now than ever, partly due to the corporatization of academia (Chan & Fisher, 2008), including increasing pressure to secure grant funding (Lilienfeld, 2017; Thyer, 2011) as well as an ever-expanding array of administrative roles in the university system (Bexley, Arkoudis, & James, 2013). Difficulty finding time for scholarly work was one of the chief complaints that Bexley et al. found among their sample of Australian academics. In my experience, senior scholars—especially full professors—are more likely to have taken on ad-ministrative roles that take time away from their scholarly work. People may also be dealing with personal and family situations that prevent them from attending to work commitments. In most cases, slow coauthors are simply overloaded and have trouble attending to all the tasks they have committed to complete. In some instances, however, slow coauthors experience difficulties with time management or are not prioritizing your paper. Perhaps the most effective course of action is to speak with the coauthor and find out what's happening in that person's life.

The chapter also covers rigidity and Machiavellianism—two traits that can lead coauthors to try to block publication of their colleagues' manuscripts or to harass, intimidate, and manipulate their colleagues. If you are working with coauthors who behave in these ways, a good strategy is to meet with your other coauthors and to develop a plan for approaching the difficult coauthor. (Of course, this approach may not be possible if the difficult coauthor is your mentor, advisor, or supervisor.) Try to understand the person's concerns and to work with them to address the concerns. Only if the person continues to be inflexible and refuses to compromise, or continues to try to undermine the other authors, should the authorship team attempt to outvote that coauthor or try to push them off the authorship. Again, as already noted, if the person is in a position of authority over you, you may have fewer options and may just have to do your best to appease the person.

Finally, the chapter considers mentor–mentee collaborations and papers where a student, postdoc, or other early-career scholar is lead author and where several faculty-level colleagues are coauthors. In both situations, men-torship is key to reducing the power imbalance and empowering the mentee to succeed. Collaborating with mentors and with other senior colleagues can be extremely beneficial for young scholars as long as the power imbalances are offset. It is essential for mentors to be available to their mentees and for mentees to be accountable to their mentors. Formal agreements between mentees and mentors can help to ensure that both parties are on the same page and that the collaboration is maximally efficient. Mentors are also essential in advocating for their mentees in larger collaborations where a mentee is lead author.

Summary

- The majority of journal articles include multiple authors.
- People who review literature or conduct statistical analyses should be listed as authors.
- Serving as a "substantive" coauthor (not including statisticians and coauthors who only review literature) involves reading manuscript drafts; adding, deleting, or modifying text; and commenting on anything that seems unclear, confusing, or troubling.
- When the first author fundamentally disagrees with a coauthor's suggestions, the two authors should have a conversation to explore the disagreement and come to a resolution.
- Authorship order and decision-making rules should be agreed upon before starting the paper.
- Active coauthoring means inserting text directly into the manuscript, whereas passive coauthoring involves providing margin comments for the first author to address.
- Mentor–mentee collaborations may require special arrangements to ensure that the coauthoring relationship will be equitable and fair.
- Large authorship teams can be challenging because of the sheer volume of comments that the first author has to incorporate into the manuscript.
- When coauthors are slow, it is important to figure out why they are slow before approaching them.
- When coauthors are difficult and resistant, it is important to try to negotiate with them before attempting to overrule or dismiss them.
- Machiavellian coauthors are those who attempt to bully or manipulate others in order to get their way. It is essential to negotiate with Machiavellian coauthors before trying to overrule or dismiss them.

References

Bexley, E., Arkoudis, S., & James, R. (2013). The motivations, values, and future plans of Australian academics. *Higher Education, 65*, 385–400.

Cals, J. W. L., & Kotz, D. (2013). Effective writing and publishing scientific papers, part IX: Authorship. *Journal of Clinical Epidemiology, 66*, 1319.

Chan, A. S., & Fisher, D. (Eds.). (2008). *The exchange university*. Vancouver: University of British Columbia Press.

Hall, K. L., Feng, A. X., Moser, R. P., Stokols, B., & Taylor, B. K. (2008). Moving the science of team science forward: Collaboration and creativity. *American Journal of Preventive Medicine, 35*, S243–S249.

Jones, D. N., & Paulhus, D. L. (2009). *Machiavellianism*. In M. R. Leary & R. H. Hoyle (Eds.), *Handbook of individual differences in social behavior* (pp. 93–108). New York: Guilford Press.

Lilienfeld, S. O. (2017). Psychology's replication crisis and the grant culture: Righting the ship. *Perspectives on Psychological Science, 12*, 660–664.

National Academy of Sciences. (2009). *On being a scientist: A guide to responsible conduct in research* (3rd ed.). Washington, DC: National Academies Press.

Oberlander, S. E., & Spencer, R. J. (2006). Graduate students and the culture of authorship. *Ethics and Behavior, 16*, 217–232.

Sandler, J. C., & Russell, B. L. (2006). Faculty–student collaboration: Ethics and satisfaction in authorship credit. *Ethics and Behavior, 15*, 65–80.

Sanfey, H., Hollands, L., & Gantt, N. L. (2013). Strategies for building an effective mentoring relationship. *American Journal of Surgery, 206*, 714–718.

Tebes, J. K. (2018). Team science, justice, and the co-production of knowledge. *American Journal of Community Psychology, 62*, 13–22.

Thyer, B. A. (2011). Harmful effects of federal research grants. *Social Work Research, 35*, 1–7.

15

Working With Public-Use and Proprietary Datasets

Chapter Objectives

When you finish reading this chapter, you should feel more comfortable with:

- The purpose of public-use and proprietary population-based datasets
- How complex sampling procedures are carried out and how the resulting data are analyzed
- Oversampling and sampling weights
- Planned missingness and missing data imputation
- Learning the codebook for a public-use or proprietary dataset
- Advantages and disadvantages of using public-use and proprietary datasets
- Whether public-use and proprietary datasets are appropriate for specific research questions

Types of Datasets

In psychology and related fields, many researchers gather their own data to test their hypotheses. However, as covered in Chapter 2, many other researchers use secondary datasets—that is, datasets that were collected for another purpose and that are effectively being "reused" to test a different set of hypotheses than they were designed to test. In some cases, students and postdoctoral fellows will use their mentors' datasets for their thesis or dissertation research. Using your mentor's dataset is clearly a type of secondary analysis. There is, however, another type of secondary data analysis—using public-use and proprietary datasets. In many cases, these datasets were collected explicitly as repositories for other researchers to use. For example, the Pew Research Center uses data from the United States Census Bureau and the American Community Survey to prepare their reports. Both data sources

The Savvy Academic. Seth J. Schwartz, Oxford University Press. © Oxford University Press 2022.
DOI: 10.1093/oso/9780190095918.003.0016

are collected to facilitate secondary data analyses—and Census and American Community Survey are free to access and download from the U.S. Census website (www.census.gov).

Public-Use Datasets

The Census and American Community Survey are examples of public-use datasets. Public-use datasets can be used to provide nationally representative samples (Herbst & Tekin, 2014), to compare results from one's own datasets to those from nationally representative samples (Freedman, Hawkes, Zimmerman, Hebel, & Magaziner, 2001), and to estimate prevalence rates (Wallin et al., 2019), among other purposes. Many public-use datasets are gathered by government agencies—for example, the National Survey on Family Growth is conducted by the Centers for Disease Control and Prevention (see https://www.cdc.gov/nchs/nsfg/index.htm). Other public-use datasets are gathered by university researchers in collaboration with government agencies. For instance, the Monitoring the Future study (http://www.monitoringthefuture.org/) is a national epidemiological study of adolescent substance use and related behaviors and is conducted by the University of Michigan in collaboration with the National Institute on Drug Abuse. Data from this survey are also available for free download.

Some disciplines, such as epidemiology, sociology, demography, and political science, rely heavily on national public-use datasets because the goals of these disciplines are to present population-based estimates of disease prevalence, population profiles, societal trends, and political ideology and behavior, respectively. In my estimation, the most effective way to learn about the public-use datasets that are available in your area of study is to look up and read recent articles and see what datasets the authors used.

Proprietary Datasets

Another kind of dataset that some people access is the proprietary dataset. Proprietary datasets are explicitly owned by a company or research group. Researchers wishing to use the data often must complete an application, pay a fee, and agree to be bound by specific terms and conditions. In some cases, even researchers who have been granted use of the dataset must submit their manuscript plans (and later the manuscript itself) to the dataset's publications committee. These publications committees have the right to request changes or to disapprove manuscripts and manuscript ideas.

One example of a proprietary dataset is the Hispanic Community Health Study/Study of Latinos (HCHS/SOL; see https://sites.cscc.unc.edu/hchs/StudyOverview). Although the HCHS/SOL study was funded by the National Institutes of Health, the study leaders maintain strict control over the dataset. However, they encourage other researchers to propose ancillary studies (sometimes including the HCHS/SOL investigators) to conduct new analyses or to collect additional data from HCHS/SOL participants. The collaborative model for the HCHS/SOL dataset is clearly different from the model used by the U.S. Census Bureau vis-à-vis the American Community Survey—whereas the Census Bureau does not restrict or constrain the use of the American Community Survey data, no one is allowed to access the HCHS/SOL data without explicit permission from the study investigators.

Note that I am not making value judgments about which collaborative model is "better" or "worse." I am simply contrasting the ways in which researchers can gain access to public-use versus proprietary datasets. It is up to individual investigators to decide which dataset they wish to use and whether they wish to (or can) undertake the procedures needed to access the dataset.

Some datasets offer both public-use and proprietary versions. The National Longitudinal Study of Adolescent Health (Add Health; https://addhealth.cpc.unc.edu/), for example, offers both public-use and restricted-use (proprietary) datasets. The public-use dataset includes half of the cases and doesn't provide potentially identifying information (e.g., ZIP codes, schools that youth attended). The restricted-use dataset includes all the cases and provides all the information collected on each participant. To access the restricted-use dataset, researchers must pay a fee and agree to follow a set of instructions necessary to protect participants' private information. For example, researchers using the restricted-use dataset are not permitted to create tables with fewer than three cases in a cell. This rule limits the risk of deductive disclosure (Sieber, 2006), where having access to several pieces of someone's demographic information can facilitate identifying that person. Later waves also include genetic information, which can also be used to identify participants (Wist, 2010). As a result, the research group that controls the restricted-use dataset needs to ensure that participant confidentiality is maintained.

In general, public-use datasets don't contain any identifying information, and the risk of breaching someone's confidentiality is therefore extremely low. Proprietary and restricted-use datasets do contain potential identifiers, such as home addresses, ZIP (postal) codes, or schools attended (this information is often used for geocoding purposes, such as calculating the number of alcohol retailers within a specific distance of someone's home address; Connor, Kypri, Bell, & Cousins, 2011). Datasets that include genetic information—such as the HCHS/SOL dataset—are also more likely to be proprietary. The inclusion of potential identifiers is a key reason why some research groups impose strict controls on who is allowed to access their datasets.

Using Public-Use and Proprietary Datasets

The first major step in using a public-use or proprietary dataset is to learn the codebook. The codebook indicates which columns in the dataset represent which variables. In principle, a codebook should be easy to interpret, but with many population-based datasets, the codebook can be quite difficult and frustrating to learn. Some reasons for this complexity include multilevel and cross-classified nesting, oversampling, and planned missingness designs. We discuss each of these issues here.

Multilevel and Cross-Classified Nesting

Classical frequentist analyses, such as *t*-tests, analyses of variance, and multiple regression, assume that each case in the sample is completely independent of every other case. For example, if we have a sample of students in a classroom and we examine the students' math grades, we might expect that their grades would be independent of one another and would be predictable based on the students' characteristics and social networks. For example, students with higher mathematical ability, whose parents monitored their homework, and who have more highly educated people in their social network would likely earn the highest math grades. Further, any difference between groups of students within the class—such as boys versus girls or students from single-parent versus two-parent families—should be attributable to the traits and social networks of the students in the class.

Another way to express the independence assumption is that, given a set of predictor variables—let's say mathematical ability, parental involvement, and the number of college graduates in a student's social network—the unexplained variability in math grades for one student should not be correlated with the unexplained variability in math grades for another student. To help clarify what I'm saying, let's look at the classical ordinary least squares

456 The Savvy Academic

(OLS) regression formula—that is, the version that is taught in introductory statistics courses:

$$Y = \alpha + \beta X + e$$

In this formula, α is the y-intercept (the point at which the regression line crosses the y-axis), β is the slope (the expected change in Y for each 1-unit change in X), and the final term in the equation, e, is the error term, which represents all of the variability in Y that is not accounted for by X (or by the set of X terms in a multiple regression equation). Note that, although we call e an error term, this labeling may be a misnomer (Keith, 2006): e represents both random error in Y and the effects of unmeasured predictors.

OLS regression models require that three assumptions be met: (1) the Y variable is normally distributed, (2) the observations are independent, and (3) homoscedasticity—namely, that the variance of e is the same for all values of X. Assumption (3) also suggests that X should not be correlated with e. That is, the explained variability (X) and the unexplained variability (e) do not vary systematically with one another. Indeed, OLS regression assumes that, if all possible predictors were entered into the model, e would represent random error, which cannot correlate systematically with anything.

Raudenbush and Bryk (2002), working primarily in educational settings, noticed that students in some classrooms tended to perform better in various academic subjects than did students in other classrooms—and that student performance appeared to vary across schools as well as between and among students (Raudenbush, 1989). Indeed, the quality of the schools and teachers, as well as individual student characteristics and social networks, explained variability in students' academic performance. Raudenbush and Bryk developed multilevel modeling to account for predictors of adolescent academic performance at both the individual level (Level 1) and the school level (Level 2).

Multilevel modeling, in essence, expands on the classic OLS regression model in at least two ways. First, the Level 1 intercept (β_{0j}) and slope (β_{1j}) are allowed to vary across Level 2 units; therefore, the Level 1 intercept and slope can be predicted by Level 2 variables. For example, the effects of mathematical ability on math grades might be different in each school, and the quality of teaching (a school-level variable) might predict the magnitude of those effects in each school. Second, the error term is broken up into three separate error terms, namely e_{ij} (Level 1) and u_{0j} and u_{1j} (Level 2). Look at the Level 1 and Level 2 equations:

Level 1: $Y_{ij} = \beta_{0j} + \beta_{1j} X_{ij} + e_{ij}$
Level 2: $\beta_{0j} = \gamma_{00} + \gamma_{01} W_j + u_{0j}$
Level 2: $\beta_{1j} = \gamma_{10} + \gamma_{11} W_j + u_{1j}$

Here X_{ij} is a Level 1 predictor, and W_j is a Level 2 predictor.

The point here is that research questions involving hierarchical nesting (e.g., students within schools, patients within hospitals, counties within states) must take this nesting into account not only in terms of the analyses that are conducted, but also in terms of the research design. Complex sampling designs, which are used in many population-based datasets, involve sampling Level 2 units (e.g., schools) and then sampling Level 1 units (e.g., students) within each Level 2 unit (Oğuz-Alper & Berger, 2020). Not only do these details need to be described in the method sections of papers you write using these datasets, but you also need to understand how the dataset is set up. Within a simple nesting design, such as students nested within schools, there will generally be two participant ID numbers—the Level 1 (student) ID and the Level 2 (school) ID. Both ID numbers must be specified within the syntax or dialog boxes that you use to conduct your analyses.

In many real-life examples, however, each case may be nested within multiple hierarchical units (Melamed & Vuolo, 2019). For example, as Meyers and Beretvas (2006) noted, students may be nested within both schools and neighborhoods. Not all students who live in the same neighborhood attend the same school, and vice versa—leading to what is called a cross-classified multilevel data structure. Each student is nested within a school and within a neighborhood, but schools and neighborhoods are not nested within one another. Meyers and Beretvas noted that analyzing cross-classified data requires a substantial amount of dummy coding (as is done in regression models with categorical predictors). If these dummy variables are created as part of the dataset you are using, you need to know what—and where— they are.

Oversampling

As is discussed in Chapter 2, when some groups represent small shares of the study population, researchers may oversample these groups so that their sample sizes are large enough to support statistical analyses. When groups have been oversampled, sampling weights must be used to account for the oversampling. Note that each group in the sample receives a sampling weight (see Chapter 2 for a more in-depth description). You therefore need to know where each sampling weight is in the dataset and what variable name is assigned to it.

Planned Missingness

Participant burden is a major concern in research studies (Lingler, Schmidt, Gentry, Hu, & Terhorst, 2014). Studies indicate that participants may respond carelessly to survey questions if the survey is too long (Bowling, Gibson, Houpt, & Brower, 2020). One way to address this problem is through planned missingness designs (Little & Rhemtulla, 2013). In a planned missingness design, the survey is divided into sections, and multiple forms of the survey are created. Within each form, one section of the survey is omitted (see Figure 15.1). In Figure 15.1, the survey is divided into three parts, and three forms of the survey are created. In Form A, sections A and B are included but section C is omitted. In Form B, sections A and C are included but section B is omitted. In Form C, sections B and C are included but section A is omitted.

So, let's assume that the survey has a total of 600 questions—200 in section A, 200 in section B, and 200 in section C. In this scenario, only 400 of those questions (i.e., 2 of the 3 sections) will be presented to any given study participant. Multiple imputation (Enders, 2010; Graham, 2012; Little, 2013) is then used to fill in the intentionally missing data within each survey form. Because sections A and B are both present in Form A—and therefore data are present

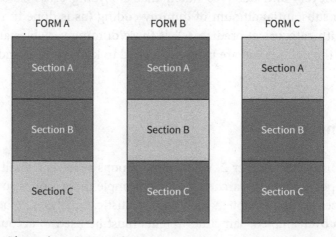

Figure 15.1 Planned missingness design.

for both section A and section C for one-third of the sample—the covariance matrix between variables in section A and variables in section B can be reliably estimated. Similar statements can be made regarding Form B (for which sections A and C are both present) and Form C (for which sections B and C are both present). As a result, we can reduce participant burden by one-third and can still reliably estimate all the parameters needed to conduct whatever analyses are needed to test one's hypotheses.

If a planned missingness design was used to collect the data you are analyzing, there should be a variable in the dataset indicating which survey form each participant completed. Note that, if the dataset is longitudinal, each participant may have completed a different survey form at each wave.

Familiarizing Yourself With the Codebook

A key principle in using public-use or proprietary datasets is that you should make sure you read the codebook (and other documentation) carefully, so you understand exactly how the study was designed and what was done at each assessment wave. Make sure you understand the dataset completely before you conduct any analyses. Many public-use datasets have websites and forums where users can post questions and interact with other users (other people using the dataset will likely be a useful resource as you learn to use the dataset). If a large number of people are using the dataset, it may be difficult to receive timely and complete answers from the people who manage or administer the dataset—other users will probably be far more responsive and helpful.

Codebooks for many public-use and proprietary datasets are quite lengthy and complex. Many public-use and proprietary datasets are based on long surveys that ask questions in many different domains. Add Health, for example, includes questions about parenting, school attendance and performance, peer affiliations, nutrition, exercise, and many other areas. A consequence of this breadth is that a large amount of data is collected from each respondent. Further, many datasets also survey large numbers of people—for example, the baseline sample size for Add Health was 90,118 (see https://addhealth.cpc.unc.edu/documentation/study-design/). The dataset is therefore massive and takes quite a bit of time to learn—and I expect that this is true of many public-use datasets.

My former PhD student and I learned firsthand how complex the Add Health dataset is. She studied the codebook intensely for more than a year, trying to match up columns of numbers and text with variable names from the codebook. Because some statistical analysis software programs don't allow file names longer that eight characters, file names are generally short. For example, youth report of mother–adolescent communication at Time 1 might be labeled YMOMCOM1. Some of these file names might be difficult to remember or keep track of, especially given the number of variables in the dataset.

Some codebooks are easier to learn than others are. For example, the Centers for Disease Control and Prevention administers the Youth Risk Behavior Surveillance Survey (YRBSS; see https://www.cdc.gov/healthyyouth/data/yrbs/data.htm), which samples adolescents and young adults and asks questions about substance use, unprotected sexual behavior, impaired driving, and other potentially dangerous behaviors. The YRBSS includes a fairly small number of items, and as a result, the codebook is short and simple. However, like most nationally representative datasets, the YRBSS studies were collected using complex, multilevel sampling strategies, and sampling weights must be used to account for oversampling of some segments of the population. In complex sampling approaches, you also must specify the primary sampling unit—that is, the level at which sampling occurred. For example, in the HCHS/SOL study, sampling was conducted at the Census block group level (LaVange et al., 2010). That is, the research team randomly sampled Census blocks rather than individuals. If you are not comfortable conducting analyses of weighted multilevel (or cross-classified) data where sampling was conducted at a level other than the individual, then I suggest that you team up with someone who does know how to analyze these types of datasets. Incorrectly using (or not using) the sampling weights and primary sampling units, and failing to specify the correct multilevel data structure, will lead to incorrect results (Raudenbush & Bryk, 2002; Winship & Radbill, 1994).

Check for Other Articles Using the Same Dataset

Because public-use datasets are often freely available, the team that manages the dataset likely does not monitor the list of papers published off the dataset. As a result, it is entirely possible that you might conduct analyses and write a manuscript that duplicates—or overlaps strongly with—something that has already been published. It is essential that you conduct a thorough literature search not only for articles on your chosen topic, but also specifically for articles using the dataset that you are planning to use. If you find an article that is similar to the one you wish to write, then you will need to present a compelling rationale for how your study contributes to the literature beyond what has already been published. For example, you might be planning to examine parenting longitudinally across a span of several years, whereas prior work might have studied parenting over only short time frames. Alternatively, you might be including predictors that prior studies have not included, or you might be comparing results across gender or ethnic groups, and other studies have not taken this step. If you cannot think of a rationale for how your planned study moves beyond prior work, then you will likely need to come up with another research idea.

Proprietary datasets often require users to submit proposals before they will be allowed to access the data. These proposals are intended to ensure that users don't duplicate prior work conducted using the dataset, that users have obtained the necessary ethical approvals to use the dataset, and that the owners of the dataset are able to maintain control over who is using the dataset. A proprietary dataset I know of has a publications committee that meets monthly to review user proposals. I have been involved in a couple of these proposals, and the publications committee is extremely rigorous and deliberative. One proposal I was involved with was reviewed by the publications committee three times, and the entire process took well over a year. On each occasion, the committee asked for additional changes to the proposal. The lead author of the proposal finally gave up and dropped the proposal after the third request for changes. Sometimes these proposals can be an exercise in persistence.

Advantages and Disadvantages of Using Public-Use and Proprietary Datasets

Advantages

Imagine being able to analyze data that will allow you to make definitive statements about a population. You can estimate prevalence rates for a given health problem, political behavior, social phenomenon, or demographic trend. Because the dataset is nationally representative, you can use it to publish articles in top journals, and you don't have to collect the data yourself. These are some of the key advantages of public-use and proprietary datasets.

Public-use and proprietary datasets also allow us to compare phenomena over time. For example, Brooks, Neeuwbeerta, and Manza (2006) used a series of population-based datasets to map changes in voting behavior across six Western countries between 1965 and 2000. Mojtabai, Olfson, and Han (2016) used data from the U.S. National Surveys on Drug Use and Health to examine trends in adolescent and young adult depressive symptoms and episodes between 2005 and 2014. Phillips and Land (2012) used nationally, state, and locally representative datasets to map the relationship between changes in unemployment and in crime rates in the United States. The analyses conducted by these author groups would likely not have been possible using datasets that the author groups collected themselves.

Disadvantages

Of course, public-use and proprietary datasets also have their disadvantages—some of which are already noted in this chapter. Because many nationally representative datasets cover a wide range of content areas, only a few items can be included for any given area. As a result, scales often must be constructed using single items (or using a small number of items). Given the importance of conceptual breadth for many constructs (Morizot, 2014), the use of single-item or extremely brief scales represents a potentially serious methodological limitation. Therefore, with many public-use and proprietary datasets, the constructs that are included in the analysis may not be as conceptually broad as we might like them to be.

A second key disadvantage of nationally representative datasets is that you don't have control of the constructs and items that are included. You also don't have control over the sampling strategy. Decisions made during data collection may not be disclosed in the documentation provided for the dataset— and errors committed during data collection may not have been caught. Collecting nationally representative datasets involves creating and managing a large team of investigators, research associates, and data collectors. With an enterprise of that size, it is almost inevitable that errors will occur and not be detected or reported. The precision and accuracy of the data therefore cannot be fully known.

A third potential disadvantage of public-use and proprietary datasets is the amount of work required to learn the codebook and familiarize yourself with the dataset. Public-use and proprietary datasets differ widely in terms of ease of use and the effort required to learn the codebook. Smaller datasets like the YRBSS may be easier to learn, whereas larger datasets like Add Health may be far more difficult to learn (as my PhD student and I found out). The learning curve involved with public-use and proprietary datasets must be factored into the timeline for completing analyses and manuscripts using these datasets.

Should You Use a Population-Based Dataset?

Population-based datasets are essential for some research questions, such as estimating prevalence rates, identifying relative risk and odds ratios vis-à-vis outcomes in the population, examining trends in population estimates across time, and other population-based objectives. Overall, if you want to draw conclusions about a population, you have to use a population-based dataset, which will generally be a public-use or proprietary dataset. Convenience and other nonprobability samples cannot be used for this purpose.

A notable exception to this principle involves hidden populations, such as undocumented immigrants, sex workers, or intravenous drug users. Because no national, state, or local registry exists for these populations, it is likely not possible to perform the complex sampling procedures needed to collect a population-based sample. However, respondent-driven sampling (Goel & Salganik, 2010) can be used to approximate a population-based sample—provided that the referral chains are long enough. Respondent-driven sampling starts with a set of seed participants. These individuals may be referred by a community partner or might be people whom the researchers know personally. Each of the seed participants is then asked to refer additional people who meet the study's inclusion criteria, and each of these additional people are asked to refer more participants. The process continues until the desired sample size is reached. Participants are compensated for each referred person who joins the study, and all the referral chains are documented (e.g., participant A referred participant E, who referred participant J, who referred participant N). A key difference between respondent-driven sampling and snowball sampling is that the referral chains are incorporated into the analyses (McCreesh et al., 2012). Snowball sampling, by contrast, does not incorporate the inherent nesting of participants within social networks (Heckathorn, 2011). If one participant refers another participant, then the two participants must know one another and may share some of their social networks in common. Their responses to the survey questions in the study may therefore be correlated because of their acquaintanceship. Respondent-driven sampling uses referral chains to correct for this correlation.

So, assuming that a population-based dataset could be gathered with our population of interest, when should we not use a population-based dataset? A first, obvious answer is that we cannot use a population-based dataset when there is no such dataset available that includes our target population, the research design we wish to use, and our variables of interest. For example, although some population-based studies are longitudinal, assessments generally occur infrequently because of the amount of effort and project co-ordination required to collect a wave of data from a population-based sample. If you are planning to conduct a daily diary study, for example—where participants are assessed every day—you will likely have to design your own study and collect your own data. If you want to utilize ecological momentary assessment methods, where participants are paged randomly and asked to answer questions on their mobile device (Shiffman, Stone, & Hufford, 2008), you will probably need to collect your own data. If you want to conduct an experimental study, you will almost certainly have to design the experiment yourself and collect your own data. If you want to conduct an in-depth quali-tative study, you will have to collect the data yourself.

Second, remember that, compared to other types of studies and datasets, population-based datasets essentially trade construct breadth and precision for representativeness and generalizability. If you are planning to test the-ories with broad constructs, and where psychometric rigor is more impor-tant than generalizability, then I advise you not to use a population-based dataset. For example, in the model of acculturation that my colleagues and I (Schwartz, Unger, Zamboanga, & Szapocznik, 2010) developed, we concep-tualized acculturation as consisting of six distinct components— heritage-cultural practices, heritage-cultural values, heritage-cultural identifications, destination-cultural practices, destination-cultural values, and destination-cultural identifications . We have conducted several studies to test this theory, all of which have utilized multi-item scales for each of the six components. No population-based dataset including these types of measures has been collected, and I am doubtful that such a dataset will ever be collected. Remember that population-based datasets are generally designed to serve as repositories—which means that small numbers of questions are included to focus on an extremely broad array of content areas. When acculturation-related articles have been published using population-based datasets, the arti-cles have generally used either proxy measures (such as birthplace or number of years spent in the destination country) or simplistic scales that don't re-flect the complexity of the acculturation construct (see Lopez-Class, Castro, & Ramirez, 2011, for a review). As Jennifer Unger and I (Schwartz & Unger, 2017) observed, construct-invalid measures are an important reason why ac-culturation research has often not lived up to the promise of the theories on which the studies are based. The fact that a population-based dataset includes a couple of questions about birthplace or language-use preferences does not mean that the dataset can support meaningful research on acculturation.

One might imagine several other constructs in psychology and other so-cial sciences that are not amenable to being assessed using single items or extremely brief scales. Some examples that come to mind include motivation, cognition, decision-making, and prejudice. If you are planning to conduct, analyze, and write up a study on constructs like these, then using a population-based dataset is likely not an option. Performance-based or experimental measures probably cannot be administered as part of a population-based data collection. Constructs that require many items probably cannot be included in population-based studies.

The point is that population-based datasets are not superior or inferior to other types of datasets—rather, they are used for different purposes. If we want to characterize a population, we should use a population-based dataset. If we want to compare trends over time, we should do so using population-based datasets. Population-based datasets are well suited for providing "broad stroke" information—such as disease prevalence, population demographics, immigration trends, and voting preferences. However, if our goal is to study a phenomenon in greater depth, such as looking at what types of activities are most likely to be experienced as intrinsically motivating, then we likely need to design our own study and collect our own data.

If you do identify a population-based dataset that might provide the desired sample, design, and variables, then you need to ask how well the constructs of interest are measured. For example, a dataset might include responses to three items focused on parent–adolescent warmth. If you are trying to decide whether to use this dataset, I suggest looking over these items and deciding whether they reflect the construct that you are seeking to measure. Chances are, the items might be different than what you would have selected for inclusion in a study that you were conducting—but are they at least reasonably reflective of what you want to include in your analyses? Can you test your hypotheses accurately using these items? (Part of the answer will probably be determined by the psychometric properties of the responses to these items—if the reliability coefficients for internal consistency are too low, then the items may not all be measuring the same construct.) If the answer is Yes, then I encourage you to consider using the dataset. On the other hand, if the dataset doesn't have the variables you need—or at least reasonable approximations of them—then you probably cannot use that dataset to test your hypotheses.

Conclusion

This chapter discusses public-use and proprietary datasets. In most cases, both types of data are collected in such a way as to be population-based—that is, representative of the city, state, country, region, or other municipality from which the data are gathered. Public-use datasets are generally available for free, whereas proprietary datasets are more tightly regulated and controlled. In either case, prevalence rates, associations, and trends obtained from population-based datasets are assumed to be more accurate than are similar estimates generated using other types of datasets. Public-use and proprietary datasets are therefore essential for making statements about a population.

However, public-use and proprietary datasets can be difficult to learn. These datasets often contain many variables, and the complex sampling procedures used result in multiple clustering, weighting, and primary sampling unit variables. Therefore, codebooks for these datasets can be complex. It is essential that you fully understand the codebook before you attempt to analyze the data—analyses conducted without the proper weighting, clustering, and sampling considerations taken into account will produce inaccurate results.

The chapter also enumerates some situations in which public-use and proprietary datasets may be necessary or advantageous, as well as some situations in which these datasets cannot (or should not) be used. Population-based datasets provide primarily descriptive information, which can be extremely useful for surveillance studies, for providing profiles of populations, and for mapping population trends and changes. Population-based datasets generally cannot be used for performance-based or experimental studies, for studies involving frequent assessments or intensive longitudinal designs, or for studies involving complex psychological constructs that cannot be easily assessed using single items or extremely brief scales. It is also critical to ensure that the constructs you wish to study can at least be reasonably approximated by the variables available in the population-based dataset that you are considering using.

Some proprietary datasets are difficult to gain access to because of burdensome application and review procedures. If you are considering using such a dataset, it's important to consider the amount of time and effort that will be required for you to obtain permission to use the data. I know of researchers who submitted, revised, and resubmitted proposals to use proprietary datasets—and who eventually gave up because the publications committee continued to ask for more and more changes to the proposal. It's a good idea to speak with someone who has already used the dataset that you are considering using—to obtain information on the ease versus difficulty of gaining access to, learning, and using the dataset.

Summary

- Disciplines like sociology, demography, political science, and public health often rely on population-based datasets to support authoritative statements about a population.
- Public-use datasets are generally collected (or supported) by government agencies and are available for free.
- Proprietary datasets are often collected by private companies and are only available for a fee—and upon approval by a data-use committee.
- Learning the codebook is essential for using public-use and proprietary datasets.
- One must also be sure to understand how the data were collected and what the sampling unit was (e.g., individual children, schools, counties).
- Many research questions can be addressed only by using population-based datasets.
- Many population-based datasets include only a few questions for each construct, so the depth of measurement is often less than in other types of datasets.
- Hidden populations (such as drug users or undocumented immigrants) often must be studied using respondent-driven sampling methods.

References

Bowling, N. A., Gibson, A. M., Houpt, J. W., & Brower, C. K. (in press). Will the questions ever end? Person-level increases in careless responding during questionnaire completion. *Organizational Research Methods*.

Brooks, C., Neeuwbeerta, P., & Manza, J. (2006). Cleavage-based voting behavior in cross-national perspective: Evidence from six postwar democracies. *Social Science Research, 35*, 88–128.

Connor, J. L., Kypri, K., Bell, M. L., & Cousins, K. (2011). Alcohol outlet density, levels of drinking, and alcohol-related harm in New Zealand: A national study. *Journal of Epidemiology and Community Health, 65*, 841–846.

Enders, C. K. (2010). *Applied missing data analysis*. New York: Guilford.

Freedman, L., Hawkes, W., Zimmerman, S. I., Hebel, J. R., & Magaziner, J. (2001). Extending gerontological research through linking investigators' studies to public-use datasets. *The Gerontologist, 41*, 15–22.

Goel, S., & Salganik, M. J. (2010). Assessing respondent-driven sampling. *Proceedings of the National Academy of Sciences, 107*, 6743–6747.

Graham, J. W. (2012). *Missing data: Analysis and design*. New York: Springer.

Heckathorn, D. D. (2011). Comment: Snowball versus respondent-driven sampling. *Sociological Methodology, 41*, 355–366.

Herbst, C. M., & Tekin, E. (2014). Child care subsidies, maternal health, and child–parent interactions: Evidence from three nationally representative datasets. *Health Economics, 23,* 894–916.

Keith, T. Z. (2006). *Multiple regression and beyond.* Boston: Allyn and Bacon.

LaVange, L. M., Kalsbeek, W. D., Sorlie, P. D., Avilés-Santa, L. M., Kaplan, R. C., Barnhart, J., . . . Elder, J. P. (2010). Sample design and cohort selection in the Hispanic Community Health Study/Study of Latinos. *Annals of Epidemiology, 20,* 642–649.

Lingler. J. H., Schmidt, K. L., Gentry, A. L., Hu, L., & Terhorst, L. A. (2014). A new measure of research participant burden: Brief report. *Journal of Empirical Research on Human Research Ethics, 9*(4), 46–49.

Little, T. D. (2013). *Longitudinal structural equation modeling.* New York: Guilford.

Little, T. D., & Rhemtulla, M. (2013). Planned missingness designs for developmental researchers. *Child Development Perspectives, 7,* 199–204.

Lopez-Class, M., Castro, F. G., & Ramirez, A. G. (2011). Conceptualizations of acculturation: A review and statement of critical issues. *Social Science and Medicine, 72,* 1555–1562.

McCreesh, N., Frost, S. D. W., Seeley, J., Katongole, J., Tarsh, M. N., Ndunguse, R., Jichi, F., . . . White, R. G. (2012). Evaluation of respondent-driven sampling. *Epidemiology, 23,* 138–147.

Melamed, D., & Vuolo, M. (2019). Assessing differences between nested and cross-classified hierarchical models. *Sociological Methodology, 49,* 220–257.

Meyers, J. L., & Beretvas, S. N. (2006). The impact of inappropriate modeling of cross-classified data structures. *Multivariate Behavioral Research, 41,* 473–497.

Mojtabai, R., Olfson, M., & Han, B. (2016). National trends in the prevalence and treatment of depression in adolescents and young adults. *Pediatrics, 138,* Article e20161878.

Morizot, J. (2014). Construct validity of adolescents' self-reported Big Five personality traits: Importance of conceptual breadth and initial validation of a short measure. *Assessment, 21,* 580–606.

Oğuz-Alper, M., & Berger, Y. G. (2020). Modelling multilevel data under complex sampling designs: An empirical likelihood approach. *Computational Statistics and Data Analysis, 145,* Article 106906.

Phillips, J., & Land, K. C. (2012). The link between unemployment and crime rate fluctuations: An analysis at the county, state, and national levels. *Social Science Research, 41,* 681–694.

Raudenbush, S. W. (1989). The analysis of longitudinal, multilevel data. *International Journal of Educational Research, 13,* 721–740.

Raudenbush, S. W., & Bryk, A. S. (2002). *Hierarchical linear models: Applications and data analysis methods.* Thousand Oaks, CA: SAGE.

Schwartz, S. J., & Unger, J. B. (2017). Acculturation and health: State of the field and recommended directions. In S. J. Schwartz & J. B. Unger (Eds.), *Oxford handbook of acculturation and health* (pp. 1–14). New York: Oxford University Press.

Schwartz, S. J., Unger, J. B., Zamboanga, B. L., & Szapocznik, J. (2010). Rethinking the concept of acculturation: Implications for theory and research. *American Psychologist, 65,* 237–251.

Shiffman, S., Stone, A. A., & Hufford, M. R. (2008). Ecological momentary assessment. *Annual Review of Clinical Psychology, 4,* 1–32.

Sieber, J. (2006). Introduction: Data sharing and disclosure limitation techniques. *Journal of Empirical Research on Human Research Ethics, 1,* 47–50.

Wallin, M. T., Culpepper, W. J., Campbell, J. D., Nelson, L. M., Langer-Gould, A., Marrie, R. A., . . . LaRocca, N. G. (2019). The prevalence of MS in the United States: A population-based estimate using health claims data. *Neurology, 92*, e1029–e1040.

Winship, C., & Radbill, L. (1994). Sampling weights and regression analysis. *Sociological Methods and Research, 23*, 230–257.

Wist, M. (2010). Caught you: Threats to confidentiality due to the public release of large-scale genetic datasets. *BMC Medical Ethics, 11*, Article 21.

16
Publishing Non-Empirical Papers

Chapter Objectives

By the time you finish reading this chapter, you should feel more comfortable with:

- Considerations to think about before you start writing a non-empirical paper
- Organizing and outlining non-empirical papers
- Types of non-empirical articles and characteristics of each type
- Protecting against certain types of reviewer comments when writing non-empirical articles

Thus far, this book has focused primarily on empirical articles. Empirical articles are largely formulaic—the introduction, method, results, and discussion headings are standard, and the ingredients that belong within each of those sections can be mapped out fairly easily. Further, because in these papers you are reporting the results of empirical research, your conclusions should be largely solid as long as they stay close to what the research design can support, and as long as the research project itself was designed, carried out, and analyzed properly.

Non-empirical papers—theoretical treatises, integrative and scoping reviews, and position papers—are considerably more difficult to write because you don't have empirical data to lean on. Furthermore, these papers don't follow a standard structure, and you are on your own in setting up, presenting, and supporting the arguments that you advance in the paper. The viability of the paper rests entirely on your ability to present the arguments in a rigorous and straightforward way and to support them with extant literature and with strong logic. Al Waterman's admonition that it can be extremely difficult to publish theory can be extended to apply to position papers and to integrative and scoping reviews. Although I define these (and other) types of non-empirical articles more fully in this chapter, let me provide brief definitions for now. Theoretical treatises introduce new theories or conceptual models; position papers advocate for new lines of research, policy initiatives,

The Savvy Academic. Seth J. Schwartz, Oxford University Press. © Oxford University Press 2022.
DOI: 10.1093/oso/9780190095918.003.0017

interventions, and the like; and integrative and scoping reviews summarize and assess the state of a body of literature.

Despite Al's warning about the difficulty involved in publishing non-empirical papers, I have managed to publish 30 theoretical, literature review, and position articles in my career. I've developed some strategies for justifying the need for a new theoretical perspective, review, or position; for laying out the tenets of your new perspective; for organizing the presentation so that readers can follow it; and for summarizing and recapping the model or conclusions proposed in the article. Two principles I follow when writing theoretical, review, and position papers are that (1) it is essential to create an outline before you start writing, and (2) headings should be used to establish a structure that the reader can follow. These principles help to prevent the logic in the paper from being AOTP (all over the place)—indeed, the AOTP trap is extremely easy to fall into when writing theoretical, review, and position papers.

Issues to Think About Before You Write

To avoid being AOTP, it is essential to have all of the tenets and principles of the new theory or position laid out before you start writing. Even before you create the outline, ask yourself:

- What are the key problems and issues that the theory, review, or position will address? In other words, what will the paper be about?
- What do we already know based on extant theory and research in the field where the new theory, review, or position will be introduced? In other words, where is the starting point for the conceptual analysis that the current paper will lay out?
- For theoretical papers, why is a new theory needed? What advantages would a new theory provide in terms of tying together ideas and concepts that have not been linked before (or have not been linked in the way that you have in mind)?
- For integrative and scoping reviews, why is the review needed? How has the field reached a place where an integrative or scoping review is necessary? How will such a review help to advance the field?
- For position papers, what will the new position advocate for that is not currently occurring? What are the advantages of adopting the position that your paper will argue for?
- How will the new theory or position help to advance future work?

Once you have the answers to these questions, you are ready to create your outline. Chapter 4 provides an outline for a theoretical paper. Notice that, in that outline, the purpose of the paper appears very early on, telling the reader what to expect. When you outline (and later write) the section on the purpose of the paper, you are offering the reader a roadmap for the arguments that you will lay out. Providing such a roadmap gives you a structure within which you can write and decreases the chances that the paper will be AOTP.

Outlining and Writing Theoretical, Review, and Position Papers

Once you lay out the roadmap for the paper, you have the headings for the sections that will follow the section on the purpose of the manuscript. In the outline provided in Chapter 4, which is for an article on rethinking acculturation and proposing an integrative acculturation theory (Schwartz, Unger, Zamboanga, & Szapocznik, 2010), we began the various section headings with the word "Rethinking." (My friend and colleague Byron Zamboanga came up with that idea.) This structure served to emphasize the theme of the article—namely, rethinking various assumptions within the acculturation literature. In this way, we were able to highlight the themes in acculturation theory that we intended to critique, rethink, and expand. The use of intentional redundancy across headings suggests the importance of using creativity to help draw the reader's attention to the primary points of the paper and of the theory, review, or position that it presents.

In theoretical, review, and position papers, it is essential to provide a thorough review of what is already known in the area represented by the manuscript. One of the primary critiques I have seen reviewers levy against theoretical and position papers (as well as against review papers) is that the theory or position being advanced is not needed. More or less, the reviewer is saying that the points being made in the manuscript have already been presented elsewhere, and there is no need to present them again. In my experience, this kind of comment often leads editors to reject theoretical, review, or position manuscripts.

By laying out what is known in the literature and indicating where the gaps are in the literature (respectfully, of course—remember José's approach where we stand on the shoulders of prior work rather than criticizing prior work for what it did not do), we can clearly articulate the need for the approach that we will present in the paper. It is important to ensure that our literature search is thorough and that we don't miss any articles that may have been published recently. Missing important articles makes authors look sloppy. I remember reviewing manuscripts where the authors claimed that no one had looked at the issues they were focusing on, but my colleagues and I had published on those issues. Needless to say, my reviews of these manuscripts were not as favorable as they could have been.

Making the case for a new theory or position is like walking a tightrope. You don't want to criticize prior work for not making the points you're making, but you also need to justify why your theory or position is necessary. Here is some of the text that we (Schwartz et al., 2010, pp. 237–238) included in our article on rethinking acculturation (I've bolded the most relevant text in this excerpt):

At least three edited books on acculturation have been published since 2003 (e.g., Berry, Phinney, Sam, & Vedder, 2006; Chun, Organista, & Marín, 2003; Sam & Berry, 2006), and a cursory search of the PsycInfo literature database, seeking journal articles with the word *acculturation* in the title, returned 107 records from the 1980s, 337 from the 1990s, and 727 from the 2000s. However, **there remain a number of important challenges regarding operational definitions, contextual forces, and relationships to psychosocial and health outcomes that must be addressed** (Rudmin, 2003, 2009). Therefore, **the purpose of this paper is to raise some of these questions and issues, and to propose an expanded, multidimensional model of acculturation and of the demographic and contextual forces that can influence the acculturation process.** As part of this objective, **we draw on and integrate various streams of literature on cultural adaptation** (specifically on cultural practices, values, and identifications), on ethnicity, on discrimination and acculturative stress, and on context of reception. Further, because the bulk of acculturation research focuses on mental or physical health indicators as correlates or outcomes of acculturation, we draw on these prior studies to illustrate some of our points. Specifically, **we use health outcomes as a way (a) to illustrate some of the limitations of the current acculturation literature, (b) to suggest ways of circumventing these limitations, and (c) to highlight potential ways to advance the conceptualization of acculturation so that we can better understand the health and well-being of international migrants.**

There are many aspects of the acculturation literature that may require rethinking, and we focus on some of those here. First, we review and contrast major acculturation models that have been developed within cultural psychology, and we outline some of the strengths and weaknesses of these approaches. Second, we discuss the role of ethnicity and heritage-receiving culture similarity in acculturation. Third, we delineate the ways in which acculturation is more or less salient, and may operate differently, for different groups or types of migrants. Fourth, we discuss the "immigrant paradox," where acculturation has been examined simplistically in relation to health outcomes, and we suggest addressing the immigrant paradox by expanding the conceptualization of acculturation. Fifth, we introduce such an expanded model of acculturation, including cultural practices, values, and identifications—which has the potential to synthesize several existing literatures and to increase the theoretical, empirical, and practical utility of the acculturation construct. Finally, we delineate context of reception as the ways in which the receiving society constrains and directs the acculturation options available to migrants, and we frame acculturative stress and discrimination under the heading of an unfavorable context of reception.

In this section, our objective was to lay out the purpose and objectives of our paper for the reader. We wanted readers to know exactly why our theory was needed and what gaps it would fill in the literature. When you write theoretical articles, you need to be similarly direct and upfront about what you are looking to do in your paper.

In 2005, I wrote an "editorial essay" (Schwartz, 2005) about expanding and refocusing the personal identity literature. This editorial essay was essentially a position paper—I was arguing that the personal identity literature was too narrow and that this narrowness did not permit the personal identity construct to live up to the promise with which Erikson (1950) and others had proposed and framed it. Here is some of the introductory text from that editorial essay (p. 293):

> In this editorial essay, I comment on some of the areas in which identity research has been lacking and on ways to expand identity research by focusing on these areas. I restrict my analysis to the literature rooted in Eriksonian and neo-Eriksonian theory because that is the area with which I am most familiar. I touch on a number of important areas, including methodological shortsightedness, reliance on a narrow and limiting theoretical approach, and lack of attention to important applied and social policy issues.

Looking back at that opening paragraph, I realize that I could—and should—have been more diplomatic in my criticisms of the personal identity literature. I should have noted the areas in which this literature had contributed, and then noted that I was aiming to stand on the shoulders of that literature and expand its reach. Had I written that editorial essay more recently,

I would have written that first paragraph quite differently than I did in 2004, when it was accepted for publication.

A key principle to apply in theoretical articles is to give an in-depth description of the theory. That is, what does the theory look like? If something is labeled as multidimensional, what are the dimensions? If variables A and B are framed as predicting or causing variables C and D, include a picture of the predictive relationships in the manuscript as a figure—or at least describe these relationships in depth in the text. If some associations apply only for certain groups or under certain conditions, make clear what those groups and conditions are. Make the postulates of your theory, review, or position as clear as you can. The reader should not be left wondering about any aspect of your theory or position—or of the conclusions you are drawing from your review.

Consider the following text from the rethinking acculturation article (Schwartz et al., 2010, pp. 242–243):

> Beyond ethnicity and cultural similarity, other factors may also determine which subgroups of migrants may face different types (and degrees) of acculturative challenges (Zane & Mak, 2003). Although there are countless permutations of factors that affect the degree of acculturative change that a migrant may face or experience, we can highlight several general patterns here. First, individuals who migrate as young children are more likely to acquire receiving-culture practices, values, and identifications easily and fluidly than those who migrate at older ages. Portes and Rumbaut (2001) referred to migrants who arrive as young children as the "1.5 generation" and noted that these individuals are, in many ways, more similar to second-generation migrants (i.e., individuals born in the receiving country and raised by foreign-born parents) than to those who migrate as adolescents or as adults. Whereas individuals who migrate as adolescents or adults likely have vivid memories of life prior to migration, this may not be the case for those who migrated as young children (Portes & Rumbaut, 2006). Second, individuals who migrate as adults—and especially those who arrive as older adults—may experience the most difficulty (or unwillingness) in adopting the practices, values, and identifications of the receiving society (Schwartz, Pantin, Sullivan, Prado, & Szapocznik, 2006). Recent migrants (and those who arrived as adults) likely have had the most direct contact with their countries of origin—which may shape the ways in which they approach their interactions with the receiving culture and with other heritage-culture individuals. Their recognizable foreign accents, or inability to speak the receiving country's language, identify them as migrant—and this may invite discrimination and scorn from native-born individuals (Yoo, Gee, & Takeuchi, 2009).

In effect, we were proposing age at arrival in the destination country as a predictor of the extent to which international migrants would experience difficulties with acculturation. We proposed three groups—those who migrate as young children, those who migrate as adolescents or young adults, and those who migrate as older adults—and we postulated that the experience of acculturation would differ markedly across these groups.

Importantly, any postulate that you propose must be testable. That is, any statement that you propose in a new theory or position, or in your analysis of the literature as part of an integrative or scoping review, needs to be able to be supported or falsified through empirical research. Sometimes it can be advantageous to suggest research designs that might be used to test the perspective or arguments you are proposing. There are at least two advantages to doing this. First, such suggestions tell readers (and reviewers) that your perspective is solid enough to be tested, and second, you are effectively setting yourself up to conduct the studies that you suggest. When you write up those studies for publication, you can cite your theoretical, position, or review article as justification for conducting the study.

Although theoretical, position, and review articles don't have to include a discussion section, they should end with a series of integrative and wrap-up statements summarizing the perspective and discussing its boundary conditions. Boundary conditions refer to the range of people, conditions, or circumstances to which the perspective applies. For example, a theory of acculturation might be framed as applying to international migrants and their immediate descendants, but not to minority groups who are not immigrants (e.g., African Americans and Native Americans in the United States, Palestinians in Israel). A theory of cognitive development might be posed as applying only to typically developing individuals, and not to those with developmental disabilities. Remember the principle that my graduate school colleague taught me many years ago about giving presentations—tell them what you're going to tell them, tell them, and then tell them what you told them. Theoretical, position, and review articles follow pretty much the same principle. The last couple of paragraphs should sum up the perspective and should set an agenda for moving forward.

In an article portraying acculturation as an identity process and framing personal identity as a stabilizing force during and after international migration (Schwartz, Montgomery, & Briones, 2006, pp. 25–26), my coauthors and I ended the article with the following two paragraphs:

In this paper, we have advanced the theses that personal identity, at least those aspects that are reasonably independent from "culturally charged" issues, can stabilize immigrant individuals and protect them from instability and distress created by the acculturation process, and that social and cultural identity guide and reflect acculturation-related change. Erikson's distinction between personal and social identity was viewed as an appropriate framework for the present analysis, given that his conceptualization included cultural and cross-cultural concerns. Our analysis of social and cultural identity involved integrating aspects of Erikson's theory and social identity theory, as social identity is taken to represent both "inner solidarity with a group's ideals" (Erikson, 1980, p. 109) and the attitudes, beliefs, and behaviors that emerge as a result of this solidarity (Tajfel & Turner, 1986).

We also advanced ideas concerning how identity interventions might be used to alleviate distress and other negative developmental outcomes in immigrant youth. Although many young people are able to successfully navigate the challenges and transitions of adolescence and emerging adulthood (Arnett, 1999), others experience various negative developmental outcomes as a result of unsupportive cultural or community contexts (Dahlberg, 1998). Immigrant youth may be at particular risk for such negative outcomes, in that they must decide how to adapt their cultural identities and maintain a personal identity—while at the same time facing unaccommodating contexts, such as poverty, disempowered status in the community, and diminished access to supportive social institutions.

When writing theoretical, position, and review articles in the social sciences, it is extremely important to stay as close to the empirical literature as possible. That is, the perspective needs to be based on research findings. It is generally not appropriate to include statements in your article that are not empirically supportable and that stray away from the current scientific research base. Such statements amount to speculation—which is not how we develop theories, positions, and research agendas in psychology and related fields.

So, if we have to stay close to existing literature, what is the point of theory? One might argue that classic psychological theorists like Erikson, Rogers, Skinner, and Maslow did not have access to empirical work, yet their theories have been well accepted and have driven scientific discourse for more than half a century. Why should we be held to a higher standard than they were?

My response is that what constitutes scientific progress has changed considerably since the classic psychological theorists published their work. Erikson, for example, based his theorizing on clinical work with World War II veterans, naturalistic observations of Native American tribes, and biographies of historical figures like Mohandas Gandhi and Martin Luther. Skinner based much of his theorizing on simple and straightforward experiments with animals and with young children. I'm not saying that these theorists' observations were not valid—rather, I'm saying that scientific research is held to a far higher standard in the 2020s than it was held to in the 1950s and 1960s. Further, the fact that we, in contrast to Erikson, Skinner, and others, do have access to solid empirical research means that we should be held to a higher standard than they were.

Most new theories involve integrating different batches of knowledge to create new ways of understanding ourselves and the world around us. For example, Phinney (1990) developed a theory of ethnic identity by integrating the concepts of exploring among, and committing to, life alternatives (from Erikson, 1950) with the concept of social identification and group self-esteem (from social identity theory; Tajfel & Turner, 1986). By integrating these two previously unconnected streams of literature, Phinney inspired a new literature on ethnic identity among international migrants and members of minority groups (Rivas-Drake & Umaña-Taylor, 2019). Similarly, in his eudaemonic theory of identity and well-being, Al Waterman (2008) drew on eudaemonist philosophers like Aristotle and Jeremy Bentham, as well as on Maslow's (1968) theory of self-actualization. There are countless other theories that have adopted similar approaches.

Types of Non-Empirical Articles

As noted already, the term *non-empirical article* is a broad umbrella that includes several variations. These include theoretical treatises, integrative literature reviews, scoping reviews, and position papers, among others. Although the structures of these articles vary somewhat, most of the principles I propose here apply across the types. Note that no article is purely theoretical or purely literature review—theoretical treatises must also review literature and stay as close as possible to the empirical literature base, and literature reviews must also draw integrative conclusions and propose directions for the field to pursue. The primary difference among the various types of non-empirical articles is the extent of emphasis placed on theorizing, reviewing and synthesizing literature, and recommending directions for future research, intervention, and policy.

Theoretical Treatises

Theoretical treatises are intended to propose new theories that can then be tested in subsequent empirical research. The treatise involves a statement of the problem that the new theory is addressing, a review of relevant theoretical and empirical work, and a set of postulates that comprise the theory that is being introduced. For example, Mathew, Hogarth, Leventhal, Cook, and Hitsman (2016) reviewed literature on the co-occurrence of cigarette smoking and depression and used this literature to support a new theoretical model of smoking motivation among depressed individuals. As part of their treatise, they suggested directions for future research and intervention development based on the model they were proposing.

In a theoretical treatise, the literature review is used to set up and support the postulates of the theory, and the extant literature is used as a springboard from which to develop the theory. Theoretical postulates generally serve as headings with which to organize the article—or, alternatively, the authors can boldface the postulates so that the reader can spot them easily. The postulates therefore serve to establish the structure of the theoretical part of the article (after the introduction and literature review). Of course, supportive literature should be provided in the section where each postulate is proposed. Just as you wouldn't build a house without a foundation, you cannot propose a theory without supportive literature—in the problem statement, in the literature review section (where you establish the literature base and the need for your new theory), and in the section where each postulate is presented.

Mathew et al. (2016, p. 405) provided an example of a theoretical postulate section with supportive literature. (Note that this article was published in a journal that follows a medical citation style that uses bracketed numbers.) Their text reads as follows:

> The unique prediction of the incentive learning account . . . is that subjective desire to smoke prompted by adverse states and goal-directed instrumental knowledge of the effective smoking response in each context are integrated to drive smoking behavior. One source of support for this claim is the finding that experimental induction of stress or negative affect provokes increases in both smoking desire and smoking behavior [79,82,131–139]. Although the mood-induced increase in smoking desire may cause the smoking behavior, as anticipated by incentive learning theory, stimulus-response-based negative reinforcement accounts would argue that the increase in smoking desire is actually epiphenomenal in relation to smoking behavior. The causal status of subjective desire in controlling behavior remains an unresolved scientific question [34,140].

Some theoretical articles also provide information on how the theory could be falsified. That is, the article provides conditions and findings that would suggest that the theory is wrong. Moffitt (1993), for example, listed criteria by which her theory could be invalidated. For example, on page 695, she stated:

If life-course-persistent and adolescence-limited delinquents, defined on the basis of their natural histories, do not show the predicted differential patterns of correlates, then the theory is wrong. . . . If life-course-persistent and adolescence-limited delinquents, defined on the basis of their natural histories, do not show the predicted differential responses to young-adulthood transitions, then the theory is wrong. . . . If adolescence-limited delinquents and abstainers, defined on the basis of their natural histories, do not differ in these predicted ways, then that part of the theory is wrong.

Remember that the scientific method requires that hypotheses must be testable and falsifiable. Theories—which are used to generate hypotheses—must also be testable and falsifiable. Suggesting specific research findings that would invalidate a theory therefore increases the testability and falsifiability—as well as the strength—of that theory.

Integrative Literature Reviews

Integrative literature reviews (also called systematic reviews) are designed to synthesize a body of literature and to advance theoretical statements about that literature and about the constructs that it represents. Integrative literature reviews are helpful when a body of literature is large, scattered, and somewhat unfocused. Torraco (2005, p. 357) noted that "As a topic matures and the size of its literature grows, there is a corresponding growth and development in the knowledge base of the topic . . . an integrative literature review of a mature topic addresses the need for a review, critique, and the potential reconceptualization of the expanding and more diversified knowledge base of the topic as it continues to develop." Torraco's point is that, as a body of literature expands in various directions, there is a need for an integrative review to tie together the various strands of literature that have developed, to extract theoretical insights from that literature, and to recommend a path forward. If written effectively, an integrative literature review can serve as a valuable resource for readers—they can consult the review article rather than having to read all of the individual studies that have been published.

Integrative literature reviews include "state-of-the-field" articles that are published in some content areas to appraise the current progress, trends, debates, and primary themes within a given area of research. For example, every 10 years, the *Journal of Marriage and Family* publishes "decade-in-review" articles on a given topic in marriage and family studies. Raley and Sweeney (2020), for instance, published a decade-in-review article on divorce, repartnering, and stepfamilies. In its first two published issues, the journal *Emerging Adulthood* published state-of-the-field articles on various topics related to the emerging adult life stage. Generally, these types of articles are invited by the journal—although many authors also publish integrative literature reviews on their own. However, as Torraco (2005) noted, integrative literature reviews are challenging to write because they require a "30,000 foot perspective" on a given field. The authors must survey the literature carefully and must develop a thesis that they will pursue as they review that literature. Said differently, integrative literature reviews don't just summarize literature—they also put forth position statements about where that literature stands, what the current state of the field signifies (e.g., Is a basic research literature ready to support intervention and policy initiatives?), what theoretical statements might best represent the where the field is and where it appears to be headed, and what future directions the authors recommend.

Authors of integrative literature reviews don't necessarily have to be senior scholars and long-standing contributors to the field represented by the review, but they should possess an intimate knowledge of the field. One of my first publications, for example, was a major review of the neo-Eriksonian personal identity literature (Schwartz, 2001). Although I had not published much within that literature prior to writing that review, I knew the literature extremely well. I was able to write the review article using my close familiarity with the neo-Eriksonian personal identity literature (including searching for recent publications that needed to be included in my analysis). Had I not known the literature well, I would probably have omitted key streams of work, misrepresented some of the work I did cite, and mischaracterized the state and needs of the field. Think of it this way—most people and groups would rather be evaluated by an "insider" (someone who understands their positions and can understand how they view the world) than by an "outsider" (see Gair, 2012, for an example related to qualitative research). Even if you are not a member of a community, summarizing a set of beliefs and assumptions in a way that accurately represents the people who hold those beliefs and assumptions is most likely to be accepted—and acted upon—by that community of people. In contrast, approaching a literature from an outsider perspective is likely to evoke defensiveness from the people and groups within that literature.

When you write an integrative literature review, I suggest that you create an outline and use themes from the literature as your headings. For example, if you were writing an integrative review of the link between peer affiliations and delinquent behavior in adolescence, you might include separate headings for the peer selection hypothesis (i.e., that teens select friends who are similar to them in terms of conventional versus deviant beliefs and attitudes; McGloin, 2009) and for the peer influence hypothesis (i.e., that deviant peers influence teens to engage in delinquent behavior; Gatti, Tremblay, Vitaro, & McDuff, 2005). You might also include headings for the specific mechanisms through which peers influence adolescent delinquency and for the ways in which parental monitoring and supervision can offset the effects of both peer selection and peer influence. Within each of these sections, you would need to include appraisals of where each of these strands of literature stands—and you should also provide an overall assessment of the literature, what the current status of the literature means theoretically, and where the literature should proceed in the future.

Scoping Review

In contrast to an integrative review, a scoping review is designed to explore a new, limited, or methodologically varied literature and to establish an agenda for that literature moving forward (Pham et al., 2014). Scoping reviews are intended to answer questions like "What is out there on the topic?" Broadly, a scoping review consists of five steps (Arksey & O'Malley, 2005): identifying a research question, searching for relevant articles and studies, selecting articles and studies for inclusion, charting the content and themes from these articles and studies, and summarizing and reporting patterns in the literature. These steps differ from those involved in integrative reviews in that the studies included for review are likely of much more varied quality and the various areas included in the review may be only loosely connected.

For example, Saigle, Séguin, and Racine (2017) conducted a scoping review of ethical challenges in suicide research. The articles that they included in their review included theoretical and review articles as well as empirical studies, to provide readers with a sense of the current thinking and empirical work on the ethics of research on suicidality. Clearly, ethical issues—where conceptual and position papers might be just as valuable as empirical studies—may represent an area where scoping reviews are especially valuable to conduct. Commentaries from ethics experts may warrant inclusion alongside research studies conducted on ethical issues.

In both integrative and scoping reviews, it is essential to specify inclusion criteria for studies that contribute to the review. The inclusion criteria generally start with keywords used in the literature search, the search engines used, and the beginning and ending dates for the search. For instance, you might conduct a search of the PsycInfo, Google Scholar, Scopus, and PubMed literature databases using the search keywords *peer, devian** or *delinquen**, and *adolescen** (note that the asterisk is a wildcard character and indicates that you are searching based on the characters that appear before the asterisk—so that both *adolescent* and *adolescence* would draw hits). You might specify that you searched for articles published between January 2005 and October 2020.

Clearly, not all of the articles that the search engine returns will qualify for inclusion in your review. You might decide, for example, that case studies are not eligible for inclusion, or that intervention studies will not be included. It is essential to report all of the criteria and limits that you placed on your search, so that someone else could repeat the search and find the same (or at least similar) results. You can create a table listing all the studies included in your review. This table is not required, but I encourage you to include it. Columns in the table would include the study authors and year of publication, the type of study or article (cross-sectional, longitudinal, experimental, position paper), the sample size, and the key findings or conclusions. If the table is too long to include in the manuscript, you can include it as online supplementary material.

Position Papers

Position papers argue for a specific viewpoint or research agenda. In most cases, empirical research is used to substantiate the argument and to present the merits of the authors' position. For example, Brody et al. (2013) published a position article arguing for the inclusion of genetics in randomized clinical trials of preventive interventions. Their contention was that, if a preventive intervention produces significantly greater effects for individuals with specific genetic profiles, then such findings suggest that those genetic profiles likely predict the etiology and prevention-related needs of individuals with varying profiles. Individuals with different genetic profiles might even require different types of interventions to prevent the outcomes of interest. In essence, Brody et al. were establishing a research agenda for genetically informed preventive intervention trials.

In a position paper, the primary thesis is presented up front, as broadly as possible, and then is broken down into parts or themes. Each of the parts or themes then becomes a heading within the paper. As an example, my colleagues and I (Schwartz, Zamboanga, & Weisskirch, 2008) argued for the need to integrate the literatures on personal and cultural identity. We provided a series of sections laying out the basic premises, assumptions, and participant populations included in the personal and cultural identity literatures.

Our goal was to illustrate that cultural identity concerns had been largely overlooked in the personal identity literature, and vice versa. Within each section, we presented the seeming incompatibilities between the two literatures and then suggested ways to overcome the incompatibilities. Indeed, the purpose of our article was to encourage theoretical and empirical efforts toward integrating the personal and cultural identity literatures.

Clinical Articles

Among the other types of non-empirical articles that are also worth mentioning are clinical articles. Clinical articles are intended to lay out a specific preventive or treatment intervention. Often, the principles of the clinical intervention are explained, and the authors may present excerpts from treatment sessions to illustrate how the intervention works. These articles are intended primarily for clinical audiences, although researchers can also use them to design studies based on the interventions presented. For example, a colleague and I (Liddle & Schwartz, 2002) published a clinical article on my colleague's treatment intervention, Multidimensional Family Therapy. In that article, we discussed how this therapy modality can be used to repair damaged attachment relationships between parents and adolescents—and we used several session excerpts to illustrate our points.

Generally, clinical articles start with an overview of the problem that the preventive or treatment intervention is designed to address. The articles then discuss some of the risk and protective factors for the target problem, after which they present the intervention as a way to promote protective factors and to offset the effects of risk factors. The various ingredients of the intervention—such as engagement strategies, developing the therapeutic alliance, and key change processes—are generally presented as separate sections or subsections. Where applicable, excerpts from intervention sessions (with identifying information changed) can be presented.

In some cases, clinical articles might conclude with a summary of empirical evidence supporting the efficacy or effectiveness of the intervention. Such evidence can include results of randomized clinical trials, single-group intervention evaluations (i.e., not including a control group), or process studies (e.g., studies linking session attendance or therapeutic alliance with outcomes). Such empirical evidence is presented as a way of strengthening the argument in favor of using the intervention.

I should note that only certain journals publish clinical articles. For example, in the field of family studies, *Family Process* publishes clinical family therapy articles, but the *Journal of Marriage and Family*, the *Journal of Family Psychology*, and the *Journal of Family Issues* generally do not. Before you submit a clinical article for publication, you should look at the contents of the last few issues of the journal you are targeting. If you cannot find any clinical articles in those issues, then you probably should not submit to that journal.

Methodological Articles

Methodological articles present new research approaches or statistical techniques. For example, Fairchild and MacKinnon (2010) summarized statistical methods for testing mediation and moderation. Raykov and Calvocoressi (2020) presented a new method for computing the proportion of explained variance in exploratory factor analysis. Farrelly et al. (2017) introduced a new heat mapping method for analyzing data from measures that are not hierarchically structured (i.e., items are not assumed to map onto latent subscale factors). Siranni, Cameron, Shi, and Heckathorn (2021) presented statistical techniques to analyze data gathered using respondent-driven sampling methods. In general, methodological articles are focused on the specific research procedures or analytic methods being proposed or reviewed, and these articles may include detailed and technical material (e.g., statistical formulas and equations).

Anticipating and Heading Off Reviewer Comments When Writing Theoretical Articles

As already noted, non-empirical articles are much more difficult to publish than empirical articles are. Because you are not basing your arguments on empirical data that you collected and analyzed, reviewers have considerably more opportunities to criticize your arguments and logic. There is also a much greater chance of being AOTP if you don't develop and follow a clear outline. As a result, thinking like a reviewer, and identifying places where a reviewer would criticize your arguments, is essential for publishing non-empirical articles.

Every statement you include in a non-empirical article must both follow from previous statements and arguments you've included and be grounded in empirical work. Contradicting yourself serves to confuse readers and to displease reviewers—neither of which is an advisable strategy when trying to publish theory, position, or review papers. Although you should not obsess over internal consistency while you're writing your first draft, you should certainly read your later drafts carefully—and encourage your coauthors to do likewise—keeping an eye out for statements that contradict other statements in the paper. Indeed, even mild contradictions are problematic—for example, saying that unaccompanied immigrant minors are highly stressed on one page, and then stating later on that these minors might be stressed, could be viewed as contradictory. The logic needs to flow smoothly and completely throughout the paper, with as few detours, sharp turns, and contradictions as possible. Remember the SLAM (specifying the limiting aspects of manuscripts) approach that van Lange (1999) observed many reviewers use—according to van Lange's argument, reviewers are often looking for weaknesses that they can mention in their reviews. Any deviation from a straight line of logic, backed up by a solid base of empirical research, is open to criticism from reviewers.

I also suggest focusing on maximizing readability as you write. For example, laying out postulates as headings (or in bolded text), and then explaining the logic undergirding them, is a strong strategy for proposing a theory. In an integrative or scoping review, including each strand of literature as a section in the paper, with integrative statements at the end of each section, can be a clear way of leading readers and reviewers through the story you are telling. When you are describing specific studies in an integrative or scoping review, be as specific as you can about how each study contributes to the themes you are laying out. Rather than describing a given study as using a deficit approach to understanding adolescent development, provide details about exactly how that study is framing adolescence in terms of problems rather than in terms of strengths. If you are citing a study suggesting that playing violent video games leads to greater aggressive behavior in adolescents and young adults, provide some information about the mechanisms that the authors of that study suggested (or examined) as being responsible for this effect. In other words, don't leave readers guessing about what you mean—tell them as clearly as possible.

Another suggestion is to make sure that every statement you make is consistent with empirical work—and cite that empirical work if possible. You do not want reviewers to accuse you of making statements that are not empirically based. Reviewers often slam theoretical, position, or review articles that are "loose," that include vague or nonspecific statements, or that include erroneous claims. My best advice is to be as clear and as specific as you can. And give the paper a critical read to make sure that every statement in the paper makes a specific, verifiable or falsifiable claim, is consistent with the rest of the paper, and stays as close to the empirical research base as possible. Your coauthors should give the paper a similar read. Submit the paper for publication only when everyone on the authorship agrees that it's ready to go out.

Further, this may sound pedantic, but make sure that you don't stray away from the primary theme of the paper. One manuscript that was submitted to my journal claimed to focus on unaccompanied immigrant minors, yet the authors included several paragraphs about general types of well-being and psychological adjustment—and unaccompanied minors weren't mentioned in any of those paragraphs. I found this paper to be AOTP, and I ultimately desk-rejected it because the logic was extremely difficult to follow. The point is that if the paper is about unaccompanied immigrant minors, then that topic needs to be kept in the reader's mind throughout the paper.

It's also essential to avoid the opposite trap—becoming so focused on small details that the larger picture is lost. I've seen authors spend so much time on small corners of their theory, position, or review that I forgot what the paper was about. In a way, being overly focused on small issues is a form of being AOTP, because the reader will have trouble following the logic underlying the paper. If you find yourself facing this problem, then introduce new headings and subheadings to help you move yourself back to the main points of the paper. Remember that outlines and headings are designed to structure the paper and to keep you from being AOTP.

One last point is related to integrative and scoping reviews, and perhaps to other types of non-empirical articles as well: it is essential to be balanced and to cover all sides of an argument. Ignoring literature you don't agree with or that doesn't support your argument generally doesn't sit well with reviewers. Even if you are arguing for a specific position, you can still acknowledge literature that approaches the issue from different perspectives than you do. You could include a sentence like "Although we are arguing in favor of Berry's (1980, 2017) approach to acculturation theory and research, we must acknowledge the critiques that other authors (e.g., Chirkov, 2009; Rudmin, 2003) have levied against Berry's approach." In this way, you are acknowledging that other perspectives exist—while at the same time telling your readers which argument you are advocating for.

However, with that said, in integrative and scoping reviews, it is essential that you state the boundaries of the review and include all articles that fall within the boundaries. Specify the search engines that you used to look for articles (and never rely on only one search engine) as well as the date range and keywords you used. You can argue in favor of imposing specific boundaries around the review and for excluding certain types of studies or articles, and in the statements where you justify these boundaries, you can acknowledge other streams of work that lie outside the boundaries of your review. But it is extremely important that you establish your position as fair and balanced.

Conclusion

This chapter outlines the principles for writing non-empirical articles. These articles are considerably more difficult to publish than standard empirical papers, which are largely formulaic and follow an established structure. In non-empirical articles, the argument needs to flow from beginning to end, with no internal contradictions and as few distractions as possible. The arguments must be empirically supported and must summarize the ideas clearly and convincingly—while also providing sufficient specificity so that the reader is able to understand your postulates, positions, or conclusions. Before starting an outline, consider why the theory, review, or position being presented in the article is necessary and what it will contribute to the literature. Carefully answering these questions will help to maximize the impact of the article on the field in which it is being written.

The chapter focuses primarily on four types of non-empirical articles—theoretical treatises, integrative reviews, scoping reviews, and position papers. All these article types involve reviewing literature and proposing new perspectives. The primary difference among the article types is the emphasis placed on surveying literature, proposing theoretical postulates, and advocating for specific research agendas or policy positions. Theoretical treatises involve some literature review to establish a literature base and a foundation for the new theory, but the emphasis is on outlining the tenets of the new theory and supporting the tenets with extant literature. Integrative literature reviews and scoping reviews also involve theorizing, offering observations and conclusions, and setting an agenda for the field, but the primary task is to identify studies (and perhaps non-empirical articles as well) and to map the state of a field of inquiry. Position papers primarily advocate for a set of directions for the field to pursue, where the suggested directions are grounded in available theories and empirical literature.

The chapter also offers guidance for writing non-empirical articles rigorously and in a way that is least likely to elicit criticism from reviewers. Issues that reviewers may be most likely to criticize in theoretical, review, and position papers include looseness (i.e., the paper includes vague and nonspecific statements); contradictions or distractions; straying too far from empirical evidence; being AOTP or focusing too much on specific corners of the theory, literature, or position; and not focusing sufficiently on the target constructs.

Because writing non-empirical papers is more challenging than writing standard empirical articles, I recommend that most beginning authors start their scholarly writing careers with empirical manuscripts. It's important to develop your writing skills with articles that are simpler and more straightforward to write. Further, I advise beginners to team up with senior colleagues the first time they write a non-empirical paper. (I'm working with a PhD student now on her first non-empirical paper, and I've had to guide her away from some of the problems that I outlined in this chapter.) Without senior colleagues and mentors to write with, it is extremely difficult for young scholars to learn how to write theoretical, review, and position papers on their own.

Summary

- Non-empirical articles include theoretical treatises, integrative and scoping reviews, and position papers.
- Outlines are essential for writing non-empirical papers.
- Early in a non-empirical paper, authors should explicitly state why the paper is necessary.
- Postulates within one's theory, review, or position should be stated clearly and explicitly.
- Integrative reviews summarize large bodies of literature, whereas scoping reviews summarize emerging literatures.
- Non-empirical articles must stay very close to what existing empirical literature can support.
- Boundaries of the theory, review, or position must be clearly stated.

References

Arksey, H., & O'Malley, L. (2005). Scoping studies: Toward a methodological framework. *International Journal of Social Research Methodology, 8*, 19–32.

Brody, G. H., Beach, S. R. H., Hill, K. G., Howe, G. W., Prado, G., & Fullerton, S. M. (2013). Using genetically informed, randomized prevention trials to test etiological hypotheses about child and adolescent drug use and psychopathology. *American Journal of Public Health, 103*, S19–S24.

Erikson, E. H. (1950). *Childhood and society.* New York: Norton.

Fairchild, A. J., & MacKinnon, D. P. (2010). A general model for testing mediation and moderation effects. *Prevention Science, 10*, 87–99.

Farrelly, C., Schwartz, S. J., Amodeo, A. L., Feaster, D. J., Steinley, D., Meca, A., & Picariello, S. (2017). The analysis of bridging constructs with hierarchical clustering methods: An application to identity. *Journal of Research in Personality, 70*, 93–106.

Gair, S. (2012). Feeling their stories: Contemplating empathy, insider/outsider positionings, and enriching qualitative research. *Qualitative Health Research, 22*, 134–143.

Gatti, U., Tremblay, R. E., Vitaro, F., & McDuff, P. (2005). Youth gangs, delinquency and drug use: A test of the selection, facilitation, and enhancement hypotheses. *Journal of Child Psychology and Psychiatry, 46*, 1178–1190.

Liddle, H. A., & Schwartz, S. J. (2002). Attachment and family therapy: Clinical utilization of adolescent-family attachment research. *Family Process, 41*, 457–478.

Maslow, A. H. (1968). *Toward the farther reaches of human nature.* New York: Penguin.

Mathew, A. R., Hogarth, L., Leventhal, A. M., Cook, J. W., & Hitsman, B. (2016). Cigarette smoking and depression comorbidity: Systematic review and proposed theoretical model. *Addiction, 112*, 401–412.

McGloin, J. M. (2009). Delinquency balance: Revisiting peer influence. *Criminology, 47*, 439–476.

Moffitt, T. E. (1993). Adolescence-limited and life-course-persistent antisocial behavior: A developmental taxonomy. *Psychological Review, 100*, 674–701.

Pham, M. T., Rajić, A., Greig, J. D., Sargeant, J. M., Papadopoulos, A., & McEwen, S. A. (2014). A scoping review of scoping reviews: Advancing the approach and enhancing the consistency. *Research Synthesis Methods, 5*, 371–385.

Phinney, J. S. (1990). Ethnic identity in adolescents and adults: A review of research. *Psychological Bulletin, 108*, 499–514.

Rivas-Drake, D., & Umaña-Taylor, A. J. (2019). *Below the surface: Talking with teens about race, ethnicity, and identity.* Princeton, NJ: Princeton University Press.

Raley, R. K., & Sweeney, M. M. (2020). Divorce, repartnering, and stepfamilies: Decade in review. *Journal of Marriage and Family, 82*, 81–99.

Raykov, T., & Calvocoressi, L. (in press). Model selection and average proportion explained variance in exploratory factor analysis. *Educational and Psychological Measurement.*

Saigle, V., Séguin, M., & Racine, E. (2017). Identifying gaps in suicide research: A scoping review of ethical challenges and proposed recommendations. *IRB: Ethics and Human Research, 39*, 1–9.

Schwartz, S. J. (2001). The evolution of Eriksonian and neo-Eriksonian identity theory and research: A review and integration. *Identity: An International Journal of Theory and Research, 1*, 7–58.

Schwartz, S. J. (2005). A new identity for identity research: Recommendations for expanding and refocusing the identity literature. *Journal of Adolescent Research, 20*, 293–308.

Schwartz, S. J., Montgomery, M. J., & Briones, E. (2006). The role of identity in acculturation among immigrant people: Theoretical propositions, empirical questions, and applied recommendations. *Human Development, 49*, 1–30.

Schwartz, S. J., Unger, J. B., Zamboanga, B. L., & Szapocznik, J. (2010). Rethinking the concept of acculturation: Implications for theory and research. *American Psychologist, 65*, 237–251.

Schwartz, S. J., Zamboanga, B. L., & Weisskirch, R. S. (2008). Broadening the study of the self: Integrating the study of personal identity and cultural identity. *Social and Personality Psychology Compass, 2*, 635–651.

Siranni, A., Cameron, C. J., Shi, Y., & Heckathorn, D. D. (2021). Bias decomposition and estimator performance in respondent driven sampling. *Social Networks, 64*, 109–121.

Tajfel, H., & Turner, J. C. (1986). The social identity theory of intergroup behavior. In S. Worchel & W. G. Austin (Eds.), *Psychology of intergroup relations* (pp. 7–24). Chicago: Nelson-Hall.

Torraco, R. J. (2005). Writing integrative literature reviews: Guidelines and examples. *Human Resource Development Review, 4*, 356–367.

Van Lange, P. A. M. (1999). Why authors believe that reviewers stress limiting aspects of manuscripts: The SLAM effect in peer review. *Journal of Applied Social Psychology, 29*, 2550–2566.

Waterman, A. S. (2008). Reconsidering happiness: A eudaimonist's perspective. *Journal of Positive Psychology, 3*, 234–252.

17
Open-Access and Pay-to-Publish Journals

Chapter Objectives

By the time you finish reading this chapter, you should feel more comfortable with:

- The difference between subscription journals and open-access journals
- Advantages and disadvantages of publishing in open-access journals
- The kinds of papers that might be best matched with open-access journals
- Using open-access journals as "backups" for manuscripts that are rejected by multiple subscription journals

Most scholarly journals are subscription journals. That is, they charge fees for accessing articles. If you want to download the full text of an article published in a subscription journal, you will have to purchase the article (or subscribe to the journal), unless you are affiliated with a university or company that has purchased access to the journal. In other words, publishing in a subscription journal is generally free of charge, but you have to pay to access articles from that journal.

In contrast, open-access journals allow users to download articles for free, but authors seeking to publish in these journals must pay an article-processing charge. These charges generally range from $1,000 to $3,000—and sometimes higher (Asai, 2021). Open-access journals are published by a range of publishers—including traditional publishers, such as Elsevier and Springer, as well as newer publishers that primarily publish open-access journals, such as BMC, Frontiers, Public Library of Sciences (PLoS), the Multidisciplinary Digital Publishing Institute (MDPI), and Hindawi. What open-access journals have in common is that authors—rather than readers—are asked to offset the costs associated with publishing.

Some traditional academic publishers offer open-access journals that are "paired" with subscription journals. For example, Elsevier publishes an open-access journal called *Addictive Behaviors Reports*, which serves as an

The Savvy Academic. Seth J. Schwartz, Oxford University Press. © Oxford University Press 2022.
DOI: 10.1093/oso/9780190095918.003.0018

open-access companion to the subscription journal *Addictive Behaviors*. Authors whose manuscripts are rejected from *Addictive Behaviors* are encouraged to submit to *Addictive Behaviors Reports*—indeed, my colleagues and I once published an article in the open-access journal after the paper was rejected by the subscription journal. Of course, an open-access journal will also send a paper out for review, but my colleagues' and my experience—as well as the experiences of many other people I know—suggests that the open-access companion journal may be easier to publish in than the subscription journal.

SAGE, another traditional academic publisher, publishes a journal called SAGE Open. SAGE Open publishes articles in all areas of scientific inquiry. Unlike traditional academic journals, this journal doesn't have an editor who handles all submissions. Rather, editors are recruited from the scholarly community, and the editors are charged with managing the review process and rendering decisions on manuscripts. Articles are published on a rolling basis, rather than being assigned to specific months and issues. SAGE also publishes a number of open-access journals—my colleagues and I published in one of them. We were asked to pay $1,500 upon acceptance for publication.

There are also some journals that are not open access but that nonetheless charge publication fees. For example, the *American Journal of Health Behavior* and *Health Behavior and Policy Review* charge publication fees as soon as a manuscript is accepted for publication. These journals are published by smaller companies that require additional funds for copyediting, processing, and hosting articles. However, readers must still pay to download articles from these journals unless authors have paid additional open-access fees.

Journals published by open-access-only publishers generally follow a different peer-review model than subscription journals do. The PLoS family of journals, for example, ask reviewers to prioritize providing an assessment of the technical accuracy of a study more than appraising potential impact (which reviewers may have difficulty assessing; Miller, 2006). The philosophy underlying this approach to peer review appears to be that the scientific community—more so than peer reviewers—is primarily responsible for judging the value of scientific articles. In my experience with the *Frontiers* family of journals, manuscripts are not necessarily rejected if reviewers disapprove of them; rather, reviewers can "withdraw" from the review process if they do not believe that a manuscript can be successfully revised in accordance with their recommendations. When reviewers withdraw, the action editor can invite new reviewers, and the process continues until at least two reviewers have approved the manuscript for publication. The names of the reviewers who approved the manuscript are then included in the published article, but reviewers who withdrew are not named.

Some of the *Frontiers* journals use a model known as "postpublication peer review" (Hunter, 2012). Within this model, submissions are published online immediately, and reviewers are then invited to comment on each article. Authors have the opportunity to revise their published articles whenever they choose to; therefore, the article represents a living document rather than an archived report in a specific volume and issue. Postpublication peer review takes advantage of the online-only format used by most open-access journals by allowing articles to be revised in real time. (Of course, a disadvantage of this approach is that writers who cite one of these articles might eventually wind up having cited an outdated version of the article and might not agree with the current version that the author has revised.)

Advantages and Disadvantages of Publishing in Open-Access Journals

You might be wondering whether you should be publishing in open-access journals, or whether subscription journals are a better option. Many senior scholars, most of whom have been active in scholarly work since before the open-access movement began, have been mistrustful of open-access journals (Xia, 2010; Xia et al., 2015). Much of this mistrust is attributable to the misbehavior of predatory open-access journals, which are discussed in Chapter 10 (Cortegiani, Misseri, Gregoretti, Einav, & Giarratano, 2019). As a reminder, predatory open access journals are fraudulent—authors are asked to pay article-processing charges and are promised extremely rapid peer review (the journals often suggest that reviews will be returned in less than a week), but the articles are often not published as agreed (e.g., copyediting may be extremely poor)—and sometimes articles are never published at all. Predatory open-access journals often list a nonexistent person as the editor-in-chief, and these journals are essentially scams intended to steal money from authors, particularly authors from developing countries (Jia et al., 2015). Unfortunately, many scholars have generalized the fraudulent business models underlying predatory open-access journals to apply to all open-access journals.

Legitimate open-access journals are actually far more similar to traditional subscription journals than they are to predatory open-access journals (Shamseer et al., 2017). There are important advantages and disadvantages to publishing in open-access journals (relative to publishing in subscription journals), and I advise you to consider these pros and cons before deciding which type of journal to send your paper to. Indeed, I argue that the two types of journals serve somewhat different functions.

Many traditional subscription journals offer name recognition and legitimacy; they have been publishing for many years, are supported by major academic publishers, and utilize standard peer review and editorial procedures. At the same time, however, articles published in subscription journals can be difficult for readers to access. Readers who are not affiliated with universities or other organizations that subscribe to a given journal must pay a fee if they wish to download articles from that journal. Some libraries access certain journals through third-party vendors (such as EBSCO, Project Muse, and Gale Academic) rather than directly through the publisher—and in many such cases, the publisher imposes an embargo (generally between 6 months and 2 years after publication) during which third-party vendors are not permitted to make articles available for download. Further, scholars are not permitted to post the final, published versions of subscription-journal articles on their personal websites or on academic social media (e.g., ResearchGate, Academia.edu). Authors are only permitted to share the final published version with someone who specifically requests it. So there are many restrictions on sharing of, and access to, articles in subscription journals because academic publishers often cover their publishing costs through subscriptions and article download fees. Authors are required to transfer the copyright for their article to the publisher, and publishers can sue authors for posting their articles on personal websites or on academic social media without permission (Jamali, 2017). Note, however, that authors can choose to pay an open-access fee (usually around $3,000) that allows them to retain the copyright and to post and share an article however they wish.

On the other hand, open-access journals allow readers to download articles free of charge. Open-access journal articles can be freely shared, posted on personal websites, and disseminated through academic social media. The authors retain the copyright for their work. However, authors finance the journal's publishing process by paying article-processing charges. In some cases, open-access journals may waive the charges for emerging scholars or for scholars from developing countries, because the charges represent a considerable impediment for writers and institutions who do not have the personal, institutional, or government funding to pay open-access fees (Nabyonga-Orem, Asamani, Nyirenda, & Abimbola, 2020). The 2020 coronavirus pandemic, which decimated researchers' and universities' budgets, also increased difficulties with paying article-processing charges (Vervoort, Ma, & Shrime, 2020). Students, postdocs, and early-career faculty members, in particular—as well as faculty at smaller colleges and universities that don't have much research infrastructure—may be effectively "priced out" of publishing in open-access journals unless they have mentors or collaborators who can pay the article-processing charges for them. Indeed, I suspect that most authors who are able to pay article-processing charges have access to grant funds or to departmental discretionary spending accounts. Young scholars and those without access to research funds may need to partner with someone who has access to grant funds or discretionary spending accounts if they need to cover an article-processing charge.

Not surprisingly, allowing readers to download articles for free immediately upon publication may lead to more downloads for open-access journals than for subscription journals (Davis, Lewenstein, Simon, Booth, & Connolly, 2008) in the first few months after publication. Open-access journals may therefore allow the newest work to be available to readers as quickly as possible. At the same time, however, citation counts for articles in subscription journals may be up to 30% greater than those for articles in open-access journals (Björk & Solomon, 2012). Although we do not know precisely why subscription-journal articles appear to have more staying power, one possible reason may involve subscription journal articles being viewed as more trustworthy. So there appears to be a trade-off between maximizing the likelihood of getting your work downloaded and read as soon as possible and maximizing the number of citations over time. For people working in "hot" fields where the primary goal is to achieve and disseminate the next major discovery as quickly as possible, open-access journals may provide a more effective venue for reaching readers immediately. In other cases—especially literature reviews, theoretical articles, and meta-analyses, where the goal is to produce a long-term influence on a field of study— subscription journals may represent a wiser choice. As already stated, open-access and subscription journals may serve somewhat different functions for authors and for readers.

Some open-access journals allow scholars to organize "article collections," which are analogous to special issues in subscription journals. My colleagues and I published in an article collection for *Frontiers in Psychology* in early 2020, and we were able to secure a waiver of the article-processing charge (that is, we didn't have to pay to publish the article). Editors of article collections receive a certain number of these waivers, which means that they can include articles from younger scholars, scholars from smaller colleges and universities, and scholars from developing countries. Although my colleagues and I didn't meet any of these criteria, none of us had enough discretionary funds to be able to pay the $3,000 article-processing charge—and I told the article collection editor that we would not be able to participate unless we received a waiver. Article collections may therefore allow scholars to publish in open-access journals even if they cannot pay the article-processing charge.

Our experience publishing in *Frontiers in Psychology* was mixed, however. The topic of the article collection was the future of cultural psychology as a field. Many cultural psychologists are eager to distinguish cultural psychology from cross-cultural psychology (Shweder et al., 2006), because cultural psychology focuses on the interplay between individuals and the cultures to which they belong, whereas cross-cultural psychology focuses on the search for "rules and exceptions" within and across cultures. Said differently, cultural psychology is concerned primarily with how individuals and cultures influence one another, whereas cross-cultural psychology is more concerned with how (and why) human thoughts, feelings, and behaviors are similar versus different across cultural contexts. The mission of our paper was to integrate cultural psychology with developmental science, using acculturation (which is inherently both cultural and developmental) as a template. We never even mentioned cross-cultural psychology in our manuscript.

Nonetheless, of the two initial reviewers who commented on our submission, one endorsed publication almost immediately, whereas the other slammed us for citing the wrong theories and invoking the wrong streams of literature. This second reviewer essentially wanted us to write a very different paper than the one we had been invited to write. The authorship group exchanged several rounds of emails about what to do, and some of my coauthors wanted to withdraw the paper from *Frontiers in Psychology* and submit to a traditional subscription journal. These coauthors believed that we would never be able to satisfy the second reviewer.

The *Frontiers* family of journals introduced a feature that they termed "interactive review." Interactive review provides a forum where authors and reviewers can dialogue with one another and come to an agreement on how a manuscript should be revised. The interactive review mechanism is intended to avoid the multiple rounds of review and revision that often occur with subscription journals. So we crafted a detailed response letter to Reviewer 2 and sent it to the reviewer through the submission site. However, the reviewer's response was even more negative than that reviewer's original review was, and the reviewer then "withdrew" from the review process. The action editor then recruited another reviewer—whose comments were even more negative than those from the reviewer who had withdrawn. The new reviewer again appeared to be defending cultural psychology against criticisms that we had not included in our paper—and the reviewer slammed us for not citing the "correct" cultural psychology theories.

The feedback we received from the second original reviewer, and from the new reviewer, is reminiscent of what is discussed in Chapter 10 as signs that you've submitted to the wrong journal. Reviewers are wondering why you are not basing your work on theories you've never heard of or don't know very well, and even the most basic assumptions underlying your manuscript are being criticized. Well, that was happening to us with *Frontiers in Psychology*, but in this case we had been invited to write the paper for an article collection. I could not figure out what was going on. After exchanging emails with the authorship group, I decided to email the action editor and ask her for guidance.

The action editor's response was not overly encouraging. She advised us to do what we could to satisfy the critical reviewer, and she even suggested that we should consider recasting the paper more in the direction that the new reviewer was suggesting. In other words, we would have to abandon the ideas that we had been invited to write about, and instead we would need to write something that a hardcore cultural psychologist would advocate for. Needless to say, I was extremely discouraged, and I emailed my coauthors and suggested that we consider withdrawing the submission from *Frontiers in Psychology* and submitting to a subscription journal. My coauthors agreed with my suggestion, but they indicated that we should let the action editor know that we were planning to pull out of the article collection.

I emailed the action editor and told her that we would not be continuing with *Frontiers in Psychology*. I thanked her for her time and effort, and I explained why we were withdrawing our submission. I asked—rhetorically—why we were invited to write a paper on the intersection of cultural psychology with developmental science but were then criticized for writing the exact paper that we had been invited to write. Something was clearly not adding up in terms of how the editorial and review process was proceeding.

The action editor's response was extremely informative regarding the *Frontiers in Psychology* review process. Although she was the action editor, she had no control over the selection of reviewers. The submission site had been automatically inviting reviewers based on the keywords we had specified when we submitted the manuscript. In the action editor's own words:

> I understand the frustration of feeling like shooting at a moving target, which I find is a byproduct of Frontiers' system. Had your manuscript been submitted to a more traditional journal, things would have proceeded quite differently. For one thing, reviewers wouldn't have been invited automatically based on keywords, and I wouldn't have invited reviewers that I know to be ideologically opposed to what you're trying to achieve in the manuscript. For another, upon receiving reviews, I would have had much more leeway in selecting the comments that I would have

encouraged you to address to make the manuscript as strong as possible, and in integrating them into a single, coherent response. As an editor, I would have had much more leverage, which would have allowed me to resolve this stalemate.

Unfortunately, Frontiers requires complete endorsement of the manuscript by at least 2 reviewers, and the "withdrawal" system makes it necessary to find additional reviewers mid-process, which adds to the feeling of a moving target. This system, which is designed to limit the editor's power, is really tying my hands, such that there is no "button" I can press to move the manuscript forward. This unfortunately results in frustrations for authors. I consulted with another editor at Frontiers with more experience, and she mentioned that these aspects of the system are the most common source of frustration working with Frontiers.

Eventually, the action editor was able to work with the *Frontiers* publisher's office to override these defaults and to invite a reviewer who was sympathetic to our objectives. We then quickly made the changes that this reviewer requested, and the manuscript was accepted for publication within less than a month.

I recount this story to provide insight into the review process used by one of the most prominent open-access publishers. Not only are *Frontiers* editors apparently required to adopt a passive approach, but also they are not even allowed to specify the reviewers they want to select! The action editor handling our submission had literally no role in the editorial process until she told the publisher's office that we were ready to withdraw our submission—and that this withdrawal would have compromised the article collection that the action editor and her colleagues were putting together. I have never asked other authors about their experiences publishing in the *Frontiers* family of journals, but the action editor's response suggests that other authors' experiences are likely similar to ours.

I also do not know whether other open-access journals and publishers use review processes like those employed by *Frontiers*. That manuscript was the only paper I have ever submitted to an open-access journal—but based on our experience with *Frontiers*, I am not certain that I will ever submit another manuscript to an open-access journal. When I looked on the *Frontiers* website, no information was posted about the action editor's role (or lack thereof) in the editorial process, or about the "withdrawal" system whereby reviewers can excuse themselves from the editorial process (and thereby require the action editor to seek new reviewers in the middle of the process). Our experience with the *Frontiers* special-collection manuscript leads me to wonder whether other open-access publishers are more (or perhaps less) transparent about their review procedures than *Frontiers* is.

Of course, my experience may be just that—my experience. It is quite possible that other authors have had much more pleasant and favorable experiences publishing in open-access journals. It's also possible that our experience might have been different had we submitted our paper as a regular manuscript rather than as part of an article collection. I really cannot say. Based on the experience that my coauthors and I had with *Frontiers in Psychology*, however, I advise you to consult with colleagues who have more experience publishing in open-access journals before you submit a manuscript to one of these journals.

Xia (2010) found that some authors submit to open-access journals because they believe that they can avoid having to go through the peer-review process. He argued that this is a misconception, and Wicherts (2016) provided evidence that many open-access journals provide rigorous peer review. However, the "postpublication peer review" model used by some open-access journals leads to very high acceptance rates (van Noorden, 2013, listed the acceptance rate for *PLoS One* as 70%). Even if peer reviewers write critical reviews of published articles, the article still appears in the literature and can be retrieved through literature searches (see Ray, 2016, for an extended critique of the open-access publishing model). Despite some evidence to the contrary, many authors (and some reviewers) continue to believe that charging authors to publish their work is likely to compromise the integrity of the peer review and editorial process—I can remember conducting a Google search on the *Frontiers* journals and coming across several comment forums where scholars reported being pressured to "tone down" their reviews of manuscripts, and to endorse publication, so that the manuscripts could be accepted and the article-processing charges could be collected. Because the people posting on these forums were anonymous, I cannot speak to the accuracy of the statements posted on these forums. However, the comments are concerning.

What Kinds of Papers Might be Best Matched with Open-Access Journals?

I caution you not to generalize the experiences and opinions of some authors and reviewers about certain open-access journals to apply to all open-access journals. There is likely a great deal of variability in quality, rigor, and author and reviewer experiences across open-access publishers, and across journals published by each open-access publisher. I've tried to present a balanced view of the open-access movement even though my own (quite limited) experience with open-access publishing was not particularly enjoyable. Indeed, as I suggest in this section, there may be certain types of papers that are best suited for the open-access publishing model, and other types of papers that may be less well suited for open-access journals.

Many research groups explicitly incorporate open-access publishing fees into their budgets, suggesting that they plan to publish articles from the project in open-access journals. Because open-access journal articles are available for download immediately upon publication, articles with urgent policy or public health importance may be strong candidates for placement in open-access journals. Papers reporting on the efficacy of coronavirus vaccines, for example, would be extremely important to disseminate as soon as possible. There are probably other time-sensitive issues that would also serve as arguments for submission to open-access journals.

Articles on controversial topics might also be ideal candidates for submission to journals that invite postpublication peer reviews and commentaries. Open-access journals that provide real-time dialogue among authors, reviewers, and readers would appear to lend themselves well to controversial topics, such as the effectiveness of masks in preventing spread of viruses, policy initiatives to regulate or ban fattening foods or carcinogenic chemicals, or the role of violent video games and media in promoting deviant behavior among children and adolescents. Indeed, although some subscription journals also invite commentaries on published articles, these commentaries often take weeks or months to appear. In contrast, real-time dialogue among authors, reviewers, and readers can contribute to policy initiatives and discussions far more quickly than the typical subscription-journal commentary model can.

At the same time, scoping reviews, integrative reviews, meta-analyses, and theoretical articles are probably best suited for traditional subscription journals because articles in these journals may have more "staying power" than articles in open-access journals. Exceptions to this might be integrative reviews and meta-analyses focused on controversial or urgent topics. For example, at the beginning of a pandemic, it might be helpful to publish a meta-analysis of the effectiveness of strategies to prevent and treat viral infections. A general rule, however, is that theoretical articles and scoping reviews—which are more "academic"—are best placed in traditional subscription journals.

It should also be noted that the majority of open-access journals focus on medicine and public health, and that far fewer focus on the social sciences. Someone seeking to publish an article on the sociology of immigration, for example, would likely experience difficulty in finding a suitable open-access journal to submit the paper to. Other than *Frontiers in Psychology*, I do not know of any open-access journals that focus specifically on social-science topics. *PLoS One* publishes articles in a variety of fields, including psychology, but the majority of its articles appear to be focused on medicine and public health. So scholars working in social-science fields may have fewer opportunities than medical and public health scholars to publish in open-access journals. Indeed, I have never seen an open-access journal article on family relationships, on ethnic discrimination, or on intrinsic motivation or well-being.

Because some open-access journals may have higher acceptance rates than many subscription journals (van Noorden, 2013), you might consider an open-access journal as an outlet for a paper that has been repeatedly rejected by subscription journals. By definition, a journal where reviewers can "withdraw," rather than simply recommending rejection, may have a greater tolerance for new ideas and for studies with interesting findings but whose methodology is somewhat flawed. Action editors can continue to seek new reviewers until they find two reviewers who are willing to endorse the paper for publication.

Conclusion

This chapter covers open-access journals and compares them to traditional subscription journals. The general principle of the open-access model is that authors, rather than readers, cover the journals' publication costs. Some traditional academic publishers maintain open-access companion journals to which authors can submit papers that have been rejected by the subscription journal. The majority of open-access journals, however, are published by specialized open-access publishers, such as *Frontiers*, *PLoS*, and *BMC*. Article-processing charges levied by these journals and publishers can range from $1,000 to above $3,000—which may result in pricing these journals out of the reach of young scholars, scholars from smaller institutions, and scholars from developing countries. Nonetheless, the open-access publishing model has resulted in faster availability of articles to the scholarly community and to the general public.

A primary message communicated in this chapter is that legitimate open-access journals—that is, those that are published by genuine publishers and that provide rigorous peer review—are neither "good" nor "bad." There are both advantages and disadvantages to publishing in open-access journals and in traditional subscription journals. The peer-review procedures maintained by many open-access journals are normally faster than those maintained by subscription journals, and the "interactive review" feature utilized by some open-access publishers reduces the likelihood that a manuscript will be sent out for review over and over again. However, many authors and readers don't completely trust the open-access publishing model—and this lack of trust might lead open-access articles to be cited less widely than articles in subscription journals. The inclusion of article-processing charges in the open-access model may lead some scholars to be suspicious and mistrustful of this model. So there are specific types of articles that might be best placed in open-access journals, such as articles with urgent and immediate importance, whereas other types of articles, such as theoretical articles, scoping reviews, and many meta-analyses and integrative reviews, would be better placed in a traditional subscription journal.

It is clear that open-access journals are here to stay, and that more and more of them will emerge over time. The majority of these journals focus on medicine and public health, but some are general and publish some social-science content. I advise readers, particularly early-career scholars, to consult colleagues who have published in a given open-access journal before submitting a paper to that journal. Whereas most subscription journals use similar peer-review procedures, open-access journals can vary widely in their peer-review philosophies (such as postpublication peer review or asking reviewers to evaluate technical merit but not overall impact). My experience with *Frontiers in Psychology* suggests that the intricacies of an open-access journal's peer-review philosophy don't always appear on that journal's website.

Finally, I should mention that all of the principles I discuss here apply only to legitimate open-access journals. Predatory open-access journals should be avoided at all costs. If a journal emails you and asks you to submit a manuscript—or promises absurdly fast peer review—I advise deleting the email. If you visit a journal's website and spot misspelled words, or if you search for the editor's name and cannot find that person at a legitimate scholarly institution, I suggest staying away from that journal. The guiding principle is that if it looks too good to be true, it probably is.

Summary

- Open-access journals charge authors to publish articles, but the articles are available to readers for free.
- Peer-review processes for open-access journals often focus on technical issues rather than on the contribution that the study makes to the literature.

- Articles published in open-access journals are often cited more quickly than articles published in traditional subscription journals, but articles published in subscription journals often have more "staying power" than articles published in open-access journals.
- Action editors for open-access journals may have less power to make decisions than action editors for subscription journals.
- Papers in "hot" fields, as well as papers addressing controversial topics, might best be placed in open-access journals. Conversely, theory and literature review papers are likely best placed in subscription journals.

References

Asai, S. (2021). An analysis of revising article processing charges for open access journals between 2018 and 2020. *Learned Publishing, 34*, 137–143.

Björk, B.-C., & Solomon, D. (2012). Open access versus subscription journals: A comparison of scientific impact. *BMC Medicine, 10*, Article 73.

Cortegiani, A., Misseri, G., Gregoretti, C., Einav, S., & Giarratano, A. (2019). The challenge of the predatory open access publishing outbreak. *European Journal of Anesthesiology, 36*, 810–813.

Davis, P. M., Lewenstein, B. V., Simon, D. H., Booth, J. G., & Connolly, M. L. (2008). Open access publishing, article downloads, and citations: Randomised controlled trial. *BMJ, 337*, Article a568.

Hunter, J. (2012). Post-publication peer review: Opening up scientific conversation. *Frontiers in Computational Neuroscience, 6*, Article 63.

Jamali, H. (2017). Copyright compliance and infringement in ResearchGate full-text journal articles. *Scientometrics, 112*, 241–254.

Jia, X., Harmon, J. L., Connolly, K. G., Donnelly, R. M., Anderson, M. R., & Howard, H. A. (2015). Who publishes in "predatory" journals? *Journal of the Association for Information Science and Technology, 66*, 1406–1417.

Miller, C. C. (2006). Peer review in the organizational and management sciences: Prevalence and effects of reviewer hostility, bias, and dissensus. *Academy of Management Journal, 49*, 425–431.

Nabyonga-Orem, J., Asamani, J. A., Nyirenda, T., & Abimbola, S. (2020). Article processing charges are stalling the progress of African researchers: A call for urgent reforms. *BMJ Global Health, 5*, Article e003650.

Ray, M. (2016). An expanded approach to evaluating open access journals. *Journal of Scholarly Publishing, 47*, 307–327.

Shamseer, L., Moher, D., Madeukwe, O., Turner, L., Barbour, V., Burch, R., . . . Shea, B. J. (2017). Potential predatory and legitimate biomedical journals: Can you tell the difference? A cross-sectional comparison. *BMC Medicine, 15*, Article 28.

Shweder, R. A., Goodnow, J. J., Hatano, G., LeVine, R. A., Markus, H. A., & Miller, P. J. (2006). The cultural psychology of development: One mind, many mentalities. In R. M. Lerner (Vol. Ed.), *Handbook of child psychology, Volume 1: Theoretical models of human development* (pp. 716–792). New York: Wiley.

van Noorden, R. (2013). The true cost of science publishing. *Nature, 495*, 426–429.

Vervoort, D., Ma, X., & Shrime, M. G. (2020). Money down the drain: Predatory publishing during the COVID-19 era. *Canadian Journal of Public Health, 111*, 665–666.

Wicherts, J. M. (2016). Peer review quality and transparency of the peer-review process in open access and subscription journals. *PLoS One, 11*, Article e0147913.

Xia, J. (2010). A longitudinal study of scholars' attitudes and behaviors toward open-access journal publishing. *Journal of the American Society for Information Science and Technology, 61*, 615–624.

Xia, J., Harmon, J. L., Connolly, K. G., Donnelly, R. M., Anderson, M. R., & Howard, H. A. (2015). Who publishes in "predatory" journals? *Journal of the American Society for Information Science and Technology, 66*, 1406–1417.

18
Books and Book Chapters

Chapter Objectives

By the time you finish reading this chapter, you should feel more comfortable with:

- The process of proposing authored and edited books
- Differences between edited books and handbooks
- Planning and writing an authored book
- Planning an edited book or handbook, and commissioning and editing chapters
- Writing book chapters

Although much scholarly work is published in journals, scholars also write and edit books. For a number of reasons that are covered in this chapter, books provide much greater opportunities to express oneself than journal articles do. Compared to the journal review process, the review process for books is less arduous, and authors have far more leeway to choose what they wish to say. Once a publisher has issued a contract for a book, it is very unlikely that the book will be rejected for publication after it has been completed. Simply put, the publisher has invested too much time and too many resources to cancel the book unless the author has committed a serious or egregious ethical breach or has produced an exceedingly poor product.

This chapter covers authored and edited books, as well as book chapters. Questions I have heard often from young scholars are generally some variant of "When in my career should I write a book? What should I write about? How much time does it take? Do I have to wait for a publisher to approach me, or can I shop an idea to a publisher?"

I answer these questions in this chapter—but first I should go over the different types of books and how each type is unique. The major types include authored books, edited books, and handbooks. There are also other types

The Savvy Academic. Seth J. Schwartz, Oxford University Press. © Oxford University Press 2022.
DOI: 10.1093/oso/9780190095918.003.0019

of books, such as encyclopedias, but we won't go over those in this chapter. Encyclopedias are very specialized and are fairly uncommon compared to authored books, edited books, and handbooks.

Authored books are just that—books that are written by a single person or group. The entire book is written by the same author (or author group), meaning that the authors must spend a great deal of time putting together the full product. This book that you are reading now took me almost 2 years to write. I have full control of the content of the book—I proposed the book concept to Oxford University Press, they approved a revised version of my proposal, and I wrote the book based on what I proposed. Although the final product was peer-reviewed (and was reviewed by Nadina Persaud, my editor at Oxford), the ideas in the book are mine, and I am solely responsible for them.

Edited books consist of chapters written by various people in the field covered by the book. For example, a colleague and I once wrote a chapter for an edited book on the lives of immigrants in the United States. Our chapter was on family relationships, but there were also chapters on school, civic engagement, peer relationships, the workplace, and several other areas. Each chapter was written by an author or author group with specific expertise in the content area covered by that chapter—and the book editor carefully reviewed each chapter, requested changes, and approved the final version once he was satisfied with it. The editor was responsible for identifying and inviting authors to write each chapter and for the content of the book as a whole—but he did not have to write the individual chapters. He also did not have full control over what was written in the book, because other people wrote each of the chapters.

Handbooks are similar to edited books, but they are far larger, more authoritative, and more far-reaching. Whereas edited books may consist of 10 to 15 chapters, handbooks can have up to 40 or 50 chapters. In 2013, my colleagues and I wrote a chapter for the *Handbook of Psychology*, which consisted of 12 volumes! The full set of volumes had more than 300 chapters. Although each volume was edited by a separate set of editors, the series editor (Irving Weiner) was responsible for the entire handbook.

Handbooks often include chapters from author groups who are major names in their respective fields. Handbook chapters are generally longer than chapters from other edited books. For example, when my PhD student Mariya Petrova and I wrote a chapter for a book on self-concept clarity, we were asked to limit our chapter to 5,000 words of text. However, the chapter that my colleagues and I wrote for the *Handbook of Psychology* consisted of almost 15,000 words of text. Handbook chapters are supposed to cover a lot of content (our chapter was on identity, including personal as well as ethnic and cultural identity)—and as a result, handbooks serve as authoritative references on a given field of study. I've edited two handbooks in my career, and I can tell you that they are a *lot* of work—far more than a regular edited book would be.

As soon as you begin to establish yourself as an important contributor to your field, you will undoubtedly be asked to write chapters for edited books. (Invitations for handbook chapters will probably begin to arrive when you become a leader in your field.) Should you accept these invitations? If so, what should you write in a book chapter? Should book chapters be reviews of existing literature? Should they report empirical findings? Should you use a book chapter as a place to report work that you have had trouble publishing in journals? If you write a set of ideas into a book chapter, does that then preclude you from publishing the ideas in a journal article later on? We cover all these issues in this chapter.

The remainder of the chapter is organized into five sections—planning an authored book, writing an authored book, planning an edited book or handbook, commissioning and editing chapters for an edited book or handbook, and writing chapters for edited books and handbooks.

Planning an Authored Book

When you decide to write an authored book, you probably will have a good idea of what you want to write about. You might even have a list of chapters in mind. My best advice is to write everything down while you are excited and enthusiastic about the ideas. Don't worry if you don't have all the chapters conceptualized—write down what you have and just write "More Here" wherever you're not sure what to include. The outline for an authored book is a living document and will be updated, edited, and revised repeatedly before it is ready to be pitched to a publisher. Again, as emphasized regarding first drafts of manuscripts, it is essential that you do not try to edit or critique the outline until you have completed a full draft of it.

Writing the Book Proposal

Once you have the full outline written, I recommend that you contact editors at various academic publishers (such as Oxford, Cambridge, APA, SAGE, Wiley, Springer, Taylor & Francis, and Elsevier) to pitch the idea. Arrange a phone call or video chat and send a copy of whatever outline you have in advance of the meeting. If an editor seems interested in what you have in mind, then you can start creating the proposal. I would not start to write a formal book proposal until you have an editor who has expressed interest.

Finding an editor to contact is not difficult. Publisher websites generally have pages for prospective book authors, and these pages will provide names and contact information for editors in each of the subject areas that the publisher covers. Just look for the editor in the area best represented by your idea and email that person. Attach your book outline (or describe the idea if the outline is still a work in progress) and ask for a meeting. Editors will probably let you know via email if your idea is not a good fit, or they will arrange a meeting with you if they want to learn more about what you have in mind.

Assuming that you've found an editor who is interested in your idea, and assuming that you have spoken with that person, it's time to create the formal book proposal. Here I list the specific questions that most publishers will ask you to answer as part of the proposal. I also provide excerpts from my answers so that you can see what a successful book proposal looks like. I also provide a checklist (Box 18.1) that you can use when writing a book proposal.

The first part of the proposal asks for your biographical information: name, affiliation, title, email, address, and phone number. You will also be asked to provide your curriculum vitae. The editor will secure peer reviews of your proposal, and one of the key questions reviewers will be asked to comment on is how well suited you are to write the book you are proposing. You don't have

Box 18.1 Checklist for Book Proposals

1. Have you made the purpose of the book clear enough so that the editor and the peer reviewers will know what the book is about?
2. Have you mapped out the list of chapters and what each chapter contributes to the book?
3. Have you justified why you are well positioned to write or edit this book?
4. Have you pinpointed the market for the book and laid out a convincing rationale for why the publisher needs to target this market?
5. Have you searched for—and listed—all similarly titled or themed books that have been published in the last 10 to 15 years? Have you argued for why your book represents a unique contribution over and above these competing titles?
6. Have you suggested people who could review your book proposal fairly and objectively?

to be a full professor to write a book, but you do have to have an established track record in the field you are proposing to write about.

The second major question is "Why write and publish a book on this particular subject right now?" You need to have a solid answer for this question. Publishers receive many more book proposals than they can contract, so you should argue persuasively for why your topic is important. Have current events highlighted the importance of your field? Is your field extremely fragmented, requiring an integrative volume to pull the various strands of literature together?

Here are some excerpts from my book proposal:

> The universe of individuals who conduct research is larger and broader than ever before. Whereas conducting and writing up research was once largely the province of professors, many others are now becoming involved in the research and publishing enterprise. Nurses, doctors, attorneys, lawmakers, agency directors, and social workers, among others, are conducting research and attempting to publish it. Not surprisingly, a number of authored and edited books have been written on the publishing process in recent years (e.g., Gutman, 2016; Henson, 2004; Jalongo & Saracho, 2016; Oermann & Hays, 2018; Rocco & Hatcher, 2011). These books are intended for various types of audiences, as noted in the Competition section.
>
> Many books on publishing focus on how to prepare the written document—the manuscript—itself. Such information, while quite useful, leaves out a key principle: before we can expect to write successfully, we must have something successful to write *about*. Conducting rigorous research is essential to the publishing enterprise; even a wonderfully written manuscript is unlikely to be published if it reports a flawed study. The value of planning and carefully executing the study, taking careful notes, partnering with statistical experts (even if one is well versed in the analytic techniques being used), and understanding the limitations of one's work are all essential steps to take before writing a single word.
>
> Other books, such as Jalongo and Saracho's (2016) authored volume and Rocco and Hatcher's (2018) edited volume, cover the functions that reviewers undertake when evaluating manuscripts; they spend far less time helping readers learn to *think* like a reviewer. Thinking like a reviewer entails critically evaluating one's own work, including recognizing major or fatal flaws that could preclude publication in higher-tier journals. Being objective about one's own research and writing is extremely difficult. I will provide concrete and accessible tips for doing this.

The next item in the book proposal template involves listing the chapters and providing an abstract for each chapter. Chapter abstracts should lay out what each chapter will cover in approximately 100 to 200 words. For example, here is one of the chapter abstracts for the book you are reading:

> This chapter will outline principles for planning research studies that will yield publishable data. I will proceed from the principle that all facets of the study must be guided by a clear set of research questions and hypotheses. Related questions are "What is the best research design for testing the questions I am proposing?" and "What research designs and methods are generally used in my field of study?" I will also discuss secondary data analyses and ways to effectively use secondary data. Key errors, such as failing to account for confounding variables, not planning for attrition in longitudinal studies, sampling problems, and use of questionable or inappropriate measurement instruments, will also be covered. The value of team science, along with some of the pitfalls of working with large research groups, will be discussed. The chapter will adopt the perspective of a journal or grant reviewer in terms of identifying potential flaws in one's work.

The next question asks for your author bio. If there are multiple authors, a bio should be provided for each author. The bio should be brief and should sketch out your credentials and justify why you are qualified to write the book you are proposing to write. Here is the bio that I provided for the book you are reading:

> Seth J. Schwartz received his master's degree in family and child sciences from Florida State University and his PhD in life-span developmental psychology from Florida International University. He is regarded as a leading scholar in the field of personal identity theory and research, and he has recently been branching out into the study of ethnic and cultural identity as well. Dr. Schwartz is also interested in the structure of identity across gender, ethnicity, and nationality, and he is interested in the ways in which social-contextual factors in the family, peer, school, and cultural contexts shape the development of identity in adolescents and emerging adults. He has published two edited books, 238 journal articles, and 27 book chapters.

Notice that I described my scholarly work briefly, and that I also talked about my scholarly output in terms of publications and books. I wanted the publisher to know that I had published enough to be taken seriously as an author of a book on writing for publication.

The next section is about the target market, which includes the primary audience for the book, other audiences who might also be interested, and societies and conferences to whom the book could be marketed, as well as whether the book could be used as a course textbook. To answer these questions, you need to have a good idea about who will buy and read your book. Will graduate students find the book interesting and useful? Will the book be directed more toward clinical professionals? Also make sure to detail why the book is a good fit for the audiences you suggest. Will you be imparting specific skills to graduate students or teaching specific clinical techniques to therapists and counselors? Remember that publishers are most likely to contract books that they believe will sell well—so the target market section is your chance to convince them that your idea will sell lots of copies.

There is also a section of the proposal on competitive titles—that is, books that have already been published and that are similar to the book you plan to write. You should make sure to do your research for this section. Go to Amazon, Barnes & Noble, and academic publisher websites, and conduct keyword searches for words related to the book you plan to write. All titles that come up, that are fairly recent (published within the last 10–15 years), and that are even tangentially relevant your work should be listed. If you don't list a competitive title and a reviewer knows about that title, you may wind up looking sloppy and unprepared.

For each competitive title you list, describe that book briefly and note how your proposed book will be sufficiently different from that existing book. For example, when I was proposing the book you are reading now, I listed some competitive titles that targeted specific fields, such as one book (Oermann & Hays, 2018) on writing for publication in the field of nursing. I also listed other titles that briefly covered how to respond to editors and reviewers (Jalongo & Saracho, 2016), but that don't go into the amount of detail that I planned to cover in my book.

Remember José's admonition about standing on the shoulders of earlier work rather than criticizing that work for what it did not do. You don't want to belittle other books for not adopting the approach you plan to adopt. I suggest objectively describing each competitive title and briefly describing what you will be doing that is different (not better or worse, just different) from what other books have done.

The final key question involves unique selling points of your book. Your response to this question is your chance to present your ideas and how they can be used to market your proposed book. Here are the answers I provided to this question:

1. I will cover the steps that occur before the paper is written—planning the study, identifying and accounting for confounding variables, carrying

out the study, and conducting the analyses. Other books about writing focus primarily on the technical aspects of writing, with far less attention to ensuring that there is *something to write about.*

2. This book will help readers learn to *think* like a reviewer and be objective about one's own research and writing.

3. Anecdotes, informative stories, and case examples will be provided from my 25-year publishing career, as well as from my experience writing with and mentoring students, postdoctoral fellows, and early-career colleagues.

4. I will discuss when (and why) authors should consider publishing their work in open-access journals that charge fees for publication.

5. The proposed book will cover strategies for responding to editors and reviewers. I will provide guidance about how to use response letters strategically, how to place responses in the letter but not in the revised manuscript, and how to "win over" difficult reviewers.

6. I will discuss specific challenges involved in publishing theoretical and policy papers—as well as ways to write theory and policy for different types of audiences.

7. I will cover book chapters—whether to write them, how to write them, how to decide what material to include, and how to use book chapters strategically to advance one's career.

8. The proposed book will guide readers in developing a scholarly network, approaching senior scholars and inviting them to collaborate, working in large writing teams, handling difficult and unresponsive coauthors, and writing with mentors and supervisors. Again, much of the guidance I provide will come from my own career experiences and how I have successfully (and sometimes unsuccessfully) handled these interactions.

Notice that this list was essentially providing the publisher with a list of excerpts that they could use to promote my book to prospective buyers. I wanted to make my editor's job as easy as possible—she could essentially take my selling points, edit them, and paste them into a promotional flyer for the book.

The final question asks for keywords for the book. You should select these in much the same way as you select keywords for journal articles. I listed four keywords—publishing journal articles, research, scholarly writing, and peer review. Technically, you can list as many keywords as you want, but I do not recommend listing more than four or five. Long lists can overwhelm readers and reviewers.

Planning and Writing the Book

The editor will secure reviews for your proposal and, if the editor decides to contract the book, you will be asked to respond to those reviews (including modifying the proposal in accordance with the reviewer feedback). Once you have made the necessary modifications, the editor will either proceed with the contract or ask you to modify the proposal further. As soon as the book is contracted, you can start writing.

Most publishing contracts are fairly standard. The copyright for the book will belong to the publisher, and the contract will list actions that you and the publisher can take if either party fails to deliver on the terms of the contract. Your royalties will be calculated as a percentage of the publisher's profits. I recommend asking a contract attorney to read over the contract before you sign it, just to ensure that you fully understand what you are signing. I've asked attorneys to read over academic publisher contracts before, and no attorney has objected to any of the terms.

Once you start writing the book, you should outline each chapter much as you would outline an empirical or theoretical article (depending on the type of material reported in the chapter). Further, you will want to ensure that the structure of the book itself—that is, how the chapters are organized—is intuitive and easy to follow. It may be wise to include section headings so that similar chapters are grouped together. The point is to ensure that the book is as readable and accessible as possible for readers.

There are many strategies for writing an authored book—but here I describe the strategy I used in writing the book you are reading. First, although I hadn't planned on including an introductory chapter to humanize myself and to give the reader a sense of who I am and what my credentials are, I decided that including a chapter like that would be a good idea. If I were reading a book on how to write for publication, I would want to know who the author was and what qualified that person to write a book on that topic. I would want some background information on why the author was recommending specific strategies for approaching the writing process. I spend a lot of time discussing the role of mentors in the writing process, so I thought it was critical to introduce my own history of mentoring and being mentored. Finally, because many of my students have told me that they could never picture themselves being able to write the way I write, I believed it was essential to outline my own history of failing and bouncing back. Without that, readers might view me as inaccessible or as someone to whom they can never match up.

Second, I chose to write the chapters sequentially. My approach was that Chapter 2 builds on principles from Chapter 1, Chapter 3 builds on principles from Chapter 2, and so on. However, you do not have to write your book that way. You may feel especially inspired to write a certain chapter on a given day—and if you do, then follow that inspiration! You can write your chapters in whatever way feels right to you—but you should make sure that readers can read the chapters sequentially without becoming confused or lost.

Third, if you are writing a book with coauthors, you might assign certain chapters to certain people. For example, if your book presents a clinical psychological approach to treating mood disorders, you might assign one person to write the chapter presenting the clinical interior of the model—that is, what happens within each session—whereas another author might write the chapter on research findings related to the model. After first drafts of all the chapters have been written, and after each author has edited their chapter as much as possible, the authors might swap chapters and edit one another's writing.

Fourth, I chose to write *all* the chapters before going back and editing *any* of the chapters. I wanted to separate the creative process of writing chapter drafts from the process of editing the drafts. I recommend this approach to other book authors as well—but keep in mind that different approaches work better for different people. Find what works for you and stay with that.

Finally, it's essential to stay in touch with your editor during the writing process. Editors can look at what you've written to ensure that you and the editor are on the same page. I find that it's more effective to solicit comments from an editor early in the process than it is to submit the full book manuscript and learn that the editor doesn't resonate with the approach you adopted. Remember that the editor needs to approve your book manuscript before it will be accepted and sent to production.

Planning Edited Books and Handbooks

Edited books and handbooks are quite different from authored books. The book editors come up with the concept for the book, sketch out the proposed list of chapters, and propose authors for each chapter. As is the case with authored books, when you are getting started, it's important to find a publisher before you do any substantive work on the book. I suggest contacting editors at major academic publishers and pitching your idea to them. Only after an editor has indicated interest and has asked you to prepare a proposal should you start developing the full list of chapters.

Note that edited books can be manageable for early-career scholars. The number of chapters is limited, and the authors don't need to be senior leaders in their respective fields. Just remember that readership and book sales will depend largely on the book's ability to appeal to a wide audience and on the recognizability of the chapter authors. (Although chapter authors don't need to be luminaries in their field, readers should be able to recognize chapter authors' names.) Chances are that an editor will not offer you a contract for a book where the chapter authors are your friends and colleagues unless all of you have solid name recognition and are writing chapters in areas that will draw interest from readers.

Let me offer you a word of caution. I remember an edited book that was published by a major academic publisher in the mid-1990s. The book was based on an international working group meeting among scholars in a small, narrow field of study. Many of the chapters consisted of verbatim dialogue among the scholars—a premise that seemed interesting—but, although I bought a copy of the book almost as soon as it was published, I knew that the readership would be limited. The book went out of print less than 3 years after it came out—because sales were extremely slow. Indeed, that was the only instance I've heard of where a book went out of print so quickly. The idea was promising, but the audience for the book was small because the field in which the book was written was extremely specialized.

Based on experiences like that one, publishers will want to know that there is an established, enduring audience for your book. That is, you need to provide credible evidence that readers will buy your book and that the book will continue to sell even after the original cohort of buyers have purchased their copies. Such evidence can take the form of library subscriptions, potential for the book to be used as a course text, and lists of conferences where the book can be displayed and sold. The issue of potential sales is important both for authored books and for edited books and handbooks, but this concern might be even more important for edited books and handbooks, given the importance of name recognition of chapter authors as well as of the book editors. Additionally, in my experience, some potential chapter authors won't commit to writing a chapter until you have the book contract from the publisher—so you may only have a list of chapters and potential authors when you propose the book.

Managing Edited Books and Handbooks

Once the book has been contracted, you need to secure authors for the chapters you have proposed. For edited books, where the scope and size of the volume are smaller than those of handbooks, many of the authors may be people you know and may have already committed to write chapters before you secured the contract. You may need to secure authors for only a handful of remaining chapters. For handbooks, however, chapter authors should be leaders in their respective fields—generally full professors—so it will likely take far more work to secure chapter authors for a handbook than for an edited book.

I've served as senior editor of two handbooks—the *Handbook of Identity Theory and Research* (with Koen Luyckx and Viv Vignoles) and the *Oxford Handbook of Acculturation and Health* (with Jennifer Unger). The identity handbook was a far larger and more ambitious project (40 chapters in total), and we were responsible for finding chapter authors across many different subfields of identity studies, including identity perspectives from developmental psychology, social psychology, sociology, anthropology, discursive analysis, political science, and public health. There is a great story behind that book, which I will recount briefly here. Just before I left Florida State University with my master's degree, Dick Dunham and I had agreed to write a "grand book" about identity. For several reasons, however, the book never came to fruition. More than 10 years later, in late 2007, I felt a flash of inspiration telling me that I should revisit the book that Dick and I had talked about. I spent part of the winter break drafting a table of contents. As luck would have it, in February 2008, an editor from Springer Publishers contacted me and told me that she had spotted a symposium I would be presenting at an upcoming conference, and that she wanted to meet to discuss turning that symposium into a book. I agreed to meet with her at the conference.

When we met, I showed her the table of contents I had written, and she was very excited. She asked me to draft a proposal, but she advised me that I would need help. One associate professor would have a very hard time editing a massive handbook alone. So, I talked with Koen, whom I already knew, and he agreed to edit the book with me. Before long, however, Koen and I—both of whom are developmental psychologists—realized that there were many other areas of identity that we didn't know much about, so we consulted with some of our colleagues, and Viv Vignoles was recommended to us as a social-psychological co-editor. We approached him with the idea, and he signed on—and our editorial team was complete.

Koen, Viv, and I spent two and a half years—no, that is not a misprint—recruiting chapter authors, working with the authors to refine their chapters, editing and reviewing chapters (we also sought external reviewers for many of the chapters), and crafting the introductory and closing chapters to tie everything together. Miraculously, we did almost all this work by email—videoconferencing software like Zoom and GoToMeeting hadn't been invented yet—and we met in person only once at the end of the process. Our accomplishment was even more remarkable given that all three of us were raising young children at that time.

When Jennifer Unger and I edited the acculturation handbook, the project was a bit smaller in scope. Almost all the authors were either psychologists or public health scholars, and we knew most of them personally or by reputation. I also had the experience with the identity handbook to draw on. Still, identifying chapter authors and securing chapter commitments weren't easy. On many occasions, a prospective chapter author would decline our invitation and recommend a colleague or a former student as a replacement. Then we would contact that person, and they would decline and recommend someone else. Sometimes a third or fourth contact would accept the invite, but on other occasions, we would wind up at a dead end after trying six or seven people. An important skill when editing books is to know when a planned chapter should be dropped from the book. If you can't find an author to write a chapter, then that chapter won't appear in the book.

Of course, one solution to this problem is to write the chapter yourself. I'm not a big fan of book editors' writing more than a couple of chapters in the book—the whole point of an edited book is for other contributors to write chapters—but sometimes writing a chapter yourself is the only way to ensure that the chapter will be included in the book. Jen Unger and I did this in our acculturation handbook—we had included a chapter on biculturalism in our table of contents, but all our colleagues who were qualified to write that chapter declined our invitation. So we decided to write the chapter ourselves and to invite our expert colleagues to coauthor it with us. Although the two people we had invited to write the chapter were not able to write it themselves, they both agreed to coauthor it with me as first author and Jen as last author. So we were able to include their perspectives and input in the book—and I had enough expertise in biculturalism to lead that chapter.

Once you have successfully recruited chapter authors, your job is only partially completed. Now you need to ensure that the authors actually write and submit their chapters. Based on my experience editing two handbooks, I can tell you that at least a couple of chapters in the book won't materialize. Authors will forget that they had agreed to write a chapter for your book, or they will be too busy to write the chapter, or they will continually promise to deliver the chapter and then never come through, or they will withdraw their agreement to write the chapter, or they may even stop responding to your attempts to contact them. All these scenarios have played out during my handbook-editing experience.

An important skill in editing books is knowing when to come to the realization that a chapter is not going to be written. If you have contacted the authors more than two or three times and they don't respond, chances are that they are not going to write the chapter. If someone promised you a chapter and then failed to deliver it more than two or three times, you can probably assume that the chapter won't materialize. If an author starts offering excuses for why they cannot write the chapter, then I suggest that you stop pursuing that chapter.

When a chapter fails to materialize, you need to ask yourself how important that chapter is to the book or handbook you are editing. If the chapter is essential, then I suggest that you start looking for someone else to write it. You might even want to ask the original author—the person who has indicated they will not be able to write the chapter—to recommend someone else who could write it. Importantly, if the book is going to be delayed because some chapter authors did not follow through with their chapters, let your editor know as soon as you can. Editors are undoubtedly accustomed to having to grant deadline extensions for edited books and handbooks—but it is nonetheless essential to stay in touch with your editor so that the editor knows that the book will not be completed on time. You do not want your editor to start promoting your book, only to learn that the book will now be delivered 6 months late.

When chapter authors submit their chapters to you, I suggest that you and your co-editors establish a system for providing feedback. For the identity handbook, where we would have many different fields and perspectives represented, Koen, Viv, and I decided on a system where one of us would serve as "editor," one of us would serve as "reviewer," and the "editor" would recruit at least one outside reviewer—often an author of another chapter—to comment on the chapter. Although this system created a lot of work for us, it ensured that each chapter received critical and rigorous feedback from two of the handbook editors and from an additional expert. When I look over the chapters in that handbook, it's clear that they benefited from our editorial approach.

For the acculturation handbook, Jen and I used a simpler approach. Because both of us were equally familiar with the material that would be covered in most of the chapters, we divided the chapters between the two of us, and each of us served as editor for our assigned chapters. On some occasions, we asked each other to comment on one another's chapters if we wanted a second perspective.

Another issue to consider is how to proceed with authors who submit chapters with spelling, grammatical, and sentence structure errors. This principle applies primarily to authors whose first language is not English, but I've also encountered some American, British, Canadian, and Australian authors whose writing needed work. I consider myself to be an obsessive-compulsive grammarian, so often I would spend many hours editing punctuation, changing words, and correcting spelling errors. You will also want the whole book to be written in a single language style, so authors who submit their chapters in British/international English might have to switch to American English, or vice versa.

You should also decide how demanding you want to be when interacting with chapter authors. As a journal editor, I can be as demanding as I want with authors because there are many more manuscripts submitted to my journal than my editorial team and I can accept. However, book chapters are different—editors are asking chapter authors to spend time writing chapter for their book, but most book chapters don't advance scholars' careers all that much. (Chapters in major handbooks are an exception, because major handbooks are likely to be read by people around the world.) Unlike journal authors, chapter authors are not so numerous that book and handbook editors can simply proceed to the next author if a current author doesn't produce the exact chapter that the editors want. My advice is to grant chapter authors a great deal of leeway and to allow them to write the chapters that they wish to write (as long as the chapters they produce are still consistent with the overall theme and mission of the book, of course). If a chapter author produces a chapter that is very different from what you were expecting and doesn't fit the theme of the book, then I advise you to contact that author, schedule a call or video chat, and try to negotiate a solution. Does the entire chapter need to be rewritten from scratch, or can the author rewrite or adjust sections of the chapter to bring it more in line with what you were hoping to receive? Make sure to be reasonable with chapter authors—remember that if a chapter author drops out of the book, you have to find another author or remove that chapter from your table of contents.

Once the chapters are finalized (or at least close to finalized), the editors should write their opening chapter. The first half of the opening chapter should introduce the subject matter that the book covers and include a series of integrative statements about that topic. Also, the first half of the opening chapter should introduce the reader to the field, set up important debates and controversies, and tell the reader why the topic of the book is important and timely. The second half of the opening chapter should briefly review and summarize the sections and chapters in the book. In the introductory chapter for the identity handbook, we (Vignoles, Schwartz, & Luyckx, 2011) sketched out connections among various approaches to identity and proposed a set of postulates about what identity is and how it operates. In the opening chapter for the acculturation handbook, we (Schwartz & Unger, 2017) laid out a number of controversies in the field of acculturation and provided our thinking on how the field should proceed in resolving those controversies. Both introductory chapters then proceeded to summarize the other chapters in each respective book.

Writing Book Chapters

Undoubtedly, many young scholars have questions about writing book chapters—whether to write book chapters at all, what to put into a book chapter, and whether material published in a book chapter can be "republished" in a journal article later on. I address these issues one at a time in this section.

Deciding Whether to Write a Chapter

When someone invites you to write a book chapter, the first step I recommend is to ask for more information about the book, who else has agreed (or is being targeted) to write a chapter, whether the authors have secured a contract from the publisher, and what the intended audience is for the book. Remember that your name will appear in the contents alongside the other chapter authors, so if you've never heard of the other authors, you might view this as a "red flag" in terms of the book's potential impact and readership.

If the book passes your "smell test," a next step might be to think about how much time you have available to write the chapter. How much time are the editors giving you to write it? Will you have enough uninterrupted time to put the chapter together? If the editors are not giving you enough time, but you are still interested in writing the chapter, then you might want to propose a delivery date that works better for you. On the other hand, if the editors are giving you too much time, it's easy to forget about the chapter as time passes. (In every instance where the editors gave me and my coauthors more than a year to write a chapter, I wound up scrambling to finish the chapter just before the deadline because I'd forgotten about it.) Propose a closer deadline that you will be able to keep in the front of your mind.

If you decide not to write the chapter, try to recommend someone else whom the book editors could approach and ask to write it. If you know the editors well and/or have a working relationship with them, they may press you even after you decline to write the chapter. Be prepared to offer reasonable justification for declining—or offer to coauthor the chapter along with someone else. I have sometimes agreed to be a chapter author as long as someone else is willing to lead the chapter—and since I became a full professor, I have often given my students and postdoctoral fellows opportunities to lead chapters that I was invited to write. But remember that setting professional boundaries is important, and if you generally do not wish to write a chapter that you have been invited to write, you are perfectly within your rights to decline the invitation. If you know you'll have trouble delivering on your promise to write the chapter if you accept the invitation, it's better to decline or to suggest someone else. Failing to deliver a chapter causes many more problems for the book editors than declining the original invitation causes.

Writing the Chapter

If you do decide to write the chapter, the question becomes what you will put in it. The handbook editors will tell you what they are looking for from you in terms of the specific content they want you to cover, but the specific type of chapter you write is largely up to you. The majority of book chapters I've seen are essentially literature reviews that provide broad coverage of a specific content area—and handbook chapters are almost always written as reviews. Chapter authors tend to cite their own work more extensively than they would in a journal article—remember that you are being asked to write about your field of study, so you are probably expected to cite your own work. Just make sure that citations to your own work are not excessive and are balanced with citations to other important work in your field.

You may also decide to include empirical work in a book chapter. I advise checking with the book editors to ensure that including empirical work is acceptable. If there is an empirical paper you have been trying to publish but that you have had trouble getting accepted in journals, you might be able to publish the paper as a book chapter. Just remember to ask the book editors whether this course of action is acceptable to them.

One question that students have asked me frequently is whether they should put their best work in a book chapter. My first answer is that you should never write or publish anything that is not your best work. I wouldn't want to put my name on subpar work. In terms of whether you should turn your best new ideas into a book chapter, the answer is that it depends on the book in which the chapter will appear. If it's a "niche" book that will attract a narrow readership, then you should write a review of existing work and save your most exciting new ideas for other articles or chapters. If the book is edited by well-known people, and if the other chapters in the book will also be written by well-known people, then consider using the chapter to introduce new ideas. Handbook chapters generally represent opportunities to introduce new and provocative ideas within the scope of a broad review of the field that you have been asked to cover in your chapter. Handbook chapters—and especially chapters in major handbooks that cover entire fields, such as the *Handbook of Child Psychology* or the *Handbook of Cross-Cultural Psychology*—are generally equivalent in prestige to articles published in top-tier journals. The material that you include in a handbook chapter, and especially the material that you write in a chapter in a major handbook, should reflect the very best work that you can produce.

What I absolutely would not do in a book chapter is recycle ideas that you've already published somewhere else. Not only is recycling existing ideas a form of self-plagiarism, but it's also intellectually dishonest. You are artificially inflating your publication count without adding anything new to the literature or to the book to which you are contributing. I'm not saying that you shouldn't draw on prior work when writing a chapter—what I am saying is that the chapter should not simply be a rehash of work you have already published somewhere else. Each piece of work you publish should represent something new—even if it's largely a different combination of ideas you have already expressed. The reader should be able to find something in your chapter that cannot be found elsewhere. If you don't have time to create something new—or if you simply don't want to—then decline the invitation to write the chapter, or else offer to coauthor it with someone else serving as lead author.

Review Process for Book Chapters

The chapter review process that most book editors utilize is less demanding than most journal review processes. Unlike journal manuscripts, book chapters are unlikely to be rejected following review. The book editors may provide rigorous feedback—as in the process that Koen, Viv, and I utilized for the identity handbook—but book chapters can generally be assumed to be "accepted" even before they are written. I've never heard of a chapter being excluded from a book after the book editors had invited the authors to write the chapter. I have seen poorly written chapters require multiple rounds of review by the book editors before the chapter was finalized, but book editors are almost always willing to work with chapter authors to improve the content and quality of the chapter. Remember that the book editors asked these authors to write the chapter, and it's generally easier to work with an existing chapter author than to search for a new author. So I would not worry about your chapter being rejected—rather, I would write the chapter as well as you can and use the book editors' feedback to help you improve and finalize the chapter.

Some book editors don't believe that it is appropriate to ask chapter authors to make major revisions to their chapters. A senior colleague of mine told me once that he generally accepted chapters "as is" and only asked for cosmetic changes. Of course, most of the books he edited were major handbooks, and authors for these handbooks are generally leaders in their fields who have lots of experience writing handbook chapters. My colleague's philosophy on reviewing handbook chapters was that, if authors required extensive editor feedback to write a good chapter, then those authors shouldn't have been invited to write a handbook chapter in the first place.

Unlike with journal editors and reviewers, with book editors you can push back against requests with which you disagree. If you wanted to write your chapter a certain way but the book editors are asking for something else, then you can set up a call or video chat and negotiate with them. A book chapter should represent what you really want to say, within the scope of the book that the book editors are putting together. Especially with handbook chapters, the book editors should give the chapter authors the freedom to write their chapters as they wish.

I know of cases where book editors have been overly meddlesome and difficult with chapter authors. A former colleague of mine adopted this kind of approach, and he even sometimes inserted himself as an author on some of the chapters. He would essentially tell chapter authors what he wanted them to say, to the point where I once asked him why he didn't just write an authored book rather than solicit chapters from other people. Not surprisingly, some authors pulled out of his book because he wouldn't allow them to write their chapters as they wanted to.

Can Ideas Expressed in Book Chapters Be Republished Elsewhere?

In my estimation, once you have expressed a set of ideas in a book chapter, you cannot write the same ideas into another publication unless the other publication is sufficiently different from the chapter. When you submit a manuscript to a journal, you are asked to verify that the paper has not been published elsewhere. When you verify this statement, you are inherently disqualifying a book chapter from being republished as a journal article. So once you put a set of ideas into a book chapter, that chapter becomes the source that should be cited for that set of ideas.

Of course, you can borrow pieces of an argument and use those pieces elsewhere, but you must cite the source where the argument was originally presented—and the primary thesis of the new article or chapter you are writing must be substantively different from that of the book chapter you are drawing from. Essentially, you should be sure that you are comfortable placing a set of ideas in a chapter before you write that chapter. As already noted, I do not suggest placing new or innovative ideas in a chapter that will be read only by a narrow audience.

One final word about book chapters—book chapters can help you "put yourself on the map" early in your career. However, if your number of book chapters exceeds your number of journal articles, hiring and tenure/promotion committees may label you as someone who is not able to publish sufficiently in peer-reviewed journals. Book chapters are not generally considered as representing peer-reviewed material—where peer review is the "gold standard" in most scholarly and scientific fields. A rule of thumb I developed early in my career was to have at least three times as many peer-reviewed articles as I had book chapters. This number is completely arbitrary, but it helped me to avoid the criticism that I was publishing too many book chapters and not enough journal articles.

So you should be careful about which book chapter invitations you accept. You don't want to accept too many book chapter invitations until you have built up your curriculum vitae with journal articles. Early in your career, book chapter invitations will likely come to you through your mentors and other senior colleagues. These chapters can help to build your career by helping you gain recognition from the book editors, from other chapter authors, and from readers. Again, however, your book chapter output should lag behind your journal article output.

Conclusion

This chapter offers principles for putting together authored books, edited books, and handbooks, as well as for writing book chapters. Books are an important part of scholarly output in most fields, and authoring or editing a book is often viewed as highly prestigious. There are many components that go into putting together an authored book, edited book, or handbook, but the first step is to find a publisher and editor who are interested in publishing your idea. You then must write a book proposal that will help the publisher decide whether to offer you a contract. Remember that scholarly publishing is a business, and publishers are most likely to offer contracts for books that will yield profits.

For an authored book, you need to produce a list of chapters and to outline each chapter as completely as you can. This strategy will make it easier for you to write the chapters later. Remember the selling points you proposed to the publisher and be sure to highlight those as you write. And if you are working with coauthors, be sure to distribute the work across the author team. Some authors may be best suited to write specific chapters.

For edited books and handbooks, you should come up with the list of chapters and target authors before you reach out to publishers. If you know some of the authors well, you can ask them whether they would be interested in writing chapters. The most important consideration for publishers when considering whether to offer a contract for an edited book or handbook is usually the expected market for the book. Books aimed toward narrow or niche audiences may go out of print quickly (although e-books may still be available even after the hard copy is out of print), and publishers may not be willing to take risks on book proposals that are unlikely to attract a wide audience. For edited books, and especially for handbooks, author name recognition is a key consideration. Readers may decide to buy a handbook, at least in part, because they are familiar with the chapter author groups and are interested in the topics that the handbook covers. Edited books are generally narrow in scope, whereas handbooks are far broader in scope and cover entire areas or fields of study. If you are proposing a handbook, be prepared for a great deal of work.

Finally, the chapter covers how to decide whether to write a book chapter and what to put into book chapters. Book chapters are easier to get published than journal articles—they are unlikely to be rejected even if the book editors utilize a rigorous review procedure—but they also are not weighted as heavily for hiring, promotion, and tenure. Book chapters can be used strategically to review existing literature, to disseminate work that you have had trouble publishing in journals, or to introduce new and innovative ideas. For edited books with somewhat smaller target audiences, I recommend reviewing literature but saving your most important ideas for a higher-impact publication. Larger edited books and handbooks are a good place to include new ideas, although handbook chapters are primarily used for providing large-scale reviews of a field of study. (You can introduce new ideas toward the end of the chapter.) Edited books—but not handbooks—can serve as outlets for papers that you haven't been able to publish as journal articles.

Perhaps the most essential idea expressed in this chapter is that it's better to decline an opportunity to write a chapter than it is to accept the invitation and then not deliver the chapter. (I have been guilty of overcommitting, and a recent instance of not being able to produce a chapter that I had promised to write was extremely embarrassing for me. The book editors would have had an easier time with finding another author than they had with my failing to produce at the end of the process.) Spending some time on book chapters is fine—but you want to be sure that journal articles comprise most of your scholarly output. A creative solution for declining an invitation to write a chapter may be to offer to coauthor the chapter with a colleague, as long as that colleague assumes first authorship.

Summary

- There are three primary types of scholarly books: authored books, edited books, and handbooks.
- Authored books are written by a single person or group. They often take multiple years to write.
- Edited books and handbooks require securing chapter commitments from people who will write those chapters. Not all the authors who agree to write chapters will deliver those chapters.
- Active scholars often receive invitations to write book chapters. The decision about whether to write the chapter should be reached in light of one's expertise on the topic as well as one's volume of current commitments. It is better to decline a chapter invitation than to fail to deliver the chapter after having agreed to write it.
- A book chapter will become the primary source for whatever material is written in it—so authors should carefully consider what they wish to put into the chapter. It is not ethical to recycle material in, or from, a book chapter.

References

Jalongo, M. R., & Saracho, O. (2016). *Writing for publication: Transitions and tools that support scholars' success.* New York: Springer.

Oermann, M., & Hays, J. (2018). *Writing for publication in nursing* (4th ed.). New York: Springer.

Schwartz, S. J., & Unger, J. B. (2017). Acculturation and health: State of the field and recommended directions. In S. J. Schwartz & J. B. Unger (Eds.), *Oxford handbook of acculturation and health* (pp. 1–14). New York: Oxford University Press.

Vignoles, V. L., Schwartz, S. J., & Luyckx, K. (2011). Introduction: Toward an integrative view of identity. In S. J. Schwartz, K. Luyckx, & V. L. Vignoles (Eds.), *Handbook of identity theory and research* (pp. 1–28). New York: Springer.

19
Conclusion

This book covers the publication process from start to finish—from coming up with a research idea, planning a study, conducting data analyses in an ethical manner, outlining sections of the manuscript, writing first drafts, and editing your work. I also provide tips for getting yourself into good writing hygiene, thinking like a reviewer about your own ideas, working with coauthors, and responding to editor and reviewer feedback. I have used my own experiences, and those of my colleagues, to illustrate many of the principles I discuss in this book. As I state many times in the book, I learned most of the skills and techniques here from my mentors and from my publishing experience. I've learned that editors and reviewers generally respond well to detailed response letters, and that they do not respond well to being blown off. (As I was writing this book, one of my coauthors submitted a revised manuscript to a moderate-prestige journal. I, along with other coauthors, told him that we were not comfortable with the revisions he had incorporated into the paper, and the response letter seemed to disregard several of the reviewer comments. Not surprisingly, the paper was rejected after the second round of review.)

One of the best pieces of advice I can offer academic writers is to take the ideas I've laid out here, adapt them to fit your own style, and use them in ways that feel most comfortable for you. You may have a specific style of working with coauthors that works for you—and if that style is producing results that you like, then stay with it. I once heard a radio host say that he was not "coming off the mountain with the tablets" when he offered his opinion on something, and I have adopted that expression as my own. I am not coming off the mountain with the tablets in this book. I am offering suggestions and strategies that have helped me to become successful in publishing. You should be the authority on what strategies produce the results you are looking for.

Happy publishing!

The Savvy Academic. Seth J. Schwartz, Oxford University Press © Oxford University Press 2022.
DOI: 10.1093/oso/9780190095918.003.0020

Index

For the benefit of digital users, indexed terms that span two pages (e.g., 52–53) may, on occasion, appear on only one of those pages.

Tables, figures and boxes are indicated by *t*, *f* and *b* following the page number

abbreviations, undefined jargon, 256–57, 277–78
abstracts
    free-form abstracts, 275–76
    for journals, 242
    meta-analytic articles and, 67
    search algorithms and, 23
    Sociological Abstracts database, 23
    structured abstracts, 276–77
    writing the abstract, 259–77
academic social media sites. *See also* Google Search
    Academia.edu, 23, 24–25, 392, 494
    following scholars on, 24–25
    ResearchGate, 23, 24–25, 97–98, 392, 494
    steps in using, 23, 232–33
academic writing, dos and don'ts, 152–65. *See also* principles of good writing
    abbreviations and acronyms, 162–63
    citing sources, 159
    contractions, 164–65
    discussion section, 162
    first-/second-person pronouns, 163–64
    introduction section, 160
    method section, 160–61
    neutral writing stance, 152–57
    offering praise for prior related studies, 157–59
    results section, 161–62
action editors
    acceptance recommendations by, 390
    addressing response letter to, 383
    appealing rejection decisions directly to, 400, 414
    assigning/choosing, 318, 334*f*, 344–47
    avoid going over the heads of, 404–5
    invitation to revise/resubmit by, 386–87, 428
    in journal review process, 334*f*
    for open-access journals, 501, 503
    rejection of manuscripts, 360–61

    requesting more space from, 368, 381
    selecting of reviewers by, 345–46, 492–93, 496
    style choices of, 348
    use of meddler strategy by, 371
    use of passive approach, 385, 388–89
    viewing of response letters by, 362
active coauthoring, 425–26, 428, 450
active/passive coauthoring strategies, 425–26, 428, 433–34, 448, 450
Adams, Gerald, 6
Add Health data set, 63, 459–60, 462
Addiction journal, 287
Addictive Behaviors Reports, open-access journal (Elsevier), 491–92
adversarial collaborations, 106
all over the place (AOTP) writing
    editing and, 227, 249, 252, 255–56, 258, 277–78
    first drafts and, 125, 144, 249
    logical leaps as symptom of, 195
    redundancy as symptom of, 249
    strategies for preventing, 471
    unjustified statements as symptom of, 252
AMA style, 220–21
American Community Survey, 453, 454
American Journal of Epidemiology, 82
American Journal of Health Behavior, 492
American Journal of Preventive Medicine, 82
American Journal of Public Health, 253
American Medical Association (AMA) citation style, 220–21
American Psychological Association (APA) Journals, 347*t*
American Psychological Association (APA) reference/citation style, 216–18
American Psychologist journal, 93–94, 135, 292–93
American Sociological Association (ASA) citation style, 218–20
anticipatory anxiety, 148–50

anxiety
anticipatory anxiety, 148–50
"blank screen" anxiety, 149, 226
coauthors and, 434
first drafts and, 232, 243–44
grant funding and, 90–91
mindfulness techniques for, 145, 146
outlining and, 230
realistic deadlines and, 243
self-judgment and, 231
Venezuelan immigrant study
example, 131–32
writer's block and, 149–50
writing self-efficacy and, 413
AOTP. *See* all over the place (AOTP) writing
APA style, 24, 216–18, 219, 233–34, 274
argument section, 170*f*
acknowledging relevant controversies, 224
creating flow and coherence, 196
creating multiple, controversy-free
sides, 211–13
"finessing" the argument, 155
first drafts and, 243
framing, for journals, 315–16
heading off major criticisms, 325–26
for journal articles, 315–16
laying out/setting up, 134–35, 253, 310
reducing distractions, confusion, 199
review by coauthors, 239–40
supportive citations/references, 213, 223
tangential text, 265–66
theoretical articles and, 242
use of acronyms, 162–63
Arnett, Jeff, 96, 151–52, 282, 292–93
articles (parts of speech), 176–77, 219
ASA style, 218–20
assembly-line approach, to publishing, 96–98
assessment of publications
new metrics, 93
Association for Psychological Science, 111, 287
authored books, 506, 507–14
book proposal checklist, 508*b*
planning and writing the book, 513–14
writing the book proposal, 507–12
authors
keeping up with, 24–25
authorship teams (large teams), 18, 418,
430–31, 433, 448–49, 450
coauthor perspective, 433–35
first-author perspective, 430–33

Bandura, Albert, xv, 413
Barr, A., 109–10
Bartholomew, R. E., 288–89

Basic and Applied Social Psychology
journal, 399
Bedeian, A. G., 91–92
Beigi, M., 413
Beretvas, S. N., 457
Berry, John, 135
Bianchi, M, 70
bias
conflicts of interest and, 88, 108–9
of grant reviewers, 114–15
of the h-index, 13–14
biculturalism daily diary study
discussion section, outline example, 133–17
introductory section, outline
example, 126–28
method section, outline example, 129–30
results section, outline example, 130–31
Big Five personality typology, 315–16
biosketches, 204–5
"blank screen" anxiety, 140, 149–47,
230, 363–64
BMC, open-access journals, 491
book chapters
deciding whether to write, 520–21
republishing ideas in one chapter
in another chapter in another
book, 523–24
review process for, 522–23
writing the chapter, 521–22
books, 505–26. *See also* authored books;
book chapters; codebooks; edited
books; handbooks
book proposals, 507–12, 508*b*
citation format, 219
handbooks, 109–10, 506–7, 514–15
managing edited books and
handbooks, 515–20
planning edited books and
handbooks, 514–15
republishing chapter ideas in other
books, 523–24
review process for chapters, 522–23
writing chapters, 520–22
Brief Strategic Family Therapy intervention,
103, 159
bring-in-money pressures, 90–92, 95, 108–9
Brody, G. H., 292, 483
Brooks, C., 461–62
Bruns, S. B., 100–1
Bryk, A. S., 456
Bryman, A., 43–44

Cameron, C. J., 485
Carnegie, Dale, 56

Centers for Disease Control and Prevention, 52, 63–64, 453, 460
Chicago citation style, 221–22
Chicago style, 24, 221–22
Child Development journal, 287, 292, 293, 407–8
Chlup, D., 413
citations
    AMA citation style, 220–21
    APA style, 24, 216–18, 219, 233–34, 274
    ASA style, 218–20
    avoidance of long strings, 214–15
    books and book chapters, 219
    in broad *vs.* narrower statements, 215–16
    Chicago style, 221–22
    citation styles, 224
    citing sources, 159–62
    classic citations, 67
    in discussion section, 162
    dos and don'ts, 159
    first drafts and, 234, 235–38
    in introduction section, 160, 215
    leading with concepts *vs.* citations, 213–14
    in method section, 160–61
    multiple sides of an argument or controversy, 211–13
    need to be current, 67
    number for a single point, 214–16
    paraphrasing and, 208
    prevalence rates, 67
    repeatedly within a paragraph, 222
    in results section, 161–62
    role in impact factor of journals, 93–94
    run-on sentences and, 183
    in scientific writing, 215
    software programs, 24, 216, 232–33
    "stretching" of, 98–100
classical test theory, 105, 107
clauses, 171, 172, 173, 174–77, 178–79, 188, 207, 266, 272–73
clinical articles, 484–85
clinical psychology journals, 293
clumsy wording, 261–62
coauthors (coauthoring), 417–50. *See also* coauthors (coauthoring), difficult situations; coauthors (coauthoring), issues for students and other mentees; collaboration
    action editors and, 318
    active/passive coauthoring strategies, 425–26, 428, 433–34, 448, 450
    ascertaining trustworthiness of, 206
    authorship agreements with, 422–23
    authorship teams, coauthor perspective, 433–35

authorship teams, first-author perspective, 430–33
    challenges of working with, 18, 417–18
    changing of their own changes by, 246–47
    drafting a list of coauthor expectations, 426
    editing and, 151–52
    getting feedback from, 138, 165, 166, 261–62, 266
    incorporating comments from, 89–90
    job description/responsibilities of, 97, 151–52, 230–31, 248, 329, 418–22, 425
    large authorship teams, 18, 418, 430–35, 448–49, 450
    leaning on, by beginning writers, 151–52
    manuscript rejection and, 301–2, 304–5
    need for reasonability and flexibility, 423–25
    outlines as agreements among, 137
    plagiarism and, 209–10
    readiness for sharing drafts with, 247–48, 257
    as resource for the primary author, 150
    selecting a target journal with, 290
    senior-junior collaborations, 407, 417, 426–29
    sharing abstract with, 274
    sharing drafts with, 17, 97, 247–48
    suspicious behavior of, 117
    "thinking like a reviewer" by, 324–25
    unresponsive coauthors, 428–29
    use of in-text edits by, 425
    use of margin comments by, 425
    working with, 150–52
    writer's block and, 238, 239
coauthors (coauthoring), difficult situations, 435–43
    difficult/resistant coauthors, 435
    harassing/intimidating other authors, 438–41
    leaving toxic collaborations, 441–43
    slow coauthors, 436–37
    trying to block publication/sabotage the manuscript, 437–38
coauthors (coauthoring), issues for students and other mentees, 443–48
    mentor-mentee collaborations, 443–46
    students leading collaborations with faculty members, 446–48
codebooks
    for proprietary data sets, 459
    for public-use data sets, 459

collaboration. *See also* coauthors
  (coauthoring)
  adversarial collaborations, 106
  benefits of, 35, 95–96
  as chance to "pay forward," 98
  coauthoring, 13
  collaborative networks, 95–96
  as early-career scholar, 407
  leaving toxic collaborations, 441–43
  Open Science Collaboration, 153
  between senior-junior scholars, 407,
    417, 426–29
  student-led, with faculty members, 417
  toxic collaborations, 417
  working with coauthors, 150–52
  on writing the results section, 34
confidence intervals, 66–67, 101–2, 399
conflicts of interest (COI), 88–99
  adopting an assembly line approach, 96–98
  bring-in-money pressures, 90–92,
    95, 108–9
  case study example, 88–89
  defined/forms of, 88–92, 108–9
  maintaining a large collaborative
    network, 95–96
  partnering with senior/junior
    colleagues, 98–99
  publish-or-perish pressures, 89–90, 95, 96,
    99, 108–9, 111, 116, 118–19
  strategies for addressing, 108–9
confounding variables, 29, 47
contents alerts, 24, 284–85
Conversations with God (Walsch), 150
Côté, Jim, 5–6, 96
cover letters, 286, 337–39, 341, 372, 383,
    384, 385
creative avoidance, 143
criticism
  heading off major criticisms, 325–29
  manuscript rejection and, 302
  plagiarism and, 204
  from reviewers, of discussion
    sections, 322–24
  from reviewers, of introductory
    sections, 320
  from reviewers, of method
    sections, 320–21
  from reviewers, of paper as a whole, 323
  from reviewers, of results sections, 322
  reviews and, 241
  of scientific process, 157–58
  self-criticism, 232, 243–44
  of unfinished thoughts, 250

Crocetti, Elisabetta, 13
cross-classified nesting, 455–57
cross-sectional studies
  examples of proper uses, 51
  limitations of, 50
  properties of, 48*t*
  purpose, advantages, disadvantages, 48*t*
  refusal by journals in using, 52
  use in estimating prevalence rates, 52
  use in mediational hypothesis, 48–50
Csikszentmihalyi, M., 145, 228
*Cultural Diversity and Ethnic Minority
    Psychology* journal, 293–94
curricula vitae, 204–5, 412
cutting length, tips for, 272–74

Dark Triad personality typology, 315–16
data sets. *See also* public-use and proprietary
    data sets
  cross-sectional data sets, 50–51, 304
  intervention data sets, 319
  longitudinal data sets, 98, 304, 412
  meta-analysis of, 68
  mixed methods/offsetting, and, 44
  national probability data sets, 64
  national/regional data sets, 63–64, 391–92
  population-based data set, 62–63, 65, 270,
    455, 457, 461–62
  proprietary data sets, 453–55
  public-use data sets, 453
  restricted-use data sets, 454
  secondary data sets, 102, 295, 318–19, 372
  statistical analysis of, 42–43, 62, 105
Davis, M. L., 66
Deferred Action for Childhood Arrivals
    (DACA) program, 53–54
Department of Defense, 113–14
desk-rejection
  description, 282, 341–43
  editor's explanations given for, 282
  initial editorial review and, 334*f*, 341–44
Developmental Psychology journal, 293
digital object identifier (DOI) numbers, 233–34
discussion section
  listing of limitations, future directions, 132–33
  overall goals, 131
  restatement of findings, 131
  review process, 322–25
  statement of "take-home points," 133
  statement of "verdict," 132
dos and don'ts, of academic writing. *See*
    academic writing, dos and don'ts
double-blind peer review process, 235–36

"drop-down" approach, to journal target selection, 289–90
Dunham, Richard (Dick), 2–3, 20–21, 96, 192, 296, 363–64, 438, 526

edited books
    comparison to handbooks, 506
    description, 506
    managing, 515–20
    planning, 514–15
editing
    avoiding self-cencoing during, 227
    being AOTP and, 227, 249, 252, 255–56, 258, 277–78
    changing changes during, 246–47
    clumsy wording, 261–62
    coauthors, feedback, and, 151–52
    comparison to carving a sculpture, 246
    of first drafts, 144–45, 165, 200
    internal inconsistencies, 257, 263–64, 277–78, 448–49
    iterative nature of, 38–39, 246
    "judgment calls" of editors, 314
    logical leaps, 134, 183–84, 193–94, 195, 200, 227, 243, 257–61
    by novice writers, 127
    overstated conclusions, 268–72
    planning edited books, 514–15
    "praying over the tables" process, 263–64
    redundancy problems, 249–50
    roadmap paragraph, 253–54
    run-on sentences, 183, 266–68
    seeking critical feedback, 248
    self-editing challenges, 240
    sharing drafts with coauthors, 247–48
    staying mindful of the outline, 248
    stream-of-consciousness process, 247
    tangents, 125, 128, 264–66
    time factors, 204–5
    tips for cutting length, 272–74
    undefined jargon, abbreviations, 256–57, 277–78
    unfinished thoughts, 250–52
    unjustified statements, 252–56, 257, 277–78, 380
    writing vs. editing phases, 244
Editorial Manager, manuscript submission site, 335
editorial styles, 348–52
    extra reviewer, 352, 353f
    interpreter, 350–52, 351f
    meddler, 352, 354f
    passive editor, 348–50, 349f

Ehrlich, E. J., 40
Eisenberg, N., 111
Elsevier, open-access journals, 491–92
Emerging Adulthood journal, 480–81
EndNote, software, 24, 216, 232–33
English language learners, 143–44
Erikson, E. H., 474, 476–77, 478
ethical data analysis, 81–120. See also research, questionable practices
    questionable research practices, 83–106
    recommendations for departmental/ univeristy adminstrations, 109–11
    recommendations for funding agencies, 113–16
    recommendations for journal editors, 112–13
    recommendations for scholars, 116–17
    researcher degrees of freedom, 81–82, 106–7, 119
    statistical power, 83–88
    strategies for avoiding questionable practices, 106–8
ethical issues. See ethical data analysis; plagiarism/plagiarizing
European Journal of Developmental Psychology, 299
EVISE, manuscript submission site, 335
experimental studies, 56–61
    consequences of not following steps, 60–61
    need for airtight methods, 56–57
    number of participation sessions, 56
    planning phases, 58–61
    properties of, 48t
    purpose, advantages, disadvantages, 48t
    random assignment as "gold standard," 57
    sample organizational chart, 59f
    staff meetings, 61
    use of Multiple Indicators, Multiple Causes method, 57–58
    use of propensity score matching, 57–58
    use of statistical methods with quasi-experimental data, 57–58
extra reviewer, editorial style, 352, 353f

Facebook, 54–56
Field, A., 66
Finley, Gordon, 14–15, 263–64, 429–30
first drafts, 226–44. See also editing
    all over the place writing and, 125, 144, 227, 242
    anxiety and, 2–17, 232
    anxiety/self-criticism/worry and, 232
    challenges of, 17

first drafts (*cont.*)
    citations and, 232–34, 235–38
    controlling over-enthusiasm, 230
    dealing with writer's block, 238–41
    expectations for, 144–45, 200
    flow state and, 146, 228
    frustrations of, 14
    getting ready, 144–45
    importance of mentors, 248
    iterations of, 246
    knowing when it's finished, 241–43
    logical leaps and, 243
    managing distractions, 229
    purpose of, 144, 200
    redundancy problems, 249–50
    reference lists and, 232–34
    role of intrinsic self-motivation, 228–29
    saving literature searches for later, 235
    self-citations and, 235–38
    self-criticism and, 232, 243–44
    self-preparation steps, 227–30
    using an outline as a template, 227, 230–31
    working up to long writing
        sessions, 229–30
Florida International University (FIU), 6
Florida State University (FSU), xiii, 2, 4,
    510, 516
flow state/allowing the words to flow, 145–46
    first drafts and, 146, 228
    within a paragraph, 193–96
    between paragraphs, 196–200
focus groups, 42–43
free-form abstracts, 275–76
frequentist analyses, 140, 455
From the Ground Up (Schultz), 1–2
Frontiers, open-access journals, 491, 492–93
    "postpublication peer review"
        model, 493
Frontiers in Psychology journal, 496–99
funding agencies, ethics-related
    recommendations, 113–16

Gillett, R., 66
Goodson, P., 413
Google Scholar, 23, 94, 482–83
    algorithms used by, 23
    clicking on "Cited By" link, 24
    h-index search on, 1, 94
    inclusion criteria, 482–83
    journal searches, 284–85
    options for obtaining cited articles, 24
    researcher profiles on, 23
    steps in using, 23, 232–33

Google search engine, 23
grammar
    common issues for writers, 171
    Native *vs.* non-Native English speakers, 16,
        143–44, 170, 179, 262
    noun-pronoun agreement and, 172
    turn-offs of poor grammar, 169–70
grants/grant writing
    anticipatory anxiety and, 148
    article in *Social Work Research,* 90–91
    awarding of grants, 35
    challenges/frustrations of, 10–11
    competition for, 110
    conflicts of interest (COI) and, 88–89
    data sets generated by, 63
    NIH research project grants, 92, 113–14
    plagiarism and, 204–5
    pressure for bringing in, 90–91
growth experiences, 3

Han, B., 461–62
handbooks, 109–10, 506–7
    comparison to edited/authored
        books, 514
    comparison to edited books, 506
    issues of potential sales, 515
    managing handbooks, 515–20
    planning handbooks, 514–15
HARKing (hypothesizing after the results are
    known), 83
    comparison to point-and-click statistical
        packages, 105
    description, 104, 105–6
    Ioannidis's view of, 104
    Kerr's labeling of, 104
    pre-registration method for preventing, 106–8
    scientific method and, 87, 120, 366
    strategies for avoiding use of, 106–8
Harter, J., 40
Head, M. L., 101
Health Behavior and Policy Review, 492
Heckathorn, D. D., 71
Heckthorn, D. D., 485
Hedges' *g* statistic, 66–67
Henkens, K., 91–92
high-prestige journals, 17–18, 287, 288,
    289–90, 291–93, 296–97, 305–6,
    318–19, 330, 335, 407–8, 412
Hindawi, open-access journals, 491
h-index
    bias/limitation of, 13–14
    description, 1, 94
    usefulness of, 95

Hispanic Community Health Study/Study of
    Latinos (HCHS/SOL), 454–55
Holman, L., 101
How to Win Friends and Influence People
    (Carnegie), 56
Huerta, M., 413
Human Development journal, 281
humility
    benefits of, C 447
    importance of, 12
    scientific humility, 17–18, 107–8,
        409–10
humor (sense of humor), importance
    of, 12
hypothesis
    association reference, 46f, 46
    causation reference, 47, 50f
    mediational hypothesis, 46f, 48–50
    prediction reference, 46f, 47

Identity journal, 278–79
if and *whether*, 178–79
impact factor, for evaluating publications
    description, 93
    h-index measure of scholars, 94
    usefulness of, 95
    weakness of, 93–94
ingroup projection theory, 69, 70
ingroups/outgroups ("us" *vs.* "them"),
    30, 215–16
Instagram, 54–56
Institute for Education Sciences, 113–14
Instructions for Authors, for
    journals, 281–82
integrative and scoping reviews. *See*
    integrative literature reviews; scoping
    reviews
integrative literature reviews, 324, 470–71,
    476, 482–83, 486, 487–88, 500
    best use for subscription
        journals, 500
    best use in traditional subscription
        journals, 501–2
    creating of an outline, 471
    importance of staying close to the
        empirical literature, 477
    inclusion of integrative/wrap-up
        statements, 476
    inclusion of literature review, 472, 488
    laying out the roadmap for, 472
    need for specifying inclusion
        criteria, 482–83
    purpose of, 488, 489

role in tying strands of literature
    together, 480–81
scoping review comparison, 482
use of outlining with, 481–82
intensive longitudinal studies, 54, 466
internal inconsistencies, 257, 263–64,
    277–78, 448–49
*International Journal of Intercultural
    Relations,* 206–7, 281, 293–94,
    343, 344–45
interpreter, editorial style, 350–52, 351f
interviews, 42–43
introductory section
    citations, 160
    dos and don'ts, 160
    of outlines, biculturalism daily diary study
        example, 126–28
    of outlines, purpose of, 126
    review process, 320
Ioannidis, John P. A., 81–82, 100–1, 104

Jaakkola, E., 21
Jarvis, B., 161
Jennions, M. D., 101
Jia, J., 288–89
job description of a reviewer, 312–15
Johnson, Earvin "Magic," 205
Journal of Adolescence, 344
Journal of Adolescent Health, 82, 253, 287
Journal of Adolescent Research, 281, 282
Journal of Child and Family Studies, 314–15
*Journal of Consulting and Clinical
    Psychology,* 293
Journal of Early Adolescence, 299
Journal of Marriage and Family, 480–81
*Journal of the American Medical
    Association,* 93–94
*Journal of the Personality and Social
    Psychology,* 292–93
Journal of Youth and Adolescence, 193,
    259, 287–88
journal prestige
    editorial selectiveness and, 285–87
    high-prestige journals, 17–18, 287, 288,
        289–90, 291, 305–6, 318–19, 330, 335,
        407–8, 412
    low-prestige journals, 287–89, 291–92,
        294–97, 298, 302–3, 305–6, 312, 319,
        355, 396–97, 406–8, 410–11
    moderate (medium)-prestige journals,
        288, 289, 291–92, 293–95, 304, 306–7,
        312, 316, 319, 330, 396–97, 406–7, 408–
        9, 412,

journal review process, 333–93. *See also*
  journal review process, initial editorial
    decisions; manuscript revision;
    manuscript revision, constructing
    the response letter; manuscript
    submission sites
  action editor/reviewer assignment, 344–47
  article formats, 335–37
  article retractions, 391–92
  asking for extensions to resubmission
    deadlines, 386–87
  author inquiries to editors, 334
  beginning authors perception of, 333–34
  copyright issues, 392
  cover letters, 337–39, 341, 372, 383,
    384, 385
  errata and corrigenda, 391
  importance of keyword choices, 339, 340*f*
  initial editorial review/desk
    rejection, 341–44
  manuscript submission sites, 335–41
  online supplemental material, 341
  provisional acceptance, 390
  provisional acceptance of manuscript, 390
  roadmap of the process, 334*f*
  second round of review, 383–86
  second round of review, outcomes, 387–89
  steps after acceptance of manuscript, 391
  submission site format-selection
    page, 336*f*
  uploading files, 341
journal review process, initial editorial
    decisions, 348–62
  easy rejections, close calls, 361–62
  editorial decisions, 355–60
  extra reviewer, 352
  extra-reviewer decision letter, 353*f*
  interpreter, 350–52
  interpreter, decision letter, 351*f*
  meddler, 352
  meddler decision letter, 354*f*
  outright rejection, 360–61
  passive editor, 348–50, 349*f*
  revise-submit recommendation, 359–60
journals. *See also* journal prestige; journal
    review process; target journal selection
  article summary template, 22*t*
  dealing with rejection, 300–5
  digital object identifier (DOI)
    numbers, 233–34
  "dumping" of manuscripts, 292
  ethics-related recommendations for
    editors, 112–13
  focus of personality journals, 315–16

framing/supporting the argument,
    315–16, 360
impact factor assessment, 93
Instructions for Authors, 281–82
keeping up with, 24–25
niche journals, 285, 287–88, 296, 307, 411
online table of content alerts, 24, 284–85
public health/medical, 82
reasons for desk-rejection, 48, 50–51, 282
refusal to use cross-sectional studies, 52
sleight of hand by editors, 82
special journal issues, 297–300
use of numbers in manuscripts, 185
word count limitations, 82

Kahn, A., 101
Kenon, Larry, 205
Kerr, N. L., 104
Kidwell, Jeannie, xiv–xv
King, Stephen, 146
Klimstra, Theo, 292
Kline, R. B., 100
Kurtines, William (Bill)
  mentoring by, xiii–xiv
  role as PhD advisor, 5–6

Laband, D. N., 300
Lakens, D., 99–100
Land, K. C., 461–62
Lanfear, R., 101
last minute approach, 203–5, 222–23, 224
laziness, 203–5, 222–23, 236, 424
Levesque, Roger, 193
literature search, 21–24
  inclusion criteria, 482–83
  key words/search terms, 23
  reference software, 24
  using search engines, 23
longitudinal designs, 28–29
longitudinal studies, 33, 38–39, 53–56
  acculturation study example, 39–41
  affiliation problems with universities,
    formal institutions, 55
  challenges of, 40, 53
  example of an error, 40–41
  intensive longitudinal studies, 54, 466
  labor intensiveness of, 53
  nonrandom attrition and, 53
  planning for retention in, 38
  properties of, 48*t*
  purpose, advantages, disadvantages, 48*t*
  quality assurance checks ("dry
    runs"), 39, 41
  reasons for choosing, 53

retention strategies, 54–56
use in testing predictive relationships, 53
voice recordings, 39–40
low-prestige journals, 287–89, 291–92, 294–97, 298, 302–3, 305–6, 312, 319, 355, 396–97, 406–8, 410–11
Luyckx, Koen, 13

Magic Johnson Principle, 205, 229
maladaptive perfection
    avoidance of, 14, 144–45
    compromises caused by, 145
    consequences/dangers of, 14–15, 144–45, 231, 243–44
    description, 14
manuscript revision. *See also* manuscript revision, constructing the response letter; rejected manuscripts
    key principles for revising, 362–63
    starting the response letter, 363–66
    turning a revise-submit into an acceptance, 362
manuscript revision, constructing the response letter, 367–83
    choosing not to revise, 381–82
    dealing with conflicting comments, 377–79
    how to address each reviewer comment, 367–71
    making revisions fit with existing text, 380–81
    responding to comments in the cover letter, 372
    responding to comments that require changes in multiple locations, 373–77
    responding to multiple iterations of the same comment, 377–79
    responding to positive comments, 373
    revising based on editorial style, 379–80
    speaking with your own voice, 382–83
    using limitations to address comments, 371–72
manuscript submission sites, 335–41
    article formats, 335–37
    asking for extensions to resubmission deadlines, 386–87
    cover letters, 337–39, 341, 372, 383, 384, 385
    formats, 335–37
    format-selection page, 336f
    keyword choices, 339, 340f
    keyword entry page, 340f
    online supplemental material, 341
    uploading files, 341

Manza, J., 461–62
meddler, editorial style, 352, 354f
mediational hypothesis
    causal sequence, 49, 50f
    predictive sequence, 49f, 49
    use in cross-sectional design, 48–50
medical journals, 82
MedLine database, 23
Mentored Scientist award, 11–12
mentors (mentoring/mentorship)
    collaborations with junior scholars, 426–29
    copy of, by mentees, 98
    expectations from scholar mentees, 151
    impact of bean counting, 90
    importance during first drafts, 248
    importance of, 240
    mentor-mentee collaborations, issues, 443–46
    obtaining feedback and support from, 226
    receiving critical feedback from, xv
    roles of, 98, 150–51, 205, 246, 248, 249, 261–62, 278, 298–99, 303, 305
    setting ground rules, 427
    skills required of, 9, 27
    toxic, unresponsive mentors, 428–29, 441
Merunka, D. R., 70
meta-analysis, in secondary data analysis, 65–68
methodological articles, 485
method section
    citations, 160–61
    dos and don'ts, 160–61
    of outline, biculturalism daily diary study example, 129–30
    of outline, information contents, 128
    review process, 320–21
Meyers, J. L., 457
Miller, A. N., 91–92
mindfulness, 145, 146, 148
mixed-methods research, 43–44. *See also* qualitative research; quantitative research
    expansion method, 44–45
    inclusion of qualitative/quantitative research, 43–44
    offsetting method, 44
    triangulation method, 43–44
moderate (medium)-prestige journals, 288, 289, 291–92, 293–95, 304, 306–7, 312, 316, 319, 330, 396–97, 406–7, 408–9, 412,
Mojtabai, R., 461–62

Monitoring the Future study (University of
Michigan), 52, 453
*Monitor of the American Psychological
Association,* 111
Montgomery, D. C., 49–50
Morgan, C., 65
Muir, J. A., 72
Mullis, Ann, 5
Mullis, Ron, 439, 5, 438
Multidisciplinary Digits Publishing Institute
(MDPI), open-access journals, 491
multilevel and cross-classified
nesting, 455–57
Multiple Indicators, Multiple Causes
(MIMIC) method, 57–58
Mummendey, A., 70

narrative storytelling, 42–43
National Institute of Alcohol Abuse and
Alcoholism, 110–11
National Institute of Child Health and
Human Development, 110–11
National Institute of Drug Abuse, 110–11
National Institute of Justice, 113–14
National Institute of Mental Health, 110–11
National Institute on Alcohol Abuse and
Alcoholism, 98
National Institutes of Health, 454
ethics-related recommendations for, 115
funding of grants, 92
grant awards from, 58
replication initiative, 32
National Longitudinal Study of Adolescent
Health (Add Health), 63
national/regional data sets, 63–64
National Science Foundation, 113–14
National Survey on Family Growth, 453
Neeuwbeerta, P., 461–62
neutral stance, in writing research
study, 152–57
*New Directions in Child and Adolescent
Development,* special issue journal, 299
New England Journal of Medicine, 93–94
Neyman-Pearson approach, to statistical
tests, 83–84, 83*t*
niche journals, 285, 287–88, 296, 307, 411
non-empirical papers, 470–89. *See also*
integrative literature reviews; position
papers; theoretical articles
clinical articles, 484–85
description, 470–71
lack of structure of, 253
methodological articles, 485

preparation for writing, 471–72
strategy for avoiding AOTP, 471–72
noun-pronoun agreement, 171, 172–73,
174, 175
noun-verb agreement, 172–73
null hypothesis, 83–84, 83*t*, 85, 87,
100, 101–2

Obama, Barack, 53–54
observational learning, xv
of and *from,* 179
Olatunji, B. O., 66
Olfson, M., 461–62
open-access journals
acceptance rates *vs.* subscription
journals, 501
action editors for, 501, 503
advantages *vs.* disadvantages, 493–99
best-matched papers for, 18, 499–501
comparison with subscription
journals, 492–93
description/review process, 406
examples of publishers, 406, 491
free downloading of articles, 491, 495
legitimate *vs.* predatory, 18, 288–89, 493–
94, 502
misconceptions about 406, 499
nonpredatory open-access journals, 406–7
pay-to-publish comparison, 296
peer review model, 492–93
Open Science Collaboration, 153
outlines/outline development, 124–38
as agreements among coauthors, 137
all over the place (AOTP) writing and, 125
creation process, 126
discussion section, 131–34
as first draft template, 227, 230–31
headlines and tangents, 125
introductory section, 126–28
method section, 128–30
outline development, 124–38
outline template, 126, 227, 230–31
planning phase, 33
reasons for creating, 17
results section, 130–31
theoretical articles, literature reviews,
position papers, 134–37
overstated conclusions, 268–72
overused words, 190

paraphrasing, citations and, 208
passive editor, editorial style, 348–50, 349*f*
passive voice, 163–64, 166, 272–73

peer-reviews
  articles, 288–89, 524
  basic function of, 313
  chances of surviving, 341–43
  delays, 346–47
  dissertations *vs.* journal
    manuscripts, 237–38
  double-blind process, 235–36, 237
  Frontiers/postpublication peer review, 493
  journals, 38, 524
  at low-prestige journals, 288–89,
    292, 305–6
  at moderate-prestige journals, 307
  NIH and, 114
  open-access *vs.* subscription
    journals, 492–93
  post-review initial editorial decisions, 393
  predatory open-access journals and, 493
  rejections, 286
*Personality and Social Psychology
  Bulletin,* 293
personality journals, 315–16
Peterson, R. A., 70
p-hacking, 99–102
  comparison with post hoc model
    modification in structural equation
    modeling, 101
  description, 99–100
  Ioannidis's view of, 104
  main problem with, 101
  misuse of *p*-value, 100
  pre-registration method for
    preventing, 106–8
  scientific method and, 87
  solutions to misuse, 101–2
  strategies for avoiding use of, 102–4,
    106–8
Phillips, J., 461–62
Phinney, J. S., 478
Piette, M. J., 300
plagiarism/plagiarizing
  commonness of, 203
  description/types of, 203
  example of accusation, 202–3
  examples, 206–7
  grant writing and, 204–5
  plagiarism checking process, 206–7
  related trust issues, 117
  research on reasons for, 203–4
  team writing approach and, 206
planned missingness designs, 455,
  458*f*, 458–59
planning a study. *See* study design

point-and-click statistical software
  HARKing and, 60
  use in statistical analysis, 42
point of diminishing returns, with
  manuscript changes, 429–30
population-based data set, 62–63, 65, 270,
  455, 457, 461–62
  codebooks, 455
  description, 63
  examples, 461–62
  reasons for/against using, 463–62
  sample recruitment, 68–69
position papers, 483–84
  challenges in writing, 242, 470–71
  critiques against, 472
  critiques of, 472
  description, 470–71, 483–84, 488–89
  establishing boundaries for, 254, 310
  ethical issues, 482
  expectations of, 253, 471
  importance of staying close to the
    empirical literature, 477
  inclusion of integrative/wrap-up
    statements, 476
  inclusion of literature review, 472, 488
  laying out the roadmap for, 472
  laying out what is already known, 472–73
  outlining of, 134–35, 138
  principles in writing, 471
  purpose of, 488
Powers, M. B., 66
"praying over the tables" editing process
  (Finley), 263–64
predatory open-access journals, 493–94, 502
preparing to write. *See* writing preparation
prepositional phrases, 171, 173–74, 175, 185
principles of good writing, 169–201
  anthropomorphisms, 183
  apostrophes, 187
  articles, 176–77, 219
  avoiding too many *ands,* 182
  big picture of writing, 170*f*
  clauses, 171, 172, 173, 174–77, 178–79,
    188, 207, 266, 272–73
  colons and semicolons, 188–89
  commas, 185–86
  conjunctions, 177–78, 219, 266
  dangling participles, 176
  distinguishing between/among
    homonyms, 190–92
  flow between paragraphs, 196–200
  flow within a paragraph, 193–96
  grammar, 16, 143–44, 170, 171, 179, 262

principles of good writing (*cont.*)
  if and *whether*, 178–79
  Native *vs.* non-native English speakers, 16,
    143–44, 170, 176, 179, 262
  noun-pronoun agreement, 171, 172–73,
    174, 175
  of and *from*, 179
  overused words, 190
  periods, 186–87
  prepositional phrases, 171, 173–74,
    175, 185
  punctuation, 185–89
  question marks, exclamation points, 185,
    188, 189
  quotation marks, 187–88
  reveal and noun-pronoun agreement, 171,
    172–73, 174, 175
  reveal and *show*, 179–80
  run-on sentences, 183, 248–49, 266–181
  split infinitives, 177
  subject and predicate, 171–72, 173–74, 182
  subject-object pronoun agreement, 173
  subject-verb agreement, 172, 175
  than versus compared to, 181
  there is sentence structure, 182
  this and *that* as indefinite references, 181
  use of *e.g.* and *i.e.*, 183–84
  use of *et cetera*, 184
  use of numbers in journal
    manuscripts, 185
  varying language, 192
  while and *since*, 180–81
pronouns, first-/second-person, 163–64
propensity score matching, 57–58
proprietary data sets, 64
  advantages of using, 461
  codebooks for, 459
  description, 453–54
  disadvantages of using, 462
  examples, 454
  gaining access to, 454, 461
  similarity to national probability data
    sets, 64
Psychological Bulletin journal, 399
Psychological Review journal, 399
Psychological Science journal, 287
psychoneuroimmunology research, 48
PsycInfo database, 23, 482–83
publications
  impact factor assessment, 93
public health journals, 82
Public Library of Sciences (PLOS),
  open-access journals, 491, 492–93, 499

public-use data sets
  advantages of using, 461
  availability of, 460–61, 465–66, 467
  codebooks for, 459
  description/examples, 453, 454–55
  disadvantages of using, 462
  gaining access to, 454
public-use and proprietary data sets. *See also*
    proprietary data sets; public-use
    data sets
  advantages of using, 461–62
  checking for articles using the same data
    set, 146–461
  codebooks, 459–60
  disadvantages of using, 462
  frequentist analyses, 140, 455
  multilevel and cross-classified
    nesting, 455–57
  oversampling, 457–58
  planned missingness designs, 455,
    458f, 458–59
publish-or-perish pressures, 89–90, 95, 96,
    99, 108–9, 111, 116, 118–19
PubMed database, 23, 482–83
punctuation, 185–89
  apostrophes, 187
  colons and semicolons, 188–89
  commas, 185–86
  periods, 186–87
  question marks, exclamation points, 185,
    188, 189

Q statistic, 66–67
qualitative research, 42–43
  purpose of, 42–43
  types of methods, 42–43
quality assurance checks ("dry runs")
  importance of, 33, 39–40, 41, 60
  in longitudinal studies, 39, 41
  planning for, 38–39
quantitative research, 43
  description/forms, 43
  example, 45
question marks, exclamation points, 185,
    188, 189

Racine, E., 482
Raudenbush, S. W., 456
redundancy
  problems in first drafts, 227, 229,
    243, 248–50
  pros of intentional redundancy, 250
  strategy for correcting, 249–50

redundancy problems, in first drafts, 249–50
reference lists, first drafts and, 232–34
Reference Manager, software, 24, 216, 232–33
reference software
    EndNote, 24, 216, 232–33
    Reference Manager, 24, 216, 232–33
registered reports, adversarial collaborations
    and, 106
rejected manuscripts, 395–415
    appealing rejected decisions, 400–5
    appealing rejected decisions,
        example, 400–3
    appealing rejected decisions, tactics to
        avoid, 404–5
    close-call rejections, 361, 389, 395
    "cursed" manuscripts, 396
    damaging impact on self-efficacy, 413
    deciding on a course of action, 410–12
    dumping vs. dropping, 319, 406–7,
        410f, 410–12
    easy rejections, 361, 395
    eventual acceptance of, 303
    reasons for rejection, 304
    repeated rejections, 405–8
    repeated rejections and self-
        confidence, 413–14
    reviewer comments "from out of left
        field," 408–9
    role of persistence in getting
        published, 408–10
rejection, dealing with, 300–5
replicability/non-replicability of study
    findings, 81–82
p-hacking/HARKING and, 104
research, questionable practices, 83–106
    conflicts of interest, 88–99
    P-hacking, 99–102
    statistical power (1 - β), 83–88
    strategies for avoiding, 106–8
researcher degrees of freedom, 81–82,
    106–7, 119
ResearchGate, 23, 24–25, 97–98, 392, 494
research hypothesis ("good" research
    hypothesis)
    characteristics of, 27–29
    choosing designs/methods, 28–29
    falsifiability component, 27–28
    including constructs, 28
    inclusion/exclusion criteria, 28
    role of theory, 29–30
resilience, importance of, 12
respondent-driven sampling methodology
    description, 40–41, 71

results section
    citations, 161–62
    dos and don'ts, 161–62
    in the outline, biculturalism daily diary
        example, 130–31
    in the outline, types of content, 130
    review process, 322
retention strategies
    acculturation study example, 55, 136
    for cross-sectional studies, 48t
    for longitudinal studies, 38, 48t, 54–55,
        321, 419
    for long-term experimental studies, 56
reveal and show, 179–80
review process (thinking like a reviewer),
    310–31. See also journal review process
    choosing action editors, 318
    citations/framing of study, 317
    confidential publication
        recommendation, 313–14
    controlling for key covariates, 318–19
    "devil's advocate" viewpoint, 311–12
    of discussion section, 322–25
    of empirical manuscripts, 311
    evaluation for fatal flaws, 316, 319
    "heading off" major criticisms, 325–29
    of introductory sections, 320
    "judgment calls" of editors, 314
    levels of review, 313
    listing of research questions,
        hypothesis, 316
    major revisions, 313, 355–56, 364–65, 367,
        371, 382–83, 424–51, 523
    of method section, 320–21
    minor revisions, 364–65, 390
    moderate revisions, 364–65
    peer review, basic function, 313
    questions for consideration, 310, 312–13
    of results section, 322
    reviewer's job description, 312–15
    scanning the editorial board, 317–18
    self-review considerations, 311,
        312, 315–25
    SLAM (stressing the limiting aspects of
        manuscripts) approach, 311–12, 486
    "30,000 feet approach," 310–11, 315, 481
revision process, 18
roadmap paragraph, 253–54
Rodriguez, Lilliana, 44
run-on sentences, 183, 248–49, 266–68

SAGE, open-access journals, 492
Saigle, V., 482

Salas-Wright, Chris, 204–5
sampling, 68–74
    Hispanic Youth Health Study
        example, 69–70
    Hurricane Maria survivors, example, 71
    importance of, 69f
    Multisystemic Therapy intervention
        example, 72–73
    qualitative/quantitative studies
        comparison, 71–72
    for randomized trials, 72
    respondent-driven sampling, 40–41, 71
    social-psychological experiments,
        example, 70
sampling weights, 64–65, 65f
SAS point-and-click statistical software, 42
Schildkraut, Deborah, 63
Schmidt, L., 101
Schneider, B., 49–50
ScholarOne, manuscript submission site, 335
scholars
    ethics-related recommendations
        for, 116–18
Schultz, Howard, 1–2
Schwartz, S. J., 70–71, 72
scientific humility, 17–18, 107–8, 409–10
scientific method
    comparison to billiards, 105–6
    HARKing and, 87, 120, 366
    hypothesizing steps component, 20, 104,
        105, 480
    p-hacking and, 87
    registered reports and, 107
    statistical analysis component, 104
    steps of, 20
scoping reviews, 482–83
    best use for traditional subscription
        journals, 500, 501–2
    ethical challenges in suicide research
        example, 482
    integrative review comparison, 482
    need for specifying inclusion
        criteria, 482–83
    purpose of, 488
    steps of, 482
Scopus database, 23, 482–83
search engines, 21, 23
    digital object identifier and, 233–34
    integrative/scoping reviews and, 487
    for literature searches, 23
    reference software and, 24
secondary data analyses, 62–64
    challenges involved in, 62–63

date collected by colleagues, 63
meta-analysis, 65–68
national/regional data sets, 63–64
population-based data sets, 62–63
proprietary data sets, 64
sampling, 68–74
sampling weights, 64–65, 65f
Séguin, M., 482
self-criticism, first drafts and, 232, 243–44
self-determination theory, 229
self-efficacy (Bandura), 413
self-motivation, role in writing first
    draft, 228–29
self-report data, 38–39, 40, 43, 105
Siranni, A., 485
Sireci, S. G., 40
Skhirtladze, Nino, 13
SLAM approach to manuscript review,
    311–12, 486
Smits, J. A., 66
social media
    academic social media sites, 23–25,
        392, 494–95
    Facebook, 54–56
    Instagram, 54–56
    Twitter, 54–56
    use in retention strategy, 55–56
Social Work Research journal, 91–92
Society for Adolescent Health and
    Medicine, 287
Society for Research on Child
    Development, 287
Society for the Study of Addiction, 287
Society for the Study of Emerging
    Adulthood, 96
Society for the Study of Identity, 5–6
Sociological Abstracts database, 23
Soto, Daniel, 55
split infinitives, 177
Springer, open-access journals, 491
SPS point-and-click statistical software, 42
"standing on the shoulders" of prior research
    approach (Szapocznik), 157–59
Stapel, Diedrik, 89
statistical analysis
    syntax/logical errors and, 41–42
    use of point-and-click statistical
        software, 42
statistical hypothesis testing
    observed/expected effect size (ES), 83–84
    sample size (N), 83–84, 85–86, 106, 107
    Type I error rate (α), 83–84, 83t, 85, 87
    Type II error rate (β), 83–84, 83t

statistical power (1 - β), 83–88
Steffens, A., 70
Steffens, M. C., 70
stream-of-consciousness editing, 247
stressing the limiting aspects of manuscripts
    (SLAM) effect, 311–12, 486
structured abstracts, 276–77
study design, 38–76. *See also*
    mixed-methods research; qualitative
        research; quantitative research
    association-prediction-causation
        relationships, 45–48, 46f
    checklist for, 48t
    choosing a research topic, 38–39
    examples of relationship associations of
        variables, 45–48, 49f
    meta-analysis, 65–68
    sampling, 68–74
    sampling weights, 64–65
    secondary data analysis, 62–64
    selection considerations, 42–61
    self-report surveys, 43
    sources of information, 38–39
    standards of scientific rigor, 43
    success factors, 38–39
    use of secondary data sets, 50
subject and predicate, 171–72, 173–74, 182
subject-object pronoun agreement, 173
subject-verb agreement, 172, 175
subscription journals
    acceptance rates *vs.* open-access
        journals, 501
    comparison to open-access journals, 491
    description, 491
    fees charged for scholarly journals, 491
    peer review model, 406, 492–93
success factors, 38
support letters, 204–5
surveys, 38–39
syntax/logical errors, 41–42
Szapocznik, José
    assistantship with, xiv–xv, 9–11, 97–98
Szapocznik, José
    advice about major publications, 90
    Brief Strategic Family Therapy
        intervention, 103, 159
    encouragement to publish in higher-
        impact journals, 95
    First Author Makes the Call strategy
        of, 137
    modeling of rigor and care in
        research, 98
    as proponent of scientific modesty, 154

"standing on the shoulders" of prior
    research approach, 157–59
tip on getting around "blank screen"
    anxiety, 149
tangents, 125, 128, 264–66
target journal selection, 281–308. *See also*
    journal prestige
    approaches, 289–97
    dealing with rejection, 300–5
    "drop-down" approach, 289–90
    focused matching approach, 290, 291
    role of journal prestige, 283–89
    self-appraisal of contributing
        work, 291–97
    sorting potential options for
        matches, 282
Taylor, S. G., 91–92
team science
    challenges of, 417–18
    described, 417
    described/advantages of, 417
    increasing emphasis on, 413–14, 415
team writing approach, 141
templates
    benefits of, 21
    book proposal template, 509–12
    first draft template, 226
    journal article summary template,
        22t, 314–21
    outline template, 126, 227, 230–31
text-messaging lingo, 16
theoretical articles, 329–30, 488
    acculturation study example, 135–36,
        473–74
    anticipating/heading off reviewer
        comments, 485–87
    best use in traditional subscription
        journals, 501–2
    challenges in writing, 134–35, 470–71
    critiques against, 472
    editorial essay example, 474–75
    importance of staying close to the
        empirical literature, 477
    inclusion of in-depth description of the
        theory, 475
    inclusion of integrative/wrap-up
        statements, 476
    inclusion of literature review, 472, 488
    laying out the roadmap for, 472
    laying out what is already known, 472–73
    outling and writing, 472–78
    purposes of, 470–71, 478–80

theory (theories)
    defined, 30–31
    role in research process, 30–31
"30,000 feet approach" review process,
    310–11, 315, 481
Thyer, B. A., 90–91
topic selection, 20–21
    discovering replication, 31–32
    identifying major contributors, 24–25
    literature searches, 21–25
    testable hypotheses/research
        question, 25–29
    thinking/planning ahead, 32–34
Torraco, R, 480–81
triangulation, 43–44
Truman, Harry, 207
Turner, S. E., 109–10
Twitter, 54–56
Type I error rate (α), 83–84, 83*t*, 85, 87
Type II error rate (β), 83–84, 83*t*

undefined jargon, abbreviations, 256–57,
    277–78
unfinished thoughts, 194–95, 200,
    250–52, 445
Unger, Jennifer, 155
University of Wales at Cardiff, xvi
unjustified statements, 252–56, 257, 277–
    78, 380
unresponsive mentors, 428–29
U.S. Census Bureau, 453, 454
U.S. National Surveys on Drug Use and
    Health, 461–62

Van Dalen, H. P., 91–92
Van Lange, P. A., 311–12

Walsch, Neale Donald, 150
Waterman, Al, 5–6, 141, 289–90, 293, 344
Weicherts, J. M., 82
while and *since,* 180–81
"Why most published research findings are
    false" (Ioannidis), 81–82
Wicherts, J. M., 499
Williams, K. D., 161
word count limitations, in journals, 82
writer's block, 149–50, 238–41, 244. *See also*
    anticipatory anxiety; "blank screen"
    anxiety
writing preparation, 140–67
    anticipatory anxiety, 148–50
    avoiding creative avoidance, 143
    "blank screen" anxiety, 140, 149–47,
        230, 363–64
    carving out time, 141–44
    challenges in getting started, 140
    choosing when to write, 146–48
    collaboration/working with
        coauthors, 150–52
    developing good writing habits, 142–44
    English language learners and, 143–44
    first draft, 138, 144–45, 146
    flow state/allowing the words to
        flow, 145–46
    maladaptive perfectionism and, 144–45
    mindfulness and, 145, 146, 148

Yang, Y., 40
Youth Risk Behavior Surveillance Survey
    (YRBSS) data set, 63–64, 460, 462
Yzerbyt, V., 70

Zamboanga, Byron, 13